LABORATORY AND DIAGNOSTIC TESTS
with Nursing Implications

TENTH EDITION

Joyce LeFever Kee, MSN, RN
Associate Professor Emerita
College of Science
University of Delaware
Newark, Delaware

330 Hudson Street, NY, NY 10013

Vice President, Health Science and TED:
  Julie Levin Alexander
Portfolio Manager: Hilarie Surrena
Portfolio Management Assistant: Taylor Scuglik
**Vice President, Content Production and Digital
  Studio:** Paul DeLuca
Managing Producer Health Science: Melissa Bashe
Content Producer: Michael Giacobbe
Operations Specialist: Maura Zaldivar-Garcia
Creative Director: Blair Brown
Creative Digital Lead: Mary Siener

Managing Producer, Digital Studio, Health Science:
  Amy Peltier
Vice President, Product Marketing: David Gesell
Executive Field Marketing Manager: Christopher Barry
Field Marketing Manager: Brittany Hammond
Full-Service Project Management and Composition:
  Sudip Sinha, iEnergizer Aptara®, Ltd.
Inventory Manager: Vatche Demirdjian
Cover Art: Shutterstock
Printer/Binder: LSC Communications, Inc.
Cover Printer: Phoenix Color/Hagerstown

Notice: Care has been taken to confirm the accuracy of information presented in this book. The author, contributors, editors, and publisher, however, cannot accept any responsibility for errors or omissions or for consequences from application of the information in this book and make no warranty, expressed or implied, with respect to its contents.

The author and publisher have exerted every effort to ensure that laboratory and diagnostic tests and drug selections and dosages set forth in this text are in accord with current recommendations and practice at time of publication. However, in view of ongoing research, changes in government regulations, and the constant flow of information relating to tests and drug therapy and drug reactions, the reader is urged to check the package inserts of all drugs for any change in indications of dosage and for added warnings and precautions. This is particularly important when the recommended agent is a new and/or infrequently employed drug.

Library of Congress Cataloging-in-Publication Data

Names: Kee, Joyce LeFever, author.
Title: Laboratory and diagnostic tests with nursing implications / Joyce
  LeFever Kee, MSN, RN, Associate Professor Emerita, College of Science,
  University of Delaware, Newark, Delaware.
Description: Tenth edition. | New York, NY : Pearson, [2018] | Includes
  bibliographical references and index.
Identifiers: LCCN 2017002010 | ISBN 9780134704463 | ISBN 0134704460
Subjects: LCSH: Diagnosis, Laboratory. | Nursing.
Classification: LCC RT48.5 .K44 2018 | DDC 616.07/5—dc23 LC record available at
  https://lccn.loc.gov/2017002010

1 17

 Pearson

ISBN 13: 978-0-13-470446-3
ISBN 10:   0-13-470446-0

This book I dedicate in loving memory of my mother and father
Esther Baker LeFever and Samuel Herr LeFever
for their years of love, encouragement, and support.

NOTICE OF PRIVACY PRACTICES

HEALTH INSURANCE PORTABILITY AND ACCOUNTABILITY PRIVACY ACT (HIPAA)

HIPAA, also known as "Notice of Privacy Practices," was first passed as an act on August 21, 1996. The details of the act and regulations were published on December 28, 2000. All agencies, including medical care personnel and facilities (physicians, care givers, institutions), laboratory and diagnostic facilities, pharmacies, and others, were required to comply with the act by April 14, 2003.

The clients sign a form to protect their medical information and laboratory test results from public disclosure without permission. This act provides the clients with more control over their health information and test results. It sets boundaries on the use and release of health records. It establishes appropriate safeguards to protect the privacy of health information. Also, this privacy act informs clients of how their health information may be used.

More information regarding HIPAA can be obtained at http://www.cdc.gov/mmwr/preview/mmwrhtml/su5201a1.htm.

CONTENTS

PREFACE

Each day hundreds of thousands of laboratory and diagnostic tests are performed, and thus nursing responsibilities are forever increasing. Nurses should understand laboratory and diagnostic tests and should provide nursing implications through nursing assessment, judgment, implementation, teaching, and interaction.

Laboratory and Diagnostic Tests with Nursing Implications, 10th edition, is designed to provide nurses and other health professionals with the necessary information regarding laboratory and diagnostic tests and corresponding nursing implications. It gives quick, pertinent information about the tests, emphasizing the purposes, procedure, and nursing implications with rationale. Reference values are given for adults and children. The tests (laboratory and diagnostic) are arranged in alphabetical order, which provides the user with quick access to the tests.

This text is appropriate for students in various types of nursing programs, including students in master's, baccalaureate, associate degree, diploma, and practical nursing programs. This book should be most valuable to the registered nurse and licensed practical nurse in hospital settings, including specialty areas such as the ICU and emergency room, clinics, health care providers' and physicians' offices, and in independent nursing practice.

NEW TO THIS EDITION

- *Fifteen New or Rewritten Laboratory and Diagnostic Tests.* These tests include the following: Zika virus; human immunodeficiency virus (HIV); antineutrophil cytoplasmic antibody; arterial blood gases (ABGs); bladder cancer/tumor markers; diabetes mellitus autoantibodies; infertility screen; placental growth factor; pregnancy-associated plasma protein-A; thyroid peroxidase (TPO); lung, lymph nodes, prostate gland, and thyroid biopsy; cardiac calcium scoring; D & C; and electroneurography.

- *Thoroughly Updated!* Updated tests include the following: arterial blood gases (ABGs), bilirubin tests, echocardiography (major revision), HIV (major revision), computed tomography (CT), magnetic resonance imaging (MRI), nuclear scan, positron emission tomography (PET), Pap smear, Pacemaker (major revision), and ultrasonography.

- *Situational Study Questions.* Practical study questions regarding common health problems, such as possible heart attack, heart failure, breast cancer, diabetes mellitus, colorectal cancer, peptic ulcer, pulmonary embolism, and others, are found at the end of Part One and Part Two. Students are given the opportunity to reflect on which tests should be considered and conducted in such instances and why.

- *Updated Part Three: Laboratory and Diagnostic Assessments of Body Function.* Laboratory and diagnostic tests have been added to the 12 categories related to organ, body structure, and clinical conditions that are within Part Three.

- *Updated! Therapeutic Drug Monitoring.* Part One has been updated to include drugs used for HIV monitoring.

- *Updated!* Appendices on abbreviations, 60 health problems with laboratory and diagnostic tests, and test values for adults and children.

- *Appendix C.* The appendix "Health Problems with Laboratory and Diagnostic Tests" includes 60 various health problems, such as Alzheimer disease, angina pectoris, and others. With each health problem, laboratory and diagnostic tests are given. This includes 20 newly added health problems since the last edition.

ORGANIZATION

Each test is discussed in seven subsections in the following sequence: (1) reference values/normal findings, (2) description, (3) purpose(s), (4) clinical problems, (5) procedure, (6) factors affecting laboratory or diagnostic results, and (7) nursing implications with rationale, including client teaching. Following the name and abbreviation for each test, there may be names of other closely associated tests. **Reference values/normal findings** are given for children and adults, including the elderly. The **description** focuses on background data and pertinent information related to the test. The general **purpose or purposes** for each test is listed. **Clinical problems** include disease entities, drugs, and foods that cause or are associated with abnormal test results. The **procedure** gives appropriate steps that the nurse and other health professionals can follow for each test. **Factors affecting laboratory or diagnostic results** alert the nurse to factors that could cause an abnormal test result. The last subsection and most valuable information for each test concerns the **nursing implications with rationale and client teaching**. For most diagnostic tests, nursing implications are given as "pretest" and "posttest." With laboratory and diagnostic tests, client teaching is included in these subsections.

There are five parts in the text: Part One, Laboratory Tests; Part Two, Diagnostic Tests; Part Three, Laboratory/Diagnostic Assessments of Body Function; Part Four, Therapeutic Drug Monitoring (TDM); and Part Five, School Health Services: Education, Screening, and Testing. There is a list of laboratory tests with page numbers at the beginning of Part One and a list of diagnostic tests with page numbers at the beginning of Part Two. In addition, general information appears in the introduction to the book, including the importance of **specimen collection** with detailed information about all types of specimen collection. Included is an explanation of the laboratory data warehouse. The value differences between men and women are presented. The **Instructions for Laboratory and Diagnostic Tests** section explains the information that will be found under the eight major subheadings for each test and gives basic information that relates to most of the laboratory and diagnostic tests.

Part Three, **Laboratory/Diagnostic Assessments of Body Function**, should be most valuable to both the practicing nurse and the student. The section consists of 12 categories related to organ system and clinical conditions. These are as follows: **Cardiac Function; Respiratory Function; Renal Function; Liver, Gallbladder, and Pancreatic Function; Gastrointestinal Function; Neurologic and Musculoskeletal Function; Endocrine Function; Reproductive Function; Arthritic, Collagen, and Infectious and Allergic Conditions; Shock; Neoplastic Conditions;** and **Hematologic Conditions.** Each category contains numerous laboratory and diagnostic tests ordered to assist in the diagnosis of disease entities and to determine organ function. These tests are briefly discussed with reference values as they relate to the organ or condition of that category. A few of the tests (e.g., enzyme tests) can be found in more than one category (cardiac, muscle, liver). **The nursing implications** are found at the end of each category.

Part Four, **Therapeutic Drug Monitoring (TDM)**, lists drugs that are monitored frequently by serum and urine for the purposes of achieving and maintaining therapeutic drug effects and for preventing drug toxicity. The TDM section includes 120 drugs and their therapeutic range, peak time, and toxic level. The current HIV drugs are given at the end of TDM, and dosing is based on the client's viral load or CD_4 counts.

Part Five, **School Health Services: Education, Screening, and Testing**, explains that school nurses are responsible for screening and testing for health problems in schoolchildren.

There are four appendices: **Abbreviations, Laboratory Test Groups** (laboratory profiles ordered for diagnosing clinical problems), **Health Problems with Laboratory and Diagnostic Tests**, and **Laboratory Test Values for Adults and Children**. Twenty new health problems have been added to Appendix C. The detailed index can assist in locating a test when the test name is different from the alphabetical listing used.

ACKNOWLEDGMENTS

I would like to extend my sincere thanks and deep appreciation to the following people who helped update the 10th edition: Ellen K. Boyda for arterial blood gases test and Pap smear; Dr. Anthony W. Clay for complete revision of echocardiography; Dr. Wesley Emmons for complete revision of HIV; Dr. Beth Ann Bilski for ultrasonography and assistance with the diagnostic tests; Katherine E. Blackhurst for assisting with the nursing implications; Dr. William Bilski for ECG (EKG); Dr. Garth Koniver for nuclear scan, positron emission tomography (PET), CT, and MRI; Leigh Silbert for her complete revisions of Pacemaker monitoring; Anne S. Biddle for the section on school health services; and Ronald J. Lefever for therapeutic drug monitoring (TDM). Thanks goes to the many professionals who had previously written, updated content, and reviewed the laboratory and diagnostic tests.

Many thanks to Hilarie Surrena, Michael Giacobbe and Sudip Sinha for their help on this edition. To my husband, Edward, go my love and appreciation for his support.

Joyce LeFever Kee, MSN, RN

PREVIOUS AND PRESENT CONTRIBUTORS AND CONSULTANTS

Anne S. Biddle, RN, BSN, NCSN
School Nurse, Newark Charter School
Newark, Delaware
Part Five: School Health Services: Education,
Screening, and Testing

Dr. Beth Ann Bilski
Newark, Delaware
Assistance with the Diagnostic Tests
Ultrasonography

Dr. William Bilski
Newark, Delaware
ECG (EKG)

Katherine Blackhurst, RN, BNS, BC, MSSI
Health Center Manager
Premise Health
Wilmington, Delaware
Assistance with Nursing Implications

Ellen K. Boyda, BSN, MSN, FNP
Family Nurse Practitioner and
Instructor, Widener College
Chester, Pennsylvania
Arterial Blood Gases
Pap Smear

Warren Butt, MD
Gastroenterology
Christiana Care Health Services
Newark, Delaware
Colonoscopy
ERCP
Esophageal Studies
Endoscopic Ultrasound
Video Capsule Endoscopy

Susan L. Chudzik, PN, MSN, CCNRP
Cardiology Department
Christiana Care Health Services
Newark, Delaware
Stress/Exercise Tests
Echocardiography
Positron Emission Tomography (PET)

Dr. Anthony W. Clay
Cardiologist
Newark and Wilmington, Delaware
Echocardiography

Laura Dechant, APN, MSN, CCRN, CCNS
Cardiac Catheterization Department
Christiana Care Health Services
Newark, Delaware
Cardiac Catheterization

Jennifer Duhon, RN, MS
Assistant Professor in Nursing
Illinois Central College
Peoria, Illinois
Reference Values Differentiation Between Men and
Women

Sharon W. Gould, MD
Director of Radiology Residency Program
Christiana Care Health Services
Newark, Delaware
Ultrasonography

Stephen Grahovac, MD
Department of Radiology
Christiana Care Health Services
Newark, Delaware
Computed Tomography (CT)
Magnetic Resonance Imaging (MRI)

Dr. Garth Koniver
Wilmington, Delaware
Computed Tomography (CT)
Magnetic Resonance Imaging (MRI)
Nuclear Scans
Positron Emission Tomography (PET)

Ronald J. Lefever, BS, RPh
Senior Pharmacist
Medical College of Virginia
Richmond, Virginia
Therapeutic Drug Monitoring (TDM)

Theresa Riggle, BS, CNMT, ARRT(N), NCT
Nuclear Medicine
Christiana Care Health Services
Newark, Delaware
Nuclear Scans

David C. Sestili, CRT, RPFT, LRCP
Technical and Research Coordinator
Pulmonary Laboratory
Temple University Hospital
Philadelphia, Pennsylvania
Pulmonary Function Tests

Leigh N. Sibert, BSN, MSN, APN ,CS
Clinical Nurse Specialist, Advanced Practice Nurse
Cardiology Consultants, P. A.
Wilmington, Delaware
Pacemaker Remote Monitoring

Helen Tang Yates, BS, MS
Professor Emerita
Medical Technology
University of Delaware
Newark, Delaware
Introduction to Laboratory Tests

ABOUT THE AUTHOR

Joyce LeFever Kee received her bachelor of science and master of science in nursing degrees from the University of Maryland and earned 36 postgraduate credits from the University of Delaware. She was an instructor at the University of Maryland for four years and instructor to associate professor at the University of Delaware for 27 years, teaching subjects including pharmacology, pathophysiology, fluid and electrolyte imbalances, and medical-surgical nursing in the classroom and clinical areas. She retired as associate professor emerita from the University of Delaware after teaching in both the undergraduate and graduate programs there.

A member of the Sigma Theta Tau Nursing Honor Society and the Phi Kappa Phi Honor Society, Kee has received the Excellence in Teaching Award and was inducted into the Mentor's Circle at the University of Delaware.

Kee gave numerous lectures and presentations throughout the United States and in Barbados from 1970 to 1990. She has written various articles, particularly on fluids and electrolytes, laboratory and diagnostic tests, and research projects, in the *American Journal of Nursing*, *Nursing Clinics of North America*, *Nursing Journal*, and *Critical Care Quarterly*. She has participated in several research studies on identification of hypertensive young adults.

Kee has authored and coauthored several texts and reference books, including *Fluids and Electrolytes with Clinical Applications* (2010); *Handbook of Fluid, Electrolyte, and Acid-Base Imbalances* (2010); *Handbook of Laboratory and Diagnostic Tests*, 8th ed. (2017); *Laboratory and Diagnostic Tests*, 10th ed. (2018); *Clinical Calculations in General and Specialty Areas*, 8th ed. (2017); and *Pharmacology: A Nursing Process Approach*, 8th ed. (2015). She has also developed a testbank booklet, instructor's manual, and study guide for some of the texts.

Consummate travelers, Kee and her husband have enjoyed visiting most parts of the world, including Australia, New Zealand, China, Japan, Great Britain, Russia, Greece, Italy, France, Turkey, Africa, South America, Egypt, Spain, India, Scandinavian countries, Mexico, the Caribbean islands, and others. They enjoy Florida in the winter.

■ INTRODUCTION

THE IMPORTANCE OF SPECIMEN COLLECTION

Nurses actively participate in laboratory testing protocols for clients. In addition to ordering laboratory tests, either on requisition slips or electronically, nurses provide input critical to obtaining valid and reliable laboratory test results. The nurse, in the role of caregiver and teacher, must communicate with the client, physician, and laboratory personnel to obtain information that might affect test results. Nursing responsibilities include explaining the laboratory test, ensuring that both the client and staff follow the procedure, assessing clinical findings with laboratory test results, noting pertinent information on the laboratory requisition slip (e.g., drugs the client is taking that might affect test results), and collecting the specimen. In some clinical settings, such as ICU, ER, and CCU, nurses also perform some laboratory procedures classified by the Clinical Laboratory Improvement Act (CLIA) as "Waivered Tests."

During the past decade, increasing numbers of point-of-care tests (POCT) have been performed by nurses. These tests have the major advantages of shortening the turnaround times for test results and of using a smaller sample of capillary blood from fingersticks. It is essential that the nurse be knowledgeable of the principle of the tests, be appropriately trained in performing the tests, and be aware of the potential errors.

Collection of specimens is the focus of this section. The following paragraphs present an overview of the various aspects of specimen collection: the types of specimens, the collection sites, the effect of the client's position and activity on test results, the importance of the time of collection, drug interference, labeling and handling of specimens, types of collection tubes, and the types of reported laboratory measurement.

Types of Specimens: The types of specimens that are used for laboratory studies are blood; urine (random or 24-hour collection); cerebrospinal fluid (CSF); feces; sputum; tissue or biopsy samples from surgery; and synovial, pleural, peritoneal, and wound exudate. Because blood is the most frequently analyzed specimen, its collection will be outlined below. When blood is withdrawn in a plain container, it clots. The fluid that can be separated from the clotted blood is called *serum*. The term *serum* is often used interchangeably with *plasma*. When an anticoagulant is added to a collection container, *no* clot is formed. The clear fluid is known as plasma, which contains the protein *fibrinogen*, a component that is converted to the substance that composes the clot, *fibrin*. Most tests (e.g., electrolyte levels) use serum from clotted blood. If a laboratory test requires plasma or whole blood, the tube used to collect the blood must contain an anticoagulant.

Drug Interference: Due to the growing number of drugs taken by clients, there is an increased chance that the laboratory results will be affected. This is especially true if drugs are taken over a period of time and at high doses. Drugs affecting test results should be noted on the laboratory slip. Drugs with a short half-life are withheld until the blood is drawn and thereby do not adversely affect the laboratory test result.

Labeling and Handling: Laboratory requisitions are designed by the institutions that use them and should include the following information: the client's full name, age, sex, room location, and possible diagnosis; the physician's name; the test being requested (indicated by a check mark); the date; the time of collection; and any special notation (such as drugs). Another type of identification, such as the client's Social Security number or medical record number, may be required. In computerized laboratories, a barcode label may be applied.

Specimen Transport: Proper handling and prompt transport of the specimen to the laboratory are vitally important. The goal for proper transport and handling is to maintain the integrity of the specimen as close to the vivo state as possible. When a blood specimen is not processed promptly, hemolysis can occur, causing inaccurate results; when a urine specimen sits longer than 30 minutes, the pH of the urine becomes alkaline as a result of bacteria growth.

Collection Tubes: Tubes have color-coded stoppers that indicate the type of additive in the tube. The additives include anticoagulants such as oxalates, citrates, ethylenediaminetetraacetic acid (EDTA), and heparin. Blood-serum specimens are obtained in a red-top tube that does not contain a chemical additive. However, there is a gel in the tube to hasten clotting and provide a separation barrier between the blood and serum. Examples of the laboratory groups and color-top tubes follow:

 Red: No additive, clotted blood. Serum is obtained from the clotted blood mass. Laboratory test groups that use red-top tubes are chemistries (electrolytes, proteins, enzymes, lipids, hormones), drug monitoring, radioimmunoassay (RIA) methods, serology, and blood banking. Hemolysis should be avoided.

 Lavender: The anticoagulant additive is EDTA. Laboratory test groups that use lavender-top tubes are hematologic tests (complete blood cell count [CBC], platelet count) and certain chemistries.

 Green: The anticoagulant additive is heparin. Laboratory test groups that use green-top tubes are arterial blood gases and the lupus erythematosus (LE) test. Although electrolyte levels are usually obtained from serum (red-top tube), a green-top tube may be substituted. In a stat situation, one need not wait for the blood to clot (red-top tube). The heparinized tube would allow the laboratory to centrifuge and separate the blood and plasma immediately.

 Blue: The anticoagulant additive is citrate. Laboratory groups that use blue-top tubes are coagulation studies (prothrombin time [PT], international normalized ratio [INR], activated partial thromboplastin time [APTT], partial thromboplastin time [PTT], and hemoglobin levels).

 Gray: The anticoagulant additive is sodium fluoride. The laboratory test for glucose uses gray-top tubes. The additive has a dual function as an anticoagulant and in preventing glycolysis, thus preserving the glucose concentration in the vivo state.

NOTE: The proper selection and usage of the color-coded collection tubes is critical for obtaining reliable test results. The additives must be compatible with the laboratory procedure. The nurse should always check with the institution's collection manual.

It would be beneficial for an institute to obtain a reference copy of the Clinical Laboratory Standards Institute (CLSI), H3-A6, Vol. 27, No. 26, sixth edition, "Procedures for Collection of Diagnostic Blood Specimens by Venipuncture." This comprehensive document provides improved safety guidelines, updated phlebotomy standards, and recommendations for order of draw for multiple-tube collections.

Types of Reported Laboratory Measurements

International System of Units: The World Health Organization (WHO) recommends that the medical and scientific community throughout the world adopt the Système International d'Unites (SI units) in order to establish a common international language for communicating laboratory measurements. Most clinical laboratories in Canada, Australia, and western Europe, and some in the United States, are now using SI units. Currently both metric and SI units are usually reported.

Reference Values: Reference values (expected values) are based on "apparently healthy" individuals and the equipment and methods used in laboratories. Due to differences in the methods and equipment used, reference values may vary among institutions.

Critical (Panic) Values: At times a client's test results may fall outside the range of reference values, and a decision must be made as to whether the physician should be notified. Most laboratories have a list of critical values. When a client's results exceed the values on this list, the physician or charge nurse must be notified immediately. The critical value policy and list are specific to each institution.

Clinical Laboratory Data Warehouse

The clinical laboratory data warehouse is created by the saving and using of data obtained from the laboratory database. Building a data warehouse provides a representation of laboratory values for the population. Test results for a few hundred people do not adequately represent the laboratory reference values for a large client population. A data warehouse of laboratory values of clients collected over numerous years is considered more effective in evaluating the population-based reference values. This method is less expensive than the traditional recruiting of volunteers for testing to determine laboratory "norms." The warehouse data include 5–10 times more people for the laboratory values/intervals. They provide a range according to age and sex better than the traditional method for obtaining laboratory values. For example, the young male has a higher alanine aminotransferase (ALT) level than the adult. Alkaline phosphatase (ALP) is usually higher in teenagers because of bone growth. By using warehouse laboratory data, accuracy for diagnosis and treatment of diseases is enhanced.

Descriptive interpretations are included for immunological procedures.

Helen Tang Yates, 2012

Instructions for Laboratory and Diagnostic Tests

This edition of *Laboratory and Diagnostic Tests with Nursing Implications* includes new and additional laboratory and diagnostic tests. Statements made in the **procedure** section, such as "there is no food or fluid restriction," will not be repeated in the **nursing implications** section. With all laboratory and diagnostic tests, the nurse needs to explain the purpose and procedure of the test, both of which can be obtained from the **description** and **procedure** sections. The following headings for laboratory and diagnostic tests help to clarify the changes.

Reference Values: Laboratory (norm) values can differ somewhat among institutions. The values given in this text are comparable to the reference values given in most institutions; however, nurses need to check the reference values at their institution.

Description: General information, such as the indications for a test or the pharmacology of a drug, is included in the description. Much of this information should be included when discussing the purpose of the test with the client.

Purpose: The general purpose is given for each laboratory and diagnostic test. If there is more than one purpose, only the most common ones are provided.

Clinical Problems: The disease entities that are associated with decreased and increased test results are listed according to decreasing frequency of occurrence. Drugs that influence test results are given for both decreased and increased levels. Drugs taken by the client that can affect test results should be listed on the laboratory requisition slip.

Procedure: The procedure is an important part of the test, and the nurse must discuss the procedure, step by step, with the client. Most of the procedures for laboratory and diagnostic tests are similar among institutions. The following are helpful suggestions applicable to most tests:

Laboratory Tests

1. Follow institutional policy and procedure.
2. Collect the recommended amount of specimen (blood, urine, etc.).
3. Avoid using the arm/hand that has an intravenous (IV) line for drawing venous blood.
4. Label clearly the specimen container with the client's identifying information.
5. Note significant drug data on the label or laboratory requisition slip or both.
6. Avoid hemolysis; do not shake blood specimens.
7. Observe strict aseptic technique when collecting and handling each specimen. Use OSHA guidelines as adopted by each institution (e.g., universal precautions).
8. Enforce food and fluid restriction only when indicated.
9. Collect 24-hour urine specimens:
   a. Have the client void prior to test, discard urine, and then save all urine for the specified time, such as 24 hours.
   b. Instruct the client to urinate into a sterile container, usually provided by the laboratory, then pour the urine into the large 24-hour container.
   c. Instruct the client to avoid contaminating the urine specimen with toilet paper or feces.
   d. Refrigerate the 24-hour urine or keep it on ice, unless preservatives are added or unless otherwise indicated.
   e. Label the urine collection bottle/container with the client's name, date, and exact time of collection (e.g., 6/21/20, 7:00 AM to 6/22/20, 7:01 AM).
10. List drugs and food the client is taking that could affect test results.
11. When possible, withhold medications and foods that could cause false test results until after the test. Before withholding drugs, check with the health care provider. This may not be practical or possible; however, if the client takes medication and the laboratory test is abnormal, this should be brought to the health care provider's attention.
12. Promptly send the specimen to the laboratory.

Diagnostic Tests

1. A signed consent form is usually requested.
2. Food and fluid restriction is frequently ordered. Check the procedure.
3. Institutional policies must be followed.

Factors Affecting Laboratory and Diagnostic Tests: Factors that affect test results should be identified and avoided when possible. When test results are abnormal, determine if factors identified could be contributing to the test results and report to the health care provider.

Nursing Diagnoses

General Basic Nursing Diagnoses: NANDA approved 2012–2014

- Activity intolerance related to diagnostic testing (e.g., angiography), pain (e.g., bone metastasis), and others.
- Anxiety related to the unknown.
- Impaired comfort related to the test procedure.
- Ineffective coping related to disease process and laboratory/diagnostic procedures.
- Disabled family coping related to numerous laboratory and diagnostic tests, hospitalization, and/or treatment.
- Deficient or excess fluid volume related to numerous laboratory and diagnostic tests and/or treatment regimen.
- Risk for injury related to allergic reactions to contrast medium (dye) because of the diagnostic test procedure.
- Deficient knowledge related to lack of understanding of laboratory and diagnostic procedures, disease process, and/or outcome.
- Noncompliance related to lack of adequate explanation and/or anxiety of the prescribed laboratory and diagnostic tests.
- Imbalanced nutrition: less than body requirements related to NPO, anorexia, vomiting, and/or diarrhea.
- Fear related to body changes, dependence, and results of the test(s).

General Basic Nursing Implications

1. Be knowledgeable about laboratory and diagnostic tests.
2. Explain the purpose(s) and procedure of each test to the client and family.
3. Provide time, and be available to answer questions. Be supportive of the client and family.
4. Follow the procedure that is stated for each test. Label specimens with client information.
5. Relate test findings to clinical problems and drugs. The test may be repeated to confirm a suspected problem.
6. Report abnormal results to the health care provider.
7. Compare test results with other related laboratory and/or diagnostic tests.
8. Encourage clients to keep medical appointments for follow-up.
9. Provide health teaching related to the clinical problem.
10. With diagnostic tests:
    a. Have the client void before premedication or before the test or both.
    b. Obtain a history of allergies to iodine or seafood. Observe for severe allergic reaction to contrast dye.
    c. Obtain baseline vital signs. Monitor vital signs as indicated following the test.
    d. If a sedative is used, instruct the client not to drive home.

DIFFERENCES IN REFERENCE VALUES BETWEEN MEN AND WOMEN*

In females, hematocrit (Hct), hemoglobin (Hgb), and red blood cell (RBC) count are less than in males. Serum ferritin is also decreased. This is due to monthly female menses. Normal values are as follows:

Hematocrit (Hct):   male: 40–54%, 0.4–0.54 (SI units)
female: 36–46%, 0.36–0.46 (SI units)

Hemoglobin (Hgb):   male: 13.5–18 g/dL, 8.4–11.2 mmol/L (SI units)
female: 12–15 g/dL, 7.45–9.31 mmol/L (SI units)

Red blood cell (RBC):   male: 4.6–6; female: 4–5

Serum ferritin: male: 15–445 ng/mL, 15–445 mcg/L
female: less than 40 years old: 10–120 ng/mL, 10–120 mcg/mL (SI units); greater than 40 years old: 10–235 ng/mL, 10–235 mcg/L (SI units); postmenopausal: 10–310 ng/mL, 10–310 mcg/L (SI units)

Apolipoprotein-A levels are increased in females due to the presence of estrogen and are decreased in males due to the presence of testosterone. Normal values are as follows:

Young adult: male: 80–155 mg/dL; 0.80–1.55 g/L (SI units)
female: 80–186 mg/dL; 0.80–1.86 g/L (SI units)

Middle-aged adult: male: 100–165 mg/dL; 1–1.65 g/L (SI units)
female: 93–200 mg/dL; 0.93–2 g/L (SI units)

Elderly: male: 85–166 mg/dL; 0.85–1.66 g/L (SI units)
female: 120–215 mg/dL; 1.20–2.15 g/L (SI units)

Apolipoprotein-B levels are increased in males due to the presence of androgens such as testosterone. Normal values are as follows:

Adult/elderly: male: 50–170 mg/dL; 0.50–1.70 g/L (SI units)
female: 46–155 mg/dL; 0.46–1.55 g/L (SI units)

Serum copper is present in increased amounts in females. Estrogen stimulates the liver to produce a compound that is responsible for transporting copper. Normal values are as follows:

Adult: male: 70–140 mcg/dL
female: 80–155 mcg/dL

The serum cholesterol in females before menopause is lower than after menopause. This is because of the presence of endogenous estrogen. Normal values are as follows:

Adult: male: less than 205 mg/dL
female: less than 190 mg/dL

---

*Written and updated by Jennifer Duhon, RN, MS, Assistant Professor, Illinois Central College, Peoria, Illinois.

The fact that females typically have less muscle mass than their male counterparts explains why females usually have decreased serum creatinine, serum myoglobin, and creatinine clearance. Normal values are as follows:

Adult serum creatinine: male: 0.5–1.5 mg/dL
        female: slightly lower than male values

Adult serum myoglobin: male: 20–90 ng/mL, 20–90 mcg/L (SI units)
        female: 12–75 ng/mL, 12–75 mcg/L (SI units)

Adult creatinine clearance: male: 85–135 mL/min
        female: slightly lower than male values

Females experience a slightly lower creatine kinase (CK), which is the result of higher muscle mass in males. Normal values are as follows:

Adult: male: 5–35 mcg/mL, 38–180 international units/L
        female: 5–25 mcg/mL, 25–150 international units/L

The erythrocyte sedimentation rate (ESR) in males is often lower than in females. This difference is caused by the female menstrual cycle and associated hormones. Normal values are as follows:

Adult less than 50 years old: male: 0–15 mm/h (Westergren method)
        female: 0–20 mm/h

Adult greater than 50 years old: male: 0–20 mm/h (Westergren method)
        female: 0–30 mm/h

Adult (Wintrobe method):   male: 0–9 mm/h
        female: 0–15 mm/h

The gamma-glutamyl transferase (for detecting hepatic disease) is usually lower in females than males. It is higher in newborns and slightly higher in the elderly than adults. Normal values are as follows.

Adult: male: 4–23 international units/L; 9–69 units/L (SI units)
        female: 3–13 international units/L; 4–33 units/L (SI units)

Females have increased levels of human growth hormone (measured as somatotrophic hormone [STH]). The presence of estrogen explains this increase. Normal values are as follows:

Adult: male: less than 5 ng/mL
        female: less than 10 ng/mL

The adrenal hormone metabolites 17-hydroxycorticosteroids (17-OHCS) and 17-ketosteroids (17-KS) are found in lesser amounts in females. 17-OHCS is lesser because males typically have more muscle mass than females. The fact that females have more estrogen than androgens explains why females have less 17-KS. Pregnanetriol is also a substance produced by the adrenal glands and is available in lower amounts in females. Normal values are as follows:

Adult 17-OHCS: male: 3–12 mg/24 h
        female: 2–10 mg/24 h

Adult 17-KS: male: 5–25 mg/24 h

female: 5–15 mg/24 h

Adult pregnanetriol: male: 0.4–2.4 mg/24 h

female: 0.5–2.0 mg/24 h

Iron (serum) level is lower in females than males. This could be due to menses. Normal value is as follows:

Adult: male: 80–180 mcg/dL

female: 69–160 mcg/dL

Leucine aminopeptidase (LAP) is an enzyme that is prescribed to detect bone disease. LAP is slightly higher in males than females. Normal values are as follows:

Adult: male: 80–200 units/mL

female: 75–185 units/mL

Osteocalcin is an indicator of bone metabolism. Elevated levels occur in females during post-menopause due to osteoporosis. The osteocalcin enters the circulation. Normal values are as follows:

Adult: male: 1.5–11.5 ng/mL; 1.5–11.5 mcg/L (SI units)

female: premenopausal: 0.5–7.8 ng/mL; 0.5–7.8 mcg/L (SI units)

postmenopausal: 1.2–11.5 ng/mL; 1.2–11.5 mcg/L (SI units)

Average serum prealbumin levels in males are higher than in females due to increased muscle mass in males and estrogen levels in females. Normal values are as follows:

Adult averages: male: 21.6 mg/dL, 216 mg/L (SI units)

female: 18 mg/dL, 180 mg/L (SI units)

Thyroxine (T_4) is the major hormone secreted by the thyroid gland. The serum value is about the same in males and females, though it can be slightly higher in females. The value is higher in newborns and in children up to the age of 6 years. Normal values are as follows:

Adult: male: 4–12 mcg/dL

female: 5–12 mcg/dL

Serum uric acid levels are higher in males than in females because estrogen promotes excretion of uric acid. Normal values are as follows:

Adult: male: 3.5–8 mg/dL

female: 2.8–6.8 mg/dL

Pulmonary function tests also differ between males and females due to factors such as age, height, weight, body type, and gender. The categories of pulmonary function tests include but are not limited to the following:

- Tidal volume
- Inspiratory capacity
- Expiratory reserve volume
- Inspiratory reserve volume
- Vital capacity
- Residual volume
- Functional residual capacity
- Forced vital capacity
- Forced inspiratory volume
- Forced expiratory volume timed
- Peak expiratory flow
- Peak inspiratory flow
- Total lung capacity

PART ONE

Laboratory Tests

Acetaminophen (serum)

Tylenol, Tempra, Datril, Liquiprin, Paracetamol, Panadol, Aceta

Reference Values

Adult: *Therapeutic:* 5–20 mcg/mL, 31–124 µmol/L (SI units). *Toxic:* Greater than 50 mcg/mL, 305 µmol/L (SI units), greater than 200 mcg/mL possible hepatotoxicity.

Child: *Therapeutic:* Same as adult. *Toxic:* Similar to adult.

Description

Acetaminophen has a similar antipyretic and non-narcotic analgesic effect to that of aspirin. Unlike salicylates (e.g., aspirin), acetaminophen does not inhibit platelet aggregation, does not produce gastric distress and bleeding, and has only a weak anti-inflammatory response.

Overdose of acetaminophen can be dangerous, since it can lead to hepatotoxicity. It is metabolized in the liver to active metabolites and is absorbed rapidly from the gastrointestinal (GI) tract. Peak time occurs ½–2 hours after oral ingestion. When there is an accumulation of acetaminophen in the body from massive dose(s) or chronic use, one of its metabolites tends to cause hepatotoxicity. Actually, a single dose of 10 g or 20–30 tablets (500/325 mg each) could cause liver damage. The half-life of acetaminophen is about 3 hours. If the half-life is greater than 4 hours, hepatic injury is likely to occur. After ingestion of a large amount of acetaminophen, either accidentally (e.g., ingested by children) or in a suicide attempt, serum concentrations are plotted on a semilogarithmic scale. If the serum value is 200 mcg/mL (1,240 µmol/L) in 4 hours, or 50 mcg/mL (310 µmol/L) in 12 hours after ingestion, hepatotoxicity could occur 3–6 days later. A suggested oral dose of acetaminophen is 2–3 g (2,000–3,000 mg) per day.

The antidote to acetaminophen toxicity is *N*-acetylcysteine (Mucomyst). It must be administered soon after acetaminophen ingestion. Liver function tests (i.e., AST [SGOT], ALT [SGPT]), bilirubin, prothrombin time (PT), and electrolytes should be closely monitored.

Purposes

- To determine if the therapeutic acetaminophen dose is within therapeutic range.
- To check for acetaminophen toxicity.

Clinical Problems

Decreased Level: High-carbohydrate meal.

Increased Level: Acetaminophen overdose, liver disease. *Drug Influence:* Phenobarbital.

Procedure

- There is no food or fluid restriction.
- Collect 3–5 mL of venous blood in a red-top tube.
- Record the dose and the time the drug was taken on the laboratory requisition slip.

Factors Affecting Laboratory Results

- None known.

A

NURSING IMPLICATIONS WITH RATIONALE

- Explain to the client that the purpose of the test is to monitor the therapeutic level or the toxic level of acetaminophen (give trade name).
- Suggest to the health care provider that liver function tests be ordered periodically for clients on long-term acetaminophen therapy. Liver damage could result when the drug is taken for weeks and/or months.
- Keep the acetaminophen bottle tightly closed and away from light.

Increased Level

- Recognize that liver disease and acetaminophen overdose could result in hepatotoxicity.
- Observe for signs and symptoms of acetaminophen toxicity (e.g., anorexia, nausea, vomiting, lethargy, generalized weakness, epigastric or abdominal pain).
- Observe for signs and symptoms of liver damage (e.g., vomiting, jaundice, right upper quadrant tenderness, abnormal liver function tests).

Client Teaching

- Inform the client about the need to take the prescribed dosage. An overdose or chronic use of acetaminophen could cause liver damage. Usually the drug should not be taken for more than 10 days at a time unless prescribed by the health care provider.
- Inform the client who consumes large amounts of alcohol of the need to consult his or her health care provider before taking acetaminophen products. This person could be prone to liver damage, and ingestion of acetaminophen would compound the liver problem.
- Instruct the client to keep acetaminophen products out of the reach of children. If a child ingests large amounts of the drug, the poison center should be called immediately, syrup of ipecac given if indicated by the center, and the child taken to the emergency room. Acetylcysteine (Mucomyst) has been used as an antidote for adults within 16 hours after drug overdose.

Acetone, ketone bodies (serum or plasma)

Reference Values

Adult: *Acetone:* Semiquantitative: Negative (less than 1 mg/dL); quantitative: 0.3–2 mg/dL, 51.6–344 µmol/L (SI units). *Ketones:* 0.5–4 mg/dL.

Child: *Newborn to 1 Week:* Slightly higher than adult. *Over 1 Week:* Same as adult.

Description

Ketone bodies are composed of three compounds—acetone, acetoacetic (diacetic) acid, and beta-hydroxybutyric acid—which are products of fat metabolism and fatty acids. Ketone bodies result from uncontrolled diabetes mellitus and starvation, causing increased fat catabolism instead of carbohydrate metabolism. In diabetic ketoacidosis, the serum acetone is greater than 50 mg/dL.

Ketones are small and excretable in the urine. However, the elevation is first apparent in the plasma or serum, then in the urine. Serum acetone (as ketones) is useful in monitoring acidosis caused by uncontrolled diabetes or starvation, since the serum level will decrease toward normal before the urine test (Acetest) does.

Purposes

- To detect the presence of ketone bodies.
- To identify the occurrence of diabetic ketoacidosis.

Clinical Problems

Increased Level: Diabetic ketoacidosis, starvation/malnutrition, vomiting and diarrhea, heat stroke, exercise.

Procedure

- There is no food or fluid restriction.
- Collect 3–5 mL of venous blood in a red-top tube.

Factors Affecting Laboratory Results

- Contamination can cause false-positive results.

NURSING IMPLICATIONS WITH RATIONALE

Increased Level

- Relate increased serum acetone levels to diabetic acidosis and starvation. Many of the diet programs call for high-protein and low-carbohydrate intake. Daily carbohydrate intake of less than 100 g can result in ketosis (excess ketone bodies) caused by the substitution of fat metabolism for energy.
- Obtain a history from the client concerning his or her diet. If the client is on a reducing diet, the increased serum level (ketosis) could be caused by a low-carbohydrate diet.
- Assess for signs and symptoms of diabetic ketoacidosis, such as rapid, vigorous breathing; restlessness; confusion; sweet-smelling breath; and a serum acetone level greater than 50 mg/dL.
- Check the urine for ketone bodies. An Acetest is usually performed and is positive.

Acetylcholine receptor antibody (AChR) (serum)

Acetylcholine Receptor Binding Antibody Test, Anti-Acetylcholine Receptor Antibody

Reference Values

Less than 0.02 to less than 0.03 nmol/L or negative.

A

Description

Acetylcholine receptor antibodies (AChRs) occur in about 85% of clients with myasthenia gravis (MG). This antibody may cause destruction of the muscle cells by binding at the acetylcholine receptors on the skeletal muscle membrane, thus preventing muscle contraction. This antibody test is most useful in the diagnosis of myasthenia gravis and in monitoring the response to drug therapy. A negative AChR test does not always increase MG. Approximately 70% of clients with ocular MG have a positive AChR test. Also, a positive result from this test confirms the autoimmune nature of the disease.

There are three AChR antibody tests, AChR-binding antibody, AChR-modulating antibody, and AChR-blocking antibody, of which the AChR-binding antibody test is the most frequently prescribed test for diagnosing MG.

Purposes

- To aid in the diagnosis of myasthenia gravis.
- To monitor the effects of drug therapy for clients with MG.

Clinical Problems

Decreased Level: *Drug Influence:* Immunosuppressive drugs.

Increased Level: Myasthenia gravis, ocular MG. *Drug Influence:* Succinylcholine.

Procedure

- There is no food or fluid restriction.
- Collect 5–7 mL of venous blood in a red-top tube.

Factors Affecting Laboratory Results

- False-positive results may occur in clients with amyotrophic lateral sclerosis (ALS).
- Clients with autoimmune liver disease may have a false-positive test result.

NURSING IMPLICATIONS WITH RATIONALE

- Obtain a history of present symptoms the client is having. Symptoms of MG may include fatigue and weakness of muscles, ptosis, diplopia, dysphagia, and difficulty in chewing. With severe MG, respiratory muscles are usually affected.
- Monitor vital signs (VS).
- Note muscle weakness in upper extremities, respiratory, eyelid.
- Answer client's questions or refer questions to other health care professionals.

Client Teaching

- Instruct client to take medication for MG as prescribed. Explain to the client that he or she should not miss scheduled drug doses.
- Inform client to keep medical appointments for monitoring MG.

Acid-base balance/imbalance
See Arterial Blood Gases (ABGs) (arterial blood)

Acid phosphatase (ACP) (serum)
Prostatic Acid Phosphatase (PAP)

Reference Values
Adult: Less than 2.6 ng/mL; 0–5 unit/L range, varies according to the method used; 0.2–13 international unit/L (SI units).

Description
The enzyme acid phosphatase (ACP) is found in the prostate gland and in semen in high concentration. It is found in lesser extent in bone marrow, red blood cells (RBCs), liver, and spleen. The highest rise in serum ACP/PAP occurs in prostate cancer. In benign prostatic hypertrophy (BPH) also, the level is above normal. A markedly elevated alkaline phosphatase level may cause a falsely high serum ACP level. Prostate-specific antigen (PSA) is a more sensitive test for diagnosing prostate cancer than ACP/PAP.

Purpose
- To compare the ACP/PAP test with other laboratory values for diagnosing prostate cancer or BPH.

Clinical Problems
Decreased Level: Down syndrome. *Drug Influence:* Fluorides, oxalates, phosphates, alcohol.

Increased Level: Carcinoma of the prostate, multiple myeloma, Paget disease, cancer of the breast and bone, BPH, sickle-cell anemia, cirrhosis, chronic renal failure, hyperparathyroidism, osteogenesis imperfecta, myocardial infarction (MI). *Drug Influence:* Androgens in females, clofibrate (Atromid-S).

Procedure
- There is no food or fluid restriction.
- Collect 3–7 mL of venous blood in a red-top tube.
- Hemolysis should be prevented, and the specimen should be taken to the laboratory immediately. ACP is heat- and pH-sensitive. If the specimen is exposed to air and left at room temperature, there will be a decrease in activity after 1 hour.

Factors Affecting Laboratory Results
- Hemolysis of the blood sample can cause an inaccurate test result.
- Certain drugs can decrease the serum ACP level (*see Drug Influence*).
- Exposure of the blood specimen to air and room temperature for longer than 1 hour can cause a decrease in the ACP level.

A

NURSING IMPLICATIONS WITH RATIONALE

Decreased Level

- Know which drugs can cause a decreased serum ACP level.

Increased Level

- Recognize clinical problems associated with an elevated serum ACP/PAP level. A high serum ACP/PAP level occurs with metastasized prostate cancer.
- Indicate on the laboratory slip if the client had a prostate examination 24 hours before the test. Prostatic massage or extensive palpation of the prostate can elevate the serum ACP/PAP.
- Check the serum ACP following treatment for carcinoma of the prostate gland. With surgical intervention, the serum level should drop in 3–4 days; following estrogen therapy (when the treatment is successful), it should drop in 3–4 weeks. If serum ACP has not been ordered, a reminder or suggestion to the physician may be necessary.
- Notify the laboratory before the serum ACP/PAP is drawn so that immediate attention will be given to the specimen.
- Encourage the client to express concerns about the prostate problem.

Activated partial thromboplastin time (APTT)

See Partial Thromboplastin Time

Adenovirus antibody (serum)

Reference Values

Adult and Child: Negative. *Positive:* Fourfold titer increase.

Description

The adenovirus is frequently present among school-aged children and military recruits; many may be asymptomatic. Adenovirus can be responsible for upper respiratory tract disease, cystitis (hemorrhagic), and keratoconjunctivitis. Transmission may be by direct or indirect contact.

Purpose

- To determine the cause of upper respiratory tract disease and pharyngitis.

Clinical Problems

Positive: Adenovirus infections of the upper respiratory tract, hemorrhagic cystitis, keratoconjunctivitis, pharyngitis.

A

Procedure

- There is no food or fluid restriction.
- Collect 3–5 mL of venous blood in a red-top tube. Avoid hemolysis. A second blood specimen is usually obtained 2–3 weeks later to determine the acute and convalescent titers. The blood specimen should be marked either acute or convalescent phase.
- A swab of the drainage from the infected area (e.g., the throat, eye, urethra) may be obtained for immunofluorescence testing to determine the presence of an adenoviral infection. The swab specimen should be labeled and taken immediately to the laboratory for testing.

Factors Affecting Laboratory Results

- Hemolysis of the blood specimen.
- Inaccurate labeling of the blood sample.

NURSING IMPLICATIONS WITH RATIONALE

- Obtain a history from the client or family concerning the infected area involved. List symptoms the client may have (such as drainage and its color).
- Check with the client about contact with other persons who have described similar symptoms.

Client Teaching

- Explain to the client the procedure for laboratory testing. There will most likely be a second blood sample taken 2–3 weeks after the first blood specimen.
- If there is a swab specimen to be obtained, explain to the client that a swab will be taken of the infected area.
- Answer the client's or family's questions or refer to appropriate health care providers.

Adrenocorticotropic hormone (ACTH) (plasma)

Corticotropin, Corticotropin-Releasing Factor (CRF)

Reference Values

7–10 AM: 8–80 pg/mL; 8–80 ng/L (SI units); highest levels occur in early morning.

4 PM: 5–50 pg/mL; 5–50 ng/L (SI units).

10 PM to Midnight: Less than 10 pg/mL; lowest levels occur at bedtime.

Description

Adrenocorticotropic hormone (ACTH), or corticotropin, is stored and released from the anterior pituitary gland (adenohypophysis) under the influence of corticotropin-releasing factor (CRF—from the hypothalamus) and the plasma cortisol from the adrenal cortex. The negative-feedback

A

mechanism controls ACTH release; when plasma cortisol is low, ACTH is released, and when plasma cortisol is increased, ACTH release is inhibited. Stress caused by surgery, infections, and physical and emotional trauma increases the ACTH level. The ACTH level follows a diurnal pattern: peaks in the early morning and ebbs in the late evening or at bedtime.

A plasma ACTH is performed to determine whether a decreased plasma cortisol level is due to adrenal cortex hypofunction or pituitary hypofunction. Two tests, ACTH suppression and ACTH stimulation, may be ordered to identify the origin of the clinical problem, either the adrenal cortex or the pituitary gland.

ACTH Suppression Test: For the ACTH suppression test, a synthetic potent cortisol, dexamethasone (Decadron), is given to suppress the production of ACTH. If an extremely high dose is needed for ACTH suppression, the cause is of pituitary origin, such as pituitary tumor producing an excess of ACTH secretion. If the plasma cortisol continues to be high with ACTH suppression, the cause could be adrenal cortex hyperfunction (Cushing syndrome). Suppressing pituitary release of ACTH will not affect a hyperactive adrenal gland.

ACTH Stimulation Test: For the ACTH stimulation test, ACTH (cosyntropin) is administered and the plasma cortisol level should double in 1 hour. If the plasma cortisol level remains the same or is lower, adrenal gland insufficiency (Addison disease) is the cause. To check for pituitary hypofunction, the drug metyrapone (Metopirone) is given to block the production of cortisol, thus causing an increase in ACTH secretion. If the ACTH level does not increase, the problem is pituitary insufficiency.

Purposes

- To determine if a decreased plasma cortisol level is due to adrenal cortex hypofunction or pituitary hypofunction.
- To evaluate the ACTH suppression test results for health problem(s) of pituitary origin.
- To check for adrenal or pituitary hypofunction.
- To utilize the ACTH stimulation test to determine the presence of adrenal gland insufficiency.

Clinical Problems

Decreased Level: Adrenocortical hyperplasia, cancer of the adrenal gland, hypopituitarism. *Drug Influence:* Steroids (cortisone, prednisone, dexamethasone), estrogen, alcohol.

Increased Level: Stress (trauma, physical or emotional), Addison disease (adrenal hypofunction), pituitary neoplasm, surgery, pyrogens, pregnancy. *Drug Influence:* Amphetamines, ethanol, estrogen, aldosterone, metyrapone, vasopressin, insulin.

Procedure

- Food and fluid may be restricted. A low-carbohydrate diet may be requested for 24 hours prior to the test.
- Collect 5–7 mL of venous blood in a lavender-top *plastic* tube or prechilled purple-top tube. Pack the tube in ice *immediately* and send it to the laboratory. Blood should not come in contact with glass. If a glass tube is used, centrifuge and transfer to a plastic vial *as soon as possible*. Additional testing may be needed because a single plasma value may be misleading.
- If adrenal hypofunction is suspected, the blood sample is taken at the peak time, in early morning. If adrenal hyperfunction is suspected, the blood sample is usually taken at low time, in the evening.

A

- Note on the laboratory label the time the blood specimen was drawn. If the test is to be repeated the next morning, the blood sample should be drawn at the same time as the first specimen.
- Restrict activity and stress (if possible) for 8–12 hours before the test. If possible, restrict drugs such as cortisone until after the test.

Factors Affecting Laboratory Results

- Certain drugs (*see Drug Influence for decreased and increased levels*).
- Stress and physical activity.
- Collection of the blood sample in a glass tube.
- Collection of the blood samples at different times of the day and not noting this on the laboratory slip.

NURSING IMPLICATIONS WITH RATIONALE

- Obtain a history of the client's clinical symptoms and drug regimen. Steroids increase the ACTH secretion.
- Compare elevated plasma ACTH levels with plasma cortisol if ordered. With adrenal gland insufficiency or a pituitary tumor, ACTH secretion will be increased.

Client Teaching

- Explain to the client undergoing ACTH suppression with dexamethasone or ACTH stimulation with ACTH or metyrapone that these drugs are used to confirm the cause of the hormonal imbalance.
- Encourage the client to avoid stress and physical exercise because they could increase plasma ACTH levels.
- Be supportive of the client and the family. Allow time for the client to ventilate his or her fears.

AIDS virus

See Human Immunodeficiency Virus (HIV)

Alanine aminotransferase (ALT) (serum)

Serum Glutamic Pyruvic Transaminase (SGPT)

Reference Values

Adult: 10–35 unit/L; 4–36 unit/L at 37°C (SI units). *Male:* Levels may be slightly higher.

Child: *Infant:* Could be twice as high as adult. *Child:* Similar to adult.

Elderly: Slightly higher than adult.

A

Description

Alanine aminotransferase (ALT)/serum glutamic pyruvic transaminase (SGPT) is an enzyme found primarily in the liver cells and is effective in diagnosing hepatocellular destruction. It is also found in small amounts in the heart, kidney, and skeletal muscle.

Serum ALT levels can be higher than levels of its sister transferase (transaminase), aspartate aminotransferase (AST)/serum glutamic oxaloacetic transaminase (SGOT), in cases of acute hepatitis and liver damage from drugs and chemicals. With its serum levels reaching 200–4,000 unit/L, ALT is used to differentiate between jaundice caused by liver disease and hemolytic jaundice. With jaundice, the serum ALT levels of liver origin can be higher than 300 units; from causes outside the liver, the levels can be less than 300 units. Serum ALT levels usually elevate before jaundice appears.

ALT/SGPT levels are frequently compared with AST/SGOT levels for diagnostic purposes. ALT is more markedly increased than AST in liver necrosis and acute hepatitis, while AST is more markedly increased in myocardial necrosis (acute myocardial infarction), cirrhosis, cancer of the liver, chronic hepatitis, and liver congestion. ALT levels are normal or slightly elevated in myocardial necrosis. The ALT levels return more slowly to normal range than AST levels in liver conditions.

Purpose

- To detect the presence of a liver disorder.

Clinical Problems

Decreased Level: Exercise. *Drug Influence:* Salicylates.

Increased Level: *Highest Increase:* Acute (viral) hepatitis, necrosis of the liver (drug or chemical toxicity). *Slight or Moderate Increase:* Cirrhosis, cancer of the liver, heart failure (HF), acute alcohol intoxication. *Drug Influence:* Antibiotics (carbenicillin, clindamycin, erythromycin, gentamicin, lincomycin, mithramycin, spectinomycin, tetracycline), narcotics (meperidine [Demerol], morphine, codeine), antihypertensives (methyldopa, guanethidine), digitalis preparations, indomethacin (Indocin), salicylates, rifampin, flurazepam (Dalmane), propranolol (Inderal), oral contraceptives (progestin-estrogen), lead, heparin.

Procedure

- There is no food or fluid restriction.
- Collect 3–5 mL of venous blood in a red-top tube. Avoid hemolysis, because RBCs have a high concentration of ALT.
- Drugs administered to the client that can cause false-positive levels should be listed on the laboratory slip along with the date last given.

Factors Affecting Laboratory Results

- Hemolysis of the blood specimen may cause false test results.
- Aspirin can cause a decrease or increase of serum ALT.
- Certain drugs can increase the serum ALT level (*see Drug Influence*).

NURSING IMPLICATIONS WITH RATIONALE

Increased Level

- Relate the client's serum ALT/SGPT to clinical problems. A high serum increase (greater than 2,000 units) can indicate liver necrosis from toxic agents or from acute viral hepatitis.
- Compare ALT and AST levels if both have been ordered. ALT is a better indicator of acute liver damage and will be at higher levels than AST in liver necrosis and acute hepatitis.
- Check for signs of jaundice. ALT levels rise several days before jaundice begins if it is related to liver damage. However, if jaundice is present and serum ALT levels are normal or slightly elevated, the liver may not be the cause of the jaundice.

Client Teaching

- Instruct the client to report signs of jaundice, such as yellow color in the sclera of the eyes.

Albumin (serum)

Reference Values

Adult: 3.5–5 g/dL; 52–68% of total protein.

Child: *Newborn:* 2.9–5.4 g/dL. *Infant:* 4.4–5.4 g/dL. *Child:* 4–5.8 g/dL.

Description

Albumin, a component of proteins, makes up more than half of plasma proteins. Albumin is synthesized by the liver. It increases osmotic pressure (oncotic pressure), which is necessary for maintaining the vascular fluid. A decrease in serum albumin will cause fluid to shift from within the vessels to the tissues, resulting in edema.

The *A/G ratio* is a calculation of the distribution of two major protein fractions, albumin and globulin. The reference value of A/G ratio is greater than 1, which is the albumin value divided by globulin value (albumin ÷ globulin). A high ratio value is considered insignificant; low ratio value occurs in liver and renal diseases. Protein electrophoresis is more accurate and has replaced the A/G ratio calculation.

Purpose

- To detect an albumin deficit.

Clinical Problems

Decreased Level (Hypoalbuminemia): Cirrhosis of the liver, acute liver failure, severe burns, severe malnutrition, preeclampsia, renal disorders, certain malignancies, ulcerative colitis, prolonged immobilization, protein-losing enteropathies, malabsorption. *Drug Influence:* Penicillin, sulfonamides, aspirin, ascorbic acid.

Increased Level (Hyperalbuminemia): Dehydration, severe vomiting, severe diarrhea. *Drug Influence:* Heparin.

A

Procedure

- There is no food or fluid restriction.
- Collect 3–5 mL of venous blood in a red-top tube.

Factors Affecting Laboratory Results

- Certain drugs could cause false negatives and false positives (*see Drug Influence*).

NURSING IMPLICATIONS WITH RATIONALE

- Check for peripheral edema and ascites when serum albumin is low. A low serum albumin decreases the oncotic pressure; thus fluid shifts from the vascular fluid to the tissue spaces, causing edema.
- Assess for skin integrity if pitted edema or anasarca is present. Implement measures to avoid skin breakdown.
- Offer foods high in protein (e.g., meats, cheese, beans).

Client Teaching

- Teach the client the importance of maintaining an adequate amount of protein in the diet with health care provider's approval. Protein should increase the serum albumin level and decrease peripheral edema unless the client has cirrhosis of the liver.

Alcohol (ethyl or ethanol) (serum or plasma)

Reference Values

No Alcohol: 0%. *No Significant Alcohol Influence:* Less than 0.05% or 50 mg/dL. *Alcohol Influence Present:* 0.05–0.10% or 50–100 mg/dL. *Reaction Time Affected:* 0.10–0.15% or 100–150 mg/dL. *Indicative of Alcohol Intoxication:* Greater than 0.15% or greater than 150 mg/dL. *Severe Alcohol Intoxication:* Greater than 0.25% or 250 mg/dL. *Comatose:* Greater than 0.30% or 300 mg/dL. *Fatal:* Greater than 0.40% or 400 mg/dL.

Description

The ethyl alcohol (ethanol) level in the blood is a frequently requested laboratory test for medical and legal reasons. In most states an alcohol level greater than 0.10% or 100 mg/dL is considered by law to be proof of alcohol intoxication. However, some states consider 0.08% or 80 mg/dL as proof of alcohol toxicity. On an empty stomach, plasma alcohol peaks in 40–70 minutes.

Serum/plasma alcohol may be used as a screening test on an unconscious client. Nurses should check for any legal ramifications (state laws) in reference to drawing blood for plasma alcohol levels.

On the roads or highways, a breathalyzer can be used by having the automobile driver breathe deeply into the breathalyzer. A conversion factor is used to estimate the amount of alcohol in the blood. Urine and saliva samples may be used to estimate the amount of alcohol in the blood.

A

Purpose

- To detect the percentage of alcohol in the bloodstream and to determine whether the client was DUI (driving under the influence).

Clinical Problems

Increased Level: Moderate to severe alcohol intoxication, chronic alcohol consumption, cirrhosis of the liver, malnutrition, folic acid deficiency, leukopenia, acute pancreatitis, gastritis, hypoglycemia, hyperuricemia. *Drug Influence:* Alcohol–drug interactions: (1) increases the effects of sedatives, hypnotics, narcotics, and tranquilizers (especially chlordiazepoxide [Librium] and diazepam [Valium]), depressing the central nervous system response; and (2) antagonizes the action of warfarin (Coumadin) and phenytoin (Dilantin).

Procedure

- Obtain a consent form if required by law.
- Cleanse the venipuncture area with benzalkonium, and then wipe the solution off with a sterile swab or sponge. *Do not use* alcohol or tincture to cleanse the area.
- Collect 3–5 mL of venous blood in a red-top tube. A green-, lavender-, or blue-top tube can be used. Avoid hemolysis.
- Write on the specimen and laboratory slip the date and time the blood specimen was drawn. The signatures of the collector and a witness may be included on the tube (only for legal cases).

Factors Affecting Laboratory Results

- Methyl alcohol (wood alcohol) and isopropyl alcohol (rubbing alcohol) can cause elevated serum alcohol levels and are very toxic.
- Cleansing the venipuncture site with alcohol or tincture can cause inaccurate results.
- Alcohol–drug interactions can affect results (*see Drug Influence*).

NURSING IMPLICATIONS WITH RATIONALE

Increased Level (Greater than 0.10% or 100 mg/dL)

- Provide safety measures to prevent physical harm to the client when the serum alcohol level is greatly increased. Side rails may be needed while the client is sleeping off the effects of alcohol.
- Follow legal ramifications in your state for drawing plasma alcohol level.

Client Teaching

- Instruct the client not to consume alcoholic beverages when taking sedatives, hypnotics, narcotics, tranquilizers (Valium, Librium), anticonvulsants (Dilantin), and anticoagulants (Coumadin). Alcohol and tranquilizers can depress respirations and might cause respiratory arrest.
- Encourage the client to attend Alcoholics Anonymous (AA) meetings for chronic alcoholism. Listen to the client's concerns.

A

Aldolase (ALD) (serum)

Reference Values

Adult: Less than 6 unit/L, 3–8 unit/dL (Sibley-Lehninger), 22–59 milliunit/L at 37°C (SI units).
Child: *Infant:* 12–24 unit/dL (4 times). *Child:* 6–16 unit/dL (2 times).

Description

Aldolase is an enzyme present most abundantly in the skeletal and cardiac muscles. This enzyme is used to monitor skeletal muscle diseases, such as muscular dystrophy, dermatomyositis, and trichinosis. It is not elevated in muscle disease of neural origin, such as multiple sclerosis, polio-myelitis, and myasthenia gravis.

Serum aldolase is helpful in diagnosing early cases of Duchenne muscular dystrophy before clinical symptoms appear. Progressive muscular dystrophy may cause elevated serum aldolase levels 10–15 times greater than normal. In late stages of muscular dystrophy, the enzyme level may return to normal or below normal. Serum aldolase is not the most effective diagnostic test for myocardial infarction, because there is only a slight rise. Following an acute MI, it peaks (two times its normal level) in 24 hours and returns to normal in 4–7 days.

Purpose

- To aid in the diagnosis of skeletal muscle diseases, such as muscular dystrophy.

Clinical Problems

Decreased Level: Late muscular dystrophy, muscle wasting disease.

Increased Level: Early and progressive muscular dystrophy; trichinosis; dermatomyositis; acute MI; acute hepatitis; cancer of gastrointestinal tract, prostate, and liver; lymphosarcoma; leuke-mia. *Drug Influence:* Alcohol, cortisone, narcotics.

Procedure

- There is no food or fluid restriction.
- Collect 3–5 mL of venous blood in a red-top tube. The serum should not be hemolyzed when measuring aldolase.

Factors Affecting Laboratory Results

- Hemolysis causes false-positive results.

NURSING IMPLICATIONS WITH RATIONALE

Increased Level

- Recognize the purpose of monitoring aldolase levels. This is a useful test for diagnosing muscular disorders.

- List on the laboratory slip any drugs the client is receiving that can elevate the serum aldolase level.
- Check serum aldolase results, and plan your nursing care according to symptoms present and psychologic needs.

Aldosterone (serum)

Reference Values

Adult: *Supine Position:* Less than 16 ng/dL. *Sitting Position:* 4–30 ng/dL.

Child: *(3–11 Years):* 5–70 ng/dL; *(11–16 Years):* 5–50 ng/dL.

Pregnancy: 2–3 times higher than adult.

Description

Aldosterone is the most potent of all mineralocorticoids produced by the adrenal cortex. Its major function is to regulate sodium, potassium, and water balance according to body needs. Aldosterone promotes sodium reabsorption from the distal tubules of the kidney and potassium and hydrogen excretion. With sodium reabsorption, water is retained. Eighty to 90% of aldosterone is inactivated in the liver.

This hormone responds to various changes in the body. When there is a sodium loss and a water loss, aldosterone is secreted to reestablish sodium and water balance. Renin promotes aldosterone secretion, which causes more sodium and water to be retained and body fluid to be increased. Stress will increase aldosterone secretion. Hypernatremia (serum sodium excess) inhibits aldosterone secretion.

Serum aldosterone is not the most reliable test, because there can be fluctuations caused by various influences. If the client is in a supine position, serum aldosterone will be lower than if he or she is in a sitting or standing position. A 24-hour urine test is considered more reliable than a random serum aldosterone collection. Several serum aldosterone levels may be requested.

Purposes

- To detect deficit or excess of aldosterone.
- To compare serum and urine aldosterone levels with other laboratory tests for determining overhydration with elevated sodium level and adrenal hypo- or hyperfunction.

Clinical Problems

Decreased Level: Overhydration with increased sodium, severe hypernatremia (sodium excess), high-sodium diet, hypokalemia, adrenal cortical hypofunction, diabetes mellitus, licorice ingestion (excessive), glucose caused by excess infusion, toxemia of pregnancy, antihypertensive therapy.

Increased Level: Dehydration, hyponatremia (sodium deficit), low-sodium diet, essential hypertension, adrenal cortical hyperfunction, cancer of the adrenal gland, cirrhosis of the liver,

A

emphysema, severe heart failure (HF), hyperkalemia, stress. *Drug Influence:* Diuretics (furosemide [Lasix] and others), hydralazine (Apresoline), diazoxide (Hyperstat), nitroprusside.

Procedure

- Food and fluids are not restricted, but excess salt and interfering substances (licorice) should not be consumed before the test. Normal salt intake is suggested.
- Collect 5 mL of venous blood in a red-top tube. A green-top tube (heparinized) may also be used.
- The client should be in a supine position for at least 1 hour before the blood is drawn.
- Write the date and time on the specimen. Aldosterone levels exhibit circadian rhythm, with peak levels occurring in the morning and lower levels in the afternoon.

Factors Affecting Laboratory Results

- A high- or low-salt diet can affect test results.
- Prolonged use of potent diuretics affects test results.
- Excessive licorice and glucose ingestion may decrease test results.
- Sitting or standing when blood is drawn may cause false-positive results.

NURSING IMPLICATIONS WITH RATIONALE

- Assess the client for signs and symptoms of dehydration when the serum aldosterone is elevated, such as poor skin turgor, dry mucous membranes, and shocklike symptoms, and for hyponatremia when the serum aldosterone is elevated.
- Compare the serum aldosterone and the 24-hour urine aldosterone results if both have been ordered.
- Record vital signs on the client. A rapid pulse and later a drop in blood pressure (BP) could be indicative of hypovolemia (fluid volume deficit).

Client Teaching

- Instruct the client to remain in a supine position for at least 1 hour before blood is drawn to prevent false test results.

Aldosterone (urine)

Reference Values

Adult: 6–25 mcg/24 h.

Description

(*See the Description for Aldosterone [serum].*)

Aldosterone causes sodium reabsorption and potassium excretion from the distal tubules of the kidney. Aldosterone secretion from the adrenal cortex influences sodium retention, fluid retention, fluid volume, and blood pressure.

A 24-hour urine aldosterone level has an advantage over a serum aldosterone level because fluctuation levels can be eliminated. Both urine and serum aldosterone will be increased by hyponatremia, a low-salt diet, and hyperkalemia. Likewise, hypernatremia, a high-salt diet, and hypokalemia will decrease urine and serum aldosterone. A urine sodium test may be ordered for comparison purposes.

Purposes

(*See Aldosterone [serum].*)

Clinical Problems

Decreased Level: Same as for serum aldosterone.

Increased Level: Tumors of the adrenal cortex or primary aldosteronism, same as for serum aldosterone.

Procedure

- Collect a 24-hour urine specimen in a large container with an acidic preservative.
- Have the client void, and discard the urine before the test begins.
- Label the container with the exact date and time for the test (e.g., 4/9/15, 7:35 AM to 4/10/15, 7:35 AM).

Factors Affecting Laboratory Results

- Failure to place all urine collected in a 24-hour period in the urine container can cause false results.
- Toilet paper and feces in the urine affect test results.

NURSING IMPLICATIONS WITH RATIONALE

- Check at specified times to determine whether the urine collection is being properly obtained.

Client Teaching

- Instruct the client on how to collect the 24-hour urine specimen. All urine should be saved after the initial urine is discarded. The urine may be kept on ice or refrigerated if indicated. Toilet paper or feces should not be in the urine.
- Answer the client's questions concerning the test and the collection procedure.

Alkaline phosphatase (ALP) with isoenzyme (serum)

Reference Values

Adult: 42–136 unit/L; ALP1: 20–130 unit/L; ALP2: 20–120 unit/L.

Child: *Infant and Child (0–12 Years):* 40–115 unit/L. *Older Child (13–18 Years):* 50–230 unit/L.

Elderly: Slightly higher than adult.

A

Description

Alkaline phosphatase (ALP) is an enzyme produced mainly in the liver and bone; it is also derived from the intestine, kidney, and placenta. The ALP test is useful for determining liver and bone diseases. In cases of mild liver-cell damage, the ALP level may be only slightly elevated, but it could be markedly elevated in acute liver disease. Once the acute phase is over, the serum level will promptly decrease, whereas the serum bilirubin will remain increased. For determining liver dysfunction, several laboratory tests are performed (i.e., bilirubin, leucine aminopeptidase [LAP], 5′-nucleotidase [5′-NT], and gamma-glutamyl transpeptidase [GGTP]).

With bone disorders, the ALP level is increased because of abnormal osteoblastic activity (bone cell production). In children, it is not abnormal to find high levels of ALP before and during puberty because of bone growth.

Isoenzymes of ALP are used to distinguish between liver and bone diseases: ALP1 indicating disease of liver origin and ALP2, bone origin.

Purposes

- To determine the presence of a liver or bone disorder.
- To compare ALP results with other laboratory tests for confirmation of a liver or bone disorder.

Clinical Problems

Decreased Level: Hypothyroidism, malnutrition, scurvy (vitamin C deficit), hypophosphatasia, pernicious anemia (PA), placental insufficiency. *Drug Influence:* Fluoride, oxalate propranolol (Inderal).

Increased Level: Obstructive biliary disease (jaundice), cancer of the liver, hepatocellular cirrhosis, hepatitis, hyperparathyroidism, leukemia, cancer of the bone (breast and prostate), Paget disease, osteitis deformans, healing fractures, multiple myeloma, osteomalacia, late pregnancy, rheumatoid arthritis (active), ulcerative disease. *Drug Influence:* IV albumin, antibiotics (erythromycin, tetracycline, lincomycin, oxacillin, penicillin), colchicine, methyldopa (Aldomet), allopurinol, phenothiazine tranquilizers, indomethacin (Indocin), procainamide, oral contraceptives (some), tolbutamide, isoniazid (INH), para-aminosalicylic acid (PAS).

Procedure

- There is no food or fluid restriction. For ALP isoenzymes, fasting overnight might be indicated.
- Collect 3–5 mL of venous blood in a red-top tube. Avoid hemolysis.
- Withhold for 8–24 hours, with health care provider's permission, drugs that can elevate the ALP level.
- List the client's age and drugs that may affect test results on the laboratory slip.

Factors Affecting Laboratory Results

- Certain drugs that increase or decrease the serum ALP levels may cause false results (*see Drug Influence*).
- Administered IV albumin can elevate the serum ALP to 5–10 times its normal value.
- Age of the client (e.g., youth and old age cause a serum increase).
- Late pregnancy to 3 weeks postpartum, which could cause a serum ALP elevation.

NURSING IMPLICATIONS WITH RATIONALE

- Know factors that can elevate serum ALP levels, such as drugs, IV albumin (can elevate serum ALP 5–10 times its normal value), age of client (elevated in children and elderly), late pregnancy to 3 weeks postpartum, and blood drawn 2–4 hours after a fatty meal.
- Record pertinent information from the procedure on the laboratory slip.
- Assess for clinical signs and symptoms of liver or bone disease.
- Check the results of other ordered liver tests to determine the significance of the elevated serum ALP in liver disease.

Client Teaching

- Inform the client that other enzyme tests may be ordered to verify diagnosis.

Allergen-specific IgE (serum)

Allergy Testing, IgE Antibody Test

Reference Values

Adult: 100 international unit/mL.

Child: *Neonates to 2 Years old*: <12 international unit/mL. *3–5 Years old*: <40 international unit/mL. *6–12 Years old*: <90 international unit/mL.

Description

Immunoglobulin E (IgE) is a protein that acts as an antibody in response to allergen stimulation. An allergen is a substance that the person is allergic to, which causes an increase in IgE. A hypersensitive reaction occurs.

This test is used to identify allergies to substances such as animal dander, foods, pollens, molds, dust, grasses, weeds, trees, insects, drugs, and miscellaneous substances. The advantage of this test is that the client does not have an allergic reaction to the allergen when induced, such as dust, because the allergen is introduced into the blood sample and not the body. A method for testing the degree of allergy to the allergen is the radioallergosorbent (RAST) test. The RAST rating is from 0 to 6. A rating of 1 or greater indicates the presence of an allergy and its severity.

Purposes

- To determine the presence of an allergy.
- To detect the type of allergen by the blood sample.
- To identify the severity of the allergy by the RAST test.

Clinical Problems

Increased Levels: Asthma, dermatitis, drug allergy, food allergy (common ones are eggs, wheat, milk, fish, shellfish, peanuts, cashew, and walnuts), and occupational allergy.
Drug Influence: Corticosteroids

Procedure

- Check with the laboratory what their policy is concerning food restriction.
- Collect 5 mL of venous blood in a red-, gray-, or gold-top (serum separator) tube.
- Take the blood sample immediately to the laboratory.

Factors Affecting Laboratory Results

- Hyposensitization treatments can decrease test results.
- Radioactive dyes within 7 days before the test can invalidate the test result.
- A parasitic infection can cause false-positive result.

NURSING IMPLICATIONS WITH RATIONALE

- Obtain a history of any previous allergies.
- Explain the procedure for the allergy test. The suspected allergen will be mixed with the client's blood sample in the laboratory. Inform the client that the allergen will not be introduced into the body.
- Ask the client if he or she is receiving hyposensitization treatments, or radioactive dye injection for a diagnostic test, or has an infection.

Client Teaching

- Inform the client that the test results can take several days.
- Instruct the client to avoid substance(s) (allergen) when it has been identified by the test.
- Be supportive to the client and answer questions or refer to appropriate health professionals.

Allergy testing

See Allergen-Specific (IgE)

Alpha-1-antitrypsin (α_1AT) (serum)

Alpha$_1$ Inhibitor, Alpha-1-Protease Inhibitor

Reference Values

Adult: 78–200 mg/dL, 0.78–2 g/L (SI units).

Child: *Newborn:* 145–270 mg/dL. *Infant:* Similar to adult range.

Description

Antitrypsin (α_1AT), or trypsin inhibitor, is a protein produced by the liver. It inhibits specific proteolytic enzymes that are released in the lung by bacteria or by phagocytic cells. A deficiency of homozygous antitrypsin (heredity linked) permits proteolytic enzymes to damage lung tissue, thus causing emphysema. Deficiency of α_1AT can be caused by genetic or environmental factors.

With inflammatory conditions, α_1AT serum level can be increased. Following the inflammatory insult that could result from a surgical wound, the serum α_1AT increases in 2–3 days and can remain elevated for 1–2 weeks. The serum level then returns to normal.

Purposes

- To determine if chronic obstructive pulmonary disease is caused by a deficiency of α_1AT.
- To detect the presence of α_1AT deficiency.

Clinical Problems

Decreased Level: Chronic obstructive lung disease (pulmonary emphysema), severe liver damage, malnutrition, severe protein-losing (nephrotic) syndrome.

Increased Level: Acute and chronic inflammatory conditions, infections (selected), necrosis, late pregnancy, exercise (returns to normal in 1 day). *Drug Influence:* Oral contraceptives.

Procedure

- Keep the client NPO (nothing by mouth), except for water, for 8 hours before drawing blood.
- Collect 3–5 mL of venous blood in a red-top tube.
- Hold oral contraceptives for 24 hours before the test, with the health care provider's permission. Any oral contraceptive taken should be listed on the laboratory slip.

Factors Affecting Laboratory Results

- Oral contraceptives can increase the α_1AT level.
- Oral intake of food before the test can cause an inaccurate result, especially if the client has an elevated serum cholesterol or serum triglyceride level.

NURSING IMPLICATIONS WITH RATIONALE

Decreased Level

- Recognize clinical problems that are associated with α_1AT deficiency (e.g., emphysema).

Client Teaching

- Explain to the client that the test is ordered to determine whether there is an antitrypsin (protein) deficiency that can cause a lung disorder (disease). A nonsmoker with an α_1AT deficiency can have emphysema. Antitrypsin inhibits proteolytic enzymes from destroying lung tissue; with a lack of this protein, the alveoli are damaged.
- Instruct the client that he or she should have nothing by mouth except water for 8 hours before the blood test; this restriction before the blood test may vary among health care providers.
- Instruct the client with an α_1AT deficit to use preventive methods in protecting his or her lungs (e.g., avoid persons with upper respiratory infection [URI], seek medical care when having a respiratory infection).
- Encourage the client to stop smoking and to avoid areas having highly polluted air. Air pollution can cause respiratory inflammation and can promote chronic obstruction lung disease.

A

Increased Level

- Check the serum α_1AT level 2–3 days after extensive surgery. Inflammation can markedly increase the serum level. A baseline serum level may be ordered before surgery for several reasons (e.g., for determining lung disease and the effects of surgery).
- Report if the serum α_1AT remains elevated 2 weeks after surgery.
- Note that serum α_1AT can be markedly elevated during late pregnancy.

Alpha fetoprotein (AFP) (serum and amniotic fluid)

Reference Values

Nonpregnancy: Less than 15 ng/mL.

Pregnancy:

SERUM		AMNIOTIC FLUID	
Weeks of Gestation	ng/mL	Weeks of Gestation	ng/mL
8–12	0–39	14	11–32
13	6–31	15	5.5–31
14	7–50	16	5.7–31.5
15	7–60	17	3.8–32.5
16	10–72	18	3.6–28
17	11–90	19	3.7–24.5
18	14–94	20	2.2–15
19	24–112	21	3.8–18
20	31–122		
21	19–124		

Description

Serum alpha fetoprotein (AFP), a screening test, is usually done between 16 and 20 weeks' gestation to determine the probability of twins or to detect low birth weight or serious birth defects, such as open neural-tube defect. If a high serum AFP level occurs, the test should be repeated 1 week later. Ultrasound and amniocentesis may be performed to confirm elevated serum levels and to diagnose neural-tube defects in the fetus.

Serum alpha fetoprotein is also the tumor marker for testicular screening and testicular cancer.

Purpose

- To identify the probability of neural-tube defects, fetal death, or other anomalies in pregnancy (*see Clinical Problems*).

Clinical Problems

Decreased Level: Down syndrome, absence of pregnancy.

Increased Level: *Nonpregnant:* Cirrhosis of the liver (not liver metastasis); hepatitis; germ-cell tumor of gonads, such as testicular cancer; metastases to liver. *Pregnant:* Neural-tube defects (spina bifida, anencephaly, myelomeningocele), fetal death, fetal distress, Turner syndrome, other anomalies (duodenal atresia, tetralogy of Fallot, hydrocephalus, trisomy 13), severe Rh immunization.

Procedure

- There is no food or fluid restriction.
- Collect 5–7 mL of venous blood in a red-top tube. Avoid hemolysis.

Factors Affecting Laboratory Results

- Fetal blood contamination could cause an elevated amniotic AFP level.
- Inaccurate recording of gestation week could affect results.
- Multiple pregnancy or fetal death could cause a false-positive test.
- Hemolysis of blood sample could affect results.
- Body weight may be a factor (although not definitely confirmed). A heavier female tends to have a lower serum AFP level.

NURSING IMPLICATIONS WITH RATIONALE

- Explain that the test is for screening purposes. If the test is positive, genetic counseling might be necessary.
- Be supportive of individuals and family.

Client Teaching

- Instruct the client that it is essential to give the correct gestation date of the pregnancy, if known, to avoid a laboratory test error. Inform the client that the test might be repeated in a week.
- If an ultrasound is performed, instruct the client that it is usually done to confirm gestational age or to confirm the positive serum AFP and amniocentesis result(s).

Alzheimer disease markers

See Amyloid Beta Protein Precursor (CSF)

Aminoglycosides (serum)

Amikacin (Amikin), Gentamicin (Garamycin), Tobramycin (Nebcin)

Reference Values

Adult:

Drug Name	THERAPEUTIC RANGE		Toxic Level
	Peak	Trough	
Amikacin	15–30 mcg/mL	<10 mcg/mL	>35 mcg/mL
Gentamicin	6–10 mcg/mL	<1.5 mcg/mL	>12 mcg/mL
Kanamycin	15–30 mcg/mL	1–4 mcg/mL	>35 mcg/mL
Netilmicin	0.5–10 mcg/mL	<4 mcg/mL	>16 mcg/mL
Tobramycin	5–10 mcg/mL	<2 mcg/mL	>12 mcg/mL

Child: Same as adult.

Description

Aminoglycosides are broad-spectrum antibiotics that are effective against gram-negative microorganisms. These agents are not well absorbed from the gastrointestinal tract and so are given parenterally. Peak action after intramuscular (IM) injection is ½ to 1½ hours, and after 30-minute IV infusion is ½ hour. Half-life is about 2 hours. Aminoglycosides cross the placental barrier but do not cross the blood-brain barrier. They are excreted mostly unchanged by the kidneys.

Ototoxicity and nephrotoxicity can result from overdose of an aminoglycoside or from long-term administration. Renal function tests (i.e., creatinine, creatinine clearance, and urinalysis) should be assessed periodically while the client is receiving these agents. If clients with renal insufficiency receive any of these drugs, dosage should be adjusted (decreased). Drug half-life is usually 24–96 hours in clients having renal damage. Gentamicin can be used in combination with ampicillin to treat certain gram-positive *Streptococci* and *Enterococci*.

Purpose

- To assess clients receiving aminoglycosides for therapeutic effect and possible toxic effect by monitoring urinary output, blood urea nitrogen (BUN), and serum creatinine levels.

Clinical Problems

Increased Levels: Overdose of aminoglycoside, renal insufficiency or failure. *Drug Influence:* Diuretics, cephalosporins (increase chance of nephrotoxicity).

Procedure

- There is no food or fluid restriction.
- Collect 3–5 mL of venous blood in a red-top tube or green-top tube (heparinized).
- Collect specimen during steady state, usually 24–36 hours after drug is started.
- Record on the laboratory requisition slip the dose, route (IM or IV), and last time drug was administered.

- Draw trough sample immediately before the next dose.
- Draw peak sample 30–60 minutes post administration of dose, depending on method of administering.

A

Factors Affecting Laboratory Results
- Renal insufficiency or failure could cause an elevated serum aminoglycoside level.

NURSING IMPLICATIONS WITH RATIONALE

- Check serum aminoglycoside (amikacin, gentamicin, tobramycin) results, and report nontherapeutic levels to health care provider immediately.
- Assess intake and output. Notify the health care provider if urine output has greatly decreased. This could be a sign of aminoglycoside toxicity.
- Monitor peak and trough levels to prevent nephrotoxicity and ototoxicity.
- Suggest renal function tests for clients receiving long-term aminoglycoside therapy and especially for those with renal insufficiency.
- Recognize that diuretics and cephalosporins coadministered with an aminoglycoside could enhance the risk of nephrotoxicity.
- Assess hearing status of the client. Any hearing impairment (loss of high-tone acuity) while the client is receiving aminoglycoside could indicate ototoxicity.

Increased Level

- Recognize that overdose of aminoglycoside or renal insufficiency could cause an elevated serum aminoglycoside level.
- Observe for signs and symptoms of nephrotoxicity (e.g., proteinuria, elevated creatinine, elevated BUN, decreased creatinine clearance test).
- Observe for signs and symptoms of ototoxicity (e.g., nausea and vomiting with motion, dizziness, headache, tinnitus, decrease in ability to hear high-pitched tones).

Amino acid (urine)

Reference Values
Normal values are age dependent; 200 mg/24 h.

Description
This test screens for elevated levels of amino acid in the urine (aminoaciduria), which can indicate inborn errors of metabolism. With abnormal metabolism, there can be an excess in one or more amino acids in the plasma and urine. The test is performed when genetic abnormalities are suspected. The amino acid screening test is positive when there is an increase in amino acid or its metabolites in the urine.

Aminoaciduria can include phenylketonuria, maple-syrup urine disease, cystinuria, and tyrosinemia. Further testing would be needed to confirm the metabolic disorder.

A

Purposes

- To screen for renal aminoacidurias.
- To detect inborn errors of metabolism.

Clinical Problems

Increased Level: Mental retardation, retarded growth, cystinuria, severe brain damage, phenyl-ketonuria, tyrosinosis, ketosis. *Drug Influence:* Penicillins, valproic acid.

Procedure

- There is no food or fluid restriction.
- Collect a clean random urine specimen. A 24-hour urine specimen may be requested.
- Pack the specimen in ice and send immediately to the laboratory. Refrigeration can be used.

Factors Affecting Laboratory Results

- Lack of protein ingestion in 48 hours can affect test results.
- Failure to ice or refrigerate the specimen.

NURSING IMPLICATIONS WITH RATIONALE

- Obtain a history of health problems that may relate to the abnormal metabolism disorder.
- Check the drug history; notify the health care provider if the client is taking a penicillin derivative.
- Allow the client and family time to express their concerns.

Ammonia (plasma)

Reference Values

Adult: 15–45 mcg/dL; 11–35 µmol/L (SI units).

Child: *Newborn:* 64–107 mcg/dL. *Child:* 29–70 mcg/dL; 29–70 µmol/L (SI units).

Description

Ammonia, a by-product of protein metabolism, is formed from the bacterial action in the intestine and from metabolizing tissues. Most of the ammonia is absorbed into the portal circulation and is converted in the liver to urea. With severe liver decompensation or when blood flow to the liver is altered, the plasma ammonia level remains elevated.

Elevated plasma ammonia is best correlated with hepatic failure; however, other conditions that interfere with liver function (heart failure, acidosis) may cause a temporary elevation of plasma ammonia.

Purpose

- To detect a liver disorder from the inability of the liver to convert ammonia to urea.

A

Clinical Problems

Decreased Level: Renal failure, malignant hypertension, essential hypertension. *Drug Influence:* Antibiotics (neomycin, tetracycline, kanamycin), monoamine oxidase inhibitors, diphenhydramine (Benadryl), potassium salts, sodium salts.

Increased Level: Hepatic failure, hepatic encephalopathy or coma, portacaval anastomosis, Reye syndrome, erythroblastosis fetalis, cor pulmonale, HF, pulmonary emphysema, high-protein diet with liver failure, acidosis, exercise. *Drug Influence:* Ammonia chloride, diuretics (thiazides, furosemide [Lasix], ethacrynic acid [Edecrin]), ion exchange resin, isoniazid (INH).

Procedure

- There is no food or fluid restriction unless indicated by the laboratory. Smoking should be avoided before the test.
- Collect 5 mL of venous blood in a green-top tube. The blood sample should be delivered immediately in packed ice to the laboratory. Ammonia levels increase rapidly after blood is drawn.
- Minimize use of tourniquet for drawing blood.
- List drugs the client is taking that could affect test results.

Factors Affecting Laboratory Results

- Failure to place the blood sample on ice and to analyze it immediately can result in a false test.
- A high- or low-protein diet can cause false test results.
- Exercise might increase the plasma ammonia level.
- Certain antibiotics (neomycin and tetracycline) decrease the ammonia level.

NURSING IMPLICATIONS WITH RATIONALE

Increased Level

- Identify clinical problems and drugs that can increase the plasma ammonia level.
- Notify the laboratory personnel when a plasma ammonia level is drawn so that it can be analyzed immediately to avoid false results.
- List antibiotics on the laboratory slip. Certain antibiotics (such as neomycin and tetracycline) can decrease the ammonia level, causing a false result.
- Observe for signs and symptoms of hepatic failure, especially when the plasma ammonia is elevated. There are many neurologic changes, such as behavioral and personality changes, lethargy, confusion, flapping tremors of the extremities, twitching, and, later, coma.
- Recognize that exercise may be a cause of an elevated plasma ammonia level.
- Know various treatments used in decreasing the plasma ammonia level. A few of these are a low-protein diet, antibiotics (such as neomycin) to destroy intestinal bacteria, enemas, cathartics (such as magnesium sulfate) to prevent ammonia formation, and sodium glutamate and L-arginine in IV dextrose solution to stimulate urea formation.

Client Teaching

- Explain to the client why he or she may be NPO 8 hours before the test: Foods containing protein may cause a higher ammonia level.

A

Amylase with isoenzymes (serum)

Reference Values

Adult: 60–160 Somogyi unit/dL, 30–170 unit/L (SI units).

Pregnancy: Slightly increased.

Child: Not usually done.

Elderly: Slightly higher than adult.

Serum Isoenzymes: *S (salivary) type:* 45–70%. *P (pancreatic) type:* 30–55%. Values may differ with method used.

Description

Amylase is an enzyme that is derived from the pancreas, the salivary glands, and the liver. Its function is to change starch to sugar. In acute pancreatitis, serum amylase is increased to twice its normal level. Its level begins to increase 2–12 hours after onset, peaks in 20–30 hours, and returns to normal in 2–4 days. Acute pancreatitis is frequently associated with inflammation, severe pain, and necrosis caused by digestive enzymes (including amylase) escaping into the surrounding tissue.

Increased serum amylase can occur after abdominal surgery involving the gallbladder (stones or biliary duct) and stomach (partial gastrectomy). Following abdominal surgery, some surgeons order a routine serum amylase for 2 days to determine whether the pancreas has been injured.

The urine amylase level is helpful in determining the significance of a normal or slightly elevated serum amylase, especially when the client has symptoms of pancreatitis. Amylase levels can also be obtained from abdominal fluid, ascitic fluid, pleural effusion, and saliva.

There are two types of amylase isoenzymes, P type (pancreatic origin) and S type (salivary origin). P-type elevation occurs more frequently in acute pancreatitis. Elevated S type can occur as a result of parotitis and ovarian and bronchogenic tumors. Amylase isoenzymes are usually ordered to rule out a nonpancreatic source of the elevated serum amylase level. A pancreatic isoenzyme kit is commercially available.

Purpose

- To assist in the diagnosis of acute pancreatitis and other health problems (*see Clinical Problems*).

Clinical Problems

Decreased Level: Intravenous 5% dextrose in water (IV D_5W), advanced chronic pancreatitis, acute and subacute necrosis of the liver, chronic alcoholism, toxic hepatitis, severe burns, severe thyrotoxicosis. *Drug Influence:* Glucose (IV D_5W), citrates, fluorides, oxalates.

Increased Level: Acute pancreatitis, chronic pancreatitis (acute onset), partial gastrectomy, peptic ulcer perforation, obstruction of pancreatic duct, acute cholecystitis, cancer of the pancreas, diabetic acidosis, diabetes mellitus, acute alcoholic intoxication, mumps, renal failure, benign prostatic hypertrophy, burns, pregnancy. *Drug Influence:* Meperidine (Demerol), codeine, morphine, bethanechol chloride (Urecholine), pentazocine (Talwin), ethyl alcohol (large amounts), ACTH, guanethidine, thiazides, salicylates, tetracycline.

Procedure

- Restrict food for 1–2 hours before the blood sample is drawn. If the client has eaten or has received a narcotic 2 hours before the test, the serum results could be invalid.
- Obtain 3–5 mL of venous blood in a red-top tube.
- List on the laboratory slip drugs that could cause a false amylase level.

Factors Affecting Laboratory Results

- Narcotic drugs can cause false-positive levels.
- IV fluids with glucose can result in false-negative levels.
- Contamination of the specimen with saliva can occur through coughing, sneezing, or talking when the tube is opened. This could cause false-positive results.

NURSING IMPLICATIONS WITH RATIONALE

Decreased Level

- Know that D_5W administered intravenously can decrease the serum amylase level, causing a false-negative result.
- Identify drugs that give false-negative levels.
- Determine when the client has ingested food or sweetened fluids. Blood should not be drawn until 2 hours after eating because sugar can decrease the serum amylase level.

Increased Level

- Know the disease entities related to increased levels, especially acute pancreatitis, abdominal surgery (partial gastrectomy, biliary resection), diabetes mellitus, cancer of the pancreas, acute alcoholic intoxication, and benign prostatic hypertrophy.
- Label the laboratory slip (for serum amylase) with the drugs the client is receiving or has received in the last 24 hours. Morphine, meperidine, codeine, pentazocine, aspirin, and hydrochlorothiazide can cause a false-positive serum amylase level.
- Check serum amylase levels for several days after abdominal surgery. Surgery of the stomach or gallbladder might cause trauma to the pancreas and cause excess amylase to be released.
- Report symptoms of severe pain when pancreatitis is suspected. The health care provider may want to draw a serum amylase level before a narcotic is given. An elevated level may indicate an acute pancreatitis.
- Explain to the client that blood is drawn for determining whether the severe pain is due to a pancreatic problem or to another cause.
- Ask the client if he or she has had pancreatitis before and has taken narcotic analgesics. A report should be given to the health care provider.
- Report elevated serum amylase results occurring beyond 3 days. If the serum amylase levels remain elevated beyond 3 days (72 hours), pancreatic cell destruction could still be occurring.

Client Teaching

- Instruct the client to assume adequate health practices, such as controlling alcohol intake and increasing protein and carbohydrates in the diet.

Amylase (urine)

Reference Values

Adult: 6.5–48 unit/h (SI units).

Description

(*See Amylase [serum].*)

Amylase is an enzyme that is produced by the pancreas, salivary glands, and liver and is excreted by the kidneys. When there is an inflammation of the pancreas or salivary gland, more amylase goes into the blood and more amylase is excreted in the urine. The urine levels of amylase could remain elevated for a week, whereas the serum amylase level tends to remain elevated for a short time (peaks in 24 hours and returns to normal in 48–96 hours).

The urine amylase test is ordered at 1-, 2-, or 24-hour timed intervals, with the 2-hour urine specimen the most commonly ordered. A 24-hour specimen may be within normal range, whereas a 2-hour specimen shows an increase.

One drawback of both urine amylase and serum amylase values is their relation to renal function. A diminished renal function could lead to a decrease in urine amylase and an increase in serum amylase.

Purpose

(*See Amylase [serum].*)

Clinical Problems

Decreased Level: Diminished renal function (*see Amylase [serum]*).

Increased Level: Acute pancreatitis, choledocholithiasis (*see Amylase [serum]*).

Procedure

- A timed urine collection is required; thus the exact beginning and end of the urine collection should be recorded (date, hour, and minute; e.g., 2/10/16, 9:02 AM to 2/10/16, 11:05 AM). First the client voids and the urine is discarded.
- The urine specimen should be refrigerated or kept on ice. No preservative is needed.

Factors Affecting Laboratory Results

- Fecal material or toilet paper contamination can affect test results.
- Diminished urine output affects test results.
- Drugs that increase or decrease amylase levels are listed at drug influence (*see Amylase [serum]*).
- Prolonged urine collection time affects test results.

NURSING IMPLICATIONS WITH RATIONALE

Decreased Level

- Check urinary output for 8 hours and 24 hours, BUN (blood urea nitrogen), and serum creatinine levels. A decrease in urine output and an increase in BUN and serum creatinine levels indicate poor kidney function. A decreased urine output could result in a decreased urine amylase.

Client Teaching

- Explain to the client the importance of collecting urine at a specified time. The client should use a urinal or bedpan and should be instructed that all urine should be saved.
- Encourage the client to drink water during the test unless water intake is restricted for medical reasons. A decreased urine output could result in no 2-hour specimen or a possible false result.

Increased Level

- Check urinary output and give fluids if the urine output is decreased. Encouraging fluids during the test should help in securing a urine specimen.
- Check the serum amylase level(s) and compare with the urine amylase level. A low serum amylase level and an increased urine amylase level could indicate that the acute problem is no longer present.
- List on the laboratory slip the drugs the client is receiving that can increase amylase levels (e.g., narcotics).
- Notify the health care provider when the client is having severe abdominal pain. The health care provider may want to order a 2-hour or 24-hour urine specimen the next day.

Amyloid beta protein precursor (CSF)

Alzheimer Disease Marker

Reference Values

Normal: Greater than 450 unit/L cerebrospinal fluid (CSF).

Description

The amyloid beta protein precursor test is a CSF test that can aid in diagnosing Alzheimer disease. The amyloid beta protein is present in the senile plaques within the brain. Amyloid can also be found in the meningeal blood vessels of clients with Alzheimer disease. It is believed that this type of protein may have neurotoxic effects on the brain cells. Small amounts

A

of amyloid can be found in the CSF of most healthy persons; however, a higher value occurs in the CSF of clients with Alzheimer, and a somewhat higher value than normal may occur in an aged client with senile dementia.

PET scan with PiB (Pittsburgh compound B) has been used to detect brain amyloid, which is a promising test for diagnosing Alzheimer disease.

Purpose

- To aid with the diagnosis of Alzheimer disease.

Clinical Problems

Increased Level: Alzheimer disease, senile dementia.

Procedure

- The client should sign a consent form.
- There is no food or fluid restriction.
- The bladder should be emptied.
- The client's position for the procedure is lying on his or her side in a "fetal" or knees-up position.
- The client should remain relaxed and still during the procedure. Taking deep breaths may help the client to relax.
- Collect at least 2 mL of CSF and place the fluid specimen in a sterile tube.

Factors Affecting Laboratory Results

- Blood in the spinal fluid can cause false test results.

NURSING IMPLICATIONS WITH RATIONALE

Client Teaching

- Explain the test procedure to the client and family. A family member may wish to be with the client during the test procedure.
- Answer the client or family member's questions, and if the answer is unknown, refer the questions to the appropriate health professional.

Posttest

- Place the client in a reclining position for 8–12 hours; the client can turn side to side. The client's head should not be raised to avoid "spinal" headache, which could occur from leaking of spinal fluid at the needle insertion site.
- Report any numbness or tingling in the extremities.
- Encourage the client to increase fluid intake for the next 24 hours.

Angiotensin-converting enzyme (ACE) (serum)

Angiotensin-1-Converting Enzyme

Reference Values

Adult greater than 20 years: 8–67 unit/L.

Child and adult less than 20 years: Test is *not* performed because they normally have elevated ACE levels.

Description

Angiotensin-converting enzyme (ACE) is found primarily in the lung epithelial cells and to a lesser extent in blood vessels and renal cells. The purpose of ACE is to regulate arterial blood pressure by converting angiotensin I to the vasoconstrictor angiotensin II, which increases blood pressure and stimulates the adrenal cortex to release aldosterone (sodium-retaining hormone). However, this test has little value for diagnosing hypertension.

High serum ACE levels are found primarily with active sarcoidosis. This test should not be performed for clients who are under 20 years of age because they normally have elevated ACE levels. Approximately 5% of the population has an elevated ACE level. The purpose for the ACE test is to diagnose and determine the severity of pulmonary sarcoidosis. Seventy to 90% of clients with active sarcoidosis have elevated serum ACE levels. Other conditions that have elevated ACE levels include Gaucher disease (disorder of fat metabolism), leprosy, alcoholic cirrhosis, active histoplasmosis, tuberculosis, pulmonary embolism, hyperthyroidism, and Hodgkin disease.

Purposes

- To assist in diagnosing various health problems, such as pulmonary sarcoidosis, related to an elevated serum ACE level.
- To compare the results of serum ACE levels with other laboratory tests for diagnosing a health problem.

Clinical Problems

Decreased Level: Therapy for sarcoidosis, diabetes mellitus, hypothyroidism, respiratory distress syndrome, severe illness. *Drug Influence:* Steroids (prednisone, cortisone).

Increased Level: Sarcoidosis, Gaucher disease, leprosy, alcoholic cirrhosis, histoplasmosis, tuberculosis, pulmonary embolism, hyperthyroidism, Hodgkin disease, myeloma, non-Hodgkin lymphoma, idiopathic pulmonary fibrosis, scleroderma.

Procedure

- The client should be NPO for 12 hours prior to the test.
- Collect 7 mL of venous blood in a red-top (preferred) or green-top tube. Check with the laboratory concerning which tube to use, the clotted blood (red-top) or heparinized (green-top) tube. Avoid hemolysis. Deliver the blood sample immediately to the laboratory.
- Record the client's age on the laboratory slip.

A

Factors Affecting Laboratory Results

- Hemolysis of the blood sample affects test results. A delay in testing the blood could cause a low serum ACE level.
- Persons under 20 years of age usually have an elevated serum ACE level; thus the test could be false positive.
- Steroids (cortisone preparations) can decrease the serum ACE level.

NURSING IMPLICATIONS WITH RATIONALE

- Check blood pressure. This test is not used to determine the cause of hypertension; however, ACE indirectly contributes to increase in blood pressure.
- Record the age of the client on the laboratory slip. Rarely is this test ordered for a client under 20 years of age.
- Suggest that the test be canceled or postponed if the client is under 20 years old.

Client Teaching

- Instruct the client that he or she should have nothing by mouth for 12 hours prior to the test. This would most likely be NPO after dinner.
- Answer questions or concerns the client may have about the test or health problems. If necessary, refer questions to other health care providers.

Anion gap

Reference Values

Adult: 10–17 mEq/L (values differ from 7 to 20 mEq/L).

Description

The anion gap is the difference between electrolytes, the positive ions (cations) of sodium and potassium, and the negative ions (anions) of chloride and bicarbonate (serum CO_2), to determine if an acid–base imbalance is present. Unmeasured anions in the serum, such as phosphates, sulfates, lactates, ketone bodies, and other organic acids, contribute to metabolic acid–base imbalances (metabolic acidosis and alkalosis). Actually, the difference between the milliequivalents of cations and anions is referred to as the *anion gap*.

Serum levels of the cations (sodium and potassium) and the anions (chloride and bicarbonate) are applied to the formula:

Anion gap = (sodium + potassium) − (chloride + HCO_3 [bicarbonate])

An elevated anion gap (greater than 17 mEq/L) indicates metabolic acidosis; a decreased anion gap (less than 10 mEq/L) indicates metabolic alkalosis.

Purpose

- To determine the presence of acidosis.

Clinical Problems

Decreased Level (less than 10 mEq/L): High electrolyte values, such as sodium, calcium, magnesium; multiple myeloma, nephrosis. *Drug Influence:* Lithium, diuretics, chlorpropamide.

Increased Level (greater than 17 mEq/L): Lactic acidosis, ketoacidosis (uncontrolled diabetes mellitus, starvation, anorexia nervosa), severe salicylate intoxication, renal failure, severe dehydration, antifreeze ingestion, paint-thinner poisoning. *Drug Influence:* Penicillin and carbenicillin in high doses, salicylates, paraldehyde, diuretics (thiazides and loop diuretics), methanol ingestion.

Normal Level Occurring in Metabolic Acidosis: Diarrhea, renal tubular acidosis, ureterosigmoidostomy, hyperalimentation, small bowel fistula, pancreatic drainage.

Procedure

- There is no food or fluid restriction.
- Obtain serum electrolyte values of sodium (Na), potassium (K), chloride (Cl), and CO_2 (bicarbonate determinant) from the laboratory slip. If not available, collect 7–10 mL of venous blood in a red-top tube.

Factors Affecting Laboratory Results

- (*See Drug Influence under decreased and increased levels.*)
- Hemolysis of blood sample increases potassium and bicarbonate levels.

NURSING IMPLICATIONS WITH RATIONALE

- Calculate the anion gap from recently obtained electrolyte values of sodium, potassium, chloride, and serum CO_2. Use the formula given in "Description" above.
- Observe for signs and symptoms of metabolic acidosis (e.g., rapid, vigorous breathing [Kussmaul breathing], increased pulse rate, flushed skin).

Anthrax

See Bioterrorism Infectious Products

Antibiotic susceptibility (sensitivity)

Reference Values

Adult: Organism is sensitive or intermediate or resistant to antibiotics.

Child: Same as adult.

A

Description

(See Cultures.)

It is important to identify not only the organism responsible for the infection but also the antibiotic(s) that will inhibit the growth of the bacteria. The health care provider orders a culture and sensitivity test (C and S) when a wound infection, urinary tract infection, or other types of infected secretions are suspected. The choice of antibiotic depends on the pathogenic organism and its susceptibility to the antibiotics.

There are two methods employed to test antibiotic susceptibility: tube dilution and disk diffusion (also called agar diffusion), with the latter being the most commonly used method. A filter paper containing small antibiotic disks is placed in a Petri dish streaked with the single type of bacteria. If bacteria surround the disk, the organism is resistant to the antibiotic. If the bacteria growth around the disk is inhibited, the organism is susceptible to the antibiotic. Recently, the term "minimal inhibitory concentration" (MIC) has been used to express (in mcg/mL) the lowest concentration of the antibiotics that will prevent visible growth of a cultured microorganism.

With the tube dilution method, bacteria are cultured in several tubes having various concentrations of antibiotic. The lowest concentration of antibiotic that inhibits the growth of the organism is the choice of antibiotic concentration for the client.

Purpose

- To check the effectiveness of selected antibiotics on a specific bacteria from a culture.

Clinical Problems

Resistant (R): The antibiotic is noneffective against the organism.

Intermediate (I): Bacterial growth retardation is inconclusive.

Sensitive (S): The antibiotic is effective against the organism.

Procedure

- It takes approximately 24 hours for bacterial growth and 48 hours for the test results.
- The specimen for C and S should be taken to the laboratory within 30 minutes of collection or else refrigerated.
- The specimen should be handled with care, preventing contamination and bacterial transmission (*see Culture Procedure*).

Factors Affecting Laboratory Results

- Antibiotics and sulfonamides could cause a false-negative reaction.

NURSING IMPLICATIONS WITH RATIONALE

- Collect specimen for C and S before preventive antibiotic therapy is started. Antibiotic therapy started before specimen collection could cause an inaccurate result.
- Record on the laboratory slip the antibiotic(s) the client is receiving, the dosages, and how long the antibiotic(s) has (have) been taken.

- Check laboratory report for C and S result. If the client is receiving an antibiotic and the report shows the organism is resistant to that antibiotic, the nurse should notify the health care provider.

Client Teaching

- Inform the client that the culture test results will be available in 48 hours.

Anticardiolipin antibodies (ACA) (serum)

Antiphospholipid Antibodies (APA), Cardiolipin Antibodies (aCL), IgG Cardiolipin Antibodies, and IgM Cardiolipin Antibodies

Reference Value

Negative.

Description

Anticardiolipin antibodies (ACA) are autoantibodies found in some clients with systemic lupus erythematosus (SLE). They occur in 45% of clients with SLE and less than 7% of clients without SLE. These antibodies were originally found in clients with SLE and were called *lupus anticoagulants (LA)*. Later it was determined that these antibodies did not act as anticoagulants and that they were found in health problems other than lupus. ACA and LA are members of the antiphospholipid family of immunoglobulins active against phospholipids. ACA may also be present in clients having thrombocytopenia, spontaneous or recurrent thrombosis, and fetal loss.

Purposes

- To aid in the diagnosis of SLE, especially in clients who have thrombocytopenia and repeated fetal loss.
- To detect ACA syndrome in clients with other health problems.

Clinical Problems

Increased Level: SLE, thrombocytopenia, thrombosis, fetal loss, infection, severe hemorrhage (rare), malignancy, acquired immunodeficiency syndrome (AIDS). *Drug Influence:* Chlorpromazine, procainamide, quinidine, penicillin, various antibiotics, phenytoin.

Procedure

- There is no food or fluid restriction.
- Collect 3–5 mL of venous blood in a red-top tube. Avoid hemolysis; send the specimen immediately to the laboratory.

Factors Affecting Laboratory Results

- Hemolysis of the blood specimen may cause a false test result.

A

NURSING IMPLICATIONS WITH RATIONALE

- Obtain a history of the client's health problem with current symptoms.
- Observe for signs and symptoms of SLE: for example, fatigue, fever, rash butterfly over nose, leukopenia.

Client Teaching

- Instruct the client to have daily rest periods, which help to decrease symptoms.
- Explain to the client the purpose of oral anticoagulant or platelet inhibitor therapy for thrombocytopenia or recurrent thrombosis if these treatments are ordered.
- Listen to the client's concerns; answer questions or refer them to other health care providers.

Anticentromere antibody

Reference Values

Normal: Negative.

Positive: *Titrated*: >1:40 for human epithelia type 2 cells (HEp-2) cells.

Description

The centromere is a region of the cell chromosomes that divides the chromosome into sections. Anticentromere antibodies are a form of antinuclear antibodies. When the cell divides, the centromere appears on the mitotic spindle. The anticentromere antibodies are found in clients with CREST syndrome, which is calcinosis, Raynaud phenomenon, esophageal dysfunction, sclerodactyly, and telangiectasia (CREST). This is associated with scleroderma disease. A large percentage of the clients with CREST syndrome have a positive anticentromere antibody titer.

Purpose

- To identify clients with CREST syndrome.

Clinical Problems

Positive Findings: CREST syndrome.

Procedure

- There is no food or fluid restriction
- Collect 7 mL of venous blood in a red-top tube. Place the blood sample tube in a biohazard bag and send to the laboratory.

NURSING IMPLICATIONS WITH RATIONALE

- Obtain a history of the client's health problem.
- Assess any clinical changes that are occurring with the client. Record the changes.

Client Teaching

- Answer client questions or refer questions to other health professionals.

Anticonvulsants (blood, serum, plasma)

Carbamazepine (Tegretol), Ethosuximide (Zarontin), Phenytoin (Dilantin), Primidone (Mysoline), Valproic Acid (Depakene)

A

Reference Values

Adult:

Drug Name	THERAPEUTIC RANGE		TOXIC LEVEL	
	mcg/mL	µmoL/L	mcg/mL	µmoL/L
Carbamazepine	4–12	16.9–50.8	greater than 12–15	greater than 50.8–69
(Child)	(Same as adult)		(Same as adult)	
Ethosuximide	40–100	283–708	greater than 100	greater than 708
(Child)	(2–4 per 1 mg/kg/day)		(Same as adult or higher)	
Phenytoin	10–20	39.6–79.3	greater than 20	greater than 79.3
Primidone	5–12	23–55	greater than 12–15	greater than 55–69
(Child <5 years) (7–10)	(30–45)		(greater than 12)	(greater than 55)
Valproic acid	50–100	347–693	greater than 100	greater than 693
(Child)	(Same as adult)		(Same as adult)	

Description

The drugs listed as anticonvulsant agents are given to control or to alleviate grand mal, psychomotor, and/or petit mal seizures. Most of them have different therapeutic ranges, peak levels, and half-life.

Carbamazepine (Tegretol): This agent is used for grand mal seizures. Peak serum level occurs 4–8 hours after oral dose; half-life is about 10–26 hours in adults and 8–20 hours in children. Steady state is reached in 2 weeks. When carbamazepine is administered with phenytoin, phenobarbital, ethosuximide, primidone, or valproic acid, serum level of the drug might decrease. A serious side effect is bone marrow depression.

Ethosuximide (Zarontin): This agent is used for petit mal seizures. Peak serum level occurs 3–5 hours after oral dose; half-life is about 60 hours in adults and 30 hours in children. Steady state is reached in 7–10 days. When administered with carbamazepine or valproic acid, ethosuximide's serum level might decrease or increase. Side effects include anorexia, nausea, vomiting, and lupus erythematosus-like syndrome.

Phenytoin (Dilantin): (*See separate listing.*)

Primidone (Mysoline): This agent is used for grand mal and psychomotor seizures. Peak serum level occurs 7–8 hours after oral dose; half-life varies from 8 to 48 hours (shorter half-life with primidone and longer with the two active metabolites, phenobarbital and phenylethylmalonamide [PEMA]). Steady state is rapidly reached. When primidone is administered with carbamazepine, its serum level may increase. Side effects include sedation, nausea, dizziness, and visual disturbance.

Valproic Acid (Depakene): This agent is used alone or with other anticonvulsants for grand mal and petit mal seizures. Peak serum level occurs 1–4 hours after oral dose; half-life is 8–15 hours.

A

Valproic acid inhibits phenobarbital metabolism. If primidone or phenobarbital is given with valproic acid, its dosage needs to be adjusted (lowered). Valproic acid can elevate ethosuximide and phenytoin levels when coadministered. It can cross the placenta. Valproic acid therapy may cause a false-positive urine ketone test. Side effects include anorexia, nausea, vomiting, fatigue, and altered liver function tests.

Purposes

- To monitor specific anticonvulsant serum levels.
- To detect the toxic level of a specific anticonvulsant.

Clinical Problems

Decreased Level: *Carbamazepine: Drug Influence:* Barbiturates, benzodiazepines, ethosuximide, phenytoin, primidone, valproic acid.

Ethosuximide: *Drug Influence:* Carbamazepine, valproic acid.

Valproic Acid: *Drug Influence:* Carbamazepine, phenytoin, phenobarbital, primidone.

Increased Level: *Carbamazepine:* Overdose of carbamazepine, liver disease, cardiovascular disease, bone marrow disease. *Drug Influence:* Phenytoin, barbiturates, propoxyphene (Darvon), erythromycin.

Ethosuximide: Overdose of ethosuximide, liver disease. *Drug Influence:* Carbamazepine, valproic acid.

Primidone: Overdose of primidone, liver disease. *Drug Influence:* Phenobarbital.

Procedure

- There is no food or fluid restriction.
- Collect 5–7 mL of venous blood in a red-top tube (valproic acid, carbamazepine), gray-top tube (primidone), or green-top tube (ethosuximide). *Check with laboratory for preferred collecting tube.*
- Record the name of drug, dose, route, and last time drug was administered on the laboratory requisition slip. Trough serum levels (drawn before next dose) are usually requested. List drugs the client is taking that might interfere with test results on requisition slip.

Factors Affecting Laboratory Results

- Drugs (*see Drug Influence*) that the client is taking could increase or decrease test results.

NURSING IMPLICATIONS WITH RATIONALE

- Administer valproic acid with meals to reduce gastrointestinal distress.
- Monitor serum drug levels (weekly, monthly, yearly) during long-term drug therapy.
- Monitor complete blood count (CBC) and platelet count prior to carbamazepine (Tegretol) therapy and at regular intervals (weekly, monthly). Bone marrow depression is rare; however, it could occur as a result of long-term carbamazepine therapy.
- Assess liver function tests (i.e., aspartate aminotransferase [AST], serum glutamic-oxaloacetic acid [SGOT], alanine aminotransferase [ALT], serum glutamic-pyruvic

transaminase [SGPT], bilirubin, alkaline phosphatase) while the client is receiving long-term anticonvulsant therapy. Compare test findings with baseline levels.

These drugs are metabolized in the liver, and hepatic damage could result.

- Assess serum amylase level while client is receiving long-term valproic acid (Depakene) therapy. Pancreatitis could result.

Client Teaching

- Inform the client not to discontinue prescribed anticonvulsant agent abruptly without the health care provider's permission. Withdrawal of any anticonvulsant drugs could precipitate seizures.
- Inform the client that photosensitivity reaction could occur when taking anticonvulsants. While in the sun, clients should wear sunglasses and sunscreen lotion.

Increased Level

- Relate clinical conditions and drugs (*see Clinical Problems*) that could elevate serum and anticonvulsant levels.
- Observe for signs and symptoms of common side effects from anticonvulsant therapy (e.g., anorexia, nausea, vomiting, fatigue, lethargy, dizziness, headache).
- Inform the diabetic client on valproic acid therapy that the drug could cause a false-positive urine ketone test.
- Report immediately symptoms of carbamazepine and primidone toxicity (e.g., diplopia, blurred vision) to the health care provider.
- Report lupus erythematosus-like symptoms resulting from long-term ethosuximide therapy.
- Assess for bleeding or bruising (petechiae, ecchymosis, epistaxis, melena) while receiving valproic acid. Report findings to the health care provider. Check the CBC for a low platelet count and blood count.

Antidepressants (tricyclics) (serum)

Amitriptyline, Desipramine, Doxepin, Imipramine, Nortriptyline

Reference Values

Adult:

Drug Name	THERAPEUTIC RANGE ng/mL	TOXIC LEVEL ng/mL
Amitriptyline HCl (Elavil)	75–225	greater than 500
Desipramine HCl (Norpramin)	125–300	greater than 500
Doxepin HCl (Sinequan)	150–300	greater than 500
Imipramine HCl (Tofranil)	150–300	greater than 500
Nortriptyline HCl (Aventyl)	75–150	greater than 300

A

Description

Antidepressants are used primarily for unipolar and endogenous depressive disorders, which are characterized by loss of interest in work or home, inability to complete tasks, and deep depression. There are three groups of antidepressants: tricyclic antidepressants (TCAs), second-generation antidepressants (newest group), and monoamine oxidase (MAO) inhibitors. Anticholinergic symptoms are common side effects of tricyclic antidepressants. With second-generation antidepressants, extrapyramidal symptoms (EPS) are common. Clients taking MAO inhibitors should avoid foods rich in tyramine (cheese, cream, chocolate, bananas, beer, red wines). Hypertensive crisis could occur when foods rich in tyramine and MAO inhibitors are combined.

Purposes

- To regulate the tricyclic drug level for obtaining a therapeutic drug level.
- To monitor the tricyclic drug dose.
- To avoid a toxic drug level.

Clinical Problems

Decreased Level: Mild, reactive, unipolar, and/or atypical depression. *Drug Influence:* Barbiturates, chloral hydrate.

Increased Level: Toxic tricyclic antidepressant. *Drug Influence:* Hydrocortisone, neuroleptics, cimetidine, oral contraceptives.

Procedure

- No food or fluid restriction is required.
- Collect 5–7 mL of venous blood in a red-top tube. Deliver blood container immediately to the laboratory.
- Obtain blood specimen 2 hours before the next drug dose.

NURSING IMPLICATIONS WITH RATIONALE

- Assess client's history related to depression.
- Record drugs that the client presently is taking. Central nervous system depressants and alcohol, if taken with antidepressants, could cause respiratory depression and hypotension.
- Monitor vital signs and urinary output. Report abnormal findings.
- Check serum tricyclic level of the drug the client is taking. Report if the level is *not* within therapeutic range.
- Assess the client's compliance to drug therapy. Report changes.
- Discuss the importance of drug compliance with the client. This is important to maintain a therapeutic drug level and possibly to avoid toxic level if the drug is taken in excess.
- Discuss possible side effects, such as dry mouth, blurred vision, fatigue, urinary retention, postural hypotension, and gastrointestinal disturbances, and report any of these to the health care provider.
- Discuss foods to avoid if the client is taking an MAO inhibitor (*see Description*).

Antidiuretic hormone (ADH) (plasma)
Vasopressor

Reference Values
Adult: 1–5 pg/mL; 1–5 ng/L.

Description
Antidiuretic hormone (ADH) is produced by the hypothalamus and stored in the posterior pituitary gland (neurohypophysis). The primary function of ADH is in water reabsorption from the distal renal tubules in response to the serum osmolality. *Antidiuretic* means "against diuresis." There is more ADH secreted from the posterior pituitary gland when the serum osmolality is increased to greater than 295 mOsm/kg (concentrated body fluids). More water reabsorption occurs, which dilutes the body fluid. When the serum osmolality is decreased to greater than 280 mOsm/kg, less ADH is secreted, and thus more water is excreted via the kidneys.

Syndrome (secretion) of inappropriate ADH (SIADH) is an excess secretion of ADH that is not influenced by the serum osmolality level. SIADH causes excess water retention. Stress, surgery, pain, and certain drugs (narcotics, anesthetics) contribute to SIADH.

Purposes
- To detect a deficit or excess in ADH secretion.
- To identify the presence of body fluid deficit or excess.

Clinical Problems
Decreased Level: Diabetes insipidus, psychogenic polydipsia, nephrotic syndrome. *Drug Influence:* Alcohol, lithium, demeclocycline, phenytoin (Dilantin).

Increased Level: SIADH, brain tumor, cancer (ectopic ADH), pulmonary tuberculosis, pain, IPPB (intermittent positive pressure breathing), surgery, pneumonia. *Drug Influence:* Anesthetics, narcotics, estrogens, oxytocin, antineoplastic (anticancer) drugs, thiazides, antipsychotics, tricyclic antidepressants.

Procedure
- The client should be NPO for 12 hours and should avoid strenuous exercise for 12 hours. Stress should be decreased or avoided.
- Collect 5–7 mL of venous blood in a lavender-top *plastic* tube or plastic syringe. A glass container can cause degradation of the ADH. If blood is drawn in glass, prechill the glass and separate immediately.
- Deliver the blood specimen immediately (within 10 minutes) to the laboratory.

Factors Affecting Laboratory Results
- Certain drugs (*see Drug Influence*), food, fluids, stress, pain, and exercise can affect test results.
- Using a glass container for blood specimen collection can cause ADH degradation.

A

- If the blood specimen is taken at night or if the client is in a standing position, the ADH level will be increased.
- A delay in the delivery of the blood specimen will affect test results. Serum should be separated from the clot within 10 minutes.

NURSING IMPLICATIONS WITH RATIONALE

- Check to determine if drugs that may affect test results should be withheld for 12 hours before the test. Drugs that must be taken before the test should be recorded on the laboratory slip.
- Record in the client's chart and on the laboratory slip if the client is having undue stress or pain. This could increase the ADH secretion and plasma level.
- Check that the blood specimen is taken immediately to the laboratory. The serum should be separated from the clot within 10 minutes.

Client Teaching

- Explain to the client the need to avoid stress and exercise before the test.
- Instruct the client to have nothing by mouth after dinner meal.
- Listen to the client's concerns.

Antiglomerular basement membrane antibody (anti-GBM, AGBM) (serum)
Glomerular Basement Membrane (GBM) Antibody

Reference Values

Negative or none detected.

Description This test is performed to detect circulating glomerular basement membrane (GBM) antibodies that can damage the GBMs in the glomeruli. The beta-hemolytic streptococcus can cause an antibody response in the renal glomeruli. Glomerulonephritis, caused by anti-GBM, is usually severe and rapidly progressive. Pulmonary hemorrhage often occurs because of cross-reactivity of anti-GBM with pulmonary vascular basement membrane.

Purpose

- To detect GBM antibodies that could cause or are causing renal disease.

Clinical Problems

Positive Result: Anti-GBM nephritis, tubulointerstitial nephritis, pulmonary capillary basement membranes.

Procedure

- There is no food or fluid restriction.
- Collect 5–7 mL of venous blood in a red-top tube. The test should be run immediately; if there will be a delay, the blood should be frozen.
- Tissue from kidney biopsy might be the specimen. Tissue should be frozen after collection.

Factors Affecting Laboratory Results

- Improper care of the specimen can result in inaccurate test results.

NURSING IMPLICATIONS WITH RATIONALE

- Obtain a history of a streptococcal throat infection.
- Monitor urine output. Because the glomeruli are damaged, oliguria usually occurs.
- Assess for signs and symptoms of renal (glomerular) disease (e.g., edema of the extremities, shortness of breath, proteinuria, hematuria, increased blood pressure, elevated serum blood urea nitrogen and creatinine, decreased urine output).

Client Teaching

- Instruct the client to follow a medical regimen of diet, drugs, and rest.

Antimitochondrial antibody (AMA) (serum)

Reference Values

Negative: At a 1:5 dilution.

Intermediate Level: 1:20–1:80.

Strongly Suggestive of Primary Biliary Cirrhosis: Greater than 1:80.

Positive for Primary Biliary Cirrhosis: Greater than 1:160.

Description

The antimitochondrial antibody (AMA) test is used to differentiate between primary biliary cirrhosis and other liver diseases. Eighty to 90% of clients with primary biliary cirrhosis have a positive titer for AMAs. A positive test result would usually rule out extrahepatic biliary obstruction and acute infectious hepatitis. To confirm biliary cirrhosis, other liver tests should be performed, such as AST/SGOT, ALT/SGPT, alkaline phosphatase, serum bilirubin, and GGT.

This test is usually performed in conjunction with antismooth muscle antibodies (ASMA, ASTHMA) test. ASMA titer is elevated with biliary cirrhosis and chronic active hepatitis. Like AMA, ASMA is seldom elevated with extrahepatic biliary obstruction. The antibodies may also be associated with autoimmune disease.

Purposes

- To aid in the diagnosis of biliary cirrhosis.
- To compare the test result with that of other liver tests.

A

Clinical Problems

Positive Titer: Primary biliary cirrhosis, chronic hepatitis, autoimmune disorders, such as systemic lupus erythematosus, rheumatoid arthritis, pernicious anemia.

Procedure

- The client should be NPO for 8 hours prior to the test.
- Collect 3–5 mL of venous blood in a red-top tube.
- Avoid hemolysis. The blood specimen should be delivered to the laboratory immediately.

Factors Affecting Laboratory Results

- Hemolysis of the blood specimen can affect test results.

NURSING IMPLICATIONS WITH RATIONALE

- Assess for the presence of jaundice.
- Check other liver tests and compare test results. If the health care provider suspects biliary cirrhosis, AMA and ASMA/ASTHMA tests are usually ordered.

Client Teaching

- Instruct the client to have nothing by mouth after midnight or 8 hours prior to the test.
- Listen to the client's concerns. Answer appropriate questions.

Antimyocardial antibody (serum)

Reference Values

Negative: None detected.

Positive: Titer levels.

Description

Antimyocardial antibody develops in response to a specific antigen in the heart muscle that can cause autoimmune damage to the heart. This antibody may be detected in the blood prior to or soon after heart disease. The antibody may be present after cardiac surgery, myocardial infarction, streptococcal infection, or rheumatic fever. This test may be used to monitor therapeutic response to treatment.

Purpose

- To identify the presence of antimitochondrial antibodies as the cause of the cardiac condition.

Clinical Problems

Positive Titer: Myocardial infarction, myocarditis, pericarditis following cardiac surgery, acute rheumatic fever, chronic rheumatic diseases, streptococcal infections, idiopathic cardiomyopathy, endomyocardial fibrosis, thoracic injury, systemic lupus erythematosus.

A

Procedure

- There is no food or fluid restriction.
- Collect 3–5 mL of venous blood in a red-top tube. Send to the laboratory immediately.

Factors Affecting Laboratory Results

- None known.

NURSING IMPLICATIONS WITH RATIONALE

- Obtain a history of heart disease.
- Check cardiac enzyme levels (creatine phosphokinase [CPK], aspartate aminotransferase [AST], and lactate dehydrogenase [LDH]). If elevated, heart disease is likely.
- Observe for signs and symptoms of heart disease, such as chest pain, dyspnea, diaphoresis, and indigestion.
- Listen to the client's concerns.

Antineutrophil cytoplasmic antibody (ANCA) (serum)
Cytoplasmic Neutrophil Antibodies

Reference Values

Negative, less than 1:20 titer

Description

The antineutrophil cytoplasmic antibodies (ANCAs) are autoimmune antibodies that respond to cytoplasmic components of neutrophil granules. There are two types of ANCAs: the cytoplasmic C-ANCA and the perinuclear P-ANCA. The P-ANCA is closely related to the antinuclear antibodies test. These two ANCAs are identified through the staining of neutrophils.

The C-ANCA test is useful in the diagnosis of Wegener granulomatosis (WG), which is found in granulomatosis vascular diseases. WG can be present in the upper and lower respiratory tracts due to granulomatosis vasculitis, glomerulonephritis that is damaged by granulomatosis, and in small vessels.

The second type, P-ANCA, is produced by a perinuclear staining of neutrophils. P-ANCA is used in diagnosing inflammatory bowel disease, such as Crohn disease and ulcerative colitis, lupus erythematosus (SLE), and liver disease.

Purposes

- To assist in the diagnosis of Wegener granulomatosis by C-ANCA staining.
- To assist in the diagnosis of inflammatory bowel disease, such as ulcerative colitis and Crohn disease, and liver diseases by P-ANCA staining.
- To monitor the response to treatment for WG.
- To monitor the response to treatment for specific inflammatory bowel and liver diseases.

Clinical Problems

Increased C-ANCA: Wegener granulomatosis; granulomatosis vasculitis in the upper and lower respiratory tracts, glomerulonephritis, small vessel vasculitis.

Increased P-ANCA: Inflammatory bowel disease (ulcerative colitis, Crohn disease), SLE, liver disease.

Procedure

- There is no food or fluid restriction.
- Collect 5 mL of venous blood in a red-top tube.
- A biopsy may be indicated. Follow procedure in assisting with biopsy.

NURSING IMPLICATIONS WITH RATIONALE

- Obtain a history of the client's health problems, which should include problems with the respiratory system, kidneys, liver, and colon.
- Record vital signs.
- Record a list of the client's medication and how frequently they are taken.
- Ask the client what over-the-counter medication he or she is taking.

Client Teaching

- Explain the test procedure.
- Allow the client time to express his or her concerns about the health problems(s).

Antinuclear antibodies (ANA) (serum)
Anti-DNA Antibody, Anti-DNP Antibody

Reference Value

Adult: Negative at 1:20 dilution.

Description

The antinuclear antibodies (ANA) test is a screening test for diagnosing systemic lupus erythematosus and other collagen diseases. ANAs are immunoglobulins (IgM, IgG, IgA) that react with the nuclear part of leukocytes. They form antibodies against deoxyribonucleic acid (DNA), ribonucleic acid (RNA), and others. Two ANAs, anti-DNA and anti–D-nucleoprotein (anti-DNP), are almost always present with SLE. Anti-DNA will fluctuate according to the disease process, with remission, and with exacerbation. It is normally present (95%) in lupus nephritis.

There is a group of ANAs to identify antibodies for specific autoimmune disease. The total ANA level can also be elevated in scleroderma, rheumatoid arthritis, cirrhosis, leukemia, infectious mononucleosis, and malignancy. For diagnosing lupus, the ANA test should be compared with other tests for lupus.

A

Purpose

- To compare the ANA test with other laboratory tests for diagnosing SLE or other collagen diseases.

Clinical Problems

Increased—Positive (greater than 1:20): SLE (most frequent cause), progressive systemic sclerosis, scleroderma, leukemia, rheumatoid arthritis, cirrhosis of the liver, infectious mononucleosis, myasthenia gravis, malignancy. *Drug Influence:* Antibiotics (penicillin, streptomycin, tetracycline), antihypertensives (hydralazine [Apresoline], methyldopa [Aldomet]), anti-TB (para-aminosalicylic acid [PAS], isoniazid [INH]), diuretics (acetazolamide [Diamox], thiazides [hydrochlorothiazide]), oral contraceptives, procainamide (Pronestyl), trimethadione (Tridione), phenytoin (Dilantin).

Procedure

- There is no food or fluid restriction.
- Collect 3–5 mL of venous blood in a red-top tube. Send to the laboratory immediately.
- List drugs the client is taking that could cause false-positive test results.

Factors Affecting Laboratory Results

- Certain drugs cause false-positive results (*see Drug Influence*).
- The aging process can cause a slight positive ANA titer.

NURSING IMPLICATIONS WITH RATIONALE

Increased—Positive Titer

- Relate clinical problems and drugs to positive ANA results. With SLE, the ANA titer may fluctuate according to the severity of the disease.
- Compare test result with other tests for lupus.
- Assess for signs and symptoms of SLE (e.g., skin rash over the cheeks and nose, joint pain).
- Promote rest during an acute phase.
- Listen to the client's concerns.

Antiparietal cell antibody (APCA) (blood)

Parietal Cell Antibody

Reference Values

Negative: Less than 1:120 titer.
Positive: 1:180 titer.

A

Description

Parietal cells in the stomach secrete hydrochloric acid (HCl), which is needed for protein catabolism. Parietal cell antibody is frequently caused by an autoimmune response.

Antiparietal cell antibody (APCA) at approximately 80–90% is sensitive for detecting pernicious anemia (PA). The APCA titer may decrease during the duration of PA. Also, this test helps in differentiating between autoimmune chronic gastritis and that of pernicious anemia. Intrinsic factor (IF) antibodies may also be found in pernicious anemia because of the disruption of the IF production caused by the autoimmune process. PA may have a genetic tendency that is not caused by an autoimmune response.

An elevated APCA may be present in other autoimmune disorders, such as myasthenia gravis and type 1 diabetes mellitus. APCA titer level may increase with age. It should not be the only test used for diagnosing pernicious anemia.

Purposes

- To screen for the presence of pernicious anemia.
- To rule out the occurrence of other autoimmune disorders, for example, myasthenia gravis, type 1 diabetes mellitus.

Clinical Problems

Positive Titer Level: Pernicious anemia, chronic gastritis, gastric ulcer, type 1 diabetes mellitus, gastric cancer, myasthenia gravis, thyroid disease.

Procedure

- There is no food or fluid restriction.
- Collect 7–10 mL of venous blood in a red-top or gray-top tube.

Factors Affecting Laboratory Results

- None known.

NURSING IMPLICATIONS WITH RATIONALE

- Obtain a history from the client related to the present health complaint. Clinical manifestations of pernicious anemia may include weakness, orthopnea, burning sensation of the tongue, dyspnea, lightheadedness, and sensitivity to temperature changes.

Client Teaching

- Encourage the client to eat a balanced diet high in protein, vitamins, and iron. Foods such as fish, red meat, eggs, and milk help to increase the daily vitamin B_{12} intake.
- Inform the client that other tests may be necessary to confirm the diagnosis (especially if pernicious anemia is suggestive).

Antiphospholipid antibodies (APA)

See Anticardiolipin Antibodies (ACA)

Antiscleroderma antibody (Scl-70) (serum)

Antibodies to Scl-70 Antigen

A

Reference Values

Negative: Borderline: 20–25 units.

Positive: Greater than 25 units.

Description

Antiscleroderma antibodies occur in 40–70% of clients with advanced or diffuse cutaneous scleroderma, interstitial pulmonary fibrosis, and peripheral vascular disease. The presence of antibodies to Scl-70 antigen is seldom present in other rheumatic disorders, such as systemic lupus erythematosus and rheumatoid arthritis.

A negative test result does not indicate the absence of sclerodermal disease. Scleroderma is considered an autoimmune collagen disorder.

Purpose

- To assist in the diagnosis of scleroderma.

Clinical Problems

Increased Levels: Scleroderma, CREST syndrome, progressive systemic sclerosis. *Drug Influence:* Aspirin, diphenhydramine HCl (Benadryl), isoniazid, methyldopa, ethosuximide, penicillin, tetracycline, streptomycin.

Procedure

- There is no food or fluid restriction.
- Collect 5 mL of venous blood in a red-top tube.

Factors Affecting Laboratory Results

- See drug list that can cause a false-positive test result.

NURSING IMPLICATIONS WITH RATIONALE

- Obtain a history of health problems. Record if client has any physical symptoms, such as a rash. There can be localized or systemic forms of scleroderma.

Client Teaching

- Explain to the client that other tests may be requested by the health care provider.
- If the client is diagnosed with systemic scleroderma, the nurse may inform the client that most systemic forms of scleroderma progress very slowly.
- Tell the client to dress warmly, including gloves, because cold weather may increase discomfort and pain.

A

Antismooth muscle antibody (ASMA, ASTHMA) (serum)

Reference Values

Negative: Less than 1:20.
Positive: Greater than 1:20.

Description

Antismooth muscle antibody (ASMA, ASTHMA) is associated primarily with autoimmune chronic active hepatitis (CAH). With CAH, the titer level is usually greater than 1:160. The titer elevation of ASTHMA occurs in more than 70% of clients with CAH, and most of the clients are females. CAH is frequently referred to as an autoimmune disease. Clients with primary biliary cirrhosis may have a slight titer elevation. Lower titer levels may be present in other conditions, such as cancer, viral infections, and acute viral hepatitis. The antimitochondrial antibody and antinuclear antibody tests may be prescribed with the ASTHMA test to differentiate the cause of the liver disorder. An elevated AMA titer is more prevalent with biliary cirrhosis, whereas ASTHMA and ANA elevations occur with chronic active hepatitis, which is referred to as lupoid hepatitis. With CAH, the ASTHMA is usually higher than the ANA.

Purpose

- To assist with the diagnosis of CAH.

Clinical Problems

Increased Levels: *High titers:* Chronic active hepatitis. *Low titers:* Primary biliary cirrhosis, cancer of the liver, infectious mononucleosis, multiple sclerosis (MS), rheumatoid arthritis, acute viral hepatitis, intrinsic asthma.

Procedure

- There is no food or fluid restriction.
- Collect 5–7 mL of venous blood in a red-top tube.
- Apply pressure to the venipuncture site to decrease bleeding. Clients with liver dysfunction tend to bleed more readily.

Factors Affecting Laboratory Results

- None known.

NURSING IMPLICATIONS WITH RATIONALE

- Obtain a history from the client related to the health problem. Jaundice may be present. Record drugs that the client is taking that may be a contributing cause of CAH.

Client Teaching

- Explain to the client that other laboratory tests may be performed—for example, ANA, AMA, bilirubin, and a liver biopsy may be requested to assure the diagnosis.
- If steroids are prescribed for CAH, explain how the steroid drug should be taken (e.g., with food). If steroid drugs are discontinued, the daily dose should be tapered over a period of days to avoid adverse effects.
- Listen to the client's concerns. Refer questions to other health professionals as needed.

Antisperm antibody test (semen, blood/serum)

Antispermatozoal Antibody, Antisperm Antibody Detection, Sperm Antibodies

Reference Values

Male: Negative for sperm agglutinating antibody Negative: 0–15% Moderately positive: 50% Strongly positive: 100%

Description

Infertility can result from antisperm antibody production. This test may be ordered to determine whether infertility could be caused by antisperm antibodies. When the sperm is blocked in the efferent testicular ducts, the formation of autoantibodies to sperm occurs in the blood. Antisperm antibodies may occur in approximately 50% of men following a vasectomy. Most of these men are infertile after repair of the ducts postvasectomy.

Using the enzyme-linked immunoabsorbent assay (ELISA), IgA and IgG antisperm antibodies can be identified. The IgA antisperm antibodies are associated with poor sperm motility. The IgG antisperm antibodies are associated with poor fusion of the sperm and ovum. By testing the sperm in the male and the cervical mucus in the female, the presence of antisperm antibodies can be identified, and the cause of infertility may be determined.

Purposes

- To determine the cause of infertility.
- To identify the presence of antisperm antibodies.

Clinical Problems

Increased Presence of Antisperm Antibodies: Infertility, blocked efferent ducts in the testes, postvasectomy.

Procedure

- There is no food or fluid restriction.

Blood/Serum

- Collect 7 mL of venous blood in a red-top tube or red/gray-top tube.

A

Semen Specimen

- Instruct the male not to have an ejaculation for 3 days prior to the test.
- Instruct the male to collect a fresh semen specimen in a clean plastic container.
- Instruct the male not to use a condom or lubricant when collecting the specimen.
- If the semen specimen is collected at home, he should take the specimen to the laboratory within 1–2 hours. The specimen should be kept warm during transport. Check with the laboratory; procedures may differ.

Vaginal Mucus Specimen

- Collect approximately 1 mL of cervical specimen in a plastic vial. Specimen should be immediately frozen.

Factors Affecting Laboratory Results

- Intercourse occurring before semen collection.
- Use of lubricants with semen collection.
- Heavy coffee consumption and smoking may decrease sperm motility.

NURSING IMPLICATIONS WITH RATIONALE

- Obtain a history of the problems concerning infertility.
- Obtain a history of drugs the clients are taking.
- Provide privacy to the male when collection of the semen occurs on-site.

Client Teaching

- Instruct the male on how to collect the semen specimen.
- Instruct the female on how the cervical specimen is obtained.
- Inform the couple when the test results will be available.
- Permit the couple to express concerns and questions about the test and possible results.
- Encourage the couple to seek genetic counseling if appropriate.

Antistreptolysin O (ASO) (serum)

Reference Values

Upper limit of normal varies with age, season, and geographic area.
Adult: Less than 100 international unit/mL; less than 160 Todd unit/mL.

Child: *Newborn:* Similar to mother's. *Two to 5 Years:* Less than 100 international unit/mL. *Twelve to 19 Years:* Less than 200 international unit/mL; less than 200 Todd unit/mL.

Description

The beta-hemolytic streptococcus secretes an enzyme known as streptolysin O, which is capable of lysing red blood cells (RBCs). Streptolysin O acts as an antigen and stimulates the immune system to develop antistreptolysin O (ASO) antibodies. A high titer of ASO indicates that

A

streptococci are present and may cause rheumatic fever or acute glomerulonephritis. Increased serum ASO levels can also indicate a recent streptococcal infection.

The ASO antibodies appear approximately 1–2 weeks after an acute streptococcal infection, peak 3–4 weeks after onset, and could remain elevated for months. Many school-aged children have a higher ASO titer level than do preschool children or adults.

Other streptococcal antigens are antideoxyribonuclease (ADNase—titer greater than 10) and antistreptococcal hyaluronidase (ASH—titer greater than 128).

Purposes

- To identify clients who are susceptible to specific autoimmune disorders (e.g., collagen disease).
- To aid in determining the effect of the beta-hemolytic streptococcus in secreting the enzyme streptolysin O.

Clinical Problems

Decreased Level: *Drug Influence:* Antibiotics.

Increased Level: Acute rheumatic fever, acute glomerulonephritis, streptococcal upper respiratory infections, rheumatoid arthritis (mildly elevated), hyperglobulinemia with liver disease, collagen disease (mildly elevated).

Procedure

- There is no food or fluid restriction.
- Collect 3–5 mL of venous blood in a red-top tube. Avoid hemolysis.
- Repeated ASO testing (once or twice a week) is advisable to determine the highest level of increase.

Factors Affecting Laboratory Results

- Antibiotic therapy decreases the antibody response.
- An increased level may occur in healthy persons (carriers).

NURSING IMPLICATIONS WITH RATIONALE

- Note that antibiotic therapy could decrease antibody response.

Increased Level

- Check serum ASO levels when the client is complaining of joint pain in the extremities. A highly elevated level could be indicative of acute rheumatic fever, and a slight elevation could be indicative of rheumatoid arthritis.
- Check the urinary output when the serum ASO is elevated. A urinary output of less than 600 mL/24 hours may be associated with acute glomerulonephritis.

Client Teaching

- Instruct the client and family that when the client has a sore throat he or she should have a throat culture taken to check for beta-hemolytic streptococcus. A throat culture might need to be repeated if the sore throat persists.

A

Antithrombin III (plasma)
AT 3, AT-III, Factor Xa Inhibitor

Reference Values

75–135% of normal/average.

Description

Antithrombin III (AT-III) is suggested to evaluate clients who have a hypercoagulable state, and especially for clients with a history of thromboembolic disease. Some clients have a genetic deficiency of AT-III, thus this predisposes the client to thrombus formation. Also, clients who are deficient in AT-III may be resistant to heparin and would require a larger dose of an anticoagulant. Usually heparin resistance does not occur unless the AT-III is less than 60%. Elevated AT-III levels may occur in clients with acute hepatitis and a deficiency in vitamin K.

Purposes

- To test for genetic deficiency of AT-III.
- To determine the effect of drugs on AT-III.

Clinical Problems

Decreased Level: Disseminated intravascular coagulation (DIC), cirrhosis, hereditary deficiency of AT-III, thrombophlebitis, chronic liver failure, pulmonary embolism, acute MI, malignancy. *Drug Influence:* Heparin, oral contraceptives, L-asparaginase.

Increased Level: Acute hepatitis, vitamin K deficiency, kidney transplant, hyperglobulinemia, *Drug Influence:* Coumarin-type anticoagulation.

Procedure

- There is no food or fluid restriction.
- Collect venous blood in a blue-top tube. A red-top tube might be used; check first.
- Send blood specimen immediately to the laboratory.
- Avoid giving heparin therapy for 2 days prior to the test.

Factors Affecting Laboratory Results

- Drugs listed under *Drug Influence* could affect test results.
- Not delivering the specimen to the laboratory immediately.

NURSING IMPLICATIONS WITH RATIONALE

- Obtain a genetic history of AT-III deficiency.
- Record the drugs the client has been taking. Heparin and oral contraceptives may affect test results. Foods that are low in vitamin K could elevate AT-III level.
- Monitor vital signs.

> **Client Teaching**
> - Inform the client not to take heparin 2 days before the test. This may cause the client to have a low AT-III level.

Apolipoproteins (Apo) (plasma)

Apolipoprotein A-1 (Apo A-1), Apolipoprotein B (Apo B), Apolipoprotein E (Apo E), Lipoprotein(a) (Lp(a))

Reference Values

Apo A-1:

Young Adult: Male: 80–155 mg/dL; 0.80–1.55 g/L (SI units)
　　Female: 80–186 mg/dL; 0.80–1.86 g/L (SI units)
Middle-Age Adult: Male: 100–165 mg/dL; 1–1.65 g/L (SI units)
　　Female: 93–200 mg/dL; 0.93–2 g/L (SI units)
Elderly: Male: 85–166 mg/dL; 0.85–1.66 g/L (SI units)
　　Female: 120–215 mg/dL; 1.2–2.15 g/L (SI units)
Child: Male: 67–150 mg/dL; 0.67–1.50 g/L (SI units)
　　Female: 60–150 mg/dL; 0.60–1.50 g/L (SI units)
Adolescent: Male: 88–148 mg/dL; 0.88–1.48 g/L (SI units)
　　Female: 83–150 mg/dL; 0.83–1.50 g/L (SI units)

Apo B:

Adult/elderly: Male: 50–170 mg/dL; 0.50–1.70 g/L (SI units)
　　Female: 46–155 mg/dL; 0.46–1.55 g/L (SI units)
5–17 years old: Male: 46–139 mg/dL; 0.46–1.39 g/L (SI units)
　　Female: 41–96 mg/dL; 0.41–0.96 g/L (SI units)
Newborn–1 year old: 11–31 mg/dL; 0.11–0.31 g/L (SI units)

Ratio, Apo A-1/Apo B:

Male: 0.82:2.20
Female: 0.92:3.20

Apo E-4:

Allele is not present.

Lipoprotein(a) (Lp(a)):

Male: Caucasian: 2.2–49 mg/dL
　　African American: 4.6–72 mg/dL
Female: Caucasian: 2–57 mg/dL
　　African American: 4.5–75 mg/dL

A

Description

Apolipoproteins are protein components of lipoproteins. The apolipoproteins are used to determine risks of atherogenic disease.

Apolipoprotein A-1 (Apo A-1) is the major component (90%) of high-density lipoprotein (HDL). As HDL increases, Apo A-1 will also increase. Apo A-1 helps to transport peripheral cholesterol to the liver for excretion. It is the "good" apolipoprotein that does not contribute to coronary artery disease (CAD) or stroke.

Apolipoprotein B (Apo B) is the major component of low-density lipoprotein (LDL) composing about 75% of the protein. Apo B exists in two forms, Apo B-100 and Apo B-48. Apo B-100 also has very low-density lipoproteins (VLDL), as well as LDL. Apo B-100 is produced in the liver, and Apo B-48 is produced in the small intestine. Apo B-100 is a better indicator of coronary artery disease than LDL. The reference values for African Americans for apolipoproteins may be 5–10% higher than for Caucasians. Also a ratio of Apo A-1 and Apo B is thought to identify atherosclerosis.

Apo B-48, the second form of Apo B, is of intestinal origin and found in chylomicrons. Apo B-48 transports lipids that have been digested in the intestines to the bloodstream.

Ratio of Apo A-1 to Apo B is thought to be more useful in identifying atherosclerotic heart disease than only LDL and VLDL. A decrease in Apo A-1 and an increase in Apo B-100 suggest an increased risk of coronary artery disease.

Apolipoprotein E (Apo E) has a role in the clearance of Apo B containing lipoproteins, including VLDL and chylomicrons. A deficit in Apo E usually produces an increase in Apo B lipoproteins. Apo E has 3 alleles: E-2, E-3, and E-4. It has been stated that E-4 contributes to coronary artery disease and Alzheimer disease. There has been some evidence that Apo E-4 allele is associated with a development of plaques, neurofibrillary tangles, and loss of brain tissue volume, which is associated with Alzheimer disease.

Lipoprotein(a) [Lp(a)] is another lipoprotein referred to as little "a" lipoprotein. The two polypeptide components of Lp(a) are Apo A-1 (dissolves fibrin clots) and Apo B-100. An increase in Lp(a) inhibits fibrin in microthrombi, thus causing atherosclerotic damage to the arterial walls. Increased levels of Lp(a) usually occurs with familial hypercholesterolemia and renal failure and in women with a decrease in estrogen levels.

Purposes

- To aid in the diagnosis of coronary artery disease.
- To identify the presence of atherosclerotic disease.

Clinical Problems

Apo A-1

Decreased Level: Coronary artery disease, ischemic coronary artery disease, MI, stroke, renal disease, chronic renal failure, nephrotic syndrome, hepatocellular disorders, smoking. *Drug Influence:* Androgens, beta-adrenergic blockers, diuretics, progestins, and synthroid.

Increased Level: Familial hyperalphalipoproteinemia. *Drug Influence:* Anticonvulsants, estrogen, hormonal replacement therapy, statin drugs, niacin, furosemide (Lasix), ethyl alcohol. *Others:* Weight reduction.

Apo B

Decreased Level: Chronic anemia, Tangier disease (alpha lipoprotein deficiency), joint inflammation, chronic pulmonary disease, Reye syndrome, malnutrition. *Others:* Weight reduction. *Drug Influence:* Synthroid, captopril, niacin, statin drugs.

Increased Level: Coronary artery disease, hyperlipoproteinemia, diabetes mellitus, MI, Cushing syndrome, familial lipidemia, nephronic syndrome, pregnancy, hepatic disease. *Drug Influence:* Beta-adrenergic blockers, corticosteroids, oral contraceptives, alcohol abuse, androgens.

Apo E-4

Increased Level: Coronary artery disease, Alzheimer disease.

Lp(a)

Decreased Level: Chronic hepatocellular disease, malnutrition.

Increased Level: Coronary artery disease, diabetes mellitus, familial hypercholesterolemia, estrogen deficit, chronic renal failure.

Procedure

- Restrict food and fluids for 12 hours before the test.
- Collect 7 mL of venous blood in a red- or lavender-top tube.
- A ratio of Apo A-1 to Apo B-100 may be ordered to predict coronary artery disease.
- Avoid smoking 1 to 3 days prior to test or check with the doctor or health facility.

Factors Affecting Laboratory Results

- Smoking may decrease Apo levels.
- Food ingested before test.
- Drugs (*see drugs that decrease or increase levels in Clinical Problems section*).
- Acute illness can increase Apo B levels.
- Diet high in fat and carbohydrates (CHO) can increase Apo B levels.

NURSING IMPLICATIONS WITH RATIONALE

- Obtain a history of client's health problems.
- Relate apolipoprotein levels with cholesterol HDL and LDL.
- List drugs client is taking that may affect test results.

Client Teaching

- Explain to the client not to eat 12 hours before test. Fluid (water) and medications are not restricted unless indicated by the health care provider.
- Encourage overweight clients with increased Apo B to reduce weight. A nutritionist may be suggested.
- Instruct client to decrease foods high in saturated fats and cholesterol.
- Encourage client to exercise if approved by the health care provider. Exercise aids with increasing the HDL.
- Explain that high alcohol consumption can affect test results.
- Encourage client to stop or decrease smoking, which can affect test results.

A

Arsenic (AS) (hair, toenails, serum, blood, urine)

Reference Values

Hair: *Normal Levels*: <1 mcg/g, 20–60 mcg/100 g, <8.7 nmol/g (SI units). *Chronic Poisoning*: >80 mcg/100g, >13 nmol/g (SI units).

Toenails: *Normal Levels*: 20–60 mcg/100g, <8.7 nmol/g (SI units). *Chronic Poisoning*: 80–180 mcg/100g, 12–24 nmol/g (SI units).

Serum: *Normal Level*: 5 mcg/mL or 0.07 μmol/L.

Blood: *Normal Level*: 2–23 mcg/L, 0.03–0.31 μmol/L (SI units). *Chronic Poisoning*: 100–500 mcg/L, 1.33–6.65 μmol/L (SI units). *Acute Poisoning*: >600 mcg/L, >8 μmol/L (SI units).

Urine: *Normal Level*: 5–50 mcg/24 h, 0.07–0.67 μmol/24 h (SI units). *Chronic Poisoning*: 50–5,000 mcg/L, 0.67–66.5 μmol/L (SI units). *Acute Poisoning*: 1,000–20,000 mcg/L, >13.3–2,666 μmol/L (SI units).

Description

Arsenic is an element found in all human tissue. It can occur during occupational exposure to paints, pesticides, herbicides, and ceramics and in environmental exposure, such as to coal burning and treated wood. However, accidental and intentional poisoning are the main causes of arsenic poisoning. Chronic exposure to arsenic can be detected in keratin, including in specimens of hair and nails (especially toenails). Chronic ingestion is associated with skin, lung, kidney, and liver damage. Chronic symptoms can include metallic taste, thrombocytopenia, leukopenia, gastrointestinal symptoms, hepatomegaly, and peripheral neuropathy.

Blood specimens are taken to determine arsenic blood levels when acute arsenic poisoning is suspected. Symptoms of acute poisoning may include abdominal pain, nausea and vomiting, bloody diarrhea, dehydration, jaundice, hypoxia, renal failure, and cardiopulmonary collapse.

Urine specimens are ordered for a fast decision of acute arsenic poisoning. Sixty-two percent of arsenic is excreted by the kidneys. Lethal dose is considered 5–50mg/kg.

Purpose

- To determine the presence of acute or chronic arsenic poisoning.

Clinical Problems

Increased Level: Accidental or intentional arsenic poisoning, occupational and environmental exposure.

Procedure

Serum and Blood:

- There is no food or fluid restriction. Client should decrease seafood intake several days before test.
- Collect 7 mL of venous blood in a red-top tube (serum collection).
- Collect 7 mL of venous blood in a green-top tube or black-top tube (blood collection).

A

Hair and Nails:

- Obtain a clip of hair or nails (preferably toenails) and place sample in a nonmetal container.

Urine:

- Collect a 24-hour urine sample in a 2–3 liter container. The container should be refrigerated.
- Discard the first morning urine specimen and collect urine in the container for 24 hours.
- List on the laboratory slip and container the client's age, date, and the exact times of urine collection (e.g., 5/10/16, 7 AM to 5/11/16, 7:03 AM).
- Avoid getting feces and toilet paper in the urine.

Factors Affecting Laboratory Results

- A diet rich in seafood prior to the test could elevate test results.

Nursing Implications with Rationale

- Obtain a history of client's contact with arsenic. This could be from an occupational or environmental exposure. If the client cannot respond, ask a person present with the client. If it is intentional arsenic poisoning, law authority should be notified.
- Check for symptoms of acute arsenic poisoning (*see Description*). Emergency treatment may be necessary.
- Collect the specimens to test for arsenic poisoning and send to the laboratory.

Client Teaching

- Explain to the client and family member(s) that it is not uncommon to have an arsenic level within normal range. The cause for the increased arsenic level should be recognized and eliminated.
- Be supportive to the client and family.

Arterial blood gases (ABGs) (arterial blood)*

Blood Gases; Acid-Base Balance and Imbalance

Reference Values

Adult: pH: 7.35–7.45; $PaCO_2$: 35–45 mm Hg; PaO_2: 75–100 mm Hg; SaO_2: Greater than 95%; SvO_2: Greater than 70%; HCO_3: 24–28 mEq/L; base excesses (BE): + 2 to –2 mEq/L.

Child: pH: 7.36–7.44. Other measurements are same as adult.

Description

Arterial blood gases (ABGs) are usually ordered to assess disturbances of acid–base (A–B) balance caused by a respiratory disorder and/or a metabolic disorder. The basic components of ABGs include the pH, $PaCO_2$, PaO_2, SO_2, HCO_3, and BE. ABGs are a diagnostic tool that reflects the client's oxygenation, ventilation, and acid–base balance.

pH: The pH, the negative logarithm of the hydrogen ion concentration, determines the acidity or alkalinity of body fluids. A pH less than 7.35 indicates acidosis, either respiratory acidosis or metabolic acidosis. A pH greater than 7.45 indicates alkalosis, either respiratory or metabolic alkalosis.

---

*Updated by Ellen K. Boyda, RN, MSN, CRNP-BC, at Widener University, Pennsylvania.

A

PaCO₂: The partial pressure of carbon dioxide ($PaCO_2$) reflects the adequacy of alveolar ventilation. When there is alveolar damage, carbon dioxide (CO_2) cannot escape. Carbon dioxide combines with water to form carbonic acid ($H_2O + CO_2 = H_2CO_3$), causing an acidotic state. When the client has alveolar hypoventilation, the $PaCO_2$ is elevated and respiratory acidosis results. Chronic obstructive pulmonary disease is a major cause of respiratory acidosis. When the client has alveolar hyperventilation (blowing off CO_2 by rapid deep breathing), the $PaCO_2$ is decreased and respiratory alkalosis results.

PaO₂: The partial pressure of oxygen (PaO_2) determines the amount of oxygen available to bind with hemoglobin. The pH affects the combining power of oxygen and hemoglobin, and with a low pH, there will be less oxygen in the hemoglobin. The PaO_2 is decreased in respiratory diseases, such as emphysema, pneumonia, and pulmonary edema; in the presence of abnormal hemoglobin (CO Hb, Meth Hb, Sulfa Hb); and in polycythemia.

SO₂: The oxygen saturation (SO_2) is the percentage of oxygen in the blood that combines with hemoglobin. It is measured indirectly by calculation of the PaO_2 and pH or measured directly by co-oximetry. The combination of oxygen saturation, partial pressure of oxygen, and hemoglobin indicates tissue oxygenation.

HCO₃ and BE: Bicarbonate ion (HCO_3) is an alkaline substance that comprises over half of the total buffer base in the blood. When there is a deficit of bicarbonate and other bases or an increase in nonvolatile acid, such as lactic acid, metabolic acidosis occurs. If a bicarbonate excess is present, then metabolic alkalosis results. The bicarbonate plays a very important role in maintaining a pH of 7.35–7.45 on an ongoing basis and also in compensation for an acidotic or alkalotic state. The base excess value is frequently checked with the HCO_3 value. A base excess of less than –2 is acidosis and greater than +2 is alkalosis.

Acid–Base Imbalances: To determine the type of A–B imbalance, the pH, $PaCO_2$, HCO_3, and BE are checked. The $PaCO_2$ is a respiratory determinant, and the HCO_3 and BE are metabolic determinants. The $PaCO_2$, HCO_3, and BE values are compared to the pH. A pH of less than 7.35 is acidosis and one of greater than 7.45 is alkalosis.

ABG Chart

THE ARTERIAL BLOOD GASES (ABG) CHART NOTES THE VALUES ASSOCIATED WITH ACIDOSIS AND ALKALOSIS		
Acidosis		Alkalosis
<7.35	pH	>7.45
>45pCO₂	(Respiratory)	<35pCO₂
<24 HCO₃	(Metabolic)	>28 HCO₃

1. If the pH is less than 7.35, the $PaCO_2$ is greater than 45 mm Hg, and the HCO_3 and BE are normal, the A–B imbalance is respiratory acidosis.
2. If the pH is greater than 7.45, the $PaCO_2$ is less than 35 mm Hg, and the HCO_3 and BE are normal, the A–B imbalance is respiratory alkalosis.
3. If the pH is less than 7.35, the $PaCO_2$ is normal, the HCO_3 and BE are less than 24 mEq/L and less than –2, the A–B imbalance is metabolic acidosis.

A

4. If the pH is greater than 7.45, the $PaCO_2$ is normal, the HCO_3 and BE are greater than 28 mEq/L and greater than $+2$, the A–B imbalance is metabolic alkalosis.

ACID–BASE (A–B) IMBALANCE	PH	PACO$_2$	HCO$_3$	BE
Respiratory acidosis	↓	↑	N	N
Respiratory alkalosis	↑	↓	N	N
Metabolic acidosis	↓	N	↓	↓
Metabolic alkalosis	↑	N	↑	↑

Purposes

- To detect metabolic acidosis or alkalosis or respiratory acidosis or alkalosis.
- To monitor blood gases during an acute illness and evaluate need for medical intervention.

Clinical Problems

Respiratory Acidosis (pH less than 7.35; $PaCO_2$ greater than 45 mm Hg): Chronic obstructive lung disease (emphysema, chronic bronchitis, severe asthma), acute respiratory distress syndrome (ARDS), obesity, drug overdose, Guillain-Barré syndrome, severe head injury, anesthesia, pneumonia, severe sleep apnea. *Drug Influence:* Narcotics, sedatives.

Respiratory Alkalosis (pH greater than 7.45; $PaCO_2$ less than 35 mm Hg): Salicylate toxicity (early phase), anxiety, hysteria, tetany, strenuous exercise (swimming, running), fever, hyperthyroidism, delirium tremens, pulmonary embolism, pregnancy.

Metabolic Acidosis (pH less than 7.35; HCO_3 less than 24 mEq/L): Diabetic ketoacidosis, severe diarrhea, starvation/malnutrition, shock, burns, kidney failure, acute myocardial infarction.

Metabolic Alkalosis (pH greater than 7.45; HCO_3 greater than 28 mEq/L): Severe vomiting, gastric suction, peptic ulcer, potassium loss (as in diuretic therapy), excess administration of bicarbonate, hepatic failure, cystic fibrosis. *Drug Influence:* Sodium bicarbonate, sodium oxalate, potassium oxalate.

Procedure

- There is no food or fluid restriction.
- If the client is receiving anticoagulant therapy or taking aspirin or has a clotting problem, the laboratory, nurse, or pulmonary technician drawing the blood should be notified.
- Collect 1–5 mL of arterial blood in a heparinized needle and syringe, remove the needle, make sure there is no air in the syringe, and apply an airtight cap over the tip of the syringe.
- Place the syringe with arterial blood in an ice-water bag (to minimize the metabolic activity of the sample) and deliver it immediately to the laboratory. Ice water is colder than ice.
- Inject plain lidocaine 1% at the site as an intervention to significantly reduce pain.
- Indicate on the laboratory slip whether the client is receiving oxygen and the flow rate, type of O_2 administration device (e.g., cannula, mask), and the client's current temperature.
- Apply pressure to the puncture site for 5 minutes, longer for persons on anticoagulants or streptokinase therapy.

A

Future Developments

Research has shown that venous pH and HCO_3 values show an excellent correlation with arterial values. While there is insufficient agreement for the correlation between venous and arterial CO_2 in determining chronic hypercarbia, soon it may be beneficial to obtain a venous blood gas (VBG). Currently, in the critically ill client, respiratory acidosis can be accurately identified using VBG sampling, reducing the need for arterial sampling in early assessment. Since arterial blood gases are the most painful lab procedure performed, being able to obtain the same information by venous blood gases is advantageous.

Factors Affecting Laboratory Results

- Improper handling of the blood sample, such as not using ice water, exposure of specimen to air, and not expelling all the heparin out of the collection syringe, causes inaccurate results.
- Hemolysis of the blood sample causes false results.
- Narcotics and sedatives can contribute to the respiratory acidotic state, and sodium bicarbonate could cause metabolic alkalosis.
- Inaccurate results can occur as a result of suctioning, changes in O_2 therapy, and ventilator use; exposure to carbon monoxide or nitrate; and blood transfusion.

NURSING IMPLICATIONS WITH RATIONALE

- First, the nurse must make an acid–base diagnosis.

Step 1: Examine the pH. A pH of less than 7.35 indicates an acidosis and a pH of greater than 7.45 indicates an alkalosis.

Step 2: Compare $PaCO_2$ level to the pH. If the pH is less than 7.35 and the $PaCO_2$ is greater than 45, the client is in respiratory acidosis. However, if the pH is greater than 7.45 and the $PaCO_2$ is less than 35, the client is in respiratory alkalosis.

Step 3: Compare the HCO_3 and the pH level. If the pH is less than 7.35 and the HCO_3 is less than 24, the client is in metabolic acidosis. However, if the pH is greater than 7.45 and the HCO_3 is greater than 28, the client is in metabolic alkalosis.

Step 4: Evaluate the signs of compensation. An example: <7.35 pH; >45 $PaCO_2$; >28 HCO_3; > +2 BE, the client is in respiratory acidosis with metabolic compensation.

Respiratory Acidosis

- Assess for signs and symptoms of respiratory acidosis, such as dyspnea, headache, disorientation, and increased $PaCO_2$ (greater than 45 mm Hg).
- Perform chest clapping to break up bronchial and alveolar secretions when applicable. Carbon dioxide can be trapped in the lungs because of excess secretions and mucous plugs.

- Administer oxygen at a low concentration (2–3 L/min) when emphysema is present.
- Check for metabolic compensatory mechanism with respiratory acidosis—HCO_3 would be elevated, greater than 28 mEq/L.

Client Teaching

- Teach the client breathing exercises to enhance CO_2 excretion from the lungs, especially diaphragmatic breathing.
- Instruct the client on how to properly use the incentive spirometer device or mini-nebulizer if ordered.
- Demonstrate the postural drainage procedure, if not contraindicated, by lowering the head of the bed or having the client lie over the side of the bed. Secretions are mobilized and excreted by gravity.

Respiratory Alkalosis

- Relate a low $PaCO_2$ value to clinical problems associated with tachypnea (rapid respiratory rate). Anxiety, hysteria, nervousness, and strenuous physical exertion can cause tachypnea. With rapid breathing, an excess of CO_2 is lost.
- Assess for signs and symptoms of respiratory alkalosis, such as tachypnea, dizziness, tingling of fingers, tetany spasms, and a $PaCO_2$ less than 35 mm Hg.
- Adjustments may need to be made if the client is receiving mechanical ventilation.

Client Teaching

- Instruct the client to breathe slowly and deeply. Breathing into a paper bag will help to decrease hyperventilation.

Metabolic Acidosis

- Relate decreased values of HCO_3 and BE to metabolic acidosis. When there is tissue breakdown from shock, malnutrition, and such, acid metabolites (e.g., lactic acid) are released. Another cause of metabolic acidosis is the presence of ketone bodies (fatty acid) from diabetic ketoacidosis.
- Assess for signs and symptoms of metabolic acidosis, such as rapid, vigorous breathing (Kussmaul breathing), flushed skin, restlessness, confusion, decreased bicarbonate (HCO_3) value of less than 24 mEq/L, and decreased BE less than –2.
- Check for respiratory compensatory mechanism with metabolic acidosis: $PaCO_2$ would be less than 35 mm Hg. The lung compensates by blowing off CO_2 through hyperventilation (Kussmaul respirations) to decrease carbonic acid in the blood and thereby decrease the acidotic state.

Metabolic Alkalosis

- Relate elevated HCO_3 and BE values to metabolic alkalosis. With severe vomiting and gastric suction, hydrogen and chloride (hydrochloric acid) are lost, causing an alkalotic state. Drugs containing sodium bicarbonate taken in excess or over a long period of time could cause metabolic alkalosis.

A

- Assess for signs and symptoms of metabolic alkalosis, such as shallow breathing, vomiting, elevated HCO_3 value of greater than 28 mEq/L, and elevated BE value of greater than $+2$.
- Stop nasogastric drainage or decrease amount of vomiting as necessary.

Client Teaching

- Instruct the client not to ingest large quantities of antacids containing base substances like bicarbonate. An alkalotic state could result.

Ascorbic acid (vitamin C) (plasma and serum)

Reference Values

Adult: 0.6–2 mg/dL (plasma), 34–114 μmol/L (SI units, plasma), 0.2–2 mg/dL (serum), 12–114 μmol/L (SI units, serum).

Child: 0.6–1.6 mg/dL (plasma).

Description

(*See Ascorbic Acid Tolerance.*)

Ascorbic acid (vitamin C) is a water-soluble vitamin found in fresh fruits and vegetables. Deficiencies of vitamin C still occur, but the severe deficiency known as scurvy is rare.

Vitamin C is important for the formation of collagen substances and certain amino acids, for wound healing, and for withstanding the stresses of injury and infection. Because vitamin C is vitally important to the body's defense mechanisms in dealing with stress caused by injury and disease, the client's ascorbic acid level should be known. This test can also be used to determine whether the ascorbic acid therapy is adequate. Excess ingestion of vitamin C is not considered toxic, as is excess ingestion of vitamins A and D (fat-soluble vitamins), because excess vitamin C is water-soluble and is excreted in the urine.

Purpose

- To determine if the ascorbic acid therapy is adequate.

Clinical Problems

Decreased Level (less than 0.6 mg/dL): Scurvy, low vitamin C diet, malabsorption, pregnancy, infections, cancer, severe burns.

Increased Level: Excess vitamin C ingestion. *Causes of False-Positive Readings:* Clinitest, serum creatinine, serum uric acid, serum bilirubin, serum ALT and AST, blood glucose, serum cholesterol. *Causes of False-Negative Readings:* Test for occult blood in stool, serum triglycerides.

Procedure

- There is no food or fluid restriction.
- Collect 5–7 mL of venous blood in a gray-top tube (plasma) or a red-top tube (serum).

Factors Affecting Laboratory Results

- High doses of ascorbic acid can cause inaccurate results.

A

NURSING IMPLICATIONS WITH RATIONALE

- Recognize the functions of ascorbic acid in maintaining the state of wellness. Ascorbic acid has been taken by persons in large doses (greater than 1 g) to prevent colds. This has not been medically proven effective.
- Answer the client's questions concerning the importance of vitamin C. It helps with the healing process.

Decreased Level

- Relate vitamin C deficit to certain clinical problems (e.g., infections, burns). Vitamin C is lost during severe infections and burns.

Client Teaching

- Encourage the client to eat foods rich in vitamin C (e.g., oranges, grapefruits, strawberries, cantaloupe, pineapple, broccoli, cabbage, spinach, kale, turnips—all excellent to good sources). Approximately 25% of the population has an ascorbic acid deficit in the body.

Increased Level

- Record on the client's chart habitual use of high doses of vitamin C. High doses of ascorbic acid can cause false-positive laboratory results.

Ascorbic acid tolerance (plasma and urine)

Vitamin C Tolerance

Reference Values

Adult: *Plasma:* Greater than 2 mg/dL. *Urine:* 4-, 5-, or 6-hour sample. *Oral:* 10% of administered amount. IV: 30–40% of administered amount.

Child: Not usually done.

Description

The ascorbic acid tolerance test is useful for determining the degree of ascorbic acid deficiency. Clients having severe burns, infections, or malignancy frequently have an ascorbic acid deficiency even when they are receiving vitamin C or have a diet adequate in vitamin C. With an ascorbic acid deficit, wound healing and recovery are prolonged.

The blood and urine tests are normally done together.

Purpose

- To detect vitamin C deficiency.

Clinical Problems

Decreased Level: Infections, burns, cancer.

Increased Level: Excess vitamin C administration.

A

Procedure

- Foods high in ascorbic acid (e.g., fruits and vegetables) should be omitted for 24 hours before the test. Water can be given.
- Have the client void and discard the urine before beginning the test.
- Administer ascorbic acid orally (11 mg/kg of body weight in a glass of water) or intravenously (10 mg/kg of body weight in saline solution).
- Collect 7 mL of venous blood in a gray-top tube 4–6 hours after the ascorbic acid is administered.
- Collect a 4-, 5-, or 6-hour urine specimen in a bottle containing acetic acid. The bottle should be kept on ice or refrigerated and taken to the laboratory immediately at the end of the specified time.

Factors Affecting Laboratory Results

- Oral high-potency vitamin supplements cause false test results.
- Ascorbic acid in IV fluids cause false test results.
- Inaccurate urine collection time and inaccurate labeling result in false test results.

NURSING IMPLICATIONS WITH RATIONALE

- Explain to the client that the purpose of the test is to determine whether there is a vitamin C deficiency in the body.
- Explain to the client that for 24 hours he or she should not eat foods high in ascorbic acid (e.g., oranges or orange juice, grapefruit, strawberries, or green vegetables). Drinking water is permissible.
- Have the client void and discard the urine.
- Administer ascorbic acid orally or intravenously according to body weight.
- Instruct the client that all urine should be saved for 4, 5, or 6 hours (according to the order or laboratory policy) in a bottle kept on ice or refrigerated. Following collection time, the urine specimen should be taken immediately to the laboratory.
- Explain to the client that blood will be drawn 4–6 hours after the ascorbic acid is administered.
- Post the time for urine collection on the chart or Kardex or by the bedside. Visitors should not discard the client's urine.

Aspartate aminotransferase (AST) (serum)
Serum Glutamic Oxaloacetic Transaminase (SGOT)

Reference Values

Adult: *Average Range:* 8–35 unit/L; 5–40 unit/mL (Frankel), 4–36 international unit/L; 15–50 unit/mL (Karmen), 8–33 unit/L at 37°C (SI units). Female values may be slightly lower than those of males. Exercise tends to increase values (values can vary among institutions).

Child: *Newborn:* Four times the normal level. *Child:* Similar to adults. *Elderly:* Slightly higher than adults.

A

Description

Aspartate aminotransferase/serum glutamic oxaloacetic transaminase (AST/SGOT) is an enzyme found mainly in the heart muscle and liver, with moderate amounts in skeletal muscle, the kidneys, and the pancreas. Its concentration is low in the blood except when there is cellular injury, and then large amounts are released into circulation.

High levels of serum AST are found following an acute MI (myocardial infarction) and liver damage. Six to 10 hours after an acute MI, AST leaks out of the heart muscle and reaches its peak in 24–48 hours after the infarction. The serum AST level returns to normal 4–6 days later if there is no additional infarction. Serum AST is usually compared with other cardiac enzymes (creatine kinase [CK], lactate dehydrogenase [LDH], troponins).

In liver disease, the serum level increases by 10 times or more and remains elevated for a longer period of time. Serum levels of AST and ALT are frequently compared.

Purposes

- To detect an elevation of serum AST, an enzyme found mainly in the heart muscle and liver that increases during an acute MI and liver damage.
- To compare AST results with CK, LDH, and troponins for diagnosing an acute MI.

Clinical Problems

Decreased Level: Pregnancy, diabetic ketoacidosis, chronic hemodialysis. *Drug Influence:* Salicylates.

Increased Level: Acute MI, hepatitis, liver necrosis, musculoskeletal diseases and trauma, acute pancreatitis, cancer of the liver, severe angina pectoris, strenuous exercise, IM injections. *Drug Influence:* Antibiotics (ampicillin, carbenicillin, clindamycin, cloxacillin, erythromycin, gentamicin, lincomycin, nafcillin, oxacillin, polycillin, tetracycline), vitamins (folic acid, pyridoxine, vitamin A), narcotics (codeine, morphine, meperidine [Demerol]), antihypertensives (methyldopa [Aldomet], guanethidine), mithramycin, digitalis preparation, cortisone, flurazepam (Dalmane), indomethacin (Indocin), isoniazid (INH), rifampin, oral contraceptives, salicylates, theophylline.

Procedure

- There is no food or fluid restriction.
- Collect 3–5 mL of venous blood in a red-top tube. Avoid hemolysis.
- Draw blood before drugs are given. The refrigerated enzyme will remain stable for 4 days.
- List on the laboratory slip drugs the client is taking that can cause false-positive levels, with the date and time last given.

Factors Affecting Laboratory Results

- IM injections could increase serum AST levels.
- Hemolysis of the blood specimen could affect laboratory results.
- Drugs increasing the serum AST level (*see Drug Influence*) could affect test results.
- Salicylates may cause false-positive or negative serum levels.

A

NURSING IMPLICATIONS WITH RATIONALE

Increased Level

- Hold drugs causing an elevated serum AST level for 24 hours prior to the blood test, with the physician's or health care provider's permission. Drugs that should not be withheld should be listed on the laboratory slip and charted.
- Compare serum AST levels with other cardiac enzyme results. Check serum ALT levels to determine if liver damage could be responsible for the abnormal value.
- Do not administer IM injections before the blood test; IM injections can increase the serum AST level. Few medications (e.g., morphine) can be given intravenously without affecting the serum level.
- Assess the client for signs and symptoms of MI (e.g., chest and arm pain, dyspnea, or diaphoresis). Changes should be reported and charted.
- Listen to the client's concerns. Answer questions or refer to appropriate health professionals.

Client Teaching

- Instruct the client to report symptoms of chest and arm pain, nausea, or diaphoresis immediately—day or night.

Aspirin

See Salicylate

Atrial natriuretic factor (ANF)

See Atrial Natriuretic Peptide (ANP)

Atrial natriuretic peptide (ANP) (plasma)

Atrial Natriuretic Factor (ANF), Atrionatriuretic Peptides

Reference Values

20–77 pg/mL; 20–77 ng/L (SI units).

Description

Atrial natriuretic peptide (ANP) is secreted from the atria of the heart and acts as an antagonist to renin and aldosterone. It is released during expansion of the atrium, produces vasodilation, and increases glomerular filtration rate. It counteracts the renin-angiotensin system by inhibiting the action of angiotensin II, thus promoting a decrease in blood pressure. ANP reduces renal reabsorption of sodium, blocks renin release by the kidney, and blocks aldosterone secretion from the adrenal glands, and thus has an antihypertensive effect. With the physiologic effects of ANP, preload, afterload, and blood volume are reduced. An elevated ANP level can be used as a diagnostic tool to detect cardiovascular disease, early asymptomatic left ventricular disorder, and HF (heart failure). However, with chronic-level HF, the ANP is decreased, whereas with acute HF, the ANP level is elevated.

Purposes

- To detect an elevated ANP level.
- To confirm cardiovascular disease, particularly HF.

Clinical Problems

Decreased Level: Chronic heart failure. *Drug Influence:* Prazosin, urapidil.

Increased Level: Acute HF, paroxysmal atrial tachycardia, early cardiovascular disease, subarachnoid hemorrhage.

Procedure

- The client should be NPO for 8–12 hours prior to the test.
- Withhold cardiac drugs, such as beta blockers, calcium blockers, diuretics, vasodilators, and digoxin, until after the blood sample has been taken. Some health care providers want these drugs withheld for 24 hours.
- Collect 5 mL of venous blood in a lavender-top tube. Ice the tube and send it immediately to the laboratory.

Factors Affecting Laboratory Results

- Cardiac drugs (*see Procedure*).
- Improper care of the blood sample.

NURSING IMPLICATIONS WITH RATIONALE

- Obtain a health and drug history from the client. List drugs that the client is currently taking. Certain cardiac drugs should be withheld until after the test because they could affect the ANP level, causing an inaccurate lab result (*see Procedure*).
- Take vital signs. Compare findings to baseline readings.
- Answer the client's questions. Be supportive of the client.

Client Teaching

- Instruct the client to keep health care appointments.
- Instruct the client to notify his or her health care provider if difficulty in breathing, shortness of breath, chest pain, and/or indigestion occurs.

Barbiturate (blood)

Reference Values

Adult:

BARBITURATE	ACTION	THERAPEUTIC	TOXIC
Secobarbital (Seconal)	Short acting	1–5 mcg/mL	greater than 8 mcg/mL
Pentobarbital (Nembutal)	Short acting	1–5 mcg/mL	greater than 8 mcg/mL
Amobarbital (Amytal)	Intermediate acting	5–14 mcg/mL	greater than 20 mcg/mL
Phenobarbital	Long acting	10–30 mcg/mL 20–40 mcg/mL (seizure control)	greater than 60 mcg/mL

Child: *Phenobarbital: Therapeutic:* 15–30 mcg/mL *Toxic:* greater than 35 mcg/mL

Description

Barbiturate toxicity is a frequent cause of unconsciousness resulting from accidental or intentional barbiturate overdose. Barbiturates have different effects, and those that are short acting tend to be more potent and toxic than the long-acting types. Phenobarbital tends to be least toxic; however, this depends on the amount taken. This long-acting barbiturate peaks in 12–18 hours, and its serum half-life is 48–96 hours.

Alcohol and tranquilizers can intensify the effects of barbiturates. Blood barbiturate levels are usually measured on unconscious/comatose clients when the cause of unresponsiveness is unknown.

Purposes

- To monitor specific barbiturate serum level.
- To detect a high serum barbiturate level.

Procedure

- There is no food or fluid restriction.
- Collect 5 mL of venous blood in a red-top (preferred) or lavender-top tube.
- Urine and gastric contents may be examined for barbiturates.

Factors Affecting Laboratory Results

- Alcohol and tranquilizers cause false results.
- Drugs such as theophyllines can elevate the barbiturate level.

NURSING IMPLICATIONS WITH RATIONALE

- Observe for signs and symptoms of barbiturate toxicity (e.g., depressed respirations, bradycardia, and loss of consciousness).
- Obtain a history from the family or a friend to determine whether the client has been taking a barbiturate and, if so, which type. Report the drug history.
- Monitor the urinary output. Renal dysfunction caused by renal ischemia and tubular damage can prolong recovery. Diuretics, especially osmotic, have been used for correcting the effects of long-lasting barbiturates.
- Report if the client is taking tranquilizers and barbiturates. The combination of these two drugs could cause respiratory distress.

Client Teaching

- Inform the client that it is important to keep medical appointments when taking barbiturates so that the health care provider can evaluate the effects of the drug and have the blood barbiturate levels checked.
- Instruct the client not to combine alcohol with barbiturates. Alcohol intensifies the effects of barbiturates, and respiratory distress could result.

Beta$_2$ microglobulin (B$_2$ M, BMG) (blood, serum, urine)

Reference Values

Blood/Serum: *Adult:* Less than 2 mcg/mL, 0.2 mg/dL, 1–2.4 mg/L, less than 170 nmol/L (SI units). *Elderly:* 0.25 mg/dL.

Urine: Less than 120 mcg/24 h, less than 10 mmol/24 h.

Description

Beta$_2$ microglobulin (B$_2$ M, BMG) is a protein of low molecular weight found on the surface of many cells; it is a component of class 1 human leukocyte antigen (HLA), particularly on lymphatic cells. B$_2$ M is filtered by the glomeruli and 95% is reabsorbed by the tubules of the kidneys. With renal disease, both blood and urine specimens are obtained for B$_2$ M, to differentiate between glomerular and tubular disease. If the blood level of B$_2$ M is increased and the urine level is decreased, then glomerular renal disease is suspected. If the blood level is low and the urine level is increased, then tubular renal disease is suggested. Blood B$_2$ M increases early with renal transplant rejection.

Other causes of an elevated B$_2$ M include lymphomas, leukemias, many neoplasms, multiple myeloma, and severe chronic inflammatory disease. It is a useful tumor marker to determine the stage of cancerous tumor—its growth rate and the prognosis.

B$_2$ M is increased in AIDS clients, especially those with opportunistic infection. It has been combined with CD$_4$ lymphocyte count for determining the probability of an HIV-infected person developing AIDS in the next 3–4 years.

Purposes

- To detect glomerular or tubular renal disease.
- To determine the stage of the tumor and prognosis.
- To determine the progression of HIV to AIDS.

Clinical Problems

Blood *Increased Level:* Glomerular renal disease; renal transplant rejection; some malignancies—lymphomas, leukemia, multiple myeloma; AIDS; Crohn disease; mercury exposure, chronic inflammatory disease; *Drug Influence:* aminoglycoside toxicity.

Urine *Increased Level:* Tubular renal disease, lymphomas, leukemia, multiple myeloma, AIDS, mercury exposure.

Procedure

Blood

- There is no food or fluid restriction.
- Collect 5 mL of venous blood in a red- or lavender-top tube.

Urine: 24 hours

- Discard the first morning urine specimen.
- Collect all urine for the next 24 hours in a large container with a preservative. Keep container refrigerated.
- Have client void at the end of the 24 hours.
- Label the urine container with the client's name, date, and the exact time of collection (e.g., 6/3/20, 7:01 AM to 6/4/20, 6:59 AM).
- No toilet paper or feces should be in the urine collection.

Factors Affecting Test Results

- Radioactive dyes given within a week before the test.
- Acid urine causing $B_2 M$ to be unstable.
- Discarding urine specimen during the 24-hour collection time.

NURSING IMPLICATIONS WITH RATIONALE

- Obtain a history of health problems.
- Determine if the client received radioactive dye within a week from a previous test. This can affect test results.

Client Teaching

- Encourage the client to express feelings and concerns by providing a private, calm environment.

Urine

- Collect urine specimen in a container with preservative during the 24 hours. Keep urine collection container in refrigerator or on ice.
- Follow strictly the date and times for the urine collection.

Bilirubin (indirect) (serum)

Van Den Bergh Test

Reference Values

Adult: 0.1–1 mg/dL, 1.7–17.1 µmol/L (SI units).

Child: Same as adult.

Description

(*See Bilirubin [total and direct].*)

Indirect-reacting or unconjugated bilirubin is protein bound and is associated with increased destruction of red blood cells (hemolysis).

Elevated indirect bilirubin can occur in autoimmune- or transfusion-induced hemolysis, in hemolytic processes caused by sickle-cell anemia, in pernicious anemia, and with malaria and septicemia. Internal hemorrhage into soft tissues and the body cavity can cause the bilirubin to rise in 5–6 hours. With certain clinical problems, heart failure, and severe liver damage, both indirect and direct bilirubin levels will increase. Indirect bilirubin frequently increases because the damaged liver cells cannot conjugate normal amounts, which leads to increased unconjugated bilirubin.

Levels of indirect serum bilirubin may increase in hemolytic disease, such as erythroblastosis fetalis, in newborns. The newborn's liver is immature, and when extremely high levels of bilirubin occur, irreversible neurologic damage, referred to as kernicterus, could result.

Purpose

- To detect the presence of unconjugated bilirubin due to hemolytic disease or liver disease.

Clinical Problems

Decreased Level: *Drug Influence:* (*See Bilirubin [total and direct].*)

Increased Level: Erythroblastosis fetalis, sickle-cell anemia, transfusion reaction, pernicious anemia, malaria septicemia, hemolytic anemias, chronic heart failure, decompensated cirrhosis, hepatitis. *Drug Influence:* Aspirin, rifampin, phenothiazines (*See Bilirubin [total and direct].*)

Procedure

- There is no laboratory test for indirect bilirubin. Indirect bilirubin is calculated by subtracting direct bilirubin from the total bilirubin:

$$\text{Total bilirubin} - \text{Direct bilirubin} = \text{Indirect bilirubin}$$

- In newborn infants, only the total is determined, and this represents the indirect bilirubin only.

Factors Affecting Laboratory Results

- (*See Bilirubin [total and direct].*)

B

NURSING IMPLICATIONS WITH RATIONALE

Increased Levels

- Check the client's indirect serum bilirubin level, and compare it with the direct bilirubin result. If the indirect bilirubin is elevated and the direct is not, then the cause is a hemolytic problem.

Client Teaching

- Instruct the client not to eat for 8 to 12 hours before blood is drawn. Carrots, yams, or foods high in fat should not be eaten the night before.

Bilirubin (total and direct) (serum)

Reference Values

Adult: *Total:* 0.1–1.2 mg/dL, 1.7–20.5 μmol/L (SI units). *Direct (conjugated):* 0.1–0.3 mg/dL, 1.7–5.1 μmol/L (SI units).

Child: *Newborn: Total:* 1–12 mg/dL, 17.1–205 μmol/L (SI units). *Child:* 0.2–0.8 mg/dL. *Panic Level* : 15 mg/dL.

Description

Bilirubin is formed from the breakdown of hemoglobin by the reticuloendothelial system and is carried in the plasma to the liver, where it is conjugated (directly) to form bilirubin diglucuronide and is excreted in the bile. There are two forms of bilirubin in the body: the conjugated, or direct-reacting (soluble), and the unconjugated, or indirect-reacting (protein bound). If the total bilirubin is within normal range, direct and indirect bilirubin levels do not need to be analyzed. If one value of bilirubin is reported, it represents the total bilirubin.

Direct or conjugated bilirubin is frequently the result of obstructive jaundice, either extrahepatic (from stones or tumor) or intrahepatic in origin. Conjugated bilirubin cannot escape in the bile into the intestine and thus backs up and is absorbed into the bloodstream. Damaged liver cells cause a blockage of the bile sinusoid, increasing the serum level of direct bilirubin. With hepatitis and decompensated cirrhosis, both direct and indirect bilirubin may be elevated.

Serum bilirubin (total) in newborns can be as high as 12 mg/dL; the panic level is greater than 15 mg/dL. Jaundice is frequently present when serum bilirubin levels are greater than 3 mg/dL.

The **transcutaneous bilirubin test** checks for the presence of hyperbilirubinemia in newborns. This small device is placed on the newborn's sternum to check the bilirubin level. It is estimated that 60% of newborns and 80% of preterm infants develop jaundice during the first week of life, and with preterm infants, most jaundice is noted while these infants are receiving nursing care. In many of these cases, the nurse will check the bilirubin level. It has been recommended by the American Academy of Pediatrics (AAP) that newborns be tested for hyperbilirubinemia by using the transcutaneous Bili-Meter (Draeger Medical's Minolta JM 103 model). By using this method, the results of the bilirubin are obtained in 7 seconds. With the serum bilirubin test for newborns, the blood is taken from the infant's heel and the sample is sent to the laboratory. The serum method can cause discomfort to the infant. It has been determined that the transcutaneous test is as accurate as the serum test and is less traumatic to the infant. At present, this form of test to determine bilirubin values is not universally used.

Purposes

- To monitor bilirubin levels associated with jaundice.
- To suggest the occurrence of a liver disorder.

Clinical Problems

Decreased Level: Iron-deficiency anemia. *Drug Influence:* Barbiturates, salicylates (aspirin)—large amounts, penicillin, caffeine.

Increased Level: Obstructive jaundice caused by stones or neoplasms, hepatitis, cirrhosis of the liver, infectious mononucleosis, liver metastasis (cancer), Wilson disease. *Drug Influence:* Antibiotics (amphotericin B, clindamycin, erythromycin, gentamicin, lincomycin, oxacillin, tetracyclines), sulfonamides, antituberculosis drugs (para-aminosalicylic acid, isoniazid [INH]), allopurinol, diuretics (acetazolamide [Diamox], ethacrynic acid [Edecrin]), mithramycin, dextran, diazepam (Valium), barbiturates, narcotics (codeine, morphine, meperidine [Demerol]), flurazepam (Dalmane), indomethacin (Indocin), methotrexate, methyldopa (Aldomet), papaverine, procainamide (Pronestyl), steroids, oral contraceptives, tolbutamide (Orinase), vitamins A, C, and K.

Procedure

- Keep the client NPO except for water for 8 to 12 hours before the procedure.
- Hold medications that would increase the serum bilirubin for 24 hours, with the health care provider's approval. If medications are given, list the drugs on the laboratory slip and the time they were last given.
- Collect 3–5 mL of venous blood in a red-top tube. Avoid hemolysis.
- *Caution:* Whenever blood is drawn for liver function tests, avoid self-contamination to prevent possible infection (such as hepatitis). Use isolation technique. Protect the blood specimen from sunlight and artificial light, as light will reduce the bilirubin content. Blood should be sent to the laboratory immediately so that separation of serum from the cells can be performed as soon as possible to avoid hemolysis. Infants can have the blood taken from the heel of the foot. Two blood microtubes should be filled.

Factors Affecting Laboratory Results

- A high-fat dinner prior to the test may affect bilirubin levels.
- Carrots and yams may increase the serum bilirubin level.
- Hemolysis of the blood specimen can give inaccurate results. The tube should not be shaken.
- A blood specimen exposed to sunlight or artificial light will degrade the bile pigment. Certain drugs (*see Drug Influence*) can increase or decrease the serum bilirubin level.

B

NURSING IMPLICATIONS AND RATIONALE

Increased Level

- Check the serum bilirubin (total), and if it is elevated, check the direct and indirect bilirubin levels.
- Check the sclera of the eyes and the inner aspects of the arm for jaundice.

Client Teaching

- Instruct the client that he or she should have nothing by mouth except water before the test. If his or her medications are withheld, an appropriate explanation should be given. The nurse should emphasize that fats, carrots, and yams should not be eaten the night before the blood test.
- Inform the parent(s) whose baby is jaundiced that the bilirubin level will be closely monitored until the level is in normal range.

Bilirubin and bile (urine)

Reference Values

Adult: *Negative:* 0.02 mg/dL.

Description

Bilirubin is not normally present in urine; however, a very small quantity could be present without being detected by routine test methods. Bilirubin is formed from the breakdown of hemoglobin and is transported to the liver, where it is conjugated and excreted as bile. Conjugated or direct bilirubin is water-soluble and is excreted in the urine when there is an increased serum level. Unconjugated or indirect bilirubin is fat-soluble and cannot be excreted in the urine.

Bilirubinuria (bilirubin in urine) indicates liver damage or biliary obstruction (e.g., stones), and a large amount has a characteristic dark-amber color. When the amber-colored urine is shaken, it produces a yellow foam. It can frequently be tested by the floor nurse with a dipstick or reagent tablet.

Purpose

- To compare the urine bilirubin level with the serum bilirubin level and other liver enzyme tests to detect liver disorder.

Clinical Problems

Increased Level: Obstructive biliary disease, liver disease (hepatitis, toxic agents), chronic heart failure with jaundice, cancer of the liver (secondary). *Drug Influence:* Phenothiazines—chlorpromazine (Thorazine), acetophenazine (Tindal); chlorprothixene (Taractan); phenazopyridine (Pyridium); chlorzoxazone (Paraflex).

Procedure

- There is no food or fluid restriction.
- Use either urine dipstick or Ictotest reagent tablets for the bilirubinuria test. The Bili-labstix is dipped in urine and after 20 seconds is compared to a color chart on the bottle. For urine dipstick and Ictotest tablets, follow the directions on the bottle.
- Test urine bilirubin within 1 hour. Keep urine away from ultraviolet light.

Factors Affecting Laboratory Results

- Certain drugs can give a false-positive result (*see Drug Influence*).
- Exposure of urine to light for 1 hour will cause deterioration of bile pigments.

B

NURSING IMPLICATIONS WITH RATIONALE

Increased Level

- Check the serum bilirubin—total and direct—and report if it is elevated. Test the urine for bilirubinuria. Compare urine and serum findings.
- Assess the color of the urine. If it is dark amber in color, shake the urine specimen and note whether a yellow foam appears.
- Record the results of a urine dipstick and the urine color on the client's chart.
- Notify the health care provider of amber urine with yellow foam and of test results.

Bioterrorism infectious products tests

Anthrax (*Bacillus anthracis*), Botulism (*Clostridium botulinum*), Smallpox (*Variola virus* [DNA virus])

Reference Values

Negative: The organism being tested.

Description

There are many products used in bioterrorism; however, three of them—anthrax, botulism, and smallpox—are presented here because these three seem to be the most common infectious agents used in bioterrorism. Discovery of any one of these agents should be reported to the Department of Public Health and the Centers for Disease Control and Prevention (CDC).

Anthrax

Anthrax is caused by *Bacillus anthracis*, which is a spore-forming gram-positive bacillus. The spores of this organism can be transmitted via inhalation, through the GI (gastrointestinal) tract, and cutaneously (through the skin) from infected animals and their products, or via intentional release for bioterrorist attack. Inhalation of the spores is the most serious transmission of anthrax and is frequently fatal. For suspected GI anthrax, culture of the blood, gastric secretions, food,

B

and feces are recommended. If cutaneous (skin) anthrax is suspected, a culture of the skin vesicle is done. Immunization is suggested for clients working directly with animals and their products and also for clients who can be contaminated with anthrax in direct warfare.

Common symptoms of anthrax include fever, fatigue, skin lesions, and/or respiratory failure. If pulmonary anthrax is present, the symptoms would include fever, dyspnea, chest pain, coughing, and cyanosis due to a lack of oxygen. Treatment for anthrax is antibiotics with repeated doses.

Botulism

Botulism is caused by *Clostridium botulinum*, which is a spore-forming anaerobic bacteria/toxin. The botulinum toxin is transmitted mainly via the GI tract and the lungs. However, the organism can pass from the person's infected wound into the bloodstream. This organism is found in the soil and in undercooked food kept at room temperature for a long period of time. It may be used as a bioterrorism agent.

Symptoms can begin 6–12 hours following the ingestion of contaminated food, and the symptoms mostly include dysphagia, blurred vision, muscle weakness, and flaccid paralysis. It is not a contagious organism. Treatment is the equine antitoxin to decrease nerve damage.

Smallpox

Smallpox is caused by a *Variola virus*, a DNA virus. It has been controlled with the smallpox vaccination. The concern today is that it can be used as a bioterrorism weapon.

There are two types of the *Variola virus*: *Variola major*, which is the most severe form of smallpox and the most common type, and *Variola minor*, which is less severe and not as common. With *Variola major*, the fever is very high and the rash is more extensive.

The early symptoms of smallpox are fever, body aches, and malaise. Rash usually begins in the mouth and then on the skin. Then it becomes a vesicular rash with fluid. Persons who are at risk of a bioterrorism attack of smallpox should be vaccinated.

Purposes

- To test for the organism/toxin that could cause anthrax, botulism, or smallpox.
- To notify the Department of Public Health and CDC of the suspected bioterrorism agent.

Clinical Problems

Anthrax: *Bacillus anthracis.*

Botulism: *Clostridium botulinum.*

Smallpox: *Variola virus*; DNA virus.

Procedure

Anthrax

- No food or fluid restriction is required.
- Obtain a culture of blood, sputum, stool, and/or fluid from the skin vesicle. Use two sterile cotton swabs to obtain the fluid from the vesicle that has been opened. The blood and sputum specimens are used for testing pulmonary anthrax.
- Take precautions as outlined by the institution when taking specimens.

Botulism
- No food or fluid restriction is required.
- Obtain gastric secretions, vomitus, and/or stool specimen when GI botulism is suspected.
- Collect 10 mL of venous blood in a red-top tube. Thirty milliliters of blood may be requested.
- Refrigerate all specimens.

Smallpox
- No food or fluid restriction is required.
- Collect vesicle fluid using sterile cotton swab(s). Remove the scab if present to obtain a culture of the vesicle fluid; however, the scab may be used for testing.
- An electron microscope can identify the brick-shaped virions of smallpox.

Factors Affecting Laboratory Results
- Insufficient amount of collected specimen.
- Contamination of specimen with other organisms.
- Not keeping the specimen iced or refrigerated as indicated.

NURSING IMPLICATIONS WITH RATIONALE

- Obtain a history related to client's contact of the infectious agent.
- Notify appropriate health officials if a bioterror agent is suspected. Further testing and isolation of the client may be necessary until the agent is identified.
- Use guidelines for client care prepared by the health department, CDC, and/or the institution. Take precautions as necessary.
- Report and document the signs and symptoms presented by the client.
- Administer medications and treatment as prescribed.

Client Teaching
- Explain to the client the types of medications and treatment he or she is to receive. If the client is being isolated, explain to the client and family the purpose for isolation.
- Answer the client and family's questions concerning isolation and the agent tested or refer to the appropriate health professionals.
- Be supportive to the client and family.

Bladder cancer/tumor markers (urine)
Bladder Tumor Associated Test, Bladder Tumor Antigen (BTA), Nuclear Matrix Proteins 22 (NMP22)

Reference Values
BTA: Negative to less than 13 units/mL

NMP22: Negative to less than 9 units/mL

B

Description

Bladder tumor antigen (BTA) and nuclear matrix protein 22 (NMP22) are antigens/proteins produced by the bladder tumor cells that can be obtained from the urine. When bladder cancer is suspected, a noninvasive urine test, BTA or NMP22, may be ordered first before ordering a cystoscopy. A cystoscopy is suggested when the BTA or NMP22 is elevated. This urine test can also be used to confirm bladder cancer after a positive bladder biopsy.

The urine test can be used at home as well as in the clinic. If used at home, the urine specimen must be refrigerated until it is transported to the laboratory. Again, if the urine test is positive, a cystoscopy is performed to obtain a biopsy.

Purposes

- To determine the presence of bladder tumor cells.
- To manage the treatment of bladder cancer.

Clinical Problems

Elevated levels: Bladder tumor, bladder malignant cells, monitoring the treatment of bladder cancer.

Procedure

- There is no food or fluid restriction
- Collect a urine specimen, approximately 30 mL, in a clean urine specimen container. The first voided urine specimen of the day is preferred.
- Refrigerate the urine specimen if it is not immediately taken to the laboratory.

Factors Affecting Laboratory Results

- Hematuria (blood in the urine) may cause a false-positive test.
- Bladder or urinary tract infection could elevate BTA levels.
- Recent bladder surgery or biopsy may cause a false-positive value.
- Kidney stones may cause an elevated level.

NURSING IMPLICATIONS WITH RATIONALE

- Obtain a history of the urinary problem(s).
- Explain the procedure for collecting the urine specimen.
- Inform the client that a positive test result would be confirmed by other tests, such as a biopsy.
- Permit the client time to express his or her concerns or fears.

Client Teaching

- Instruct the client on how to collect the urine specimen if taken at home.
- Answer any of the client's questions or concerns about the test and possible positive results.

Bleeding time (blood)

Reference Values

Adult: *Ivy Method:* 1–9 minutes. *Panic Level:* >15 minutes. *Duke Method:* 1–3 minutes. SI units for the Ivy and Duke methods are the same. (Duke method is seldom performed.)

B

Description

Two methods, Ivy and Duke, are used to determine whether bleeding time is normal or prolonged. Bleeding time is lengthened in thrombocytopenia (decreased platelet count, less than 50,000). The test is frequently performed when there is a history of bleeding (easy bruising), familial bleeding, or preoperative screening. The Ivy technique, in which the forearm is used for the incision, is the most popular method. Aspirin and anti-inflammatory medications can prolong the bleeding time.

Purpose

- To check bleeding time for various health problems.

Clinical Problems

Decreased Rate: Hodgkin disease.

Prolonged Rate: Thrombocytopenic purpura, platelet abnormality, vascular abnormalities, leukemia, severe liver disease, disseminated intravascular coagulation, aplastic anemia, factor deficiencies (V, VII, XI), Christmas disease, hemophilia. *Drug Influence:* Salicylates (aspirin, others), dextran, mithramycin, warfarin (Coumadin), streptokinase (streptodornase; fibrinolytic agent).

Procedure

Ivy Method

- Cleanse the volar surface of the forearm (below the antecubital space) with alcohol and allow it to dry. Inflate the blood pressure cuff to 40 mm Hg, and leave it inflated during the test. Puncture the skin 2.5 mm deep on the forearm; start timing with a stopwatch. Blot blood drops carefully every 30 seconds until bleeding ceases. The time required for bleeding to stop is recorded in seconds.
- The test should *not* be performed while the client is taking anticoagulant or aspirin; withhold medications for 3–7 days.

Duke Method

- There is no food or fluid restriction.
- The area used is the earlobe.

Factors Affecting Laboratory Results

- Method used; improper technique—the puncture wound might be deeper than required. Blotting the incision area and not the blood drops can break off fibrin particles, prolonging the bleeding time.
- Aspirin and anticoagulants increase the bleeding time.

B

NURSING IMPLICATIONS WITH RATIONALE

Prolonged Rate

- Relate prolonged bleeding time to clinical problems and drugs. The nurse should be familiar with the methods used to obtain the bleeding time.
- Obtain a drug history of the last time (date) the client took aspirin or anticoagulants. Aspirin prevents platelet aggregation, and bleeding can be prolonged by taking only one aspirin tablet (5 grains, or 325 mg) 3 days prior to test. A history of taking "cold medications" should be recorded, because many cold remedies contain salicylates.
- Note whether the client has been consuming alcohol. Alcohol increases bleeding time, and the bleeding may be difficult to stop.
- Apply a dressing to the puncture wound site (Ivy method) to stop the bleeding.

Client Teaching

- Instruct the client not to take aspirin and over-the-counter (OTC) cold remedies for 3 days before the test. If the client takes aspirin or anticoagulants, the laboratory should be notified and the drug names should be written on the laboratory slip.
- Explain to the client how the test is performed. In the Ivy method the forearm is used, and in the Duke method the earlobe is used. The step-by-step method of the procedure should be explained (*see Procedure*). The nurse should check with the laboratory for changes in procedure.
- Listen to the client's concerns.

Blood gases
See Arterial Blood Gases

Blood smear
Blood Study of Erythrocytes and Leukocytes

Reference Values

Normal red blood cells (RBCs) size (7–8 um), shape (normocytes), color, and content, and white blood cells (WBCs) with differentials.

Description

Blood smear is another blood test used to determine abnormalities associated with blood cells. A drop of blood is examined microscopically for the cause of a hematologic disease, especially anemia and leukemia. A stain is applied to the blood smear. The size, shape, color, and content of the cells are examined by a pathologist.

RBC indices (see page 380) can also identify the size, shape, and volume of RBCs. The blood smear and RBC indices can be a part of the CBC test.

Purpose

- To identify a cause of the hematologic disorder.

Clinical Problems

Abnormal Findings: Iron-deficiency anemia (small RBCs, crescent shape, pale color), folic acid and vitamin B_{12} deficiency (large-size RBCs), hereditary and acquired immunohemolytic anemia (small, round RBCs), thalassemia (small RBCs with less hemoglobin), leukemia (increased number of immature WBCs), infection (increased number of WBC count), chronic disease (decreased WBC count). *Drug Influence:* antineoplastic drugs.

B

Procedure

- There is no food or fluid restriction.
- Collect a drop of blood from the finger and place it on a slide, *or* collect 7–10 mL of venous blood in a lavender-top tube.

NURSING IMPLICATIONS WITH RATIONALE

- Obtain a history of client's health problem.
- Assess client's vital signs.
- Observe for any physiological abnormal changes. This could include color (paleness), breathing, and other clinical signs.
- Determine client's dietary intake that may contribute to his or her hematologic health problem.

Client Teaching

- Suggest foods from the food pyramid or food plate that may improve the client's health.
- Answer client's questions or refer to appropriate health professionals.
- Instruct client to keep medical appointments.

Blood urea nitrogen (BUN) (serum)

Reference Values

Adult: 5–25 mg/dL.

Child: *Infant:* 5–15 mg/dL. *Child:* 5–20 mg/dL. *Newborn:* 3–12 mg/dL.

Elderly: Could be slightly higher than adult.

Description

Urea is formed as an end product of protein metabolism and is excreted by the kidneys. An elevated blood urea nitrogen level could be an indication of dehydration, prerenal failure, or renal failure. Dehydration from vomiting, diarrhea, and/or inadequate fluid intake can cause an

B

increase in the BUN (up to 35 mg/dL). With dehydration, the serum creatinine level would most likely be normal or high normal. Once the client is hydrated, the BUN should return to normal; if it does not, prerenal or renal failure would be suspected. Nephrons (kidney cells) tend to decrease during the aging process, and so older persons may have a higher BUN. Digested blood from gastrointestinal bleeding is a source of protein and can cause the BUN to elevate. A low BUN value usually indicates overhydration (hypervolemia).

The **BUN/creatinine ratio** is a calculation with reference value of 10:1–15:1. A decreased BUN/creatinine ratio occurs with malnutrition, liver disease, low-protein diet, excessive IV fluids, dialysis, or overhydration. An elevated BUN/creatinine ratio, greater than 15:1, is found in renal disease, inadequate renal perfusion, shock, dehydration, GI bleeding, and drugs such as steroids and tetracyclines. See separate listing for BUN/creatinine.

Purpose

- To detect a renal disorder or dehydration associated with increased BUN levels.

Clinical Problems

Decreased Level: Severe liver damage, low-protein diet, overhydration, malnutrition (negative nitrogen balance), IV fluids (glucose). *Drug Influence:* Phenothiazines.

Increased Level: Dehydration; high-protein diet; GI bleeding; prerenal failure (low renal blood supply caused by heart failure, diabetes mellitus, acute myocardial infarction, renal insufficiency/failure from shock, sepsis, kidney diseases [glomerular nephritis, pyelonephritis]), licorice (excessive ingestion). *Drug Influence:* Nephrotoxic drugs; diuretics (hydrochlorothiazide [HydroDIURIL], ethacrynic acid [Edecrin], furosemide [Lasix], triamterene [Dyrenium]); antibiotics (bacitracin, cephaloridine [high doses], gentamicin, kanamycin, chloramphenicol [Chloromycetin], methicillin, neomycin, vancomycin); antihypertensive agents (methyldopa [Aldomet], guanethidine [Ismelin]); sulfonamides; propranolol; morphine; lithium carbonate; salicylates.

Procedure

- It is preferable to have the client remain NPO for 8 hours.
- Collect 3–5 mL of venous blood in a red-top tube. Avoid hemolysis.

Factors Affecting Laboratory Results

- The hydration status of the client should be known. Overhydration can give a false-low BUN level, and dehydration can give a false-high BUN level.
- Drugs (e.g., antibiotics, diuretics, and antihypertensive agents) raise the BUN level.

NURSING IMPLICATIONS WITH RATIONALE

- Compare serum BUN and serum creatinine results. If both BUN and creatinine are elevated, kidney disease should be highly suspected.

Decreased Level

- Assess the client's dietary intake. A low-protein intake and a high-carbohydrate intake can decrease the BUN level.
- Report on clients receiving continuous dextrose intravenously without protein intake.
- Check the client for signs and symptoms of overhydration (irritated cough, dyspnea, neck-vein engorgement, and chest rales) when the BUN is decreased. Overhydration (hypervolemia) causes hemodilution, diluting the urea in the blood.

Increased Level

- Report urinary output less than 25 mL/hour or 600 mL/day. Urea is excreted by the kidneys, and with a decreased urine output, urea accumulates in the blood.
- Check vital signs. A fast pulse, decreased blood pressure, and increased respiration could indicate dehydration and, if severe enough, could lead to shock.
- Determine the hydration status of the client. If dehydration is present, the elevated BUN may be attributed to hemoconcentration. Hydrating with IV fluids should correct the problem.
- Avoid overhydration with IV fluid. Rapid administration of IV fluids can overload the vascular system, especially in the aged, in children, and in heart patients, resulting in hypervolemia. This can lead to pulmonary edema.
- Assess the client's dietary intake. A high-protein diet will increase the serum BUN. Individuals on a high-protein diet for dieting purposes will have an elevated BUN level unless adequate fluids are taken.
- Recognize drugs that increase the BUN (e.g., antibiotics, diuretics, antihypertensive agents, and others; *see Drug Influence*).

Client Teaching

- Instruct clients with a slightly elevated BUN to increase fluid intake. Care should be taken in forcing fluids in clients with heart and kidney problems.

Blood urea nitrogen/creatinine ratio (serum)
Urea Nitrogen/Creatinine Reference Values

Reference Values

Adult: 10:1–20:1 (BUN:creatinine). *Average:* 15:1.

Description

The blood urea nitrogen (BUN)/creatinine ratio is an effective test primarily for determining renal function. BUN level can increase because of dehydration as well as renal dysfunction. The creatinine level does not increase with dehydration but definitely increases with renal dysfunction. This ratio test is more sensitive to the relationship of BUN to creatinine than separate tests of BUN and creatinine. However, liver function, dietary protein intake, and muscle mass may affect test result.

A decreased ratio can occur from acute renal tubular necrosis and low protein intake. The ratio may be increased because of reduced renal perfusion, glomerular disease, obstructive uropathy, or high protein intake.

Purpose

- To determine renal function.

Clinical Problems

Decreased Ratio: Acute renal tubular necrosis, low protein intake, malnutrition, pregnancy, liver disease, hemodialysis (urea loss). *Drug Influence:* Phenacemide.

Increased Ratio: Reduced renal perfusion (dehydration, heart failure), glomerular disease, tissue or muscle destruction, high protein intake, obstructive uropathy, azotemia. *Drug Influence:* Tetracycline, corticosteroids.

Procedure

- No food or fluid restriction is required.
- Collect 5–7 mL of venous blood in a red-top tube.

Factors Affecting Laboratory Results

- Variations in protein intake; liver disease.

NURSING IMPLICATIONS WITH RATIONALE

- Assess the client's renal function, including urine output, BUN, and serum creatinine level. Urine output should be at least 600 mL per day.
- Place a note in client's chart or Kardex that urine needs to be measured.
- Assess the client's dietary intake. Record increase or decrease in protein intake.
- Check the client's hydration status. Dehydration may cause an increase in the BUN/ creatinine ratio.

Client Teaching

- Inform the client that urine needs to be measured, and instruct the client to urinate in a urinal or bedpan. Inform the health care personnel after each voiding so that urine can be measured. Tell the client not to put toilet paper in the urine.

Blood volume

Reference Values

Adult: *Total Blood Volume:* 55–80 mL/kg. Male: 7.5% body weight. Female: 6.5% body weight. *Red Cell Volume:* Male: 25–35 mL/kg. Female: 20–30 mL/kg. *Plasma Volume:* Male: 32–46 mL/kg. Female: 30–45 mL/kg.

Description

The blood volume determination is commonly used to determine the total blood, red blood cell, and plasma volumes. Two radioactive substances can be used for measurement: Cr-51–tagged red cells for RBC volume and I-131– or I-125–tagged human serum albumin for plasma volume. The client's blood is mixed with the radioactive substance.

This test is useful for monitoring blood loss during surgery, evaluating gastrointestinal or uterine bleeding, determining the cause of hypotension, determining the blood component lost (e.g., RBCs, plasma) for replacement therapy, and diagnosing polycythemia vera.

B

Purposes

- To determine total blood volume (RBC and plasma).
- To monitor blood loss during surgery.
- To evaluate GI or uterine bleeding.

Clinical Problems

Decreased Volume: Dehydration (total and plasma volume), hypovolemic shock, hemorrhage.

Increased Volume: Dehydration (RBC volume), polycythemia vera, overhydration (total volume).

Procedure

- Obtain the height and weight of the client.
- Obtain a blood sample.
- Personnel from the nuclear medicine laboratory will obtain a blood sample and mix a radio-isotope (radionuclide, i.e., I-131, I-125, Cr-51) with the blood. After 15–30 minutes, the blood containing the radioactive substance will be reinjected into the client.
- Collect another blood sample in 15 minutes.

Factors Affecting Diagnostic Results

- IV fluids can affect the test results.
- Prolonged time for blood sample collection can affect results. If I-131–tagged albumin is used, it will leave the plasma (intravascular fluid compartment) after 15 minutes and enter the extravascular fluid compartment.

NURSING IMPLICATIONS WITH RATIONALE

- Explain the procedure to the client.
- Start IV therapy, if ordered, after the blood volume determination test has been completed.
- Explain to the client that the radioactive substance he or she will receive is of low amount and should be harmless.
- Answer the client's questions or refer to the appropriate health professionals.
- Observe for signs and symptoms of dehydration (e.g., dry mucous membrane, poor skin turgor, and shocklike symptoms).
- Observe for signs and symptoms of shock (e.g., tachycardia; tachypnea; pale, cold, clammy skin; and later a drop in blood pressure).

Brain natriuretic peptide (BNP) (plasma)

Triage BNP, N-terminal Pro-brain Natriuretic Peptide (NT-proBNP)

B

Reference Values

Desired Values: Less than 100 pg/mL; less than 100 ng/L (SI units).

Positive Values: Greater than 100 pg/mL; greater than 100 ng/L (SI units).

Severe Heart Failure: Greater than 400 pg/mL; greater than 400 ng/L (SI units).

Description

Brain natriuretic peptide, or B-type natriuretic peptide (BNP), is a neurohormone secretion primarily in the cardiac ventricles and will increase in response to volume expansion and pressure overload. BNP does not exist in the brain but was labeled BNP because it was first found in the brain of pigs. It exists in the cardiac ventricular muscle. It is the second type of the natriuretic peptide group; atrial natriuretic peptide (ANP), being the first, exists in the cardiac atrial muscle. The BNP test has been approved by the FDA to aid in the diagnosis of heart failure (HF). Heart failure is difficult to diagnose among persons with lung disease, those who are obese, and the elderly. BNP is ordered to determine heart failure and is considered a more sensitive test than ANP for diagnosing heart failure.

The BNP is more highly elevated in clients with HF than those with a lung disease. Frequently the BNP is higher than 100 pg/mL in women who are 65 years old or older. For example, an 80-year-old woman's BNP may be 160 pg/mL; however, with heart failure, the BNP is markedly higher and can be greater than 400 pg/mL. This test does not replace other clinical findings and tests for diagnosing HF, but if HF is suspected, BNP is helpful for confirming the diagnosis. If the BNP is within normal range for a client having difficulty breathing, the client's condition is most likely noncardiac dyspnea.

N-terminal pro-brain natriuretic peptide (NT-proBNP, triage BNP) is a rapid bedside immunoassay test that measures the level of brain natriuretic peptide. The test is readable in 15 minutes and is used to aid in the diagnosis of heart failure. Also the NT-proBNP can indicate milder cardiac dysfunction. The test is used in emergency rooms to receive quick BNP results.

Purpose

- To aid in the diagnosis of heart failure.

Clinical Problems

Increased Level: Heart failure, left ventricular hypertrophy, myocarditis, early rejection of heart transplant, prolonged systemic hypertension, acute myocardial infarction (AMI), Cushing syndrome, renal failure.

Procedure

- No food or fluid restriction is required.
- Collect 5 mL of venous blood in a red-top tube.

Factors Affecting Laboratory Results

- Older persons and women usually have higher BNP levels.
- Elevated BNP in clients having had recent heart surgery.

NURSING IMPLICATIONS WITH RATIONALE

- Assess the client for signs and symptoms of heart failure (e.g., dyspnea, coughing, edema).
- Obtain a history of previous health problems, such as heart failure.
- Obtain NT-proBNP test results (if available) to identify the presence of heart failure.

Client Teaching

- Tell the client to report difficulty breathing, swelling of the extremities, and/or coughing.
- Inform the client that more than one laboratory test may be needed to diagnose the health problem.
- Instruct the client to keep health/medical appointments, which are necessary to decrease or control the problem of heart failure if diagnosed.
- Instruct the client to take the prescribed medications for heart failure. At times, clients will stop taking the medications for heart failure when they feel better, and, unfortunately, heart failure will reoccur.

Breast cancer genetic testing (BRCA-1, BRCA-2) (blood)

Reference Values

Adult: Negative findings of genetic mutation of BRCA-1 and BRCA-2.

Description

Predisposition to breast and ovarian cancers can be determined by the mutations in BRCA-1 and BRCA-2. Approximately 22% of families have inherited the BRCA-1 gene, and another 20% of families have the BRCA-2 gene. The genetic defect is an autosomal dominant gene. The BRCA-1 and BRCA-2 can be passed on to children by the female or male. Males who carry the BRCA-1 and BRCA-2 genes are susceptible to breast cancer, and they have a higher risk for developing prostate or colon cancer. However, genetic testing is ordered mostly for women who are at risk of breast or ovarian cancer.

Women who carry the BRCA gene and have a strong family history of breast cancer have a 50% risk of developing breast cancer by age 50, and a 70–90% risk by the age of 70. If the woman already has breast cancer, she would have a 65% chance of developing breast cancer in the other breast during her lifetime.

BRCA genetic testing can also indicate if the woman is susceptible to ovarian cancer. Only 2% of women develop ovarian cancer by the age of 70. However, if the woman has a strong familial history of ovarian cancer and has the BRCA-1 gene, her risk for developing ovarian cancer by the age of 50 is 30%. By the age of 70, her risk for developing ovarian cancer would be 25–45%.

B

Purposes

- To identify clients who are at risk for developing breast cancer.
- To identify clients who are at risk for developing ovarian cancer.

Clinical Problems

Increased Level: Risk for breast cancer, risk for ovarian cancer.

Procedure

- Food and fluids are not restricted.
- Collect 5 mL of venous blood in a lavender- or blue-top tube.
- Do not freeze the blood specimen.

Factors Affecting Laboratory Results

- Frozen blood specimen.

NURSING IMPLICATIONS WITH RATIONALE

- Obtain a family history of breast or ovarian cancer.

Client Teaching

- Inform the client that BRCA genetic testing may or may not be covered by medical insurance.
- Suggest that the client receive genetic counseling regardless of whether the test is negative or positive.
- Encourage the client to ventilate his or her feelings and concerns in a private environment.

Breast cancer tumor prognostic markers

Estrogen Receptor Assay (ER Assay), DNA Ploidy, S-Phase Fraction, Cathepsin D, HER-2/c-erb-B 2/neu Oncoprotein, p53 Protein

---

Findings

Favorable and unfavorable.

ER Assay: *Favorable:* Greater than 11% of cell nuclei stained. *Unfavorable:* Less than 10% of cell nuclei stained.

DNA Ploidy: *Favorable:* Diploid. *Unfavorable:* Aneuploid (rapid cell replication and tumor growth).

S-Phase Fraction: *Favorable:* Less than 5%. *Unfavorable:* Greater than 5% (higher S-phase fraction).

Cathepsin D: *Favorable:* Less than 10%. *Unfavorable:* Greater than 10%.

HER-2/neu Oncoprotein: *Favorable:* Less than 10% partial staining in cancer cells. *Moderately Unfavorable:* 10–20% partial staining in cancer cells. *Strongly Unfavorable:* Greater than 20% partial staining in cancer cells.

p 53 Protein: *Favorable:* Less than 10%. *Unfavorable:* Greater than 10%, mutated p 53 protein in tumor cells.

Description

Thirty percent of clients whose tumors have been removed and have no evidence of lymph node involvement will have a recurrence of malignancy. There are new tumor markers that can predict if more extensive therapy is needed.

Estrogen Receptor Assay (ER Assay): Tumors with a positive ER assay are more responsive to antiestrogen therapy (estrogen deprivation) and/or removal of the ovaries than the tumors that have a negative ER assay. On primary breast cancer tumors, estrogen receptor assay should be performed. Postmenopausal women are more likely to have breast tumors that are mostly estrogen-positive tumors than premenopausal women.

DNA Ploidy: This test determines cell replication. Aneuploid cells (rapidly replicating cells) have a poorer prognosis. Unfortunately, 65% of breast cancer cells are aneuploid. Those with a diploid tumor have a more favorable prognosis.

S-Phase Fraction: Tumors that have high S-phase fractions have a poorer survival rate than those with a low S-phase fraction and diploid tumors. More aggressive cancer cells that divide more rapidly are in the S-phase stage.

Cathepsin D: Clients with an increase in Cathepsin D protein in the breast cancer cells have an unfavorable prognosis. Increased Cathepsin D has been associated with tumor invasion, metastatic cancer, and recurrence of breast cancer.

HER-2/neu Oncoprotein: The presence of a high level of HER-2/neu oncoprotein in the tumor is associated with poor prognosis. HER-2/neu oncoprotein may be identified in the blood. A high level is associated with low estrogen and progesterone receptor concentration; thus the client has little to no response to hormonal therapy. The clients with HER-2/neu oncoprotein may benefit from trastuzumab (Herceptin), a chemotherapy (monoclonal antibody) drug. Herceptin may control the cancer when the client has not responded to other treatment.

P 53 Protein: Increase in p 53 protein is present in more aggressive breast cancer. Mutant p 53 protein occurs on the surface of cancer cells. Increased levels indicate poor prognosis. This test is frequently done along with the lymph nodes testing.

Purposes

- To determine the prognosis of breast cancer from the biopsy of the tissue or entire tumor.
- To determine if the cancer has recurred.
- To determine if the cancer has metastasized.

Clinical Problems

Increased Level: Favorable and unfavorable prognosis of breast cancer, recurrence of breast cancer, breast cancer that has metastasized.

B

Procedure

- Obtain a signed consent form.
- No food or fluid restriction with a needle biopsy. With an incision, NPO may be required.
- Cleanse the breast area.
- Obtain a sample of the breast tumor tissue. A needle biopsy of the tumor may be used to aspirate tissue and fluid.
- The sample of tumor tissue is placed in formalin.
- The container with the tissue is marked with the client's name and date. Indicate on the container the location of the tissue.
- The tissue may be frozen. Check with the laboratory.
- Apply a dressing to the incisional site.

Factors Affecting Diagnostic Results

- Inadequate amount of tissue specimen.
- Improper preservative agent in the container.

NURSING IMPLICATIONS WITH RATIONALE

- Check that the consent form is signed.
- Obtain a familial history of breast cancer.
- Obtain from the client the location of the lump. The mammogram is usually available.
- Indicate which breast, right or left, and mark the location of the lesion.
- Obtain vital signs.

Client Teaching

- Permit client to express her concerns with the procedure and the probability of having breast cancer. Emotional support may be needed. Allow her to vent her feelings.
- Monitor vital signs. Compare VS with the baseline VS.
- Instruct the client to report excessive bleeding or redness at the incisional area.
- Instruct the client to take analgesics and antibiotics if ordered. Tell the client if antibiotics are ordered, all of the tablets/capsules should be taken as prescribed.
- Inform the client that the test results should be back in 1 week.
- Instruct the client how and when to clean the incisional area.
- Tell the client to call for a follow-up appointment.

Bromide (serum)

Reference Values

Adult: *Toxic Levels:* Greater than 100 mg/dL.
Child: Same as adult.

B

Description

The use of bromides as a prescription drug for depression and sedation is seldom ordered; however, today many bromide-containing compounds in patent medicines are available to the public. Because of the cumulative effect of bromides, chronic bromide intoxication is becoming a common occurrence. Acute bromide intoxication is rare, since bromide can cause gastrointestinal irritation.

The half-life of bromide is 12 days. Bromide is slowly excreted by the kidney, and the treatment for chronic bromide intoxication is to accelerate urinary excretion by chloride administration and mercurial diuretics.

Purpose

- To check for possible bromide toxicity.

Procedure

- There is no food or fluid restriction.
- Collect 5 mL of venous blood in a green-top tube.
- A colorimetric test using gold chloride is an old but still useful test. The gold chloride reacts with the bromide in the plasma/serum, forming a yellow/red/orange color, depending on the bromide concentration.

Factors Affecting Laboratory Results

- An extremely high bromide level will cause a decreased chloride level, because both are anions.

NURSING IMPLICATIONS WITH RATIONALE

- Observe for signs and symptoms of chronic bromide intoxication (e.g., anorexia, fever, skin rash, motor incoordination, tremors, delirium, impaired intellectual function, constipation, and weight loss).
- Obtain a history of over-the-counter drugs taken: when, for how long, and the daily quantity taken. If the bottle is available, read the label of the ingredients contained in the medicine.
- Check urine output. Bromides are excreted slowly by the kidneys, so "good" kidney function is extremely important.

Client Teaching

- Teach clients to read labels on patent medicines. Explain the importance of contacting a health care provider before taking most patent medicines.

Calcitonin (Hct) (serum)

Reference Values

Adult: *Male:* Less than 40 pg/mL, less than 40 ng/L (SI units). *Female:* Less than 25 pg/mL, less than 25 ng/L (SI units).

Child: *Newborn:* Usually higher than in adults. *Child:* Less than 70 pg/mL, less than 70 ng/L (SI units).

Description

Calcitonin, a potent hormone secreted by the C cells of the thyroid gland, aids in maintaining normal serum calcium and phosphorus levels. This hormone is secreted in response to an elevated serum calcium level. It inhibits calcium reabsorption by the osteoclasts and osteocytes of the bones and increases calcium excretion by the kidneys. Calcitonin acts as an antagonist to the parathyroid hormone (PTH) and vitamin D, lowering serum calcium levels to maintain calcium balance in the body.

Excess calcitonin secretion occurs in medullary carcinoma of the thyroid. A serum calcitonin level is frequently ordered to aid in the diagnosis of thyroid medullary carcinoma (greater than 500–2,000 pg/mL [probable] and greater than 2,000 pg/mL [definite]) and ectopic calcitonin-producing tumors of the lung and breast. Monitoring calcitonin levels after medullary carcinoma removal will help predict if the tumor will recur.

When the serum calcitonin level is slightly to moderately elevated (100–500 pg/mL), a *calcitonin stimulation test* might be performed in diagnosis of thyroid medullary carcinoma. This test consists of either a 4-hour calcium infusion or a 10-second pentagastrin infusion with measurement of serum calcitonin before and after the infusion.

Purpose

- To aid in the diagnosis of thyroid medullary carcinoma or parathyroid hyperplasia or adenoma.

Clinical Problems

Increased Level: Medullary carcinoma of the thyroid, carcinoma of the lung or breast, chronic renal failure, parathyroid hyperplasia or adenoma, pernicious anemia, Zollinger-Ellison syndrome, acute or chronic thyroiditis, islet cell tumors, pheochromocytoma.

Procedure

- The client should be NPO after midnight. A small amount of water could be given if needed.
- Collect 5–7 mL of venous blood in a green- or lavender-top tube or in a chilled red-top tube (preferred). Avoid hemolysis. Send the blood specimen immediately to the laboratory for analysis or freeze to avoid deterioration.

Calcitonin Stimulation Test

- Draw serum calcitonin level before administering IV calcium or IV pentagastrin.

- Administer IV calcium (15 mg/kg) over 4 hours to provoke calcitonin secretion.

OR

- Administer IV pentagastrin (0.5 mcg/kg) over 5–10 seconds.
- After IV calcium infusion, draw serum calcitonin level 3–4 hours postinfusion. After pentagastrin infusion, draw serum calcium level at 2 minutes, 5 minutes, and 10 minutes.

Factors Affecting Laboratory Results

- Hemolysis could increase serum calcitonin level.
- Levels may be increased during pregnancy and lactation.

NURSING IMPLICATIONS WITH RATIONALE

- Obtain a history of familial thyroid carcinoma. Record and report a positive history.
- Observe for signs and symptoms of hypercalcemia (e.g., lethargy, headaches, weakness, muscle flaccidity, nausea and vomiting, and anorexia).

Client Teaching

- Instruct the client to remain NPO after midnight.
- Explain the calcitonin stimulating test (if ordered) to the client. Refer to the procedure.
- Inform the client that test results may take several days.

Calcium (Ca) and ionized calcium (serum)

Reference Values

Adult Total Ca: 4.5–5.5 mEq/L, 9–11 mg/dL, 2.3–2.8 mmol/L (SI units). *Ionized Ca:* 4.25–5.25 mg/dL, 2.2–2.5 mEq/L, 1.1–1.24 mmol/L.

Child: *Newborn:* 3.7–7 mEq/L, 7.4–14 mg/dL. *Infant:* 5–6 mEq/L, 10–12 mg/dL. *Child:* 4.5–5.8 mEq/L, 9–11.5 mg/dL.

Description

Calcium is found most abundantly in the bones and teeth. Approximately 50% of the calcium is ionized, and only ionized calcium can be used by the body. Protein and albumin in the blood bind with calcium, thus decreasing the amount of free, ionized calcium. The ionized calcium level can be determined by using formulas that estimate the ionized calcium from total calcium. These formulas have been disputed. Only a few laboratories have the equipment to perform serum-ionized calcium level tests. In acidosis, more calcium is ionized, regardless of the serum level, and in alkalosis, most of the calcium is protein bound and cannot be ionized.

The *serum-ionized calcium* (iCa) level is not affected by changes in serum protein/albumin concentration, and it reflects calcium metabolism better than total calcium values. A decrease in ionized calcium, less than 2.2 mEq/L or less than 4.25 mg/dL, might lead to neuromuscular irritability or tetany symptoms (tingling, twitching, spasmodic contractions).

Calcium is necessary for the transmission of nerve impulses and contraction of the myocardium and skeletal muscles. It causes blood clotting by converting prothrombin into thrombin. It strengthens capillary membranes. With a calcium deficit, there is an increased capillary permeability, which causes fluid to pass through the capillary.

A low serum-calcium level is called *hypocalcemia*, and an increased level is called *hypercalcemia*. Calcium imbalances require immediate attention because serum calcium deficit can cause tetany symptoms, unless acidosis is present, and serum calcium excess can cause cardiac dysrhythmias.

Purposes

- To check for serum calcium excess or deficit.
- To monitor calcium levels.
- To detect calcium imbalance.

Clinical Problems

Decreased Level: Diarrhea, malabsorption of calcium from the gastrointestinal tract, extensive infections, burns, lack of calcium and vitamin D intake, hypoparathyroidism, chronic renal failure caused by phosphorous retention, alcoholism, pancreatitis. *Drug Influence:* Cortisone preparations, antibiotics (gentamicin, methicillin), magnesium products (antacids), laxatives (excessive use), heparin, insulin, mithramycin, acetazolamide (Diamox).

Increased Level: Hypervitaminosis D; hyperparathyroidism; malignant neoplasm of the bone, lung, breast, bladder, or kidney; multiple myeloma; prolonged immobilization; multiple fractures; renal calculi; exercise; alcoholism (alcoholic binge); milk-alkali syndrome. *Drug Influence:* Alkaline antacids, estrogen preparations, calcium salts, vitamin D.

Procedure

- There is no food or fluid restriction, unless SMA_{12} or similar group test is ordered.
- Collect 3–5 mL of venous blood in a red-top tube.

Factors Affecting Laboratory Results

- Drugs (*see Drug Influence*) can cause calcium excess or deficit.
- A diet low in calcium or high in calcium and vitamin D can affect results.
- IV saline (NaCl) solution can promote calcium loss.

NURSING IMPLICATIONS WITH RATIONALE

Decreased Level

- Observe for signs and symptoms of hypocalcemia (e.g., tetany symptoms: muscular twitching and tremors, spasms of the larynx, paresthesia [tingling in and numbness of fingers], facial spasms, and spasmodic contractions).

- Check serum calcium values, and report abnormal results to the health care provider, especially if tetany symptoms are present.
- Assess for positive Chvostek and Trousseau signs of hypocalcemia. To test for positive Chvostek sign, tap the area in front of the ear and observe for spasms of the cheek and the corner of the lip. To test for positive Trousseau sign, inflate the blood pressure cuff for several minutes and observe for carpal spasms.
- Administer oral calcium supplements before or 1–1½ hours after meals.
- Observe for symptoms of hypocalcemia when the client is receiving massive transfusions of citrated blood. Citrates prevent calcium ionization. The serum calcium level may be affected.
- Monitor the pulse regularly if the client is receiving a digitalis preparation and calcium supplements. Calcium excess enhances the action of digitalis and can cause digitalis toxicity (nausea, vomiting, anorexia, bradycardia—arrhythmias).
- Administer IV fluids with 10% calcium gluconate slowly. Calcium should be administered in 5% dextrose in water and not in a saline solution, since sodium promotes calcium loss. Calcium should not be added to solutions containing bicarbonate because rapid precipitation will occur.
- Monitor the electrocardiogram during hypocalcemia for prolonged ST segments and lengthened QT intervals.

Client Teaching

- Instruct the client to avoid overuse of antacids and to prevent the chronic laxative habit. Excessive use of certain antacids could cause alkalosis, decreasing calcium ionization. In addition, many antacids contain magnesium, which could lower the serum calcium level. Many laxatives contain phosphates (phosphorous), which have an opposing effect on calcium, causing calcium loss. Chronic use of laxatives will decrease calcium absorption from the GI tract. Suggest fruits for improving bowel elimination.
- Encourage the client to consume foods high in calcium (milk and milk products) and/or high in protein. Protein is needed to enhance calcium absorption.
- Teach the client with hypocalcemia to avoid hyperventilation and crossing his or her legs, which could cause tetany symptoms.

Increased Level

- Observe for signs and symptoms of hypercalcemia (e.g., lethargy, headaches, weakness, muscle flaccidity, heart block, anorexia, nausea, and vomiting).
- Promote active and passive exercises for bedridden clients. This will prevent calcium loss from the bone.
- Identify symptoms of digitalis toxicity when the client has an elevated serum calcium level and is receiving a digitalis preparation.
- Notify the health care provider if the client is receiving a thiazide diuretic, because this will inhibit calcium excretion and promote hypercalcemia.
- Check the urine pH. Calcium salts are more soluble in acid urine (pH less than 6) than in alkaline.
- Handle clients with long-standing hypercalcemia and bone demineralization gently to prevent pathologic fractures.

Client Teaching

- Instruct the client to avoid foods high in calcium, to be ambulatory when possible, and to increase oral fluid intake. Increased fluid intake dilutes calcium in the serum and urine and prevents calculi formation.
- Encourage the client to eat acid-ash foods, such as cranberry juice, meats, fish, poultry, eggs, cheese, and cereals, to keep the urine acidic.

C

Calcium (Ca) (urine)

Reference Values

Adult: *24 Hours:* Low-calcium diet: Less than 150 mg/24 h, less than 3.75 mmol/24 h (SI units); average-calcium diet: 100–250 mg/24 h, 2.50–6.25 mmol/24 h; high-calcium diet: 250–300 mg/24 h, 6.25–7.50 mmol/24 h.

Child: Same as adult.

Description

Urine calcium reflects the dietary intake of calcium, the serum calcium level, and the effects of disease entities (hypo- or hyperparathyroidism, multiple myeloma, bone tumors, etc.). Hypercalciuria (increased calcium levels in the urine) usually accompanies an increased serum calcium level. Calcium excretion fluctuates and is lowest in the morning and highest after meals.

A 24-hour urine specimen for calciuria is useful for determining parathyroid gland disorders. In hyperparathyroidism, hyperthyroidism, and osteolytic disorders, the urinary calcium excretion is usually increased; it is decreased in hypoparathyroidism.

Purpose

(*See Calcium [serum].*)

Clinical Problems

Decreased Level: Hypoparathyroidism, vitamin D deficiency, hypothyroidism, chronic renal failure, malabsorption syndrome. *Drug Influence:* Thiazide diuretics.

Increased Level: Hyperparathyroidism, osteoporosis, hyperthyroidism, malignancies (bone, breast, bladder), multiple myeloma, leukemias, hypervitaminosis D, amyotrophic lateral sclerosis (ALS), renal calculi acid–base imbalance. *Drug Influence:* Cholestyramine resin, sodium- and magnesium-containing drugs, parathyroid injection, vitamin D.

Procedure

- Label the bottle with the exact date and the times that the urine collection started and ended.
- Acidic preservatives are required by most laboratories.
- Indicate on the laboratory slip whether the client's calcium intake has been limited in the last 3 days or whether the client has had an average or high calcium intake.

Factors Affecting Laboratory Results

- Discarded urine—all urine should be saved for the 24-hour urine collection.
- High or low calcium content of diet may affect test results.
- Thiazide diuretics can decrease the urine calcium level, and drugs containing sodium and magnesium can elevate the urine calcium level.

C

NURSING IMPLICATIONS WITH RATIONALE

Decreased Level

- Observe for tetany symptoms if the client's urine calcium level is low (*see Calcium [serum] for tetany symptoms*).
- Have available a 10% solution of calcium gluconate for emergencies. When administered, IV calcium should be diluted in 5% dextrose in water and not in saline solution.
- (*See Calcium [serum] for other nursing implications.*)

Increased Level

- Observe clients for symptoms of renal calculi, especially if there is a history of renal calculi. Strain the urine, if indicated, and report severe low-back pain.
- Prevent the possibility of a pathologic fracture by moving the client gently. The client should be encouraged to do active exercises.
- (*See Calcium [serum] for other nursing implications.*)

Client Teaching

- Instruct the client and family members that urine is to be saved. Tell the client not to put toilet paper or feces in the urine.

Calcium channel blockers (serum)

Verapamil (Calan, Isoptin), Nifedipine (Procardia), Diltiazem (Cardizem)

Reference Values

Adult:

DRUG NAME	THERAPEUTIC RANGE	TOXIC LEVEL
Verapamil	100–300 ng/mL	300 ng/mL
	0.08–0.3 mcg/mL	0.3 mcg/mL
Nifedipine	50–100 ng/mL	100 ng/mL
Diltiazem	50–200 ng/mL	200 ng/mL

Note: Dosage is calculated according to mg/kg.

C

Description

Calcium channel blockers inhibit slow-channel calcium influx into the myocardial cells and vascular smooth muscle. As the result of these actions, a decrease in myocardial contraction and myocardial oxygen consumption and coronary and systemic vasodilation can occur. Calcium channel blockers were commercially available in the United States in the late 1970s for treating ischemic heart disease, or angina pectoris. Of the three calcium channel blockers, nifedipine (Procardia) is the most potent vasodilator, then verapamil (Calan, Isoptin), and, least, diltiazem (Cardizem). Calcium channel blockers are being prescribed more frequently for their antianginal actions.

Verapamil (Calan, Isoptin): This agent can be administered orally or intravenously. Verapamil has a negative inotropic effect and should be used with caution in clients with heart failure. Ninety percent is bound to plasma proteins; 70% of the metabolized drug is excreted in the urine, 15% is excreted in feces, and 4–5% is excreted unchanged in the urine. The peak serum level is 5 hours for an oral dose and 10–15 minutes for an IV bolus. The half-life is 3–7 hours and after chronic therapy, 8–10 hours.

Nifedipine (Procardia): This agent has potent coronary and peripheral vasodilator effects. Ninety percent of the drug is absorbed and bound to plasma proteins. About 75% of the metabolized drug is excreted in the urine and 15% through the gastrointestinal tract. The peak serum level is 2 hours after the oral dose. The half-life is 4–5 hours.

Diltiazem (Cardizem): This calcium channel blocker is not as potent as verapamil or nifedipine. It is absorbed rapidly in the GI tract, and 80% is bound to plasma protein. Metabolites of diltiazem are excreted in the urine and feces. The peak serum level is 2 hours.

Purposes

- To monitor a specific calcium channel blocker level for maintaining a therapeutic range.
- To detect the toxic level for a specific calcium channel blocker, such as verapamil, nifedipine, or diltiazem.

Clinical Problems

Increased Level: Overdose of verapamil, nifedipine, or diltiazem; liver or renal diseases.

Drug Influence: Beta blockers (e.g., propranolol [Inderal]).

Procedure

- There is no food or fluid restriction.
- Collect 3–5 mL of venous blood in a red-top tube. Check with your laboratory for the preferred collecting tube.
- Record on the laboratory requisition slip the name of the drug, and the dose, route, and last time the drug was administered.

Factors Affecting Laboratory Results

- None known.

NURSING IMPLICATIONS WITH RATIONALE

- Check the client's pulse rate and BP (blood pressure) before each administered dose. The vasodilation effect of verapamil and diltiazem lowers pulse rate and BP. Nifedipine can decrease BP substantially without decreasing pulse rate.
- Observe for signs and symptoms related to calcium channel blocking agents (e.g., nausea, abdominal distress, headache, dizziness, lightheadedness, flushing hypotension, bradycardia).
- Monitor BP every 15 minutes for 1 hour after administering an IV bolus of verapamil. Transient asymptomatic hypotension could occur.
- Monitor urine output. Decreased output could indicate renal insufficiency; toxicity could result.
- Recognize that a calcium channel blocker administered with a beta blocker could cause severe hypotension.

Client Teaching

- Teach the client how to take a radial pulse. Inform the client that the pulse rate should be checked before each dose and changes reported to the health care provider.
- Instruct the client not to abruptly discontinue a calcium channel blocking agent. Withdrawal symptoms (e.g., severe hypotension) could result.
- Instruct a client having constipation (verapamil induced) to eat foods high in fiber or to take a mild laxative.
- Instruct a client having palpitations and/or peripheral ankle or leg edema (nifedipine induced) to rest and to elevate the leg(s). Report changes to the health care provider.

Cancer tumor markers (CA 15-3, CA 19-9, CA 27.29, CA 50, CA 125, CA 549) (serum)

Cancer Antigen 15-3, CA 19-9, CA 27.29, CA 50, CA 125, CA 549

Reference Values

CA 15-3: Less than 30 units/mL; less than 30 kU/L (SI units).

CA 19-9: Less than 37 units/mL; less than 37 kU/L (SI units).

CA 27.29: Less than 37 units/mL; less than 37 kU/L (SI units).

CA 50: Less than 17 units/mL; less than 17 kU/L (SI units).

CA 125: Less than 35 units/mL; less than 35 kU/L (SI units).

CA 549: Less than 10 units/mL; less than 10 kU/L (SI units).

Description

Tumor markers is a term used to refer to molecules that can be detected in a blood sample. Common clinical uses of tumor markers are for cancer detection. These markers are frequently used to screen and diagnose the presence of possible cancer, to monitor the response of cancer treatment, and to determine the recurrence of cancer. Some of these cancer tumor markers are specific to a type of cancer, for example, CA 15-3 for breast cancer. A single test value should not be the only method used to determine if cancer is or is not occurring. Several tumor markers taken, which could be over a period of time, are more useful for diagnostic and monitoring purposes.

CA 15-3 is a marker for identifying breast cancer and monitoring clients' response to treatment. It is a more sensitive test for breast cancer than CEA (carcinoembryonic antigen). Greater than 80% of clients with metastatic breast cancer have an elevated CA 15-3 level. Elevated CA 15-3 may occur with ovarian, lung, pancreatic, colon, and prostate cancers.

CA 19-9 is a cancer antigen in aiding the diagnosis of pancreatic, hepatobiliary, gastric, and colorectal cancers. About 70–75% of clients with pancreatic cancer and 60–65% of clients with hepatobiliary cancer have an elevated CA 19.9 level. A minimal elevation of CA 19.9 levels may indicate pancreatitis, cirrhosis, or inflammatory bowel disorder, but *not* pancreatic and hepatobiliary cancer. This is also useful for monitoring the success of treatment and for detecting recurrence of the cancer.

CA 27.29 is a tumor marker to detect breast cancer recurrence in clients with stage II or III. Approximately 64% of clients with metastatic breast cancer have an elevated CA 27.29 level. This test is not approved for screening of breast cancer.

CA 50 is found in clients with gastrointestinal tumors and biliary tract tumors. It tends to be a more sensitive marker as the disease progresses and not when the disease regresses. CA 50 can also be used in diagnosing pancreatic cancer.

CA 125 is an indicator of nonmucinous epithelial ovarian cancer. About 80% of women with an elevated CA 125 greater than 35 units/mL are positive for ovarian cancer. Women with less than 55 units/mL tend to have a better survival rate. Approximately 25% of women with benign ovarian tumors have elevated CA 125. CA 125 is useful to monitor the client's response to chemotherapy and to check if the cancer is recurring. It is better not to repeat CA 125 level until after 3 weeks of chemotherapy.

CA 549 is a new cancer marker to detect breast cancer recurrence and to monitor the response to treatment of breast cancer. It can be used in combination with another cancer screening test, CA 15-3, in detecting moderate to advanced breast cancer. The CA 549 test result could be normal if the breast cancer is in the early stage. The CA 549 may be increased in ovarian and gastric cancer.

Purposes

- To identify clients with elevated serum cancer markers.
- To monitor the effects of treatment for the cancer.
- To determine the recurrence of the cancer.

Clinical Problems

Decreased Level: Effective response to treatment, benign disease.

Increased Levels:

CA 15-3: Breast cancer (most common); metastatic cancer; ovarian, lung, pancreas, colon, prostate cancers; chronic hepatitis; cirrhosis.

CA 19-9: Cancer of the pancreas (most common), colon, liver, GI tract; pancreatitis; cholecystitis; cirrhosis.

CA 27.29: Breast cancer, recurrence of breast cancer, metastatic breast cancer, benign disease.

CA 50: Gastrointestinal tumor, biliary tract tumors.

CA 125: Ovarian cancer (most common); benign ovarian tumors; uterine tumors; cancer of the pancreas, breast, colon, lung; pregnancy; endometriosis; cirrhosis; pancreatitis.

CA 549: Moderate to advance breast cancer, breast cancer metastasis, ovarian and gastric cancer.

Procedure

- No food or fluid restriction is required.
- Collect 5–7 mL of venous blood in a red-top tube.
- Blood sample should be refrigerated immediately.

Factors Affecting Laboratory Results

- Benign breast and ovarian disease may cause an increase in CA 15-3, CA 27.29, CA 125.
- Menstruation may cause a slight elevation of CA 125.
- Radioisotopes given 30 days prior to CA 15-3, CA 19-9, CA 50, CA 125, CA 549.
- False-positive increase level of CA 50 may occur with benign liver disease.

NURSING IMPLICATIONS WITH RATIONALE

- Explain the test procedure to the client.
- Instruct the client to call the health care provider or physician for the test results.
- Have blood sample refrigerated unless it is immediately tested.

Client Teaching

- Be available for client to express feelings or concerns about a specific cancer tumor marker test.
- Be available to answer client's questions about the test results or have the questions answered by another health care professional.

Candida antibody test

Reference Values

Negative

Positive: Greater than 1:8 titer.

Description

This antibody test is to identify systemic candidiasis most often caused by *Candida albicans*, a yeast infection. Candidiasis frequently occurs in the immunocompromised person, and if untreated, the condition can become life threatening. *Candida* infection accounts for approximately 80% of all major systemic fungal infections. It is the fourth most common organism found in bloodstream infections. Nosocomial candidiasis increased about fivefold in the last 10 years, which contributed to the prolongation of hospitalization.

Vulvovaginal candidiasis may result from prolonged use of potent broad-spectrum antibiotics (oral or intravenously administered) and glucocorticoid therapy. This type of candidiasis is associated with debilitating diseases, uncontrolled diabetes mellitus, and pregnancy. If untreated, it can lead to systemic candidiasis. Usually candidiasis occurs to the skin and mucous membrane.

Purpose

- To diagnose systemic candidiasis that cannot be determined by culture or by tissue specimen.

Clinical Problems

Increased Level: Systemic candidiasis.

Procedure

- There is no food or fluid restriction.
- Collect 5 mL of venous blood in a red-top tube. Avoid hemolysis by not shaking the tube.

Factors Affecting Laboratory Results

- Hemolysis of the blood specimen.

NURSING IMPLICATIONS WITH RATIONALE

- Obtain a history of the client's health complaint. Determine if the client is immunocompromised because of HIV or a debilitating disease.
- Record the drugs that the client is taking.
- Check vital signs. Report abnormal findings.

Client Teaching

- Instruct the client to remain on the drug treatment regimen for candidiasis. Stopping the therapy could cause a relapse.
- Listen to the client's concerns. Answer questions, and if answers are unknown, refer the client to other health professionals.

Cannabinoid (marijuana) (urine)

Reference Value

Negative: Less than 50 ng/mL (cutoff concentration).

Description

Marijuana is a mixture of dried leaves and flowering tops of the plant *Cannabis sativa L.* The agents that produce the hallucinogenic and biological effects of marijuana are called cannabinoids. A positive test for cannabinoids indicates the presence of cannabinoid metabolites, of which carboxy THC is the major one.

Peak plasma levels of carboxy THC occur within 10 minutes of inhalation and approximately 1 hour after ingestion. Excretion in the urine begins within 72 hours after exposure and the length of detection can be 30–60 days. With chronic users, carboxy THC may accumulate in fatty tissue, which leads to a longer detection time in the urine because they are released from these sites slowly over time.

Purposes

- To evaluate the use of marijuana.
- To determine if marijuana toxicity has occurred.

Clinical Problems

Increased Level: Presence of carboxy THC, use of marijuana, marijuana toxicity.

Procedure

- There is no food or fluid restriction.
- Collect 20 mL of urine specimen. Repeat urine collection in 1 or 2 days or more if needed.
- Chain-of-custody documentation may be required if testing is for legal purposes.

Factors Affecting Laboratory Tests

- Early urine specimen collection.

NURSING IMPLICATIONS WITH RATIONALE

- Obtain a history of the use of marijuana.
- Monitor vital signs.
- Have another health professional verify or check urine collection for legal purposes. Complete necessary forms for the urine specimen according to the policy of the health department or institution if needed.

Client Teaching

- Be supportive to the client and family. Refer test results requested by family to appropriate health professionals.
- Do not express judgment about marijuana use to client or family.

Carbon dioxide combining power (serum or plasma)

CO_2 Combining Power

Reference Values

Adult: 22–30 mEq/L, 22–30 mmol/L (SI units).

Panic Range: Less than 15 mEq/L and greater than 45 mEq/L.

Child: 20–28 mEq/L.

Description

The serum carbon dioxide (CO_2) test, usually included with the electrolyte test, is performed to determine metabolic acid–base abnormalities. The serum CO_2 acts as a bicarbonate (HCO_3) determinant. When serum CO_2 is low, HCO_3 is lost, and acidosis results (metabolic acidosis). With an elevated serum CO_2, HCO_3 is conserved and alkalosis results (metabolic alkalosis).

Purpose

- To check for the presence of metabolic acidosis or alkalosis.

Clinical Problems

Decreased Level: Metabolic acidosis, diabetic ketoacidosis, starvation, severe diarrhea, dehydration, shock, acute renal failure, salicylate toxicity, exercise. *Drug Influence:* Diuretics (chlorothiazide [Diuril], hydrochlorothiazide [HydroDIURIL], triamterene [Dyrenium]), antibiotics (methicillin, tetracycline), nitrofurantoin (Furadantin) paraldehyde.

Increased Level: Metabolic alkalosis, severe vomiting, gastric suction, peptic ulcer, hypothyroidism, potassium deficit, emphysema (hypoventilation). *Drug Influence:* Barbiturates, steroids (hydrocortisone, cortisone), diuretics (mercurial agents, ethacrynic acid [Edecrin]).

Procedure

- There is no food or fluid restriction.
- Collect 3–5 mL of venous blood in a green-top tube. A tourniquet should be used for a short time.

Factors Affecting Laboratory Results

- Drugs that can increase or decrease the serum CO_2 level (*see Clinical Problems*).

NURSING IMPLICATIONS WITH RATIONALE

Decreased Level

- Know that a decreased serum CO_2 level is related to an acidotic state. Whenever there is excess acid in the body and the kidneys cannot excrete it, metabolic acidosis results. There are many causes of acidosis (*see Clinical Problems above*).

- Assess for signs and symptoms of metabolic acidosis when the client's serum CO_2 level is decreased, especially when it is less than 15 mEq/L. Symptoms include deep, vigorous breathing (Kussmaul breathing), and flushed skin.
- Report clinical findings of metabolic acidosis to the health care provider.

Increased Level

- Know that an increased serum CO_2 level is related to an alkalotic state. Whenever there is an excess of HCO_3 in the body or a loss of acid, metabolic alkalosis occurs. There are many causes of alkalosis (*see Clinical Problems above*).
- Assess for signs and symptoms of metabolic alkalosis when the client has been vomiting or has undergone gastric suctioning for several days. Signs and symptoms include shallow breathing, a serum CO_2 level greater than 30 mEq/L, and a base excess greater than +2.

C

Carbon monoxide, carboxyhemoglobin (blood)

Reference Values

Adult: *Nonsmoker:* Less than 2.5% of hemoglobin. *Smoker:* 4–5% saturation of hemoglobin. *Heavy Smoker:* 5–12% saturation of hemoglobin. *Toxic:* Greater than 15% saturation of hemoglobin. **Child:** Similar to adult nonsmoker.

Description

Carbon monoxide (CO) combines with hemoglobin to produce carboxyhemoglobin, which can occur 200 times more readily than the combination of oxygen with hemoglobin (oxyhemoglobin). When CO replaces oxygen in the hemoglobin in excess of 25%, CO toxicity occurs.

Carbon monoxide is formed from incomplete combustion of carbon-combining compounds, as in automobile exhaust, fumes from improperly functioning furnaces, and cigarette smoke. Continuous exposure to CO, increasing carboxyhemoglobin by greater than 60%, leads to coma and death. The treatment for CO toxicity is to administer a high concentration of oxygen.

Purpose

- To determine the percentage of CO in the hemoglobin; if high, it could be fatal.

Clinical Problems

Increased Level: Smoking and exposure to cigarette smoke, automobile exhaust fumes, and defective gas-burning appliances.

Procedure

- There is no food or fluid restriction.
- Collect 7 mL of venous blood in a lavender-top tube.
- The most common method of analysis is performed with an IL-CO oximeter, a direct-reading instrument.

Factors Affecting Laboratory Results

- Heavy smoking.

C

NURSING IMPLICATIONS WITH RATIONALE

- Determine from the client's history (obtained from the client, family, or friends) whether CO inhalation could have occurred.
- Assess for mild to severe CO toxicity. Symptoms of mild CO toxicity are headache, weakness, malaise, dizziness, and dyspnea with exertion. Symptoms of moderate to severe toxicity are severe headache, bright-red mucous membranes, and cherry-red blood. When carboxyhemoglobin exceeds 40%, the blood's residue is brick red.
- Identify individuals who might be a candidate for CO poisoning. Persons complaining of continuous headaches or who are living (24 hours a day) in a house with an old heating system in the winter should have a blood CO test performed.

Carcinoembryonic antigen (CEA) (serum, plasma)

Reference Values

Adult: *Nonsmokers:* Less than 2.5 ng/mL. *Smokers:* Less than 5 ng/mL. *Acute Inflammatory Disorders:* Greater than 10 ng/mL. *Neoplasms:* Greater than 12 ng/mL.

Child: Not normally done; assumed to be low (level) after the child is several months old.

Description

Carcinoembryonic antigen (CEA) has been found in the GI epithelium of embryos and has been extracted from tumors in the adult gastrointestinal tract. Originally the CEA test was used to detect colon cancer, especially adenocarcinoma. Elevated levels might occur when inflammation and tissue destruction are present. CEA should never be used as the sole criterion for diagnosis.

The CEA test is a nonspecific test. However, elevated levels have been found in approximately 70% of clients with known cancer of the large intestine and pancreas. The primary role of the CEA test is to monitor the treatment of colon and pancreatic carcinoma. It is also used for follow-up studies once cancer has been diagnosed. If the levels fall after treatment, the cancer is most likely under control. A CEA test may be ordered at 30- to 90-day intervals, and if a significant CEA level recurs, the physician may resume chemotherapy treatments or consider another form of therapy.

Purposes

- To monitor the treatment for colon or pancreatic carcinoma.
- To compare with other laboratory tests for diagnosing an inflammatory condition or GI or pancreatic cancer.

Clinical Problems

Increased Level: *Cancer:* GI tract (esophagus, stomach, small and large intestine, rectum), liver, pancreas, lung, breast, cervix, bladder, testes, kidney; leukemia; pulmonary emphysema; cirrhosis of the liver; bacterial pneumonia; chronic ischemic heart disease; acute pancreatitis; acute renal failure; ulcerative colitis; chronic cigarette smoking; neuroblastoma; inflammatory diseases; surgical trauma.

Procedure

- There is no food or fluid restriction.
- Collect 5–7 mL of venous blood in a red-top or lavender-top tube (preferred). Avoid hemolysis.
- Heparin should not be administered for 2 days before the test. It interferes with the results.

Factors Affecting Laboratory Results

- Heparin interferes with the result of the CEA test.
- Hemolysis can affect test results.

NURSING IMPLICATIONS WITH RATIONALE

Increased Level

- Relate clinical problems to elevated CEA levels. CEA levels greater than 12 ng/mL do not always indicate cancer, nor do levels less than 10 ng/mL indicate an absence of cancer. The CEA test is useful for management of cancer treatment.
- Be supportive of client and family while awaiting test results.
- Hold heparin injections for 2 days before the test, with the health care provider's permission. If heparin is given, this fact should be noted on the laboratory slip.

Cardiolipin antibodies (IgG, IgM) (serum)

See Anticardiolipin Antibodies

Cardiovascular disease (CVD) genetic test (serum, blood)

Angiotensinogen (AGT) Gene

Reference Values

Negative: Absence of angiotensinogen (AGT) gene.

Description

Many clients with cardiovascular disease (CVD) do not have risk factors of CVD, for example, hypercholesterolemia, high blood pressure (hypertension), diabetes mellitus, and/or obesity. The angiotensinogen (AGT) gene is a strong indicator of CVD. AGT is an autosomal recessive gene, and when the client has a pair of elevated AGT genes, he or she has a greater chance of developing CVD at an early age. These clients have a risk of life-threatening angina pectoris, myocardial infarction, hypertension, and cardiomegaly. With a high risk for CVD, the client should be monitored frequently for signs and symptoms of CVD, for example, chest pain, dyspnea, fluid retention, high blood pressure, elevated lipids, and diabetes mellitus. Treatment might include lipid-lowering drugs, antihypertension drugs, diuretics, and management of diabetes. Genetic counseling may be suggested.

Purposes

- To identify the client who is at risk of CVD, for example, familial history of CVD.
- To monitor signs and symptoms of CVD.

Clinical Problems

Increased Level: Elevated angiotensinogen (AGT) gene, hypercholesterolemia, hypertension, diabetes mellitus, angina pectoris, myocardial infarction.

Procedure

- No food or fluid restriction is required. Some institutions may have a restriction.
- Collect 5–7 mL of venous blood in a red- or lavender-top tube.

Factors Affecting Laboratory Results

- None known.

NURSING IMPLICATIONS WITH RATIONALE

- Obtain a history of familial CVD and signs and symptoms of CVD.
- Assess laboratory results, for example, AGT, lipid profile, electrolytes. These laboratory tests are needed as well as other tests to diagnose cardiovascular disease.
- Take baseline VS (vital signs). Monitor VS as indicated.

Client Teaching

- Suggest that the client seek genetic counseling when the AGT levels are elevated.
- Be available to answer questions that the client may have or refer the questions to other health professionals.
- Be supportive of the client during and following testing for genetic CVD.

Carotene (serum)

Reference Values

Adult: 60–300 mcg/dL, 0.74–3.72 µmol/L (SI units) (varies with diet).

Child: 40–130 mcg/dL.

Description

Carotene is a fat-soluble vitamin found in yellow and green vegetables and fruits. After absorption from the intestine, carotene is stored in the liver and can be converted to vitamin A, according to body needs. When fat absorption is decreased, the serum carotene level is decreased, which is indicative of fat malabsorption syndrome. Causes of serum carotene deficit include poor diet, malabsorption, high fever, and pancreatic insufficiency.

Purpose

- To determine the cause of malabsorption syndrome or liver disease.

Clinical Problems

Decreased Level: Malabsorption syndrome, pancreatic insufficiency, protein malnutrition, febrile illness, severe liver disease, cystic fibrosis.

Increased Level: Hyperlipidemia, diabetes mellitus, chronic nephritis, hypothyroidism, diet high in carrots, hypervitaminosis A (slight elevation), pregnancy, hypocholesterolemia.

Procedure

- Foods rich in carotene—yellow and green vegetables, vegetable juice, and fruits—should be omitted for 2–3 days before the test (check laboratory procedure). If the health care provider wishes to check the serum carotene level for determining the absorption ability, a diet high in carotene will be ordered for several days. Water is permitted.
- NPO, a diet low in carotene, or a diet high in carotene should be recorded on the laboratory slip.
- Collect 7 mL of venous blood in a red-top tube. Protect from light.

Factors Affecting Laboratory Results

- Mineral oil will interfere with carotene absorption.
- Foods rich in carotene can affect the serum results.

NURSING IMPLICATIONS WITH RATIONALE

Client Teaching

- Explain to the client that diet will be high or low in carotene, depending on the health care provider's clinical assumptions and orders. Drinking water is permitted.
- Explain to the client that the test is to determine whether there is a vitamin (carotene) deficiency.
- Answer the client's questions concerning what foods to avoid or to eat before the test. Vegetables and fruits are rich in carotene.

Catecholamines (plasma)

Reference Values

Epinephrine: *Supine:* Less than 50 pg/mL. *Sitting:* Less than 60 pg/mL. *Standing:* Less than 90 pg/mL.

Norepinephrine: *Supine:* 110–410 pg/mL. *Sitting:* 120–680 pg/mL. *Standing:* 125–700 pg/mL.

Dopamine: *Supine and Standing:* Less than 87 pg/mL.

Pheochromocytoma: *Total Catecholamines:* Greater than 1,000 pg/mL.

Description

The three main catecholamines are epinephrine (adrenaline), norepinephrine, and dopamine, which are hormones secreted by the adrenal medulla. These catecholamines respond to stress, fear, hypoxia, hemorrhage, and strenuous exercise by increasing the blood pressure. Catecholamines can be measured from plasma or by a 24-hour urine collection specimen. Catecholamine levels can vary according to time of day, body posture, and stress. The 24-hour urine catecholamine collection has the advantage of determining the daily secretion of hormones. A single plasma catecholamine level could be misleading because of catecholamine fluctuation, but it is considered 75% effective in diagnosing pheochromocytomas. Incorrect collection of a plasma catecholamine level can cause an inaccurate test result.

Fractional analysis of catecholamine levels (epinephrine, norepinephrine, dopamine) is helpful for identifying certain adrenal medullary tumors suspected in hypertensive clients. A comparison of the plasma catecholamine level with a 24-hour urine catecholamine test can aid in diagnosing pheochromocytoma.

Purpose

- To assist in the diagnosis of the health problem related to the abnormal amount of catecholamines in the plasma and urine.

Clinical Problems

Decreased Level: *Norepinephrine:* Anorexia nervosa, orthostatic hypotension. *Dopamine:* Parkinsonism.

Increased Level: *Epinephrine and Norepinephrine:* Pheochromocytoma (continuous elevation with epinephrine); ganglioneuroblastoma, ganglioneuroma, and neuroblastoma (higher elevations with norepinephrine); diabetic ketoacidosis; kidney disease; shock; thyrotoxicosis; acute myocardial infarction; strenuous exercise. *Drug Influence:* Epinephrine, norepinephrine, bronchodilators, amphetamines, selected beta-adrenergics.

Procedure

- Foods rich in amines, such as chocolate, cocoa, wine, beer, tea, aged cheese, nuts (especially walnuts), and bananas, should be avoided 2 days prior to test.
- Selected drugs, such as over-the-counter cold medications that contain sympathomimetics, diuretics, and antihypertensives, should be avoided for 2 days prior to the test.

- Strenuous exercise and smoking should be avoided prior to the test.
- NPO (food and fluids) 12 hours prior to the test.
- An indwelling venous catheter may be inserted for collection of blood samples. Having an IV in place helps to avoid a surge in catecholamine release when a venipuncture is performed during collection of the blood sample. The test may require a blood sample while the client is in a supine position and a sample while in a standing position. Blood should be collected early in the morning.
- Collect 7–10 mL of venous blood in a green- or lavender-top tube. Place the blood sample immediately in an ice bath and take it to the laboratory. The laboratory should be notified when the specimen is obtained because the test should be run within 5–10 minutes after being drawn.

Factors Affecting Laboratory Results

- Not following the test procedure.
- Not putting the blood sample on ice or not running the test immediately.
- Plasma catecholamine levels decrease rapidly if red blood cells are not separated from the plasma within 5–10 minutes.

NURSING IMPLICATIONS WITH RATIONALE

- Monitor the client's BP. Report BP that remains elevated and responds poorly to drug therapy.
- Check urine output. Report abnormal decreases in urine output.
- Ascertain if the client is extremely apprehensive or has given indications of stressful situation(s). Catecholamine levels are increased during stressful conditions.
- Alert the laboratory of the order for plasma catecholamine. This is necessary so that the test can be processed in the laboratory within 5 minutes after the blood sample is obtained.

Client Teaching

- Explain the procedure to the client. An explanation should be given at least 24 hours before the test (in most cases, 48 hours). Writing out the procedure for the client may be helpful in relieving anxiety.
- Emphasize the importance of not exercising or smoking before the test. Encourage the client to relax as much as possible prior to the test.
- Listen to the client's concerns. Refer questions to other health care providers as needed.

Catecholamines (urine)

Reference Values

Adult: Less than 100 mcg/24 h (higher with activity), less than 0.59 μmol/24 h (SI units), 0–14 mcg/dL (random), epinephrine less than 20 ng/24 h, norepinephrine less than 100 ng/24 h.

Child: Level less than adult because of weight differences.

Description

Catecholamines are hormones (epinephrine and norepinephrine) secreted by the adrenal medulla. Catecholamine production increases after strenuous exercise; however, urinary levels are 3–100 times greater than normal in cases of pheochromocytoma (tumor of the adrenal medulla). In some psychiatric clients, the urine catecholamine level increases only slightly. In children, this test may be used to diagnose malignant neuroblastoma.

Certain drugs, coffee, and bananas cause elevated catecholamine levels. The urine catecholamine test is considered a more reliable test than a serum catecholamine test.

Purposes

(*See Catecholamines [plasma].*)

Clinical Problems

Increased Level: Pheochromocytoma, severe stress (septicemia, shock, burn, peritonitis), malignant neuroblastoma, acute myocardial infarction (first 48 hours), chronic ischemic heart disease, cor pulmonale, carcinoid syndrome, bipolar disorder, depressive neurosis, strenuous exercise. *Drug Influence:* Antibiotics (ampicillin, demeclocycline, erythromycin, tetracyclines), antihypertensives (methyldopa [Aldomet], hydralazine [Apresoline]), vitamins (ascorbic acid [vitamin C], B complex), chlorpromazine (Thorazine), quinine, quinidine, isoproterenol (Isuprel) or epinephrine by inhalation.

Procedure

- Food and fluids other than those mentioned below are not restricted.
- Drugs, chocolate, coffee, and bananas should not be taken for 3–7 days before the test. The number of days may vary among laboratories.
- Collect urine for 24 hours in a large container with a preservative (10 mL of concentrated hydrochloric acid), and keep the bottle refrigerated. The pH of the urine collection should be below 3.
- Label the large container with the client's name and the dates and exact times of the 24-hour urine collection (e.g., 4/10/20, 7:30 AM to 4/11/20, 7:30 AM).

Factors Affecting Laboratory Results

- Foods such as bananas, coffee, chocolate, and vanilla could cause an inaccurate test result.
- Certain drugs can affect test results (*see Drug Influence*).

NURSING IMPLICATIONS WITH RATIONALE

Client Teaching

- Explain to the client and family that all urine should be saved in the refrigerated container. Inform the client that toilet paper and feces should not be put in the urine.
- Explain to the client that there is a strong acid that acts as a preservative in the urine container and that he or she should not urinate directly into the container.
- Explain that fasting can increase catecholamine levels. Foods are not restricted except for those listed in the procedure.

Increased Level

- Recognize the causes of an elevated urine catecholamine level other than pheochromocytoma. These include severe stress, strenuous exercise, and acute anxiety and other psychiatric disorders. The highest levels occur in pheochromocytoma.
- Check vital signs and report rising blood pressure readings.
- Report if the client has been involved in strenuous activity or has suffered from severe anxiety.

C

Cerebrospinal fluid (CSF)

[Color, Pressure, Cell Count, Protein, Chloride, Glucose, Culture] Spinal Fluid

Reference Values

	COLOR	PRESSURE (mm H$_2$O)	CELL COUNT (LEUKOCYTES) (mm^3, μL)	PROTEIN (mg/dL)	CHLORIDE (mEq/L)	GLUCOSE (mg/dL)
Adult	Clear, colorless	75–175	0–8	15–45	118–132	40–80
Child	Clear, colorless	50–100	0–8	14–45	120–128	35–75
Premature infant			0–20	less than 400		
Newborn	Clear		0–15	30–200	110–122	20–40
1–6 months				30–100		

Description

Cerebrospinal fluid (CSF), also known as spinal fluid, circulates in the ventricles of the brain and through the spinal cord. Of the 150 mL of CSF, approximately 100 mL are produced by the blood in the brain ventricles and are reabsorbed back into circulation daily.

Spinal fluid is obtained by a lumbar puncture (spinal tap) performed in the lumbar sac at L3–4, or at L4–5. First CSF pressure is measured, then fluid is aspirated and placed in sterile test tubes. Data from the analysis of the spinal fluid are important for diagnosing spinal cord and brain diseases.

The analysis of spinal fluid usually includes color, pressure, cell count (leukocytes, or white blood cells [WBCs]), protein, chloride, and glucose. In addition, the pH of the CSF is usually checked; it is usually slightly lower, about one-tenth (0.1) of a point, than the pH of the serum. The CSF protein and glucose levels are lower than the blood levels; however, the CSF chloride level is higher than the serum chloride level. Normally a culture is done to detect any organism present in the fluid.

Purpose

- To detect color, pressure, leukocyte count, protein, glucose, and presence of bacteria in the CSF.

Clinical Problems

CSF	DECREASED LEVEL	ELEVATED LEVEL	COMMENTS
Color		Abnormal color	
		1. Pink or red—subarachnoid or cerebral hemorrhage; traumatic spinal tap	
		2. Xanthochromia (yellow color)—previous sub-arachnoid hemorrhage	Yellow color indicates old blood (4–5 days after a cerebral hemorrhage), mixture of bilirubin and blood, or extremely elevated protein levels; fluid discoloration normally remains for 3 weeks.
Pressure	Dehydration, hypovolemia	Intracranial pressure due to meningitis, subarachnoid hemorrhage, brain tumor, brain abscess, encephalitis	Slight elevation can occur with holding breath or tensing of muscles.
Cell count (lymphocytes)		Less than 500 mm^3 (μL): viral infections—poliomyelitis, aseptic meningitis, syphilis of CNS; multiple sclerosis; brain tumor; abscess; subarachnoid hemorrhage (40% or more monocytes)	WBC differential count may be ordered to identify the types of leukocytes.
		Greater than 500 mm^3 (μL): ↑ granulocytes, purulent infection	
Protein		Meningitis: tuberculosis, purulent, aseptic Guillain-Barré syndrome Subarachnoid hemorrhage Brain tumor Abscess Syphilis	Protein and cell counts usually increase together.
		Drug influence anesthetics acetophenetidin (phenacetin) chlorpromazine (Thorazine) salicylates (aspirin) streptomycin sulfonamides	

CSF	DECREASED LEVEL	ELEVATED LEVEL	COMMENTS
Chloride	Tubercular meningitis Bacterial meningitis		IV saline or electrolyte infusion could cause an inaccurate result. Syphilis, brain tumors and abscess, and encephalitis do not affect the CSF chloride level.
Glucose	Purulent meningitis Presence of fungi, protozoa, or pyogenic bacteria Subarachnoid hemorrhage Lymphomas Leukemia	Cerebral trauma Hypothalamic lesions Diabetes (hyperglycemia)	Brain abscess or tumor and degenerative diseases have little effect on the CSF glucose. The CSF glucose is usually two thirds of the blood glucose. The blood glucose level is determined for comparative reasons.
Culture		Meningitis	Generally done when meningitis is suspected.

Procedure

- There is no food or fluid restriction.
- Collect a sterile lumbar puncture tray, an antiseptic solution (e.g., povidone-iodine or iodine), a local anesthetic (e.g., lidocaine), sterile gloves, and tape.
- Place the client in a "fetal" position, with the back bowed, the head flexed on the chest, and the knees drawn up to the abdomen.
- Label the three test tubes 1, 2, and 3.
- The physician checks the spinal fluid pressure, using a manometer attached to the needle. The physician collects a total of 9–12 mL of spinal fluid—3 mL in no. 1 tube, 3 mL in no. 2 tube, and 3 mL in no. 3 tube. The first tube could be contaminated (with blood from the spinal tap) and should *not* be used for cell count, culture, or protein determination.
- Label the tubes with the client's name and room number and the date. Take the test tubes immediately to the laboratory.

Queckenstedt Procedure: The Queckenstedt procedure is performed during a lumbar puncture when spinal block is suspected. Temporary pressure is applied to the jugular veins while the CSF pressure is monitored. Normally the CSF pressure will rise when the jugular veins are compressed. In partial or total CSF block, the pressure fails to rise with jugular vein compression, or it takes 15–30 seconds for CSF pressure to drop after compression is released.

Factors Affecting Laboratory Results

- Refrigeration may affect the results of the culture.
- A traumatic spinal tap could cause the presence of blood in the fluid specimen, which could be mistaken for a clinical problem.
- Certain drugs could cause a false, increased, CSF protein level (*see Clinical Problems: Drug Influence*).
- IV fluid containing chloride could invalidate the CSF chloride level determination.
- Hyperglycemia could increase the CSF glucose level.

NURSING IMPLICATIONS WITH RATIONALE

- Explain the procedure for the lumbar puncture to the client by giving a step-by-step detailed explanation.
- Collect the specimen in numerical order of tubes. Do not mix the numbers. The first tube may have some red blood cells because of the needle insertion. For culture, the second or third test tube is used. For protein and cell count, the third specimen tube is used.
- Check the vital signs before the procedure and afterward at specified times (e.g., ½, 1, 2, and 4 hours).
- Assess for changes in the neurologic status after the procedure (e.g., increased temperature, increased blood pressure, irritability, numbness and tingling in the lower extremities, and nonreactive eye pupils).
- Administer an analgesic as ordered to relieve a headache if it occurs.
- Be supportive of the client before, during, and after the lumbar puncture.

Client Teaching

- Instruct the client to relax and to take deep and slow breaths with his or her mouth open. Hold the client's hand to give reassurance, unless this is opposed by the client.
- Instruct the client to remain flat in bed in the prone or supine position for 4–8 hours following the lumbar puncture. Headaches are common because of spinal fluid leaking from the site of the lumbar puncture, which can occur if the client is in an upright position.

Ceruloplasmin (Cp) (serum)

Reference Values

Adult: 18–45 mg/dL, 180–450 mg/L (SI units).

Child: *Infant:* Less than 23 mg/dL, or may be normal. *Child:* 30–65 mg/dL.

Description

Ceruloplasmin (Cp) is a copper-containing glycoprotein known as one of the alpha-2-globulins in the plasma. Ceruloplasmin is produced in the liver and binds with copper. The principal role of ceruloplasmin is not clearly understood, except that when there is a serum deficit, there is an increased urinary excretion of copper and increased depositing of copper on the cornea, brain, liver, and kidney, causing damage and destruction of the organs. A deficit of ceruloplasmin or hypoceruloplasmin can result in Wilson disease (hepatolenticular degeneration), commonly seen between the ages of 7 and 15 and in early middle age.

Purpose

- To detect Wilson disease or a liver disorder.

Clinical Problems

Decreased Level: Wilson disease (hepatolenticular degeneration), protein malnutrition, nephrotic syndrome, newborns, and early infancy.

Increased Level: Cirrhosis of the liver; hepatitis; pregnancy; Hodgkin disease; cancer of the bone, stomach, lung; myocardial infarction; rheumatoid arthritis; infections and inflammatory process; exercise. *Drug Influence:* Oral contraceptives, estrogen drugs.

Procedure

- There is no food or fluid restriction.
- Collect 3–5 mL of venous blood in a red-top tube.
- Withhold drugs containing estrogen for 24 hours before the blood test, with the health care provider's permission.

Factors Affecting Laboratory Results

- Estrogen therapy, pregnancy, and exercise could cause an elevated serum ceruloplasmin level.
- In Wilson disease with severe liver damage, a normal serum level could result.

NURSING IMPLICATIONS WITH RATIONALE

Decreased Level

- Relate hypoceruloplasmin (serum ceruloplasmin deficit) to Wilson disease; serum level below 15 mg/dL after the age of 7.
- Assess for signs and symptoms of Wilson disease (e.g., abnormal muscular rigidity [dystonia], tremors of the fingers, dysarthria, and mental disturbances).
- Check the cornea of the eye for a discolored ring (Kayser-Fleischer ring) from copper deposits.

Increased Level

- Relate clinical problems of liver disorders, cancer, infections, inflammations, and drugs to hyperceruloplasmin (serum ceruloplasmin excess).
- Note whether the client has been exercising in the last 24 hours, because a slight elevation could be due to strenuous exercise.

Chlamydia (serum and tissue smear or culture)

Reference Values

Normal Titer: Less than 1:16.

Positive Titer: Equal to or greater than 1:64.

C

Description

Chlamydia is a bacteria-like organism and has some features of a virus. There are two species of chlamydia: *C. psittaci*, which can cause psittacosis in birds and humans, and *C. trachomatis*, which appears in three types (lymphogranuloma venereum [LGV, venereal disease], genital and other infections, and trachoma [eye disorder]).

The occurrence of *C. psittaci* is more common in persons working in pet stores who may have contact with infected birds such as parakeets and in those working in the poultry industry who may come in contact with infected turkeys. A respiratory infection may result and could cause chlamydial pneumonia. Serologic testing or tissue culture may be performed for diagnosis.

The *C. trachomatis* strain, LGV, is transmitted through sexual intercourse. It can occur in both males and females, causing enlargement of the inguinal and pelvic lymph nodes. Pregnant women can pass chlamydia infection to the newborn during birthing. This can cause trachoma ophthalmia neonatorum in the infant, which may lead to blindness later if untreated. Untreated genital infections caused by *C. trachomatis* could lead to sterility.

With psittacosis and LGV, the serum titer level is greater than 1:64 (more than four times the reference value). The titer level for genital infection caused by *C. trachomatis* is usually between 1:16 and 1:64. Normally the general population has a titer level of less than 1:16. Tissue culture may be used to confirm test results with the titer level. Tetracycline and erythromycin, not penicillin, are usually the antibiotics used to treat chlamydia.

Purpose

- To identify the presence of a chlamydial infection, *C. psittaci* or *C. trachomatis*.

Clinical Problems

Positive Titer: Psittacosis; LGV; genital infections—pelvic inflammatory disease (PID), endometriosis, salpingitis; trachoma ophthalmia neonatorum; chlamydial pneumonia.

Negative Titer: Antibiotic therapy.

Procedure

- There is no food or fluid restriction.
- Collect 3–5 mL of venous blood in a red-top tube. Avoid hemolysis.
- Tissue smear or culture may be obtained from the cervix or other areas.

Factors Affecting Laboratory Results

- Hemolysis of the blood specimen.
- Antibiotic therapy taken before tests could cause negative test results.

NURSING IMPLICATIONS WITH RATIONALE

- Obtain a history from the client of any contact with birds that may be infected with *C. psittaci*. Clients who work in pet shops or the poultry industry may be infected with *C. psittaci* and have psittacosis.

- Check for signs and symptoms of psittacosis, which include a nonproductive or slightly productive cough, chills, fever, headache, gastrointestinal symptoms, bradycardia, and mental changes.
- Assess if the woman is pregnant and has enlargement of the pelvic or inguinal lymph nodes. Genital infection from chlamydia could be passed to the infant during vaginal birthing process. Prenatal screening of pregnant women for chlamydial infection is being considered. Symptoms can be vague. The incidence of chlamydial infection in infants is 28 out of 1,000 live births.

Client Teaching

- Encourage the client with *C. trachomatis* infection to give name(s) of sexual partner(s). Certain antibiotic therapies can eliminate the organism and prevent passing the infection to others. The sexual partner(s) may also need treatment.
- Explain to the mother with a chlamydial infection that the infant should be checked.
- Inform clients with a titer less than 1:16 that an acute chlamydial infection is unlikely.
- Listen to the client's concerns. Respond to questions and/or refer to other health professionals as needed.

Chlordiazepoxide (serum)

Librium, Librax

Reference Values

Adult: *Therapeutic Range:* 1–5 mcg/mL. *Peak Time:* 1–3 h. *Toxic Level:* Greater than 5 mcg/mL.

Description

Chlordiazepoxide (Librium), a benzodiazepine and anxiolytic, is used mostly for the treatment of anxiety and alcohol withdrawal effects. It also suppresses seizure activity.

Purposes

- To monitor chlordiazepoxide levels for the treatment of anxiety or alcohol withdrawal.
- To detect a chlordiazepoxide toxic level.

Clinical Problems

Decreased Level: *Drug Influence:* Phenothiazine drug group.

Increased Level: Overdose of chlordiazepoxide.

Procedure

- There is no food or fluid restriction.
- Collect 7 mL of venous blood in a red-top tube.

Factors Affecting Laboratory Results

- Phenothiazines and taking other benzodiazepines with chlordiazepoxide could cause central nervous system depression.

C

NURSING IMPLICATIONS WITH RATIONALE

- Observe for side effects of chlordiazepoxide (e.g., lethargy, drowsiness, slurred speech, tremors, transient hypotension, dizziness, bradycardia, dry mouth).

Client Teaching

- Instruct the client to report side effects. Many of the side effects will disappear after taking the drug for a few days.
- Advise the client that if dizziness occurs he or she should rise slowly from a lying position.
- Inform the client to avoid heavy smoking, because it could cause side effects. Heavy smoking can enhance the effect of chlordiazepoxide.
- Explain to the client that antacids might delay absorption of Librium. Inform the health care provider if the client is taking antacids.

Chloride (Cl) (serum)

Reference Values

Adult: 95–105 mEq/L, 95–105 mmol/L (SI units).

Child: *Newborn:* 94–112 mEq/L. *Infant:* 95–110 mEq/L. *Child:* 98–105 mEq/L.

Description

Chloride is an anion found mostly in the extracellular fluid. Chloride plays an important role in maintaining body water balance, osmolality of body fluids (with sodium), and acid–base balance. It combines with the hydrogen ion to produce the acidity (hydrochloric acid) in the stomach.

For maintaining acid–base balance, chloride competes with bicarbonate for sodium. When the body fluids are more acidic, the kidneys excrete chloride and sodium, and bicarbonate is reabsorbed. In addition, chloride shifts in and out of red blood cells in exchange with bicarbonate.

Most of the chloride ingested is combined with sodium (sodium chloride [NaCl] or "salt"). The daily required chloride intake is 2 g. *Hypochloremia* means serum chloride deficit; *hyperchloremia* means serum chloride excess.

Purpose

- To check the chloride level in relation to potassium, sodium, and acid–base balance.

Clinical Problems

Decreased Level: Vomiting, gastric suctioning, diarrhea, hypokalemia (decreased potassium), hyponatremia (decreased sodium), low-sodium diet, continuous IV 5% dextrose in water (D_5W), gastroenteritis, colitis, adrenal gland insufficiency (Addison disease), diabetic acidosis, heat exhaustion, hyperaldosteronism, acute infections, burns, excessive diaphoresis (sweating/perspiration), metabolic alkalosis. *Drug Influence:* Diuretics (mercurials, thiazides, loop), bicarbonates.

Increased Level: Dehydration, hypernatremia (increased sodium), hyperparathyroidism, cancer of the stomach, multiple myeloma, adrenal gland hyperactivity, head injury, eclampsia, cardiac decompensation, excessive IV saline (0.9% NaCl), kidney dysfunction (glomerulonephritis, acute renal failure, pyelonephritis), hyperventilation, metabolic acidosis. *Drug Influence:* Acetazolamide, ammonium chloride, boric acid, cortisone preparations, ion exchange resins, prolonged use of triamterene (Dyrenium).

Procedure

- There is no food or fluid restriction. This test may be combined with other tests (e.g., for serum electrolytes), so the client may be NPO. Check with the laboratory.
- Collect 3–5 mL of venous blood in a red- or green-top tube.

Factors Affecting Laboratory Results

- Drugs (*see Drug Influence*).

NURSING IMPLICATIONS WITH RATIONALE

Decreased Level

- Assess for signs and symptoms of hypochloremia (hyperexcitability of the nervous system and muscles, tetany [twitching, tremors], slow and shallow breathing, and decreased blood pressure resulting from fluid and chloride loss).
- Inform the health care provider when the client is receiving IV D_5W continuously. If no other solutes are given, the body fluids will be diluted, and the client will not receive the daily required chloride intake.
- Check the serum potassium and sodium levels. Chloride is frequently lost with sodium and potassium (plentiful in the gastrointestinal tract). With vomiting, potassium, hydrogen, and chloride are lost, causing hypokalemic–hypochloremic alkalosis. Both potassium and chloride must be replaced, for if potassium is given and not chloride, hypokalemic alkalosis will persist.
- Observe for symptoms of overhydration when the client is receiving several liters of normal saline (0.9% NaCl) for sodium and chloride replacement. Sodium holds water, and if there is a history of a heart or kidney disorder, water accumulation could occur. Symptoms of overhydration include a constant, irritated cough; dyspnea; neck and hand vein engorgement; and chest rales.

Client Teaching

- Instruct the client *not* to drink only plain water if there is a serum chloride deficit. Encourage the client to drink fluids containing sodium and chloride (e.g., broth, tomato juice, cola drinks).
- Instruct the client to drink and eat foods rich in chloride (e.g., broth, seafood, milk, meats, eggs, and table salt).

Increased Level

- Assess for signs and symptoms of hyperchloremia (similar to acidosis)—weakness, lethargy, and deep, rapid, vigorous breathing.
- Notify the health care provider if the client is receiving IV fluids containing normal saline. Check for symptoms of overhydration.
- Monitor daily weights and intake and output to determine whether fluid retention is present because of sodium and chloride excess.

Client Teaching

- Instruct the client to avoid drinking or eating salty foods. Encourage the client not to use the salt shaker and some salt substitutes.
- Instruct the client to read labels, because some salt substitutes contain calcium chloride or potassium chloride.

Chloride (sweat)

Screening (Silver Nitrate); Iontophoresis (Pilocarpine)

Reference Values

Adult: Less than 60 mEq/L.

Child: Less than 50 mEq/L; marginal: 50–60 mEq/L; abnormal: greater than 60 mEq/L (possible cystic fibrosis).

Description

Sodium and chloride concentrations in sweat are higher in persons with cystic fibrosis, even though there usually is not an increased amount of sweat. Sweat chloride is considered more reliable than sweat sodium for diagnostic purposes. Some falsely negative sweat sodium levels have been reported in persons with cystic fibrosis.

Two types of sweat chloride tests are used: (1) screening tests, which use silver nitrate on agar or filter (special) paper and require contact with the hand (palm or fingers), and (2) iontophoresis, in which pilocarpine is placed on the forearm to increase sweat gland secretion. A positive screening test is usually validated with iontophoresis, because the chloride level in the palm of the hand is usually higher than anywhere else. Some health care providers believe that the screening should be routine in all children; however, others disagree.

Purpose

- To aid in the detection of cystic fibrosis.

Clinical Problems

Increased Level: Cystic fibrosis, asthma.

Procedure

Screening Test (Silver Nitrate)
- Wash the child's hand and dry it. For 15 minutes, keep the hand from contacting any other part of the body.
- Moisten the test paper containing silver nitrate compound with distilled water (*not saline*).
- Press the child's hand on the paper for 4 seconds.
- A positive result occurs when the excess chloride combines with the silver nitrate to form white silver chloride on the paper.
- A heavy hand imprint is left by the child with cystic fibrosis.

Iontophoresis (Pilocarpine): Usually performed by laboratory personnel.
- There is no food or fluid restriction.
- Electrodes are placed on the skin of the forearm to create a small electric current for transporting pilocarpine (a stimulating drug) into the skin to induce sweating.
- Sweat is collected and weighed. Chloride is measured.

Factors Affecting Laboratory Results

- Unwashed hands for the screening test affect test results.
- Use of saline solution to moisten the test paper causes inaccurate test results.

NURSING IMPLICATIONS WITH RATIONALE

- Explain the procedures (screening or iontophoresis or both) to the child and family. Answer questions if possible, or refer them to appropriate health professionals.
- Explain to the child and family that the tests are not painful.
- Remain with the child during the procedure. Give comfort and reassurance as needed.

Increased Level

- Associate an elevated sweat chloride level with cystic fibrosis. With cystic fibrosis, sweat chloride levels could be 2–5 times greater than normal.
- Obtain a familial history of cystic fibrosis, when indicated.
- Determine whether the child has washed and dried his or her hands before the screening test is performed. Dried sweat can leave a chloride residue, thus causing a false-positive result.

Cholesterol (serum)

Reference Values

Adult: *Desirable Level:* Less than 200 mg/dL. *Moderate Risk:* 200–240 mg/dL. *High Risk:* Greater than 240 mg/dL. *Pregnancy:* High risk levels but a return to prepregnancy values 1 month after delivery.

Child: *Infant:* 90–130 mg/dL. *Child (2–19 Years): Desirable Level:* 130–170 mg/dL. *Moderate Risk:* 171–184 mg/dL. *High Risk:* Greater than 185 mg/dL.

Description

Cholesterol is a blood lipid synthesized by the liver and is found in red blood cells, cell membranes, and muscles. About 70% of cholesterol is esterified (combined with fatty acids), and 30% is in the free form. Cholesterol is used by the body to form bile salts for fat digestion and for the formation of hormones by the adrenal glands, ovaries, and testes. Thyroid hormones and estrogen decrease the concentration of cholesterol and an oophorectomy increases it.

Serum cholesterol is used as an indicator of atherosclerosis and coronary artery disease. Hypercholesterolemia causes plaque deposits in the coronary arteries, thus contributing to myocardial infarction. High serum cholesterol levels can be due to a familial (hereditary) tendency, biliary obstruction, and/or dietary intake. Approximately one third of Americans have a serum cholesterol level below 200 mg dL, which is desirable.

Purposes

- To check the client's cholesterol level.
- To monitor cholesterol levels.

Clinical Problems

Decreased Level: Hyperthyroidism, Cushing syndrome (adrenal hormone excess), starvation, malabsorption, anemias, acute infections. *Drug Influence:* Antilipids (Zocor, Mevacor, Lipitor), thyroxine, antibiotics (kanamycin, neomycin, paromomycin, tetracycline), nicotinic acid, estrogens, glucagon, heparin, salicylates (aspirin), colchicine, oral hypoglycemic agents.

Increased Level: Acute myocardial infarction; atherosclerosis, hypothyroidism, biliary obstruction; biliary cirrhosis; cholangitis; familial hypercholesterolemia; uncontrolled diabetes mellitus; nephrotic syndrome; pancreatectomy; pregnancy (third trimester); types II, III, and V hyperlipoproteinemia; heavy stress periods; high-cholesterol diet (animal fats). *Drug Influence:* Aspirin, corticosteroids, steroids (anabolic agents and androgens), oral contraceptives, epinephrine and norepinephrine, bromides, phenothiazines (chlorpromazine [Thorazine]), trifluoperazine [Stelazine], vitamins A and D, sulfonamides, phenytoin (Dilantin).

Procedure

- Keep the client NPO (food, fluids, and medications) for 12 hours. The client may have water.
- Collect 3–5 mL of venous blood in a red-top tube. Avoid hemolysis.
- List drugs the client is taking that are not withheld on the laboratory slip.

Factors Affecting Laboratory Results

- Aspirin and cortisone could cause decreased or elevated serum cholesterol levels.
- A high-cholesterol diet before the test could cause elevated serum cholesterol levels.
- Severe hypoxia could increase the serum cholesterol level.
- Hemolysis of the blood specimen may cause an elevation of the serum cholesterol level.

NURSING IMPLICATIONS WITH RATIONALE

Increased Level

- Relate clinical problems and drugs to hypercholesterolemia. An elevated cholesterol level can indicate liver disease as well as coronary artery disease.
- Hold drugs that could increase the serum level for 12 hours before the blood is drawn, with the health care provider's permission.

Client Teaching

- Explain to the client and family what is considered a normal serum cholesterol level and the effects of an elevated cholesterol level.
- Encourage the client to lose weight if overweight and hypercholesterolemic. Losing weight if obese can decrease serum cholesterol level.
- Instruct the client with hypercholesterolemia to decrease the intake of foods rich in cholesterol (e.g., bacon, eggs, butter, fatty meat, certain seafood, coconut, and chocolate).
- Instruct the client with severe hypercholesterolemia to keep medical appointments for follow-up care.

Cholinesterase (blood [RBCs] or plasma)

Acetylcholinesterase (True Cholinesterase of Blood Nerve Tissue—RBC); Pseudocholinesterase (Serum)

Reference Values

Adult: 0.5–1 unit (RBC), 3–8 unit/mL (plasma), 6–8 international unit/L (RBC), 8–18 international unit/L at 37°C (plasma).

Child: Similar to adult.

Description

There are two different cholinesterases (CHS): *acetylcholinesterase* (true cholinesterase), found in the red blood cells (erythrocytes) and nerve tissue, and *pseudocholinesterase*, or serum cholinesterase (PCHE). Cholinesterase is an enzyme that breaks down acetylcholine at the nerve synapse and neuromuscular junction.

Decreased cholinesterase levels may indicate insecticide poisoning caused by excessive exposure to organic phosphate agents, liver disorders (hepatitis and cirrhosis), or an acute infection. This test is not used for assessment of liver function.

Purpose

- To detect a decrease in plasma cholinesterase level due to insecticide poisoning or other health problems.

Clinical Problems

Decreased Level: Insecticide poisoning, liver disorders (hepatitis, cirrhosis, obstructive jaundice), malnutrition, acute infections, anemias, carcinomatosis.

Increased Level: Nephrotic syndrome.

Procedure

- There is no food or fluid restriction.
- Collect 5–7 mL of venous blood in a green- or lavender-top tube.

Factors Affecting Laboratory Results

- Nonheparinized tube for cholinesterase-RBC test affects test result.

NURSING IMPLICATIONS WITH RATIONALE

Decreased Level

- Obtain a history of the client's exposure to insecticides—kind, length of time, and amount. Excessive exposure to organic phosphate can cause acute or chronic toxicity, and the acetylcholinesterase level would be decreased.
- Report if the client has not been eating or has an acute infection.

Chromosomal analysis (blood)

Chromosome Karyotype, Chromosome Studies

Reference Values

Normal: 46 chromosomes. *Men*: 44 autosomes + XY (totaling 46 chromosomes). *Women*: 44 autosomes + XX (totaling 46 chromosomes).

Description

Chromosomal analysis aids in the diagnosis of chromosomal abnormalities, leading to disorders such as mental retardation. With chromosomal analysis, karyotyping is done by arranging the chromosomes in order of the largest to the smallest and analyzing for structural changes with each chromosome. A normal karyotyping includes 22 pairs of autosomal chromosomes and a pair of sex chromosomes (XY for male and XX for female). Any change in the karyotyping of the chromosomes because of duplication, deletion, translocation, or genetic rearrangement will cause an abnormality.

C

Chromosomal karyotyping is useful for detecting not only Down syndrome resulting from Trisomy 21 chromosome but also abnormal sex chromosomes. In females, instead of the XX (double pair of X), with Turner syndrome it could be X0 or X/XX or X/XXX. The characteristics of the female with Turner syndrome are short stature, webbed neck, streak ovaries, amenorrhea, infertility, and cardiac defects. In males, instead of XY, with Klinefelter syndrome, the sex chromosomes would be XXY. The characteristics of the male with Klinefelter syndrome are long arms and legs; lack of beard, body, and pubic hair; gynecomastia; testicular atrophy; and infertility. Chromosomal karyotyping can be useful in determining the causes of infertility, delayed puberty, primary amenorrhea, recurrent miscarriage, and selected cancers.

Other methods for performing chromosomal analysis are from amniotic fluid, placenta tissue, bone marrow, buccal smear, skin, and with other types of body tissues.

Purposes

- To determine the presence of a chromosomal abnormality.
- To identify the risk for developing a disease or a fetal anomaly.
- To detect causes of infertility, delayed puberty, amenorrhea, and others.

Clinical Problems

Chromosomal Anomalies: Down syndrome (Trisomy 21), Edward syndrome (Trisomy 18), Patau syndrome (Trisomy 13), Turner syndrome (female sex chromosome defect), Klinefelter syndrome (male sex chromosome defect), growth retardation, amenorrhea, delayed puberty, infertility, stillbirths or miscarriages associated with malformation, hypogonadism, selected cancer, chronic myelogenous leukemia, Tay-Sachs disease, and sickle-cell anemia.

Procedure

- NPO for 4 hours before test. No fatty foods for 12 hours before the test.
- A signed consent form may or may not be required. Check with the policy at your institution.
- Collect 7–10 mL of venous blood in a green-top tube. The specimen may be obtained from the bone marrow by using a heparinized syringe. Do not shake the tube to avoid hemolysis of the specimen. Invert the green-top tube several times.
- For fetuses, the specimen may be collected by amniocentesis.
- Send the specimen immediately to the laboratory or refrigerate until testing. Testing should be within 48 hours.

Factors Affecting Laboratory Results

- Hemolysis of the blood specimen.
- Blood specimen not sent to the laboratory immediately or not refrigerated.

NURSING IMPLICATIONS WITH RATIONALE

- Obtain a history from the client and/or family of any known genetic disorders.
- Obtain a history of the client's health problems.
- Ask if the client has made any dietary changes recently. Anorexia could cause amenorrhea.

Client Teaching

- Advise the client that the test results may not be available for days or weeks, which depends on the type of specimen.
- Listen to the client's concerns. Answer questions or refer questions to other health care providers. The test and the results can be a cause of emotional upset for the client and family.
- Explain to the client that genetic counseling (if appropriate) may be needed.

C

Clostridium difficile toxin assay (stool)

Clostridium Difficile

Reference Values

Negative: No *Clostridium* toxin.

Description

Clostridium difficile (*C. difficile*) is a gram-positive bacteria that can release necrotizing toxins. *C. difficile* infection occurs in the intestine especially in those who are immunocompromised or who have been taking broad-spectrum antibiotics, such as ampicillin, cephalosporins, or clindamycin. The normal flora of the intestine contains organisms that normally do not multiply. However, with certain antibiotic therapy, *C. difficile* bacteria increases, resulting in *Clostridium difficile* toxin. As the result of *C. difficile* infection in the bowel, watery and voluminous diarrhea occurs. It is referred to as *Clostridium difficile* enterocolitis. It is a common cause of diarrhea in hospitals. Clients with diarrhea from this bacteria usually have fever, abdominal cramps, abdominal bloating, and an increase in leukocyte count. Symptoms generally occur between 5 and 10 days after antibiotic therapy.

The toxin from *C. difficile* can be diagnosed from a stool specimen. A stool culture for *C. difficile* can be taken, but the results take longer than the *C. difficile* toxin assay.

Purpose

- To diagnose the cause of severe diarrhea.

Clinical Problems

Increased Level: Diarrhea from *Clostridium difficile* toxin.

Procedure

- There is no food or fluid restriction.
- Obtain a fresh stool specimen (solid or liquid) in a sterile sealed plastic container with a lid. The order may be for more than one stool specimen.
- Urine and toilet paper should not be mixed with the stool.

Factors Affecting Laboratory Results

- Insufficient amount of stool collection.
- Urine and toilet paper with the stool.

NURSING IMPLICATIONS WITH RATIONALE

- Note when antibiotic therapy was started and diarrhea occurred.
- Record vital signs, for example, temperature, blood pressure, and pulse.

Client Teaching

- Explain to the client about how to collect a stool specimen. Urine and toilet paper should not be a part of the stool specimen. Stool specimen should be placed in a sterile container.
- Tell the client to record the number of watery stools and their frequency.
- Inform the client to describe his or her symptoms, such as abdominal cramps and/or bloating, stool consistency, and color.
- Be available to answer client's questions.

Clot retraction (blood)

Reference Values

Adult: 1–24 hours (retraction of clot).

Child: Similar to adult.

Description

The clot retraction (shrunken clot) test is useful in determining whether bleeding disorders are due to a decreased platelet count. In this simple test, the rate and degree of contraction of a blood clot are measured; the clot of blood in the test tube will diminish in size as fluid (serum) separates from the red cells. Platelets are responsible for the shrinkage of the blood clot. Frequently, when there is a platelet deficit, clot retraction will be slower and the clot formation will be softer.

In 1 hour the clot should be one half its original size (volume). The retraction should be near completion in 4 hours and definitely completed in 24 hours.

Purpose

- To determine if the bleeding disorder is due to a decreased platelet count.

Clinical Problems

Decreased Clot Formation: Thrombocytopenia (decreased platelets), thrombasthenia (abnormal platelets), anemia (pernicious, folic acid, aplastic), Waldenström macroglobulinemia.

Procedure

- There is no food or fluid restriction.
- Collect 5 mL of venous blood in a red-top tube.

Factors Affecting Laboratory Results

- A high hematocrit can cause poor clot retraction.

- Decreased fibrinogen can cause RBCs to spill out of the serum when retraction begins, resulting in poor cell retraction.
- Anticoagulants can inhibit clot formation.

C

NURSING IMPLICATIONS WITH RATIONALE

Decreased or Poor Clot Formation

- Report to the health care provider if bleeding time is prolonged.
- Note when the blood clot begins to separate from the tube wall. This usually begins to happen within 30 minutes to 1 hour. Note the length of time required for clot retraction (clot shrinking and fluid release).
- Check the consistency of the clot. Soft clots and shapeless clots may be due to abnormal or decreased platelets.
- Check the client's hemoglobin, hematocrit, and platelet count. A high hematocrit resulting from hemoconcentration or polycythemia may cause decreased clot retraction. Clot retraction is influenced by the number of functional platelets and not necessarily by the total count.

Coagulation factors (plasma)

See Factor Assay

Cold agglutinins (serum)

Cold Hemagglutinin

Reference Values

Adult: 1:8 antibody titer, greater than 1:16 significantly increased, greater than 1:32 definitely positive.

Child: Similar to adult.

Elderly: Values are increased more than adults.

Description

Cold agglutinins (CAs) are antibodies that agglutinate red blood cells at temperatures between 0°C and 10°C. Elevated titers (greater than 1:32) are found frequently in clients with primary atypical pneumonia or with other clinical problems, such as influenza, pulmonary embolism, and cirrhosis. The cold agglutinins test is often done during the acute and convalescence phases of illness.

Purposes

- To determine the presence of an increased antibody titer, significant for atypical pneumonia, influenza, or leukemia.
- To compare test results with other laboratory tests.

Clinical Problems

Increased Level: Primary atypical pneumonia, influenza, cirrhosis of the liver, lymphatic leukemia, multiple myeloma, pulmonary embolism, acquired hemolytic anemias, malaria, infectious mononucleosis, frostbite, viral infections (cytomegalovirus), tuberculosis.

Procedure

- There is no food or fluid restriction.
- Collect 5–7 mL of venous blood in a red-top tube. Keep the specimen warm. Take it immediately to the laboratory. The blood sample should not be refrigerated.
- The laboratory may rewarm the sample for 30 minutes before the serum is separated from the cells.

Factors Affecting Laboratory Results

- Antibiotic therapy may cause inaccurate results.
- Increased cold agglutinins may interfere with typing and crossmatching.
- Improper blood collection procedure may affect results.

C

NURSING IMPLICATIONS WITH RATIONALE

Increased Level

- Relate increased cold agglutinin levels to clinical problems, particularly primary atypical pneumonia.
- Answer the client's questions concerning the significance of the test. Answers might include "most persons have an antibody titer level, but some have higher levels, such as older adults and those with viral infections; high titers may persist for years, and the test may be repeated at a later date."

Complement: total (serum)

CH50

Reference Values

Adult: 75–160 unit/mL, 75–160 unit/L (SI units).

Description

Total complement plays an important role in the immunologic enzyme system reacting to an antigen–antibody response. The complements make up about 10% of the serum globulins. The complement system has over 20 components, including 9 major components numbering C1–C9. C3 and C4 are the most abundant complements and are discussed separately in the text. The total complement may be referred to as *total hemolytic complement,* or CH50. CH50 assesses the function of the complement system. When the complement system is stimulated, it increases phagocytosis, lysis, or destruction of bacteria, and produces an inflammatory response to infection.

Most assays for CH50 are most sensitive to changes in C2, C4, and C5. Assay should be used as a screen for overall complement function and not as a quantitative measure of C1 activation during the course of disease states.

Purposes

- To identify the effects of the immunologic enzyme system regarding the presence of inflammatory condition(s) or tissue rejection.
- To compare serum complement tests with serum immunoglobulins to determine the cause of the health problem.

C

Clinical Problems

Decreased Level: Allograft rejection, hypogammaglobulinemia, acute poststreptococcal glomerulonephritis, acute serum sickness, systemic lupus erythematosus, lupus nephritis, hepatitis, subacute bacterial endocarditis, hemolytic anemia, rheumatic fever, multiple myeloma, advanced cirrhosis.

Increased Level: Acute rheumatic fever, rheumatoid arthritis, acute myocardial infarction, ulcerative colitis, diabetes mellitus, thyroiditis, Wegener granulomatosis, obstructive jaundice.

Procedure

- There is no food or fluid restriction.
- Collect 3–5 mL of venous blood in a red-top tube. Allow it to clot at room temperature. Spin at 4°C. Transfer the serum and freeze immediately. This test may be sent to a large reference laboratory.

Factors Affecting Laboratory Results

- Hemolysis of the blood sample caused by rough handling.

NURSING IMPLICATIONS WITH RATIONALE

- Obtain a history from the client of an infectious process or abnormal response to infection. Complement deficiency may occur to those persons susceptible to infection and with certain autoimmune diseases.
- Assess the client's vital signs and urine output. Report abnormal findings.
- Compare total complement results with serum immunoglobulins. Complement results give information about the client's immune system.

Complement C3 (serum)

C3 Component of the Complement System

Reference Values

Adult: *Male:* 80–180 mg/dL, 0.8–1.8 g/L (SI units). *Female:* 76–120 mg/dL, 0.76–1.2 g/L (SI units).

Child: Usually not performed.

Description

Complement C3 is the most abundant component of the complement system (a group of 11 proteins). The complement system has an important role in the immunologic system, and the complements' components are activated when IgG and IgM antibodies are combined with their specific antigens.

The total complement system and C3 are decreased in systemic lupus erythematosus, glomerulonephritis, and acute renal transplant rejection. Following onset of an acute or chronic inflammatory process or acute tissue destruction (necrosis), the total complement may be temporarily elevated. C3 and C4 of the complement system are best known, and the others (C1, C2, and C5–C9) are still under study and intense research.

Purposes

- To assist in the detection of acute inflammatory disease (e.g., rheumatoid arthritis) and other health problems (elevated level), and SLE, glomerulonephritis (decreased level) (*see Clinical Problems*).
- To compare the test results with other laboratory data to determine health problems.

Clinical Problems

Decreased Level: Systemic lupus erythematosus, glomerulonephritis, acute poststreptococcal glomerulonephritis, acute renal transplant rejection, cirrhosis of the liver, multiple sclerosis (slightly lower), protein malnutrition, anemias (pernicious, folic acid), septicemia (gram negative), bacterial endocarditis.

Increased Level: Acute rheumatic fever, rheumatoid arthritis, early SLE, and malignant neoplasms of the esophagus, stomach, colon, rectum, pancreas, lungs, breast, cervix, ovary, prostate, and bladder.

Procedure

- There is no food or fluid restriction.
- Collect 3–5 mL of venous blood in a red-top tube.
- Take the blood sample to the laboratory immediately.

Factors Affecting Laboratory Results

- Heat can destroy complement components.
- C3 is unstable, and the serum value may decrease if the sample is left standing for 1–2 hours at room temperature.

NURSING IMPLICATIONS WITH RATIONALE

- Compare the serum C3 and C4 results.
- Be supportive of client and family.

Decreased Level

- Relate a decreased C3 level to clinical problems such as SLE and kidney disorders.
- Check the serum C3 value with other laboratory studies that are ordered and related to the disease process.

Increased Level

- Relate an elevated C3 level to an acute or chronic inflammatory process and tissue necrosis, such as rheumatic fever, rheumatoid arthritis, and malignancies with metastasis.

Complement C4 (serum)

C4 Component of the Complement System

Reference Values

Adult: 15–45 mg/dL, 0.15–0.45 g/L, or 150–450 mg/L (SI units).

Child: Usually not performed.

Description

(*See Complement C3 [serum].*)

Complement C4 is the second most abundant component of the complement system. A decrease in the C4 as well as the C3 levels is commonly found in diseases such as systemic lupus erythematosus (SLE), glomerulonephritis, and renal transplant rejection.

An elevated serum C4 level is indicative of an acute inflammatory process; however, a well (healthy) person may have an elevated C4 level. With cancer, the C4 level is usually increased (with links to the stage of the disease), but the serum level drops significantly in the terminal phase of the malignancy.

Purposes

(*See Complement C3 [serum].*)

Clinical Problems

Decreased Level: Lupus nephritis, SLE (C4 decreased time is longer than C3 decreased time), acute poststreptococcal glomerulonephritis (C4 level usually lower than C3 level), cirrhosis of the liver, bacterial endocarditis.

Increased Level: Rheumatoid spondylitis; juvenile rheumatoid arthritis; cancer of the esophagus, stomach, colon, rectum, pancreas, lung, breast, cervix, ovary, prostate, and bladder.

Procedure

- There is no food or fluid restriction.
- Collect 3–5 mL of venous blood in a red-top tube.
- Take the blood sample to the laboratory immediately.

Factors Affecting Laboratory Results

- Heat will decrease the complement C4 level.
- C4 is unstable and the serum level will decrease if it remains at room temperature for more than 1–2 hours.

NURSING IMPLICATIONS WITH RATIONALE

Decreased Level

- Relate a decreased serum C4 level to clinical problems. With lupus nephritis and post-streptococcal glomerulonephritis, the serum C4 level is extremely low.
- Compare the serum C3 and C4 results to determine which component of the complement system is involved.

C

Coombs direct (blood [RBCs])

Direct Antiglobulin Test

Reference Values

Adult: Negative.

Child: Negative.

Description

The direct Coombs test detects antibodies attached to red blood cells that may cause cellular damage. This test can identify a weak antigen–antibody reaction even when there is no visible RBC agglutination. A positive Coombs test reveals antibodies present in RBCs, but the test does not identify the antibody responsible.

This test is useful for diagnosing early erythroblastosis fetalis (hemolytic disease of newborns), autoimmune hemolytic anemia, hemolytic transfusion reaction, and some drug sensitizations (e.g., to levodopa and methyldopa).

The direct Coombs test is also known as the direct antiglobulin test, a method of detecting in vivo sensitization of RBCs.

Purpose

- To detect antibodies on RBCs.

Clinical Problems

Positive (+1 to +4): Erythroblastosis fetalis, acquired hemolytic anemia (autoimmune), transfusion reactions (blood incompatibility), leukemias (lymphocytic, myelocytic), systemic lupus erythematosus. *Drug Influence:* Antibiotics (cephaloridine [Loridine], cephalothin [Keflin], penicillin, streptomycin, tetracycline), chlorpromazine (Thorazine), phenytoin (Dilantin), ethosuximide (Zarontin), hydralazine (Apresoline), isoniazid (INH), levodopa (Dopar), methyldopa (Aldomet), procainamide (Pronestyl), quinidine, rifampin (Rifadin), sulfonamides.

Procedure

- There is no food or fluid restriction.
- Collect 5–7 mL of venous blood in a lavender-top tube. A red-top tube could be used, but a serum separator tube should not be used. Venous blood from the umbilical cord of a newborn may be used. Avoid hemolysis.

Factors Affecting Laboratory Results

- Certain drugs may cause a positive test result (*see Drug Influence*).

NURSING IMPLICATIONS WITH RATIONALE

Positive Test

- Report the drugs the client is receiving that could produce a positive direct Coombs test (e.g., antibiotics, phenytoin, sulfonamides, chlorpromazine, methyldopa, and others [*see Drug Influence*]).
- Observe for signs and symptoms of whole-blood transfusion reactions (e.g., chills, fever [slight temperature elevation], and rash).
- Observe the newborn for symptoms of erythroblastosis fetalis, especially if the condition is suspected. The main symptom is jaundice of the skin, nails, and sclerae.

Coombs indirect (serum)

Reference Values

Adult: Negative.

Child: Negative.

Description

The Coombs indirect test can detect free circulating antibodies in the client's serum. This test is done in crossmatching blood for transfusions to prevent transfusion reaction to incompatible blood caused by minor blood-type factors. As a result of previous transfusions, a recipient's blood may contain specific antibody (antibodies) that could cause a transfusion reaction.

The indirect Coombs test is also known as the indirect antiglobulin test, a method of detecting in vitro sensitization of red blood cells.

Purpose

- To check the recipient's and the donor's blood for antibodies prior to blood transfusion.

Clinical Problems

Positive (+1 to +4): Incompatible crossmatched blood, specific antibody (previous transfusion), anti-Rh antibodies (detected during pregnancy), acquired hemolytic anemia. *Drug Influence:* Same as for the direct Coombs test (*see Coombs Direct*).

Procedure

- There is no food or fluid restriction.
- Collect 5–7 mL of venous blood in a red-top tube. Do not use a serum separator tube. The blood bank will use the serum from the recipient's blood and select the compatible blood for proper transfusion.

Factors Affecting Laboratory Results

- Certain drugs can cause positive results (*see Clinical Problems: Drug Influence under Coombs Direct*).

NURSING IMPLICATIONS WITH RATIONALE

- Obtain a history of previous transfusions and report any previous transfusion reactions.
- Report any drugs the client is receiving that could cause a positive result. Record drug information on the client's chart in the nurse's notes or progress notes.

Client Teaching

- Explain to the client that the donor's and the recipient's blood are checked for antibodies prior to a blood transfusion to avoid a transfusion reaction.

Complete blood count (CBC) (blood)

Reference Values

See individual tests for children and newborns.

Adult

RBC Count: *Male*: 4.6–6 million/µL, 4.6–6 $\times 10^{12}$/L (SI units). *Female*: 4–5 million/µL, 4–5 $\times 10^{12}$/L (SI units).

Hemoglobin (Hgb, Hb): *Male*: 13.8–18 g/dL. *Female*: 12–15 g/dL.

Hematocrit (Hct): *Male*: 40–54%. *Female:* 36–46%.

    RBC Indices, see page 380
    Mean corpuscular volume (MCV): 80–98 µm³, 80–98 fl (SI units).
    Mean corpuscular hemoglobin (MCH): 27–31 pg.
    Mean corpuscular hemoglobin concentration (MCHC): 32–36% (0.32–0.36 g/dL).
    Red blood cell distribution width (RDW): 11.5–14.5%

WBC Count: 4,500–10,000 µL (mm³)

WBC Differential Count
    Neutrophils: 50–70%, 2,500–7,000 µL (mm³)
    Eosinophils: 1–3%, 100–300 µL (mm³)
    Basophils: 0.4–1%, 40–100 µL (mm³)
    Lymphocytes: 25–35%, 1,700–3,500 µL (mm³)
    Monocytes: 4–6%, 40–100 µL (mm³)

Platelet Count: 150,000–400,000 µL, 0.15–0.4 $\times 10^{12}$/L (SI units).

Description

The complete blood count (CBC) is a group of tests that evaluate the hematologic system and possible health problems—for example, anemias and acute illness—that are associated with blood cells. It is a valuable screening test that gives information about the client's blood cell values with the laboratory reference values. It basically includes the red blood cells and their indices, hemoglobin and hematocrit, white blood cells with differential WBC, and platelets. The CBC is usually prescribed at least once a year along with the physical examination and before surgery. The reference values could differ slightly among institutions and age groups.

Purposes

- To detect low red blood cell count and RBC indices of clients who may have anemias.
- To determine abnormal CBC results associated with infections and minor and severe health problems, such as cancer.
- To assess CBC before a surgical intervention.
- To prescribe CBC as part of a physical examination.

Clinical Problems

Decreased Level: Anemias, cancer, chronic kidney disease, pregnancy, acute blood loss, lupus (SLE). *Drug Influence:* Antibiotics, antineoplastic agents, sulfonamides (*see individual lab tests*).

Increased Level: Dehydration, infections, cancer, polycythemia vera (*see individual lab tests*).

Procedure

- Collect 7–10 mL of venous blood in a lavender-top tube. Invert the tube to mix with the anticoagulant.
- There is no food or fluid restriction.
- Blood sample should be tested within 10 hours. The tube can be refrigerated up to 20 hours, but the blood sample should *not* be frozen.

Factors Affecting Laboratory Results

- The blood sample *not* mixed with the anticoagulant in the tube.
- Dehydration and overhydration could affect test results.
- Certain medications can affect test results.

NURSING IMPLICATIONS WITH RATIONALE

- Explain the reason for the CBC test. The test might be ordered before a physical examination, surgery, or for assistance with diagnosing a health problem.
- Check if vital signs are in order.
- Assess the results of the CBC test.

Client Teaching

- Discuss the results of the CBC test with the client.
- Answer the client's questions concerning the CBC test, such as why the test was ordered.

Copper (Cu) (serum and urine)

Reference Values

Adult: *Male:* 70–140 mcg/dL, 11–22 μmol/L (SI units). *Female:* 80–155 mcg/dL, 12.6–24.3 μmol/L (SI units). *Pregnancy:* 140–300 mcg/dL.

Child: *Newborn:* 20–70 mcg/dL. *Child:* 30–190 mcg/dL. *Adolescent:* 90–240 mcg/dL. *Urine:* *Adult and Child:* 0–60 mcg/24 h, 0.095 μmol/24 h.

Description

Copper is required for hemoglobin synthesis and for activation of respiratory enzymes. Approximately 90% of the copper is bound to alpha 2-globulin, referred to as ceruloplasmin, which is the means of copper transportation in the body. In hepatolenticular disease (Wilson disease), the serum copper level is less than 20 mcg/dL, and the urinary copper level is greater than 100 mcg/24 hours. There is a decrease in copper metabolism with Wilson disease, and excess copper is deposited in the brain (basal ganglia) and liver, causing degenerative changes. Wilson disease is more likely to be found in the Italian and Sicilian populations and in the Eastern European Jewish people. A low-copper diet and D-penicillamine will promote copper excretion.

Hypercupremia (excess copper) can be observed during pregnancy, anemias, leukemia, collagen disease, and thyroid diseases. Serum copper and serum ceruloplasmin tests are frequently ordered together and compared. Both show decreased levels with Wilson disease, and the urine copper level is elevated.

Purposes

- To detect if there is a serum copper excess or deficit.
- To aid in the diagnosis of Wilson disease (hepatolenticular disease).

Clinical Problems

Decreased Level: Hepatolenticular disease (Wilson disease), protein malnutrition, chronic ischemic heart disease.

Increased Level: Cancer (bone, stomach, large intestine, liver, lung), Hodgkin disease, leukemias, hypothyroidism, hyperthyroidism, anemias (pernicious and iron deficiency), rheumatoid arthritis, systemic lupus erythematosus, pregnancy, cirrhosis of the liver. *Drug Influence:* Oral contraceptives.

Procedure

A serum and a urine specimen may be requested simultaneously.

Serum

- There is no food or fluid restriction.
- Collect 5 mL of venous blood in a red-top tube or a royal blue-top tube (used for trace metal).

Urine:
- Discard the first morning urine specimen and then begin a 24-hour urine collection in a container specified for this test.

Factors Affecting Laboratory Results

- A diet low or high in copper before the blood test may cause inaccurate results.
- Metallic contamination of collection tubes or equipment affects test results.

C

NURSING IMPLICATIONS WITH RATIONALE

- Assess for signs and symptoms of hepatolenticular disease (Wilson disease—e.g., rigidity, dysarthria, dysphagia, incoordination, and tremors).
- Check for a Kayser-Fleischer ring (dark ring) around the cornea. This is a copper deposit that the body has not been able to metabolize.
- Compare the serum copper level with the serum ceruloplasmin level if both have been ordered. If hepatolenticular disease is present, the serum copper and ceruloplasmin levels would be decreased and the urine copper level would be increased.

Client Teaching

- Explain to the client with Wilson disease that foods rich in copper (e.g., organ meats, shellfish, mushrooms, whole-grain cereals, bran, nuts, and chocolate) should be avoided. Canned foods should be omitted. A low-copper diet and D-penicillamine promote copper excretion.

Cortisol (plasma)
Hydrocortisone, Compound F

Reference Values

Adult: 8 AM–10 AM: 5–23 mcg/dL, 138–635 nmol/L (SI units). 4 PM–6 PM: 3–13 mcg/dL, 83–359 nmol/L (SI units).

Child: 8 AM–10 AM: 15–25 mcg/dL. 4 PM–6 PM: 5–10 mcg/dL.

Description

Cortisol is a potent glucocorticoid released from the adrenal cortex in response to ACTH stimulation. Cortisol affects carbohydrate, protein, and lipid metabolism; acts as an anti-inflammatory agent and helps with the maintenance of blood pressure; inhibits insulin action; and stimulates glucogenesis in the liver.

Levels of plasma cortisol are higher in the morning and lower in the afternoon. When there is adrenal or pituitary dysfunction, the diurnal variation in cortisol function ceases.

Purposes

- To determine the presence of an elevated or decreased plasma cortisol level.
- To associate a decreased cortisol level with an adrenocortical hypofunction.

Clinical Problems

Decreased Level: Anterior pituitary hypofunction, adrenal cortical hypofunction (Addison disease), respiratory distress syndrome (low-birth-weight newborns), hypothyroidism, exercise (slight decrease). *Drug Influence:* Androgens, phenytoin (Dilantin).

Increased Level: Cancer of the adrenal gland, benign tumor on the adrenal cortex, adrenal cortical hyperfunction (Cushing syndrome), stress, pregnancy, obesity, acute myocardial infarction, acute alcohol intoxication, diabetic acidosis, hyperthyroidism. *Drug Influence:* Oral contraceptives, estrogens, spironolactone (Aldactone), triparanol.

Procedure

- There is no food or fluid restriction.
- Collect 5–7 mL of venous blood in a red-top or green-top (heparinized) tube.
- Write the date and time the blood was drawn on the laboratory slip. If the client has taken estrogen or oral contraceptives in the last 6 weeks, the drug(s) should be listed on the laboratory slip. *Recommendation:* Stop medication 2 months before test.
- Advise the client to rest in bed for 2 hours before the blood is drawn.

Factors Affecting Laboratory Results

- Certain drugs can affect cortisol levels (*see Drug Influence*).
- Physical activity prior to the blood test might decrease the cortisol level.
- Obesity can cause an elevated serum level.
- Inaccurate labeling of the blood specimen (e.g., with the wrong time) can affect results.

NURSING IMPLICATIONS WITH RATIONALE

- Obtain a history of drugs taken prior to hospital admission or the test. Oral contraceptives and estrogen taken within 6 weeks of the test can cause false-positive results.

Decreased Level

- Observe for signs and symptoms of Addison disease (adrenal cortical insufficiency). Symptoms are anorexia, vomiting, abdominal pain, fatigue, dizziness, trembling, and diaphoresis.

Increased Level

- Observe for signs and symptoms of Cushing syndrome (excess adrenal cortical hormone). Symptoms are fat deposits in the face (moon face), neck, and upper back; irritability; mood swings; bleeding under the skin; muscle wasting; and weakness.

Client Teaching

- Instruct the client that he or she should be on bed rest for 2 hours prior to the test. Physical activity affects the cortisol level.

C-peptide (serum)

Connecting Peptide Insulin, Pro-Insulin C-Peptide

C

Reference Values

Adult: *Fasting:* 0.8–1.8 ng/mL; 0.27–0.63 nmol/L (SI units).

Description

C-peptide is an inactive amino acid formed during the conversion of pro-insulin to insulin in the beta cells of the pancreas. The C-peptide levels can indicate the beta cell activity in the production of insulin. Normally, C-peptide levels correlate with the insulin levels because both are released from the beta cells of the pancreas in similar amounts. C-peptide has a longer half-life than insulin, so C-peptide levels can be increased in blood circulation.

The C-peptide levels can indicate the presence of insulin antibodies in a diabetic client receiving (exogenous) insulin. When exogenous insulin increases the serum insulin levels, C-peptide levels remain unaffected or decreased. The C-peptide levels are high with insulinoma.

Purposes

- To identify excess insulin administration in the diabetic or nondiabetic; insulin level is increased and the C-peptide level is decreased.
- To assist in the diagnosis of insulin antibodies.
- To assist in the diagnosis of insulinoma.
- To evaluate the insulin reserve in insulin-dependent diabetic or type 1 diabetes mellitus.
- To detect the cause of hypoglycemia.

Clinical Problems

Decreased Level: Type 1 diabetes mellitus, pancreatectomy. *Drug Influence:* Atenolol, calcitonin, rosiglitazone, troglitazone.

Increased Level: Insulinoma, type 2 diabetes mellitus, beta cell transplants, renal failure. *Drug Influence:* Sulfonylurea and glyburide (oral hypoglycemic drug groups); cortisone drugs, for example, prednisone, betamethasone; oral contraceptives; estrogen drugs; chloroquine; terbutaline.

Procedure

- NPO, except some water, for 8–10 hours before the test.
- Collect 5–7 mL of venous blood in a red-top tube. Blood sample of insulin may also be collected. Insulin specimen should be placed on ice.

Factors Affecting Laboratory Results

- Hemolysis of the blood sample.
- Liver dysfunction can cause an increased C-peptide level.
- Renal failure can cause an increased C-peptide level.
- Drugs (*see Decreased and Increased Levels, Clinical Problems*).
- Radioisotope testing before the blood is drawn for C-peptide.

NURSING IMPLICATIONS WITH RATIONALE

- Obtain a history of client's health problems related to diabetes mellitus, for example, symptoms related to hypoglycemia.
- Obtain a list of medications the client is taking.

Client Teaching

- Explain to the client that he or she should adhere to the American Dietetic Association (ADA) diet. Have a nutritionist speak to the client.
- Explain to the client the importance of insulin regulation, diet, and weight control.
- Listen to the client's concerns. Answer questions or refer them to other health professionals.

C

C-reactive protein (CRP) (serum) and N high sensitivity CRP (hs CRP)

Reference Values

Adult: Not usually present: *Qualitative:* Greater than 1.2 titer. *Positive:* Quantitative: 20 mg/dL.

Child: Not usually present.

N High Sensitivity CRP (hs CRP)

Adult: Less than 0.175 mg/L.

Description

C-reactive protein (CRP) is produced in the liver in response to tissue injury and inflammation. It appears in the blood 6–10 hours after an acute inflammatory process and tissue destruction and peaks within 48–72 hours. The serum CRP usually decreases after the third day of injury. Serum CRP is also found in many body fluids (e.g., pleural, peritoneal, and synovial fluids).

This type of protein is needed to fight injury and infection. Inflammation can cause the protein to become an inflammatory protein. Many references state that the inflammatory protein is an important factor in cardiovascular disease.

Chronic infection, fat cells, hypertension, smoking, cardiovascular and peripheral disease, stroke, and rheumatoid arthritis can produce these inflammatory proteins, which weaken the fatty plaques and cause eruption. The pieces of plaques become clots, which lead to decreased blood flow and even heart attacks. Higher levels of inflammatory proteins in the blood indicate a higher potential for atherosclerosis.

N High Sensitivity CRP (hs CRP): This test is a highly sensitive test for detecting the risk of cardiovascular and peripheral vascular diseases. It is frequently combined with cholesterol screening. Approximately one third of those who have had a heart attack have normal cholesterol levels and normal blood pressure. A positive hs CRP test may indicate that the client is at a high risk for coronary artery disease and stroke. The CRP does not elevate in cases of angina pectoris. This test can detect an inflammatory process that is caused by the build-up of plaque (atherosclerosis) in the arterial system, particularly the coronary arteries. Positive serum hs CRP values are much lower than the standard serum CRP, which makes it a more valuable test for predicting coronary heart disease.

Purposes

- To associate an increased CRP titer with an acute inflammatory process.
- To detect the risk of coronary heart disease (hs CRP).
- To compare test results with other laboratory tests, for example, erythrocyte sedimentation rate (ESR), antistreptolysin O, cholesterol, and serum lipoprotein tests.

Clinical Problems

Increased Level: Chronic infections, cardiovascular and peripheral diseases, acute myocardial infarction, stroke, inflammatory bowel disease, rheumatoid arthritis, rheumatic fever, systemic lupus erythematosus, bacterial infections, bacterial meningitis, late pregnancy, intrauterine contraceptive devices, cancer with metastasis. *Drug Influence:* Oral contraceptives.

Decreased Level: *Drug Suppression:* Steroids (cortisone, prednisone), salicylates (aspirin).

Procedure

- Restrict food and fluids, except water, for 8–12 hours before the test.
- Collect 3–5 mL of venous blood in a red-top tube. Avoid heat since CRP is thermolabile.

Factors Affecting Laboratory Results

- Pregnancy (third trimester) could elevate the CRP level.
- Oral contraceptives and intrauterine contraceptive devices might elevate the CRP level.

NURSING IMPLICATIONS WITH RATIONALE

- Recognize that an elevated serum CRP level is associated with an active inflammatory process and tissue destruction (necrosis). The CRP and hs CRP may be elevated in cardiovascular and peripheral diseases, stroke, rheumatoid arthritis, chronic infections.
- Assess for signs and symptoms of an acute inflammatory process, such as pain and swelling in joints, heat, redness, or increased body temperature.
- Assess for signs and symptoms of cardiovascular and peripheral diseases and for chest pain associated with coronary artery disease.
- Compare the serum hs CRP with serum cholesterol and serum lipoprotein tests. An elevated serum hs CRP and serum cholesterol profile may indicate a high risk of coronary artery disease.
- Compare the results of the serum CRP level. If the titer is decreasing, the client is responding to treatment and/or the acute phase is declining. The CRP titer may be compared to the ESR. The serum CRP level will elevate and return to normal faster than the ESR.
- Notify the health care provider of a recurrence (exacerbation) of an acute inflammation. The health care provider may wish to order a serum CRP test or a serum hs CRP level.

Creatine phosphokinase (CPK) (serum), CPK isoenzymes (serum)

Creatine Kinase (CK)

C

Reference Values

Adult: *Male:* 5–35 mcg/mL, 30–180 international unit/L, 55–170 unit/L at 37°C (SI units). *Female:* 5–25 mcg/mL, 25–150 international unit/L, 30–135 unit/L at 37°C (SI units).

Child: *Newborn:* 65–580 international unit/L at 30°C. *Child: Male:* 0–70 international unit/L at 30°C. *Female:* 0–50 international unit/L at 30°C.

CPK Isoenzymes:

CPK-MM:	94–100%	(muscle)
CPK-MB:	0–6%	(heart)
CPK-BB:	0%	(brain)

Most labs have replaced CPK isoenzymes with CPK-MB fraction only.

Description

Creatine phosphokinase (CPK), also known as creatine kinase (CK), is an enzyme found in high concentration in the heart and skeletal muscles and in low concentration in the brain tissue. Serum CPK/CK is frequently elevated by skeletal muscle disease, acute myocardial infarction, cerebrovascular disease, vigorous exercise, intramuscular (IM) injections, and electrolyte imbalance-hypokalemia. CPK/CK has two types of isoenzymes: M, associated with muscle, and B, associated with the brain. Electrophoresis separates the isoenzymes into three subdivisions: MM (in skeletal muscle and some in the heart), MB (in the heart), and BB (in brain tissue). When CPK/CK is elevated, a CPK electrophoresis is done to determine which group of isoenzymes is elevated. Increased isoenzyme CPK-MB could indicate damage to the myocardial cells.

Serum CPK/CK and CPK-MB rise within 4–6 hours after an acute MI, reach a peak in 18–24 hours (greater than 6 times the normal value), and then return to normal within 3–4 days, unless new necrosis or tissue damage occurs. If medication for acute MI has to be given parenterally (for instance, morphine), it would be better to give it intravenously than intramuscularly so that mild muscle injury (from IM) would not elevate the CPK level; however, injections have little or no effect on CPK-MB. Draw blood for a serum CPK/CK level before giving an IM injection.

Purposes

- To suggest myocardial or skeletal muscle disease.
- To compare test results with aspartate aminotransferase/serum glutamic oxaloacetic transaminase and lactate dehydrogenase levels to determine myocardial damage.

Clinical Problems

Increased Level: Acute myocardial infarction, skeletal muscle disease, cerebrovascular accident (CVA), and with all, elevated CPK isoenzymes. *Drug Influence:* IM injections, dexamethasone (Decadron), furosemide (Lasix), aspirin (high doses), ampicillin, carbenicillin, clofibrate.

CPK-MM Isoenzyme: Muscular dystrophy, delirium tremens, crush injury/trauma, surgery and postoperative state, vigorous exercise, IM injections, hypokalemia, hemophilia, hypothyroidism.

CPK-MB: Acute MI, severe angina pectoris, cardiac surgery, cardiac ischemia, myocarditis, hypokalemia, cardiac defibrillation.

CPK-BB: CVA, subarachnoid hemorrhage, cancer of the brain, acute brain injury, Reye syndrome, pulmonary embolism and infarction, seizures.

Procedure

- There is no food or fluid restriction.
- Collect 5–7 mL of venous blood in a red-top tube. Avoid hemolysis.
- Note on the laboratory slip the number of times the patient has received IM injections in the last 24–48 hours.

Factors Affecting Laboratory Results

- IM injections can cause an increased serum level of total CPK/CK.
- Vigorous exercise elevates the levels.
- Trauma and surgical intervention elevate serum levels.

NURSING IMPLICATIONS WITH RATIONALE

- Avoid giving IM injections until after blood is drawn for CPK.

Increased Level

- Relate increased serum (CPK/CK and isoenzymes [CPK-MM, CPK-MB, and CPK-BB]) to clinical problems. The CPK-MB is useful in making the differential diagnosis of myocardial infarction.
- Indicate whether the client has received an IM injection in the last 24–48 hours on the laboratory slip and chart.
- Assess the client's signs and symptoms of an acute MI. Symptoms include pain; dyspnea; diaphoresis (excess perspiration); cold, clammy skin; pallor; cardiac dysrhythmia.
- Check the serum CPK/CK level at intervals, and notify the physician of serum level changes. The serum CPK/CK may be repeated every 6–8 hours during the acute phase. When the CPK/CK and CPK-MB are highly elevated, there may be extensive muscle damage to the myocardium. For acute MI, also check results of the AST (SGOT) and LDH tests.
- Compare serum AST/SGOT and LDH levels with CPK and CPK-MB.
- Provide measures for alleviating pain.

Creatinine (serum)

Reference Values

Adult: 0.5–1.5 mg/dL, 45–132.3 μmol/L (SI units). Females may have slightly lower values because of their lesser muscle mass.

Child: *Newborn:* 0.8–1.4 mg/dL. *Infant:* 0.7–1.7 mg/dL. *Child (2–6 Years):* 0.3–0.6 mg/dL, 27–54 μmol/L (SI units). *Older Child:* 0.4–1.2 mg/dL, 36–106 μmol/L (SI units). Values increase slightly with age relative to muscle mass.

Elderly: May have decreased values relative to decreased muscle mass and decreased creatinine production.

Description

Creatinine, a by-product of muscle catabolism, is derived from the breakdown of muscle creatine phosphate. The amount of creatinine produced is proportional to the muscle mass. Creatinine is filtered by the glomeruli and is excreted in the urine.

Serum creatinine is considered a more sensitive and specific indicator of renal disease than blood urea nitrogen (BUN). It rises later and is *not influenced by diet or fluid intake.* A slight BUN elevation could be indicative of hypovolemia (fluid volume deficit); however, a serum creatinine of 2.5 mg/dL could be indicative of renal impairment. BUN and creatinine are frequently compared. If BUN increases and serum creatinine remains normal, dehydration (hypovolemia) is present; and if both increase, then renal disorder is present. Serum creatinine is especially useful in evaluation of glomerular function.

Purpose

- To diagnose renal dysfunction.

Clinical Problems

Decreased Level: Pregnancy, eclampsia.

Increased Level: Acute and chronic renal failure, shock (prolonged), systemic lupus erythematosus, cancer (intestine, bladder, testes, uterus, prostate), leukemias, Hodgkin disease, essential hypertension, acute myocardial infarction, diabetic nephropathy, heart failure (long standing), diet rich in creatinine (e.g., beef [high], poultry and fish [minimal] effect). *Drug Influence:* Amphotericin B, cephalosporins (cefazolin [Ancef], cephalothin [Keflin]), gentamicin, kanamycin, methicillin, ascorbic acid, barbiturates, lithium carbonate, mithramycin, methyldopa (Aldomet), glucose, protein, ketone bodies (increased), triamterene (Dyrenium).

Procedure

- There is no food or fluid restriction. Red meats should be avoided the night before the test.
- Collect 3–5 mL of venous blood in a red-top tube.
- List any drugs the client is taking that could elevate the serum level on the laboratory slip.

Factors Affecting Laboratory Results

- Certain drugs (*see Drug Influence*) may increase the serum creatinine level.
- Red meat consumed in large quantities may affect results.

C

NURSING IMPLICATIONS WITH RATIONALE

- Relate the elevated creatinine levels to clinical problems. Serum creatinine may be low in clients with small muscle mass, in amputees, and in clients with muscle disease. Older clients may have decreased muscle mass.
- Hold medications (*see Drug Influence*) for 24 hours before the test, with the health care provider's permission. Certain medications that cannot be withheld should be listed on the laboratory slip and noted on the client's chart.
- Check the amount of urine output in 24 hours. Less than 600 mL/24 hours can indicate renal insufficiency. Creatinine is excreted by the kidneys, and a continuous decrease in urine output could result in an increased serum creatinine level.
- Compare the BUN and creatinine levels. If both are increased, the problem is most likely kidney disease.

Client Teaching

- Instruct the client to eat less beef, poultry, and fish if the serum creatinine level is extremely elevated. Normally food does not have an effect on the serum creatinine level.

Creatinine clearance (urine)

Creatinine (urine)

Reference Values

Adult: 85–135 mL/min. Females may have somewhat lower values.

Child: Similar to adult. *Newborn:* 40–60 mL/min.

Elderly: Slightly decreased values than adult due to decreased glomerular filtration rate (GFR) caused by reduced renal plasma flow.

Urine Creatinine: 1–2 g/24 h.

Description

Creatinine is a metabolic product of creatine phosphate in skeletal muscle, and it is excreted by the kidneys. Creatinine clearance is considered a reliable test for estimating GFR. With renal insufficiency, the GFR is decreased, and the serum creatinine is increased. GFR decreases with age, and with the older adult, the creatinine clearance may be diminished to as low as 60 mL/minute.

The creatinine clearance test consists of a 12- or 24-hour urine collection and a blood sample.

The formula for calculating the creatinine clearance test is:

$$\text{Creatinine clearance} = \frac{\text{Urine creatinine (mcg/dL)} \times \text{Urine volume (dL)}}{\text{Serum creatinine (mcg/dL)}}$$

A creatinine clearance less than 40 mL/minute is suggestive of moderate to severe renal impairment.

Purposes

- To detect renal dysfunction.
- To monitor renal function.

Clinical Problems

Decreased Level: Mild to severe renal (kidney) impairment, hyperthyroidism, progressive muscular dystrophy, amyotrophic lateral sclerosis. *Drug Influence:* Phenacetin steroids (anabolic), thiazides.

Increased Level: Hypothyroidism, hypertension (renovascular), exercise. *Drug Influence:* Ascorbic acid, steroids, levodopa, methyldopa (Aldomet), phenolsulfonphthalein (PSP) test.

Procedure

- Hydrate client before test.
- Instruct the client to avoid meats, poultry, fish, tea, and coffee for 6 hours before the test and during test, with the health care provider's permission.
- List drugs the client is taking that could affect test results on the laboratory slip.

Blood: Collect 3–5 mL of venous blood in a red-top tube the morning of the test.

Urine: Have the client void and discard the urine before the test begins. Note the time. Save all urine during the specified time (12 or 24 hours) in a urine container without any preservative, and keep it refrigerated or on ice.

- Encourage water intake hourly during the test to have sufficient urine output.
- Label the container with the exact time and date the urine collection started and ended.

Factors Affecting Laboratory Results

- Phenacetin decreases the creatinine clearance.
- Toilet paper and feces will contaminate the urine.

NURSING IMPLICATIONS WITH RATIONALE

- Inform the health care provider of medications the client is receiving that could cause false test results.

Client Teaching

- Explain to the client the procedure for blood and urine collection. Blood is drawn in the morning. The client voids and the urine is discarded. Then all urine is saved for 12 hours or 24 hours in a urine container. Toilet paper and feces should not be in the urine.

- Instruct the client not to consume meats, poultry, fish, tea, or coffee for 6 hours before the test or during the test, according to the health care provider's orders.
- Encourage water intake throughout the test—approximately 100 mL/hour.
- Instruct client not to do strenuous exercise during the test.

C Crossmatching (blood)
Blood Typing Tests, Compatibility Test for RBCs, Type and Cross Match

Reference Values
Adult: Compatibility; absence of agglutination (clumping) of cells.
Child: Same as adult.

Description
The four *major* blood types (A, B, AB, and O) belong to the ABO blood group system. Red blood cells have either antigen A, B, AB, or none on the surface of the cells. Type A has A antigen, B has B antigen, AB has A and B antigens, and O does not contain an antigen. These antigens are capable of producing antibodies. The AB blood person is the universal recipient (can accept all blood), because there are no antibodies; the O blood person is the universal donor (can give blood to all types).

ABO blood type and Rh factor are first determined, then the compatibility of donor and recipient blood is determined by major crossmatch. The major crossmatch is between the donor's RBCs and the recipient's serum, and the test is performed to determine if the recipient has any antibodies to destroy the donor's RBCs.

Purpose
- To determine blood type.

Procedure
- There is no food or fluid restriction.
- Collect 7–10 mL of venous blood in a red-top tube (not a serum separator tube).

Factors Affecting Laboratory Results
- Previously received incompatible blood can make blood crossmatching difficult.

NURSING IMPLICATIONS WITH RATIONALE
- Observe the client for signs and symptoms of fluid volume deficit (hypovolemia), such as tachycardia (pulse greater than 100), tachypnea (rapid breathing), pale color, clammy skin, and low blood pressure (late symptoms). Crystalloid solutions (saline, lactated Ringer's) might be given rapidly to replace fluid volume until a transfusion can be administered. Usually 15–45 minutes are required to type and crossmatch blood.

- Check the date of the unit of blood. Usually blood should be used within 28 days. Blood that is older than 28 days should not be given to a client having hyperkalemia.
- Monitor the recipient's vital signs before and during transfusions. Signs and symptoms of transfusion reaction include a rise in temperature greater than 1.1°C, chills, and dyspnea.
- Start the blood transfusion at a slow rate for the first 15 minutes; stay with the client and observe for adverse reactions.
- Flush the transfusion set with normal saline if other IV solutions are ordered to follow the blood.

C

Cryoglobulins (serum)

Reference Values

Adult: Negative.

Child: Negative.

Description

Cryoglobulins are abnormal immunoglobulins (Ig) that are in the blood and will precipitate at low temperatures and dissolve at warm temperatures. They are present in IgG and IgM groups. When they are exposed to very cold temperatures, they precipitate in the smaller blood vessels, such as the fingers, and can cause Raynaud phenomenon with symptoms of pain, coldness of the fingers, cyanosis, and purpura. These abnormal Ig proteins occur in other disease entities, such as autoimmune disorders (e.g., rheumatoid arthritis, systemic lupus erythematosus); acute and chronic infections (e.g., infectious mononucleosis, streptococcal glomerulonephritis, endocarditis); and lymphoid malignancies (e.g., leukemia, lymphoma, multiple myeloma). They can also occur in hepatitis C and Sjögren syndrome.

Cryoglobulins are classed as 1, 2, or 3. Type 2 cryoglobulinemia is the most common, occurring in Raynaud phenomenon, rheumatoid arthritis, nephrotic syndrome, and sensory-motor neuropathy. Type 1 cryoglobulin is associated with lymphocytic leukemia, lymphoma, and multiple myeloma. The cryoglobulin level could be equal to or greater than 5 mg/mL. Type 3 cryoglobulin is found with streptococcal glomerulonephritis, endocarditis, SLE, chronic infections, infectious mononucleosis, and rheumatoid arthritis.

Purposes

- To assist in diagnosing certain autoimmune disorders, lymphoid malignancies, acute and chronic infections, and Raynaud phenomenon.
- To compare the test results with other laboratory tests.

Clinical Problems

Increased Level: Raynaud phenomenon, autoimmune disorders (rheumatoid arthritis, SLE), acute and chronic infections (infectious mononucleosis, streptococcal glomerulonephritis, endocarditis), certain malignancies (leukemia, lymphomas, multiple myeloma), Sjögren syndrome, hepatitis C, certain renal dysfunctions (nephrotic syndrome), and sensory-motor neuropathy.

Procedure

- There is no food or fluid restriction unless indicated. Some institutions' protocols require food and fluid restriction for 4–8 hours.
- Collect 10 mL of venous blood in a syringe/tube prewarmed to 37°C or 98.6°F in a red-top tube to prevent loss of cryoglobulins.
- Transport blood specimen immediately in a warm container.
- In the laboratory, the blood specimen is then refrigerated and checked periodically for precipitation. If precipitation occurs, the blood specimen is rewarmed, and if the precipitation is dissolved, cryoglobulin is present.

Factors Affecting Laboratory Results

- Collecting blood in a red-top tube that has not been prewarmed.
- Not transporting the blood specimen immediately to the laboratory in a warmed container.
- Refrigerating the blood specimen before transporting the blood sample to laboratory.

NURSING IMPLICATIONS WITH RATIONALE

- Obtain a history of client's clinical problems.
- Observe for signs and symptoms of SLE (e.g., "butterfly" rash on cheeks and bridge of the nose, arthritis, and urinary insufficiency).
- Observe for signs and symptoms of rheumatoid arthritis (e.g., pain and stiffness in the joints; swollen, red, tender joints; joint deformities; and inability to make a fist and flexion contractures).
- Compare serum cryoglobulins with other laboratory tests.

Client Teaching

- Instruct the client to remain NPO as indicated (some institutions state NPO for 4–8 hours) before the test. Check with your health facility.
- Explain the test procedure. The result of the test takes several days.
- Advise the client with Raynaud symptoms to avoid cold temperatures and to dress warmly, including hat and gloves.
- Answer questions the client may have or refer the questions to appropriate health professionals.

Cultures (blood, sputum, stool, throat, wound, urine)

Reference Values

Adult: Negative or no pathogen.

Child: Same as adult.

Description

(*Also see Antibiotic Susceptibility.*)

Cultures are taken to isolate the microorganism that is causing the clinical infection. Most culture specimens are obtained using sterile swabs with medium (solid or broth), a sterile container (cup) with a lid, and a sterile syringe with a sterile bottle of liquid medium. The culture specimen should be taken immediately to the laboratory after collection (no longer than 30 minutes), because some organisms will die if not placed in the proper medium and incubated.

Most specimens for culture are blood, sputum, stool, throat secretions, wound exudate, or urine. It usually takes 24–36 hours to grow the organisms and 48 hours for the growth and culture report.

Purpose

- To isolate the microorganism in body tissue or body fluid.

Clinical Problems

SPECIMEN	CLINICAL CONDITION OR MOST COMMONLY ISOLATED ORGANISM
Blood	Bacteremia, septicemia, postoperative shock, fever of unknown origin
Sputum	Pulmonary tuberculosis, bacterial pneumonia, chronic bronchitis, bronchiectasis
Stool	*Salmonella* species, *Shigella* species, enteropathogenic *Escherichia coli*, *Staphylococcus* species, *Yersinia*
Throat	Beta-hemolytic streptococci (rheumatic fever), thrush (*Candida* species), tonsillar infection, *Staphylococcus aureus*
Wound	*Staphylococcus* species: *S. aureus*, *Pseudomonas aeruginosa*, *Proteus* species, *Bacteroides* species, *Klebsiella* species, *Serratia* species
Urine	*Escherichia coli*, *Klebsiella* species, *Pseudomonas aeruginosa*, *Serratia* species, *Shigella* species, yeasts: *Candida* species

Procedure

- It is essential to wash your hands both before and after collecting the specimen.
- Send the specimen for culture to the laboratory *immediately* after collection.
- Obtain the specimen before antibiotic therapy is started. If the client is receiving antibiotics, the drug(s) should be listed on the laboratory slip.
- Collection containers or tubes should be sterile. Aseptic technique should be used during collection. Contamination of the specimen could cause false-positive results and/or transmission of the organisms.
- Check with the laboratory for specific techniques used.

Blood: Cleanse the client's skin according to the institution's procedure. Usually the skin is scrubbed first with povidone-iodine (Betadine). Iodine can be irritating to the skin, so it is removed and an application of benzalkonium chloride or alcohol is applied. Cleanse the top(s) of the culture bottle(s) with iodine and leave it to dry. The bottle(s) should contain a culture medium. Collect 5–10 mL of venous blood and place in the sterile bottle. Special vacuum tubes containing a culture medium for blood may be used instead of a culture bottle.

Sputum: *Sterile container or cup:* Obtain sputum for culture early in the morning, before breakfast. Instruct the client to give several deep coughs to raise sputum. Tell the client to avoid spitting saliva secretion into the sterile container. Saliva and postnasal drip secretions can contaminate the sputum specimen. Keep a lid on the sterile container. The container *should not* be completely filled and should be taken immediately to the laboratory. The sputum sample should not remain for hours by the client's bedside unless one needs a 24-hour sputum specimen (in this case, an extra sterile container should be left). *Acid-Fast Bacilli (TB Culture):* Follow the instructions on the container. Collect 5–10 mL of sputum, and take the sample immediately to the laboratory or refrigerate the specimen. Three sputum specimens may be requested, 1 each day for 3 days. Check for proper labeling.

Stool: Collect an approximately 1-inch-diameter feces sample. Use a sterile tongue blade and place the stool specimen in a sterile container with a lid. The suspected disease or organism should be noted on the laboratory slip. The stool specimen should not contain urine. The client should not be given barium or mineral oil, which can inhibit bacteria growth.

Throat: Use a sterile cotton swab or a polyester-tipped swab. The sterile culture kit could be used. Swab the inflamed or ulcerated tonsillar and/or postpharyngeal areas of the throat. Place the applicator in a Culturette tube with its culture medium. Take the throat culture specimen immediately to the laboratory. Do *not* give antibiotics before taking the culture.

Wound: Use a culture kit containing a sterile cotton swab or a polyester-tipped swab and a tube with culture medium. Swab the exudate of the wound and place the swab in the tube containing a culture medium. Wear sterile gloves when there is an excess amount of purulent drainage.

Urine: *Clean-caught (midstream) urine specimen:* Clean-caught urine collection is the most common method for collecting a urine specimen for culture. There are noncatheterization kits giving step-by-step instructions. Catheterizing for urine culture is seldom ordered. Usually the client collects the urine specimen for culture, so a detailed explanation should be given, according to the instructions. The penis or vulva should be well cleansed. At times, two urine specimens (2–10 mL) are requested to verify the organism and in case of a possible contamination of the urine specimen. Collect a midstream urine specimen early in the morning, or as ordered, in a sterile container. The lid should fit tightly on the container and the urine specimen should be taken immediately to the bacteriology laboratory or be refrigerated. Label the urine specimen with the client's name, the date, and the exact time of collection (e.g., 7/22/20 @ 8:00 AM). List any antibiotics or sulfonamides the client is taking on the laboratory slip.

Factors Affecting Laboratory Results

- Contamination of the specimen causes inaccurate results.
- Antibiotics and sulfonamides may cause false-negative results.
- Urine in the stool collection may cause false test results.

NURSING IMPLICATIONS WITH RATIONALE

- Explain the procedure for obtaining the culture specimen. Answer questions. If the client participates in the collection of the specimen (e.g., urine), the procedure should be reviewed several times.
- Hold antibiotics or sulfonamides until after the specimen has been collected. These drugs could cause false-negative results. If these drugs have been given, they should be listed on the laboratory slip and recorded on the client's chart.
- Deliver all specimens immediately to the laboratory or refrigerate the specimen.

- Handle the specimen(s) with extreme care. Aseptic technique should be used. Prevent contamination of the specimen(s) or transmission of the organism to other clients or yourself. Observe strict aseptic techniques.
- Keep lids on sterile specimen containers. Sputum cups should not be uncovered by the bedside.
- Suggest a culture if a pathogenic organism is suspected. Check the client's temperature.

C

Cyanide (serum, blood)

Reference Values

Serum: *Lethal:* >0.1 mg/L, >3.7 µmol/L (SI units). *Smoker:* 0.006 mg/L.

Blood: *Lethal:* >1 mg/L, >36 µmol/L (SI units). *Smoker:* 0.04 mg/L.

Description

Cyanide is a very toxic chemical that stops cellular respiration, causing death by asphyxia. One of the main causes of cyanide poisoning is suicide. Other causes include toxic fumes from burning nitrogen-containing products (a hazard for firefighters), industrial exposure to pesticides and metallurgy, and accidental poisoning from ingestion.

Purposes

- To test for cyanide poisoning.
- To check smokers for the risk of cyanide poisoning.

Clinical Problems

Increased Level: End products of combustion from metal and plastic refineries, cigarette smoking, and organic solvent of methyl cyanide.

Procedure

- Collect 7 mL of blood in a lavender-top or green-top tube.
- Give 15 mL of oxygen by mask.

Factors Affecting Laboratory Results

- Insufficient blood specimen can cause false results.

NURSING IMPLICATIONS WITH RATIONALE

- Obtain a history of work-related possible cyanide toxicity from client, family, or worker.
- Provide oxygen to the client if breathing is labored. Cyanide poisoning can cause shortness of breath (SOB) and dyspnea.
- Monitor respiratory and neurologic status of the client.

- Assess client for symptoms related to cyanide poisoning, such as labored breathing, dizziness, syncope, tachycardia, convulsion, and unresponsiveness.
- Loss of consciousness, metabolic acidosis, and respiratory failure are late stages of cyanide poisoning.

Client Teaching

- Answer client's family questions or refer them to appropriate health professionals.
- Be supportive to client and family.

C

Cytokines

Reference Values

Varies with the cytokines.

Description

Cytokines are a group of proteins from many cells, for example, T cells and B cells, lymphocytes, monocytes, and eosinophils that produce immune responses. These groups of cells protect the body from inflammation, infection, allergies, and tumor. A cytokine might act differently from another cytokines in different types of cells.

Leukocytes (lymphocytes and monocytes) produce interleukins that are effective against many disease processes, such as asthma, interstitial cystitis, rheumatoid arthritis, multiple sclerosis, tumors, and others. The research on cytokine assay is ongoing. This test can determine the progression of AIDS. Also, it may be used to determine the immune function and response.

Purposes

- To determine the immune response to various health problems.
- To obtain cytokine assay for research.

Clinical Problems

Increased Level: Various health problems, for example, rheumatoid arthritis, cancer, AIDS, inflammatory diseases, multiple organ failure, bone marrow suppression, and others.

Procedure

- Collect 7 mL of venous blood in a red-top tube.
- Other fluids can be used in this test, for example, joint fluid, cerebrospinal fluid.
- Specimen should be immediately refrigerated or frozen.

Factors Affecting Laboratory Results

- Degradation of the cytokines in the collection tube.
- Changes occurring to cytokines by stimulating or inhibiting other cytokine while in the collection tube.

NURSING IMPLICATIONS WITH RATIONALE

- Obtain a history of the health problems, which may vary.
- Explain the purpose and procedure for the cytokine test. If the main purpose is not known, refer to the physician or other health care provider.
- Have the client sign a permission form for a spinal test in order to obtain the cerebrospinal fluid.

Client Teaching

- Be available to the client and family to express any concerns. If answers are unknown, refer to the health care provider.

C

Cytomegalovirus (CMV) antibody (serum)

Reference Values

(Enzyme immunoassay [EIA] for IgG and IgM.)

Adult or Child: Negative to less than 0.30: no CMV IgM Ab detected. 0.30–0.59: weak positive for CMV IgM Ab (suggestive of a recent infection in neonates. Significance of this low level in adults is not determined). Greater than 0.60: positive for CMV IgM Ab.

Description

Cytomegalovirus (CMV) belongs to the herpes virus family and causes the most common congenital infection in infants. CMV can be found in most body secretions (saliva, cervical secretions, urine, breast milk, and semen). If the pregnant woman is infected with CMV, it crosses the placenta, infecting the fetus. In infants, this virus can cause cerebral tissue malformation and damage. Urine specimens for CMV bodies or throat swabs may be used to detect CMV, but they frequently are not as helpful in detection as the serology test.

Many adults have been exposed to the virus and have developed immunity to CMV. Transmission of the CMV virus to immunocompromised persons such as persons with the acquired immunodeficiency syndrome (AIDS) is serious, because these people tend to acquire this virus readily. Also, transmission of CMV can be via blood transfusions from CMV-seropositive donors. Serologic studies (CMV-IgM antibodies and CMV-IgG antibodies) yield results in a shorter period than by culture. Cultures may be used to confirm the findings.

Purpose

- To identify the CMV in possibly infected childbearing or pregnant women, infants, or immunocompromised persons.

Clinical Procedure

Increased Levels: Prone to CMV infection are childbearing women, infants, persons with AIDS or other immune deficiency, posttransplant organ recipients, and those who have had open heart surgery or hepatitic syndromes.

Procedure

- There is no food or fluid restriction.
- Collect 5–7 mL of venous blood in a red-top tube. Two blood samples are usually requested; the first is drawn during the acute phase, and 10–14 days later the second specimen is drawn for the convalescent phase.

Factors Affecting Laboratory Results

- A false-positive test result may occur for those with the rheumatoid factor in the serum or those exposed to the Epstein-Barr virus.
- Serum CMV test performed on infants who are younger than 6 months old. These infants could have the maternal CMV antibodies in their blood.

D

NURSING IMPLICATIONS WITH RATIONALE

- Obtain a history from the client of possible herpes-like viral infection.
- Assess the client for chronic respiratory infection or changes in vision. CMV retinitis can occur, which may result in blindness. Antiviral drugs may be used to treat CMV.
- Use aseptic technique when caring for clients infected with CMV.

Client Teaching

- Explain to the client that a blood sample is taken during the acute phase and again in approximately 2 weeks during the convalescent phase to determine the effectiveness of the treatment.
- Listen to the client's concerns about the possible effects of this virus on self or infant. Refer questions to appropriate health professionals as necessary.

D-dimer test (blood)

Fragment D-Dimer, Fibrin Degradation Fragment

Reference Values

Negative for D-Dimer Fragments: Greater than 250 ng/mL, greater than 250 mcg/L (SI units).

Description

D-dimer, a fibrin degradation fragment, occurs through fibrinolysis. This test measures the amount of fibrin degradation that occurs. It confirms the presence of fibrin split products (FSPs) and is more specific for diagnosing DIC (disseminated intravascular coagulation) than FSPs. However, both D-dimer and FSP tests are frequently used to determine DIC in a client.

D-dimer levels are increased when a fibrin clot is broken down by the thrombolytic drug, tissue plasminogen activator (tPA), or streptokinase.

Purpose

- To detect the presence of DIC in a client.

Clinical Problems

Increased Levels: Disseminated intravascular coagulation; pulmonary embolism; arterial, coronary, and venous thrombosis; possibly myocardial infarction; neoplastic disease, surgery up to post second day; late pregnancy; sickle-cell crisis.

Procedure

- There is no food or fluid restriction.
- Collect 7 mL of venous blood in a blue-top tube. Avoid hemolysis; invert tube gently, and do not shake the tube.
- Apply pressure to the venipuncture site, especially if the client has a bleeding tendency. Pressure may need to be applied for up to 5 minutes.
- Blood specimen should be taken to the laboratory within 4 hours.

Factors Affecting Laboratory Results

- Hemolysis of the blood specimen.

D

NURSING IMPLICATIONS WITH RATIONALE

- Obtain a history of unexplained bleeding or any condition that is included in the Clinical Problems.
- Note signs of sweating, cold and mottled fingers and toes, petechiae, and bleeding. Report adverse signs and symptoms immediately.
- Check and monitor vital signs.

Client Teaching

- Explain to the client and family the purposes of the test.

Dexamethasone suppression test (DST)
ACTH Suppression Test

Reference Values

Greater than 50% reduction of plasma cortisol and urine 17-hydroxycorticosteroids (17-OHCS). *Rapid* or *Overnight Screening Test:* Plasma cortisol: 8 AM less than 10 mcg/dL, 4 PM less than 5 mcg/dL. Urine 17-OHCS (5-hour specimen): Less than 4 mg/5 h.

Increased Dexamethasone Dose: *Low Dose:* Plasma cortisol; one half of client's baseline level. Urine 17-OHCS: Less than 2.5 mg/24 h/second day. *High Dose:* Plasma cortisol; one half of client's baseline level. Urine 17-OHCS: one half of client's baseline level.

Note: The high dose test is done if results do not change with a low dose of dexamethasone.

Description

Dexamethasone (Decadron) is a potent glucocorticoid. The dexamethasone suppression test distinguishes between adrenal hyperplasia and adrenal tumor as the cause of adrenal hyperfunction, such as Cushing disease, and is used to diagnose and to manage depression.

When given dexamethasone, there is a reduction (suppression) in adrenocorticotropin hormone (ACTH) secretion (negative feedback), thus causing a lower plasma and urine cortisol. Low-dose and high-dose dexamethasone are used to distinguish between adrenal hyperplasia and adrenal tumor (nonsuppressed at low or high doses). Adrenal hyperplasia will suppress at high doses but not at low doses. With adrenal cancer, cortisol secretion continues; and with ectopic ACTH-producing tumor (e.g., lung cancer), the tumor (ectopic) will continue to secrete ACTH regardless of a high cortisol level.

In psychiatry, the test is useful in diagnosing affective diseases, such as endogenous depression (melancholia). In approximately 50% of these clients, suppression of plasma cortisol and ACTH do not occur with a low dose of dexamethasone. Also, this test is helpful to identify if the depressed client responds to antidepressants rather than psychologic therapy.

The test could be a rapid or overnight screening test or a 2-day test (eight doses of dexamethasone) with low and/or high doses of the drug.

Purpose

- To distinguish between adrenal hyperplasia and adrenal tumor as the cause of adrenal hyperfunction.

Clinical Problems

Adrenal Hyperplasia (Cushing Disease)

Low Dose: No changes in plasma cortisol or 17-OHCS level.
High Dose: 50% reduction of plasma cortisol or 17-OHCS level.

Adrenal Cancer or Ectopic Tumor

Low Dose and High Dose: No changes in plasma cortisol or 17-OHCS level.

Procedure

- Obtain a baseline plasma cortisol and urine 17-OHCS level 24 hours before the test.
- Avoid tea, caffeinated coffee, chocolates. No other food or fluid restriction is required.
- Refrigerate urine for 17-OHCS levels.

Rapid or Overnight Screening Test

- NPO after midnight. Check with laboratory policy.
- Give dexamethasone 1 mg or 5 mcg/kg PO at 11 PM.
- Obtain baseline plasma cortisol and urine 17-OHCS levels. Draw blood at 8 AM for plasma cortisol level. Obtain a urine OHCS level at 12 noon.

Increased Dexamethasone Dose: Two days of low or high doses of dexamethasone (Decadron).

Low Dose

- Give dexamethasone 0.5 mg every 6 hours for 2 days (total of 4 mg).
- Obtain a plasma cortisol level at 8 AM, 4 PM, and 11 PM and a 24-hour urine 17-OHCS level after a 2-day low-dose test. If no suppression is found, the high-dose test may be recommended.

- Give dexamethasone 2 mg every 6 hours for 2 days (total of 16 mg).
- Obtain a plasma cortisol level at 8 AM, 4 PM, and 11 PM and a 24-hour urine 17-OHCS level after a 2-day high-dose test.

Factors Affecting Laboratory Results
- Ingestion of excess coffee, tea, and chocolates could increase steroid release.
- Not refrigerating urine for 17-OHCS test could affect results.
- Drugs that may cause false negatives include synthetic steroid therapy and high doses of benzodiazepines.
- Drugs that may cause false positives include phenytoin (Dilantin), barbiturates, meprobamate, carbamazepine.

D

NURSING IMPLICATIONS WITH RATIONALE

- Report anxiety, stress, fever, or infection to the health care provider.
- Obtain baseline plasma cortisol and urine 17-OHCS levels 24 hours before the test. For the screening test, a plasma cortisol level should be obtained at 8 AM and a urine 17-OHCS level at 12 noon. For the 2-day dexamethasone test, a plasma and urine level should be obtained after 2 days of low or high dexamethasone dosage.
- Administer dexamethasone at specified times *on time*. Milk or antacids may be required to decrease gastric irritation.
- Provide ample time for the client to ask questions. Refer unknown answers to appropriate health professionals.
- Assess for side effects of dexamethasone resulting from high doses (e.g., weight gain, gastric discomfort).
- Monitor electrolytes during the test. Steroid causes serum potassium loss and serum sodium excess.
- Check blood glucose for hyperglycemia while the client is taking high doses of dexamethasone. This drug is a glucocorticosteroid and can elevate blood glucose levels.
- Be supportive to client and family members during the test. This is a time-consuming test procedure. Cooperation from client and family members is needed for accurate results.

Client Teaching
- Instruct the client to avoid caffeinated coffee, tea, and chocolate.

Diabetes mellitus autoantibodies (serum)
See also Insulin Antibodies

Reference Values
No antibody detection.

Description

Type 1 diabetes mellitus (Type 1 DM; DM 1) or insulin-dependent diabetes mellitus (IDDM) is an autoimmune disease that results in destruction to the pancreatic B cells, causing a loss of insulin. It is described in the insulin antibodies section. Autoimmune diabetes could be the result of a genetic or environmental occurrence. These antibodies occur in type 1 DM (DM type 1), but they do not occur in type 2 DM (DM type 2). Usually the antibodies occur years before the symptoms.

Some clients who had gestational diabetes mellitus will eventually require insulin. Those clients most frequently have antibodies present.

Purposes

- To identify clients with type 1 DM (DM1) that have diabetes mellitus autoantibodies.
- To identify clients who have diabetes mellitus autoantibodies that may require insulin in the future.

Clinical Problems

Increased Level: Type 1 diabetes mellitus (DM1), gestational diabetes mellitus.

Procedure

- There is no food or fluid restriction.
- Collect 5 mL of venous blood in a red- or lavender-top tube.

Factors Affecting Laboratory Results

- Radioactive scans that were done 1 to 7 days before the diabetes mellitus autoantibody test can interfere with test results.

NURSING IMPLICATIONS WITH RATIONALE

- Obtain a history from the client of his or her symptoms that relate to diabetes mellitus.
- Obtain a client history of genetic, environmental, and recent illnesses, such as hepatitis or other infectious diseases.
- Permit the client time to express his or her concerns about the test results.
- Answer client questions or refer the questions to a health care provider.

Diazepam (serum)

Valium

Reference Values

Therapeutic: *Adult:* 0.5–2 mg/L, 400–600 ng/mL.
Toxic: *Adult:* 3 mg/L, greater than 3,000 ng/mL.

Description

Diazepam (Valium), a benzodiazepine, has been one of the most commonly prescribed antianxiety agents in the United States. The clinical uses of diazepam include treatment of status epilepticus; alcohol withdrawal; induction of anesthesia for minor surgical procedures and endoscopic procedures; cardioversion; and muscle relaxation, especially in paraplegia, cerebral palsy, and tetanus.

Diazepam is absorbed from the gastrointestinal tract and is metabolized in the liver to a large number of metabolites. The peak blood level occurs 1–2 hours after the oral dose. After a single oral dose of 10–15 mg, peak value level usually is 200–300 ng/mL. Half-life is 10–40 hours (40 hours with continuous use). The major metabolite, *N*-desmethyldiazepam, has a half-life of 50–90 hours. Onset of action is 30–60 minutes after oral dose, 15–30 minutes after IM injection, and 1–5 minutes after IV dose. Diazepam is excreted in the urine as metabolites. This drug can cross the placenta and might cause teratogeny (birth defects).

A steady state for the serum diazepam level may take 1–2 weeks to attain. Monitoring the serum diazepam level should be continued once the steady state is reached and especially when daily dose is changed.

D

Purposes

- To monitor diazepam levels.
- To detect toxic levels of diazepam.

Clinical Problems

Decreased Level: Smoking.

Increased Level: Diazepam overdose, liver disease, alcohol. *Drug Influence:* Cimetidine (Tagamet), isoniazid (INH), valproic acid (Depakene).

Procedure

- There is no food or fluid restriction.
- Collect 3–5 mL of venous blood in a red-top tube 2 hours after an oral dose or at trough level (before the next dose).
- Record the dose, route, and last-administered dose on the laboratory requisition slip.

Factors Affecting Laboratory Results

- Drugs (*see Drug Influence above*) might cause an increased diazepam level.
- Taking other benzodiazepines (e.g., chlordiazepoxide [Librium], chlorazepate dipotassium [Tranxene]) along with diazepam will interfere with correct test results, because these agents contain many of the same active metabolites.

NURSING IMPLICATIONS WITH RATIONALE

- Record the dose, route, and last time the drug was given on the requisition slip. Usually the blood specimen is drawn 2 hours after taking diazepam.
- Elicit from a female client if she is pregnant or intends to become pregnant before giving diazepam. This drug may have teratogenic effects.

■ Monitor frequently serum diazepam levels in children, in the elderly, and in debilitated adults. Small doses of diazepam should be given to these individuals to avoid diazepam toxicity.

■ Recognize that erratic absorption of diazepam could result from IM administration. Diazepam toxicity could occur after numerous injections.

Decreased Level

■ Recognize that smoking can decrease the diazepam level.

■ Avoid administering diazepam in IV fluids. This drug could precipitate in the fluids or adhere to the IV bag or tubing, thus decreasing prescribed dosage.

Increased Level

■ Recognize that diazepam overdose, liver disease, or alcohol could elevate the serum diazepam level.

■ Check for signs and symptoms of diazepam toxicity (e.g., drowsiness, ataxia, confusion, headache, slurred speech, tremors, hypotension, tachycardia, and circulatory collapse).

Client Teaching

■ Instruct the client not to ingest alcohol or other central nervous system depressants while taking diazepam. The effects of taking these substances together could cause severe drowsiness, respiratory distress, or respiratory arrest.

■ Explain to the client that diazepam should never be abruptly discontinued. Diazepam is tapered to lower doses over 1–2 weeks to avoid withdrawal symptoms (e.g., confusion, tremors, paranoia, ataxia, visual hallucinations, sweating, and abdominal and muscle cramps).

Differential white blood cell (WBC) count

See WBC Differential

Digoxin (serum)

Lanoxin

Reference Values

Therapeutic: *Adult:* 0.5–2 ng/mL, 0.5–2 nmol/L (SI units). *Infants:* 1–3 ng/mL. *Child:* Same as adult.

Toxic: *Adult:* Greater than 2 ng/mL, greater than 2.6 nmol/L (SI units). *Infants:* Greater than 3.5 ng/mL. *Child:* Same as adult.

Description

Digoxin, a form of digitalis, is a cardiac glycoside agent given to increase the force and velocity of myocardial contraction. More than 75–95% of the drug is absorbed through the gastrointestinal tract, and a large amount of digoxin is excreted unchanged through the kidneys. The half-life of digoxin is 35–40 hours, with a shorter half-life in neonates and infants and a longer time in short-term infants/premature infants.

Serum plateau levels of digoxin occur 6–8 hours after an oral dose, 2–4 hours after IV administration, and 10–12 hours after IM administration. The most frequent routes used for administering digoxin are by mouth (oral) and IV.

Electrolyte imbalance (hypokalemia or hypomagnesemia), acid–base disturbances, and certain drugs predispose the person to digitalis toxicity. Common signs and symptoms of digitalis toxicity include pulse rate less than 60 per minute, anorexia, nausea, vomiting, headaches, and visual disturbance.

D

Purpose

- To monitor digoxin levels.

Clinical Problems

Decreased Level: Decreased GI absorption, decreased GI motility. *Drug Influence:* Antacids, Kaopectate, metoclopramide (Reglan), barbiturates, cholestyramine (Questran), spironolactone (Aldactone).

Increased Level: Digoxin overdose, renal disease, liver disease. *Drug Influence:* Amphotericin B, diuretics (ethacrynic acid [Edecrin], furosemide [Lasix], thiazides), chlorthalidone (Hygroton), quinidine, reserpine (Serpasil), succinylcholine, sympathomimetics, corticosteroids.

Procedure

- There is no food or fluid restriction.
- Collect 3–5 mL of venous blood in a red-top tube.
- Obtain a blood sample 6–10 hours after administration of oral digoxin, or, frequently preferred, take sample prior to next dose.

Factors Affecting Laboratory Results

- Administering digoxin intramuscularly might cause the absorption rate to be erratic, especially in a debilitated or elderly person with poor tissue perfusion.
- A low serum potassium or magnesium level could cause digitalis toxicity, and a high serum calcium level could cause digitalis toxicity.
- Hypothyroidism, severe heart disease, and renal function abnormalities may predispose a client to digitalis toxicity.

NURSING IMPLICATIONS WITH RATIONALE

- Do not confuse digoxin with other digitalis glycosides (e.g., digitoxin). Digitoxin has a longer half-life and cumulative effect.

- Check serum digoxin results and report nontherapeutic levels to the physician immediately.
- Keep the digoxin bottle away from light.
- Obtain a blood sample for serum digoxin determination during predicted plateau levels for oral, IV, and IM administration.
- Take the apical pulse for 1 minute prior to administering digoxin. If the pulse rate is less than 60 per minute, do not give the digoxin, and notify the health care provider.

Decreased Level

- Associate GI disturbance and certain drugs (e.g., antacids, Kaopectate, barbiturates, cholestyramine, spironolactone) with a decreased therapeutic serum digoxin level. The digoxin dose might need to be increased if those drugs are being taken. If the digoxin dose has been increased while the client is on the drug(s) and later the drug has been discontinued, the digoxin dosage should be decreased.
- Inform the health care provider which drugs the client is taking that might decrease the effectiveness of the prescribed digoxin dose.

Increased Level

- Check serum potassium, magnesium, and calcium levels. Hypokalemia, hypomagnesemia, and hypercalcemia enhance the action of digoxin and could cause digitalis toxicity.
- Observe for signs and symptoms of digitalis toxicity (e.g., pulse rate less than 60 per minute, anorexia, nausea, vomiting, headache, visual disturbance).

Client Teaching

- Instruct the client to take his or her pulse before taking digoxin and to call the health care provider if the rate is less than 60 per minute in adults; in children a rate of less than 70 per minute should be reported.

Dilantin

See Phenytoin

D-xylose absorption test (blood and urine)

Reference Values

Adult: 25 grams: *Blood:* 25–75 mg/dL/2 h (average 45 mg/dL/2 h). *Urine:* Greater than 3.5 g/5 h; greater than 5 g/24 h. *Blood:* 8–28 mg/dL (= 15.7 mg/dL). *Urine:* 1.2–2.4 g/5 h (= 1.8 g)

Child: *Blood:* 30 mg/dL/1h

Description

The D-xylose absorption test determines the absorptive capacity of the small intestine. After ingestion of D-xylose, a pentose sugar, serum and urine D-xylose levels are measured. Usually a low serum D-xylose level (less than 25 mg/dL) and a low urine D-xylose level (less than 3 g) are indicative of malabsorption syndrome.

Abnormal test results occur in celiac disease, small-bowel ischemia, Whipple disease, Zollinger-Ellison syndrome, enteritis, massive intestinal resection, and intestinal bacterial overgrowth.

Various clinical problems, such as vomiting, hypomotility, dehydration, alcoholism, rheumatoid arthritis, severe heart failure, ascites, and poor renal function, could cause low urine D-xylose levels that are not secondary to intestinal malabsorption. Endoscopic examination and biopsy frequently are necessary to confirm the diagnosis of malabsorption.

Purpose

- To aid in the diagnosis of gastrointestinal disturbance/disorder.

Clinical Problems

Decreased Level: Celiac disease, small-bowel ischemia, Whipple disease, Zollinger-Ellison syndrome, radiation enteritis, multiple jejunal diverticula, diabetic neuropathy, diarrhea, lymphoma, amyloidosis, scleroderma, massive intestinal resection, bacterial overgrowth.

Procedure

- Restrict foods for 8 hours for adults and for 4 hours for children prior to test. Foods that contain pentose, such as fruits, jams, jellies, and pastries, should be withheld for 24 hours prior to the test.
- The client ingests 25 g of D-xylose dissolved in 8 oz (240 mL) of water. An additional 8 oz of water should follow the mixture of D-xylose and water. Some institutions use a 5-g dose instead of 25 g. Child dose is based on weight: 0.5 g/kg but not more than 25 g.
- Collect 7 mL of venous blood in a red-top tube. Blood specimens are drawn at 30, 60, and 120 minutes or at 2 hours only after D-xylose ingestion.
- Discard the urine specimen prior to the urine collection. Keep all urine refrigerated; at the end of 5 hours, send the urine collection to the laboratory.
- Check the order for the length of collection time (i.e., 5 hours or 24 hours). Note on the laboratory slip the period of urine collection and the age of the client. Older adults with mild renal impairment can have a decreased 5-hour test result and a normal 24-hour test.
- Indicate on the laboratory slip any drugs the client is taking that could affect test results. Nonsteroidal anti-inflammatory drugs (NSAIDs) such as aspirin, Motrin, Advil, and indomethacin (Indocin), should be withheld for 24 hours. Note the drug dose and the last time it was taken on the laboratory slip.

Factors Affecting Laboratory Results

- Drugs such as aspirin, indomethacin (Indocin), and atropine can decrease intestinal absorption.
- Foods high in pentose (e.g., fruits, jams, jellies, and pastries) can affect serum and urine D-xylose results.
- Hemolysis of the blood sample could cause inaccurate test results.

- Renal impairment or insufficiency could decrease urine output, thus affecting urine test results.
- Vomiting, dehydration, hypomotility, alcoholism, and other conditions (*see Description*) could cause a decreased urine D-xylose level that is not due to malabsorption.

NURSING IMPLICATIONS WITH RATIONALE

- Explain the blood and urine test procedures to the client.
- Assess communications for verbal and nonverbal expressions of anxiety and fear concerning tests or the potential or actual problem.
- Report to the health care provider if the client is having severe diarrhea, vomiting, and dehydration. These clinical problems could cause a decreased urine D-xylose level.
- Provide ongoing assessment before, during, and after the procedure. Document and communicate alterations.
- Be supportive to the client and to family members. They might be most anxious about the test procedure and the unknown test results. Client compliance during the procedure is essential for accurate test results.

Client Teaching

- Inform the client that food is restricted, but fluids are not. Instruct the client not to eat foods high in pentose (jellies, jams, fruits) for 24 hours before the test.
- Instruct the client to save all urine during the 5- or 24-hour urine test. Refrigerate urine collection.
- Instruct the client to withhold aspirin, indomethacin (Indocin), and atropine or atropine products, with the health care provider's approval, for 24 hours before the test. Aspirin could decrease D-xylose excretion and indomethacin and atropine could decrease intestinal absorption. Note on the laboratory slip the last drug dose and dosage that the client received.
- Be prepared to repeat information to the client and family if the anxiety or fear level is determined to be high. Provide written instructions to reinforce verbal instructions.

Encephalitis virus antibody (serum)

Reference Values

Titer: Less than 1:10. Definite confirmation of the virus: a fourfold rise in titer level between the acute and convalescent blood specimens.

Description

Encephalitis is inflammation of the brain tissue, which is frequently due to an arbovirus transmitted by a mosquito after the mosquito has been in contact with an animal host. There are several groups of arbovirus causing encephalitis. The animal host varies according to location.

Eastern Equine Encephalitis Virus: It is mainly found in the eastern United States from New Hampshire to Texas. Transmission is by the mosquito from the animal hosts: birds, ducks, fowl, and horses. Symptoms include fever, frontal headaches, drowsiness, nausea and vomiting, abnormal reflexes, rigidity, and bulging of the fontanelle in infants. The mortality rate of 65–75% is one of the highest for viral encephalitis.

California Encephalitis Virus: Incidence is highest in children in the north central United States. It is transmitted by infected mosquitoes and ticks. Symptoms include fever, severe headaches, stiff neck, and sore throat.

St. Louis Encephalitis Virus: This virus occurs most frequently in the southern, central, and western United States. It is a Group B arbovirus and is transmitted by an infected mosquito. The animal host is the bird. The symptoms of headache, stiff neck, and abnormal reflexes may be mild or severe.

Venezuelan Equine Encephalitis Virus: The incidence of this virus is highest in South America, Central America, Mexico, Texas, and Florida. It is a Group A arbovirus and is transmitted by an infected mosquito. The animal hosts are the rodent and horse. Symptoms can be mild such as flulike symptoms or severe such as disorientation, paralysis, seizures, and coma.

Western Equine Encephalitis Virus: Occurrence is primarily west of the Mississippi, particularly California, in the summer months and early fall. The virus is transmitted by mosquitoes infected by animal hosts: birds, squirrels, snakes, and horses. Symptoms include sore throat, stiff neck, lethargy, stupor, and coma in severe cases.

E

Purposes

- To detect the presence of an elevated encephalitis virus antibody titer, which indicates an inflammation of the brain tissue caused by an arboviral infection.
- To screen for an arbovirus.

Clinical Problems

Increased Titer: Viral encephalitis (identified strain), meningoencephalitis.

Procedure

- There is no food or fluid restriction.
- Collect 3–5 mL of venous blood in a red-top tube. Two blood specimens should be taken at least 2–3 weeks apart, first during the acute phase of the viral infection and second during the convalescent phase.
- Cerebrospinal fluid can be used to identify the virus.

Factors Affecting Laboratory Results

- Not obtaining a blood sample during both the acute and the convalescent phases.

NURSING IMPLICATIONS WITH RATIONALE

- Obtain a history of the client's contact with mosquitoes. Ascertain when the client first became ill.
- Assess for symptoms associated with encephalitis, such as fever, frontal headaches, sore throat, stiff neck, and lethargy.

Client Teaching

- Explain to the client that there will be two blood samples taken 2–3 weeks apart.
- Listen to the client's concerns. Answer the client's questions or refer to other professional health care providers.

Enterovirus group (serum)

Reference Values

Norm: Negative.

Positive: Fourfold rise in titer between the acute and convalescent periods.

Description

The enterovirus group includes many types of viruses that are found in the alimentary tract. Examples of these serotype viruses include Coxsackie A and B, echovirus, and poliomyelitis viruses. Testing for the enterovirus group is usually indicated when there is an epidemic outbreak of one of these viruses. Other methods for enteroviral testing include specimens from oropharynx, stool, and cerebrospinal fluid.

Purpose

- To identify the presence of an enterovirus associated with an epidemic outbreak such as Coxsackie A and B.

Clinical Problems

Positive Titer: Enteroviral infections.

Procedure

- There is no food or fluid restriction.
- Collect 3–5 mL of venous blood in a red-top tube. Usually two blood specimens are required; one at the acute phase and the second one during the convalescent phase (2–3 weeks between the two phases).

Factors Affecting Laboratory Test

- Not collecting two blood samples, one during the acute phase and one during the convalescent phase.

NURSING IMPLICATIONS WITH RATIONALE

- Obtain a history of an alimentary tract infection. Symptoms may vary, so the client's description of the symptoms should be recorded.
- Assess the client's vital signs. Report abnormal findings.

Erythrocyte osmotic fragility

See Osmotic Fragility

Erythrocyte sedimentation rate (ESR) (blood)

Sedimentation (SED) Rate

Reference Values

Adult: *Westergren Method: Male:* Less than 50 Years: 0–15 mm/h. *Female:* Less than 50 Years: 0–20 mm/h. *Male:* Greater than 50 Years: 0–20 mm/h. *Female:* Greater than 50 Years: 0–30 mm/h. *Wintrobe Method: Male:* 0–9 mm/h. *Female:* 0–15 mm/h.

Child: *Newborn:* 0–2 mm/h; *4–14 Years:* 0–10 mm/h.

E

Description

The erythrocyte sedimentation rate (ESR) (known also as the sedimentation rate or SED rate) is the rate at which red blood cells settle in unclotted blood in millimeters per hour (mm/hour). The ESR is nonspecific. The rate can be increased in acute inflammatory process, acute and chronic infections, tissue damage (necrosis), rheumatoid arthritis, collagen diseases, malignancies, and physiologic stress situations (e.g., pregnancy). To some hematologists, the ESR is unreliable because it is nonspecific and is affected by physiologic factors that cause inaccurate results.

The C-reactive protein test is considered more useful than the ESR because CRP increases more rapidly during an acute inflammatory process and returns to normal faster than the ESR. The ESR is still an old standby used by many physicians as a rough estimate of the disease process and for following the course of illness. With an elevated ESR, other laboratory tests should be conducted to properly identify the clinical problem.

Purpose

- To compare with other laboratory values for diagnosing inflammatory conditions (*see Clinical Problems*).

Clinical Problems

Decreased Level: Polycythemia vera, heart failure, sickle-cell anemias, infectious mononucleosis, factor V deficiency, degenerative arthritis, angina pectoris. *Drug Influence:* Ethambutol (Myambutol), quinine, salicylates (aspirins), cortisone, prednisone.

Increased Level: Rheumatoid arthritis, rheumatic fever, acute myocardial infarction, cancer (stomach, colon, breast, liver, kidney), Hodgkin disease, multiple myeloma, lymphosarcoma, bacterial endocarditis, gout, hepatitis, cirrhosis of the liver, acute pelvic inflammatory disease, syphilis, tuberculosis, glomerulonephritis, systemic lupus erythematosus, hemolytic disease of newborns (erythroblastosis fetalis), pregnancy (second and third trimesters). *Drug Influence:* Dextran, methyldopa (Aldomet), methysergide (Sansert), penicillamine (Cuprimine), procainamide (Pronestyl), theophylline, oral contraceptives, vitamin A.

Procedure

- There is no food or fluid restriction.
- Collect 7 mL of venous blood in a lavender-top tube. Keep the specimen in a vertical position.
- Take the blood specimen to the laboratory immediately. Blood should not stand, because the ESR could increase.
- If the blood specimen is refrigerated, it should be allowed to return to room temperature before it is tested.
- Hold medications that can cause false-positive results for 24 hours before the test, with health care provider's permission.

Factors Affecting Laboratory Results

- Factors increasing the ESR—pregnancy (second and third trimesters); menstruation; drugs (*see Drug Influence*); the presence of cholesterol, fibrinogen, and globulins.
- Factors decreasing the ESR—newborns (decreased fibrinogen level); drugs (*see Drug Influence*); high blood sugar, serum albumin, and serum phospholipids.

E

NURSING IMPLICATIONS WITH RATIONALE

Increased Level

- Relate an elevated ESR to clinical problems and drugs. The ESR is a nonspecific test, but it can indicate an inflammatory process occurring.
- Answer the client's questions about *the significance* of an increased ESR. An answer could be that other laboratory tests are usually performed in conjunction with the ESR for adequate diagnosis of a clinical problem.
- Compare ESR with CRP test results.

Estetrol (E$_4$) (plasma and amniotic fluid)

Reference Values

Pregnancy:

PLASMA		AMNIOTIC FLUID	
Week of Gestation	pg/mL	Week of Gestation	ng/mL
20–26	140–210	32+	0.8
30	greater than 350	40+	13
36	greater than 900		
40	greater than 1,050		

Description

Estetrol (E$_4$) is an effective indicator of fetal distress during the third trimester of pregnancy. Estetrol increases during gestation. At term, estetrol consists of .05–2% of the total unconjugated estrogen.

One test alone should not determine fetal distress. Several values, such as estriol (E₃) and human placental lactogen, are usually obtained to verify the possible diagnosis.

Purpose

- To detect the occurrence of fetal distress.

Clinical Problems

Decreased Level: Fetal distress, intrauterine fetal death, anencephalic fetus, fetal malformations.

Procedure

- There is no food or fluid restriction.
- Collect 5–7 mL of venous blood in a red-top tube.

Factors Affecting Laboratory Results

- Unknown.

E

NURSING IMPLICATIONS WITH RATIONALE

- Obtain a history of current problems related to the pregnancy.
- Monitor fetal heart rate.
- Compare serum estetrol with estriol and human placental lactogen levels. Report laboratory values to the health care provider.
- Listen to the client's and family's concerns. Refer questions to appropriate health professionals as necessary.

Estradiol (E₂) (serum)

Reference Values

Adult: *Female:* Follicular phase: 20–150 pg/mL. Midcycle: 100–500 pg/mL. Luteal phase: 60–260 pg/mL. Postmenopausal: Less than 30 pg/mL. *Male:* 15–50 pg/mL.

Child: 3–10 pg/mL.

Description

Estradiol (E₂) is a more potent estrogen than estrone (E₁) and estriol (E₃). This serum test is ordered for determining the presence of gonadal dysfunction. It is useful for evaluating menstrual and fertility problems in the female. It is not used to evaluate fetal well-being in pregnant females. Estradiol is produced mostly by the ovaries and also by the adrenal cortex and the testes. The serum estradiol levels are likely to be increased in males who have testicular or adrenal tumors and in females with estrogen-secreting ovarian tumors. Because serum estradiol level of prepubertal children may not be accurate, the serum test may need to be repeated.

Purposes

- To determine the presence of gonadal dysfunction.
- To evaluate menstrual and fertility problems in the female.

Clinical Problems

Decreased Level: Primary amenorrhea, anorexia nervosa, ovarian failure, pituitary insufficiency (hypopituitarism), menopause.

Increased Level: Ovarian tumors, testicular tumors, adrenal hyperplasia or tumors.

Procedure

- There is no food or fluid restriction.
- Collect 5–7 mL of venous blood in a red-top tube. For females, the blood sample may be drawn before ovulation occurs or at midcycle in the morning.
- Include on the laboratory slip the phase of the menstrual cycle the client is currently in.

Factors Affecting Laboratory Results

- Incorrect listing of the menstrual phase could affect the test result.

E

NURSING IMPLICATIONS WITH RATIONALE

- Obtain the phase of the menstrual cycle from the client. Record on the laboratory slip.
- Ascertain the client's concern about the test result. Be supportive.

Estriol (E₃) (serum and urine)

Reference Values

Pregnancy

SERUM		URINE	
Weeks of Gestation	ng/dL	Weeks of Gestation	mg/24 h
25–28	25–165	25–28	6–28
29–32	30–230	29–32	6–32
33–36	45–370	33–36	10–45
37–38	75–420	37–40	15–60
39–40	95–450		

Description

Estriol (E_3) is a major estrogenic compound produced largely by the placenta. It increases in maternal serum and urine after 2 months of pregnancy and continues at high levels until term. If toxemia, hypertension, or diabetes is present after 30 weeks of gestation, estriol levels are monitored. A decline in serum or urine estriol levels suggests fetal distress caused by placental malfunction. Serum estriol is replacing urine estriol because specimen collection is easier and there is no 24-hour waiting period. The advantage of the 24-hour urine estriol is avoidance of estriol value variations that usually occur within the day. A urine estriol averages out the "within-day" fluctuations of estriol. Repeated serum and/or urine estriol are frequently ordered.

Purposes
- To monitor estriol levels.
- To determine fetal distress after 30 weeks' gestation.
- To compare test results with estetrol test results regarding fetal distress.

Clinical Problems
Decreased Level: Fetal distress, placental dysfunction, diabetic pregnancy, pregnancy with hypertension, impending toxemia.

Increased Level: Urinary tract infection, glycosuria. *Drug Influence:* Antibiotics (ampicillin, neomycin), hydrochlorothiazide (HydroDIURIL), cortisone preparations.

Procedure
- There is no food or fluid restriction.

Serum
- Collect 5–7 mL of venous blood in a red-top tube.

Urine
- Collect urine for 24 hours in a large container with preservative.
- Label the client's name, date, and the exact times of collection (e.g., 3/28/20, 8 AM to 3/29/20, 8:03 AM).
- Two 24-hour urine specimens (taken a day apart) are usually ordered for more valid results.

Factors Affecting Laboratory Results
- Multiple pregnancy can increase levels.
- Incorrect gestation week can cause a false test result.
- Glycosuria and urinary tract infection could give false urine estriol results.

NURSING IMPLICATIONS WITH RATIONALE
- Monitor the fetal heart rate, the patient's blood pressure, and sugar in the urine. Hypertension and diabetes could cause placental dysfunction, leading to fetal distress.
- Report glycosuria and urinary tract infection during pregnancy; both could cause a false result.
- Be supportive of the client and family.

Client Teaching
- Inform the client that several blood samples may be taken. If a urine collection is ordered, inform the client that all urine should be saved and that there may be more than one 24-hour urine specimen requested.

Estrogen (serum)

Reference Values

Adult: *Female:* Early menstrual cycle: 60–200 pg/mL. Midmenstrual cycle: 120–440 pg/mL. Late menstrual cycle: 150–350 pg/mL. Postmenopausal: Less than 30 pg/mL. *Male:* 40–115 pg/mL.
Child: *1–6 Years:* 3–10 pg/mL; *8–12 Years:* Less than 30 pg/mL.

Description

Estrogens are produced by the ovaries, adrenal cortex, and testes. There are over 30 estrogens identified in the body, but only three measurable types of estrogens: estrone (E_1), estradiol (E_2), and estriol (E_3). Total serum estrogen reflects estrone, mostly estradiol, and some estriol. For fetal well-being during pregnancy, serum E_3 is used.

Purpose

- To diagnose ovarian dysfunction and other health problems (*see Clinical Problems*).

Clinical Problems

Decreased Level: Ovarian failure or dysfunction, primary hypogonadism, Turner syndrome, intrauterine death in pregnancy, pituitary insufficiency, postmenopausal symptoms, anorexia nervosa, psychogenic stress.

Increased Level: Ovarian tumors, precocious puberty, adrenal hyperplasia or tumors, testicular tumor, cirrhosis of the liver.

Procedure

- There is no food or fluid restriction.
- Collect 5–7 mL of venous blood in a red-top tube. Avoid hemolysis.
- Indicate on the laboratory slip the phase of the client's menstrual cycle.

Factors Affecting Laboratory Results

- Oral contraceptives can increase the estrogen level; steroids can affect test results; and clomiphene, an estrogen antagonist, could decrease the estrogen level.
- Shaking the blood sample could cause hemolysis.

NURSING IMPLICATIONS WITH RATIONALE

- Indicate on the laboratory slip if the client is taking steroids, oral contraceptives, or estrogens.
- Note on the laboratory slip the phase of client's menstrual cycle.
- Assess communications for verbal and nonverbal expressions of anxiety and fear concerning tests or the potential or actual problem.
- Encourage ventilation of feelings through provision of a private, calm environment. Use quiet, steady speech patterns when interacting with the client. Employ touch if appropriate.

Decreased Level

- Note and record if the client is postmenopausal.

Increased Level

- Recognize clinical problems that can increase the estrogen level. Men can have an increased estrogen level caused by adrenal or testicular tumors.
- Assess for signs and symptoms of estrogen excess in men (e.g., enlarged breasts, voice change).
- Be supportive to clients, female and male, having excessive estrogen levels. Encourage them to express their concerns.

Estrogens (total) (urine—24 hours)

E

Reference Values

Adult: *Female:* Preovulation: 5–25 mcg/24 h. Follicular phase: 24–100 mcg/24 h. Luteal phase: 22–80 mcg/24 h. Postmenopause: 0–10 mcg/24 h. *Male:* 4–25 mcg/24 h.

Child: *Less than 12 Years:* 1 mcg/24 h. *Postpuberty:* Same as adult.

Description

Estrogens—hormones composed of estrone, estradiol, and estriol—are produced by the ovary, by the adrenal gland, and in pregnancy by the placenta. (*Also see Estriol.*) This 24-hour urine test is useful for diagnosing ovarian disorders and for the analysis of tumor tissue in breast cancer. To evaluate ovarian dysfunction, the age of the client and the phase of the menstrual cycle should be known.

Purpose

(*See Estrogen [serum].*)

Clinical Problems

Decreased Level: Ovarian dysfunction, ovarian agenesis, infantilism, pregnancy (intrauterine death), menopausal and postmenopausal symptoms. *Drug Influence:* Phenothiazines (in some cases), tetracyclines (in some cases), vitamins.

Increased Level: Adrenocortical tumor, adrenocortical hyperplasia, ovarian tumor, some testicular tumors, pregnancy (gradual increase from the first trimester on). *Drug Influence:* Phenothiazines, tetracyclines, vitamins (in some cases).

Procedure

- There is no food or fluid restriction.
- Collect a 24-hour urine sample in a refrigerated container. A preservative is usually added.

- Label the urine bottle with the client's name, the date, and the exact time of collection (e.g., 5/24/20, 7:02 AM to 5/25/20, 7:01 AM). Toilet paper or feces should not be in the urine.
- Record the client's age and phase of the menstrual cycle on the laboratory slip.

Factors Affecting Laboratory Results

- Certain drugs may cause a decrease or an increase in the estrogen level (*see Drug Influence*).
- Saving only part of the 24-hour urine sample may cause an inaccurate result.

E

NURSING IMPLICATIONS WITH RATIONALE

- Check to see that a preservative is in the urine container. If not, notify the laboratory.
- Inform the client and family that all urine should be saved and placed in the refrigerated container. Toilet paper and feces should not be in the urine.

Decreased Level

- Obtain a history of menstrual problems and the present menstrual cycle (e.g., 14 days since the last menstrual period). The phase of the menstrual cycle has an influence on the test result.

Client Teaching

- Instruct the client to keep accurate monthly records on the time of menstruation, how long each menstrual period lasts, and the amount of menstrual flow.

Estrone (E_1) (serum and urine)

Reference Values

SERUM	URINE
Adult:	
Female:	Female:
Follicular phase: 30–100 pg/mL	Follicular phase: 4–7 mcg/24 h
Ovulatory phase: greater than 150 pg/mL	Ovulation: 11–30 mcg/24 h
Luteal phase: 90–160 pg/mL	Luteal phase: 10–22 mcg/24 h
Postmenopausal: 20–40 pg/mL	Postmenopausal: 1–7 mcg/24 h
Male: 10–50 pg/mL	
Less than 10 pg/mL	

Description

Estrone (E$_1$) is a potent estrogen; however, estrone and estriol (E$_3$) are not as potent as estradiol (E$_2$). Estrone is a metabolite of estradiol. During the third trimester of pregnancy, the estrone levels can increase up to tenfold the level for a nonpregnant female. Estrone is the major estrogen present after menopause. The serum estrone test is frequently ordered with other estrogen tests.

Purposes

- To determine ovarian failure.
- To check occurrence of menopause.
- To compare test results with other laboratory estrogen tests.

Clinical Problems

Decreased Level: Ovarian failure or dysfunction, intrauterine death in pregnancy, menopausal and postmenopausal symptoms. *Drug Influence:* Digoxin, estrogens.

Procedure

- Note on the laboratory slip the phase of the client's menstrual cycle.

Serum
- There is no food or fluid restriction.
- Collect 7–10 mL of venous blood in a red-top tube.

Urine
- Collect a 24-hour urine sample in a collection container that contains a boric acid preservative. Before the urine collection begins, the client should urinate and discard that urine.
- Label the urine bottle with the client's name, date, and exact time of collection (e.g., 3/14/20, 7 AM to 3/15/20, 7 AM). Toilet paper and feces should not be in the urine.

Factors Affecting Laboratory Results

- Feces and toilet paper in the urine collection container will contaminate the specimen.

NURSING IMPLICATIONS WITH RATIONALE

- Obtain a history of signs and symptoms related to the clinical problem.
- Report laboratory value(s) of estrone and other estrogen factors to the health care provider. Compare the serum estrone and/or urine estrone results with the serum total estrogen results.
- Be supportive to the client and family. Refer the client's and family's questions to appropriate health professionals.

Client Teaching

- Instruct the client and/or family to save all urine and place in the container and to avoid putting toilet paper and feces in the urine specimens and collecting container.

E

Euglobulin lysis time (plasma)

Reference Values

No lysis in 1–1½ h; normal lysis: 1.5–3 h.

Description

This test measures fibrinogen activity by measuring the interval between clot formation and euglobulin precipitation. Euglobulin is an acid-insoluble fraction of plasma. The time for which the clot is dissolved (lysis) is recorded. If a clot lysis is less than 1 hour, pathologic fibrinolysis is occurring.

Purpose

- To detect abnormal fibrinolysis.

Clinical Problems

Shortened Lysis Time: Disseminated intravascular coagulation, pathologic fibrinolysis, hemorrhage, cirrhosis, septic abortion, incompatible blood transfusions. *Drug Influence:* Clofibrate, epinephrine, streptokinase, urokinase, tissue plasminogen activator.

Procedure

- There is no food or fluid restriction.
- Do not massage the vein to be used for blood sample.
- Collect 4.5 mL of venous blood in a blue-top tube. Mix thoroughly with the anticoagulant in the tube. A control tube may be requested.
- Pack the blood sample in ice and send it to the laboratory immediately. Blood should be centrifuged within 30 minutes.

Factors Affecting Laboratory Results

- Tourniquet that has been applied over a prolonged time.
- Excess pumping of the fist will shorten lysis time.
- Hemolysis of the blood sample.
- Failure to deliver the blood sample immediately to the laboratory.

NURSING IMPLICATIONS WITH RATIONALE

- Obtain a history of possible abnormal bleeding.
- Notify the laboratory when blood will be drawn so it can be tested immediately.
- Check for bleeding or hematoma at the venipuncture site.
- Be available to answer the client's and/or family's questions. Allow the client time to express his or her concerns.

Client Teaching

- Instruct the client to avoid strenuous physical activity 1 hour before the blood is drawn.

Factor assay (plasma)

Factors I through XIII, Coagulation Factors, Blood Clotting Factors

Reference Values

Factor I (Fibrinogen): 200–400 mg/dL; minimal for clotting 75–100 mg/dL.

Factor II (Prothrombin): Minimal hemostatic level: 10–15% concentration.

Factor III (Thromboplastin): Variety of substances.

Factor IV (Calcium): 4.5–5.5 mEq/L or 9–11 mg/dL.

Factor V (Proaccelerin): 50–150% activity; minimal hemostatic level: 5–10% concentration.

Factor VI: Not used.

Factor VII (Proconvertin Stable Factor): 65–135% activity; minimal hemostatic level concentration.

Factor VIII (Antihemophilic Factor [AHF], VIII-A): 55–145% activity; minimal hemostatic level: 30–35% concentration.

Factor IX (Christmas Factor, IX-B): 60–140% activity; minimal hemostatic level: 30% concentration.

Factor X (Stuart Factor): 45–150% activity; minimal hemostatic level: 7–10% concentration.

Factor XI (Plasma Thromboplastin Antecedent [PTA] XI-C): 65–135% activity; minimal hemostatic level: 20–30% concentration.

Factor XII (Hageman Factor): Minimal hemostatic level: 0% concentration.

Factor XIII (Fibrin Stabilizing Factor [FSF]): Minimal hemostatic level: 1% concentration.

Description

Factor assays are ordered for identification of defects in the blood coagulation mechanism because of a lack of one or more of the 12 plasma factors (excluding factor VI). These 12 factors are important for clot formation, and these have been numbered according to the sequence of their discovery. To standardize clotting factors, the International Committee on Nomenclature of Blood Clotting Factors was established in 1954, and 12 clotting (coagulation) factors were given Roman numerals, named, and described.

Purpose

- To identify the blood factor that is causing the bleeding or blood disorder.

Functions of Coagulation Factors

FACTOR	NAME	SOURCE, FUNCTION
I	Fibrinogen	Manufactured by the liver; essential plasma protein; split by thrombin to produce fibrin strands necessary for clot formation.
II	Prothrombin	Produced in the liver and requires vitamin K for its synthesis. Prothrombin is converted to thrombin by the action of extrinsic and intrinsic thromboplastin.

(Continued)

Functions of Coagulation Factors

FACTOR	NAME	SOURCE, FUNCTION
III	Thromboplastin	Thromboplastic activity is found in most tissues; this factor converts prothrombin to thrombin.
IV	Calcium	Absorbed in the gastrointestinal tract from food. Inorganic ion is required in all stages of coagulation—thromboplastin generation, enzymatic conversion of prothrombin to thrombin, and stabilization of the fibrin clot.
V	Proaccelerin (labile factor)	Formed by the liver; for acceleration of thromboplastin generation; prompt conversion of prothrombin to thrombin; deteriorates rapidly in plasma at room temperature.
VI		Not used.
VII	Proconvertin (stable factor)	Manufactured in the liver and requires vitamin K for its synthesis; not destroyed or consumed in the clotting process; stable in heat; accelerates the conversion of prothrombin to thrombin. Use of anticoagulants depresses factor VII in the plasma.
VIII	Antihemophilic factor (A)	Produced by the reticuloendothelial cells; unstable at room temperatures; required for the generation of thromboplastin; essential for the conversion of prothrombin to thrombin; sex linked.
IX	Plasma thromboplastin component (PTC) (Christmas factor, antihemophilic factor B)	Manufactured in the liver and requires vitamin K for its synthesis; stable in plasma and serum; not destroyed or consumed in the clotting process; essential for generating thromboplastin; sex linked.
X	Stuart factor	Manufactured in the liver and requires vitamin K for its synthesis; stable in plasma and serum; not consumed in the clotting process; helps produce the thromboplastin-generating system.
XI	Plasma thromboplastin antecedent (PTA) (antihemophilic C)	Synthesis unknown; present in serum and plasma; consumed during the clotting process; essential for plasma-thromboplastin formation.
XII	Hageman factor	Synthesis unknown; activated in contact with glass and following injury; activated factor XII stimulates factor XI to continue the clotting process; converts plasminogen to plasmin in fibrinolysis.
XIII	Fibrinase (fibrin stabilizing factor [FSF])	Synthesis unknown; enzyme (fibrinase) present in blood, tissue, and platelets and helps to stabilize fibrin strands to form a firm clot.

Clinical Problems

A deficiency in one or more factors usually causes bleeding disorders. The associated clinical problems and the causes of these problems are outlined in the following table.

Coagulation Factor Deficiencies

FACTOR	CLINICAL PROBLEMS (DECREASED LEVELS)	RATIONALE
I	Hypofibrinogenemia Leukemia Severe liver disease Disseminated intravascular coagulation	Deficiency of fibrinogen and fibrinolysis
II	Hypoprothrombinemia Severe liver disease Vitamin K deficiency Drugs: salicylates (excessive), anticoagulants, antibiotics (excessive), hepatotoxic drugs	Impaired liver function, vitamin K deficit
III	Thrombocytopenia	Low platelet count
IV	Hypocalcemia Malabsorption syndrome Malnutrition Hyperphosphatemia Multiple transfusions containing citrate	Low calcium intake in diet
V	Parahemophilia (congenital) Severe liver disease Disseminated intravascular coagulation	Congenital problem, impaired liver function
VII	Hepatitis Hepatic carcinoma Hemorrhagic disease of newborn Drugs: antibiotics (excessive), anticoagulants	Impaired liver function, certain drugs affecting the clotting time, vitamin K deficit
VIII	Hemophilia A von Willebrand disease Disseminated intravascular coagulation Multiple myeloma Lupus erythematosus	Congenital disorder (sex linked) occurring mostly in males; circulating factor VIII inhibitors
IX	Hemophilia B (Christmas disease) Hepatic disease Vitamin K deficiency	Congenital disorder (sex linked) occurring mostly in males; circulating factor IX inhibitors
X	Severe liver disease Hemorrhagic disease of newborns Disseminated intravascular coagulation Vitamin K deficiency Drugs: anticoagulants	Impaired liver function; vitamin K deficit
XI	Hemophilia C Congenital heart disease Intestinal malabsorption of vitamin K Liver disease Drugs: anticoagulants	Congenital deficiency in both males and females; circulating factor XI inhibitors
XII	Liver disease	
XIII	Agammaglobulinemia Myeloma Lead poisoning Poor wound healing	Circulating factor XIII inhibitors; mild bleeding tendency

F

Procedure

- There is no food or fluid restriction.
- Collect 5–7 mL of venous blood in a blue-top tube (tube tops used may differ among laboratories).
- Mix the blood with an anticoagulant solution thoroughly, and avoid air bubbles.
- The tubes should be delivered to the laboratory immediately.

Factors Affecting Laboratory Results

- Clotted blood cannot be used for this laboratory test.
- The factor assay results (factors I, V, and VIII) could be affected if the blood samples do not receive immediate attention in the laboratory.

NURSING IMPLICATIONS WITH RATIONALE

- Obtain a familial history of bleeding disorders and a history of the client's bleeding tendency.
- Observe the venipuncture site for seeping of blood. Apply pressure to the site.
- Observe for signs of bleeding (e.g., purpura, petechiae, or frank, continuous bleeding). Report your observations, and record them on the client's chart.

F

Fasting blood sugar (FBS)

See Glucose—Fasting Blood Sugar

Febrile agglutinins (serum)

Reference Values

Adult (febrile, titers): *Brucella:* Less than 1:20, less than 1:20–1:80 (individuals working with animals). *Tularemia:* Less than 1:40. *Widal (Salmonella):* Less than 1:40 (nonvaccinated). *Weil-Felix (Proteus):* Less than 1:40.

Child: Same as adult.

Description

Febrile agglutination tests (febrile group) identify infectious diseases causing fever of unknown origin. Isolating the invading organism (pathogen) is not always possible, especially if the client has been on antimicrobial therapy, so indirect methods are used to detect antibacterial antibodies in the serum. Detection of these antibodies is determined by the titer of the serum in highest dilution that will cause agglutination (clumping) in the presence of a specific antigen. The test should be done during the acute phase of the disease (maybe several times) and then done again about 2 weeks later. A single agglutination titer is of minimal value. These tests can be used to confirm pathogens already isolated or to identify the pathogen present late in the disease (after several weeks).

Diseases commonly associated with febrile agglutination tests are brucellosis (undulant fever), salmonellosis, typhoid fever, paratyphoid fever, tularemia, and certain rickettsial infections (typhus fever).

Purpose

- To detect increased titer caused by febrile agglutinins denoting a specific pathogen.

Clinical Problems

TEST	PATHOGEN(S) ANTIGEN(S)	INCREASED LEVELS
Brucella	*Brucella abortus* (cattle)	Brucellosis titer greater than 1:160
	B. suis (hogs)	
	B. melitensis (goats)	
Pasteurella (tularemia)	*Pasteurella tularensis*	Tularemia (rabbit fever) titer greater than 1:80
Widal	*Salmonella* O (somatic)	Salmonellosis
	Salmonella H (flagellar)	Typhoid fever
	O and H portions of the organism act as antigens to stimulate antibody production	Paratyphoid fever titer: O antigen—greater than 1:80 suspicious, greater than 1:160 definite; H antigen—greater than 1:40 suspicious, greater than 1:80 definite
	Salmonella vi (capsular)	Nonvaccinated or vaccinated over 1 year before
Weil-Felix	*Proteus* X	Rickettsial diseases
	Proteus OX19	Epidemic typhus
		Tickborne typhus (Rocky Mountain spotted fever)
	Proteus OX2	Boutonneuse tick fever
		Queensland tick fever
		Siberian tick fever
	Proteus OXK	Scrub typhus titer—greater than 1:60 significant, greater than 1:80 definite

Procedure

- There is no food or fluid restriction.
- Collect 5–7 mL of venous blood in a red-top tube. Avoid hemolysis.
- Draw blood before starting antimicrobial therapy if possible. If the client is receiving drugs for an elevated temperature, write the names of the drugs on the laboratory slip.
- The blood sample should be refrigerated if it is not tested immediately or frozen if it is to be kept 24 hours or longer.

Factors Affecting Laboratory Results

- Vaccination could increase the titer level.
- Antimicrobial therapy could decrease the titer level.
- Leukemia, advanced carcinoma, some congenital deficiencies, and general debilitation could cause false-negative results.

NURSING IMPLICATIONS WITH RATIONALE

- Obtain a history of the client's occupation, geographic location prior to the fever, and recent vaccinations. Exposure to animals and ticks could be suggestive of the causative organism.
- Record on the laboratory slip and in the client's chart whether the client has been vaccinated against the pathogen within the last year. Vaccinations can increase the antibody titer.
- Monitor the temperature every 4 hours, when elevated.
- Remind the health care provider of the need to repeat the tests when the fever persists and/or when the titer levels are suspicious. Titer levels could rise fourfold in 1–2 weeks.
- Check to determine whether the blood sample has been taken before you give antibiotics or other drug agents to combat fever and the suspected organism. Antibiotic therapy could depress the titer level.

Client Teaching

- Instruct the client to keep a record of temperatures and to notify the health care provider of changes in body temperature.

F

Fecal fat (stool)

Reference Values

Quantitative

Adult: 2–7 g/24 h; 7–25 mmol/day (SI units).

Child: Less than 1 year old: less than 1 g/24 h.

Qualitative

Adult: Neutral fat: Less than 50 globules/high-power field (HPF). Fatty acids: Less than 100 globules/HPF.

Description

Fecal fat test is conducted to confirm the diagnosis of steatorrhea (malabsorption of fat). Clients having steatorrhea have a higher fat content in the stools. The cause of steatorrhea may be due to an impairment of intestinal absorption of fat, deficiency of pancreatic digestive enzymes, or a decrease in bile production. Causes of fat absorption impairment could be Crohn disease, celiac disease, or Whipple disease. Causes of maldigestion could be pancreatic duct obstruction or bile duct obstruction that may be due to gallstones or a tumor. The pancreatic enzymes, such as amylase, lipase, and trypsin, are not able to mix with the food to promote fat digestion. Without digestion, the fats cannot be absorbed.

Collection of stool specimen is usually for 24 hours; however, a 2- or 3-day stool collection may be ordered. Also, a random specimen may be ordered for a qualitative test.

Purposes

- To determine the presence of high fat content in the stool.
- To determine the cause of the high fat content in the stool.
- To confirm the diagnosis of steatorrhea.

Clinical Problems

Increased Levels Because of Malabsorption: Celiac disease, Whipple disease, cystic fibrosis, Crohn disease, radiation enteritis.

Increased Levels Because of Maldigestion: Pancreatic obstruction, bile duct obstruction, gallstones, cancer, surgical removal of a section of the intestine.

Drugs that May Increase Steatorrhea: Colchicine, neomycin, kanamycin, lincomycin, methotrexate.

Procedure

- There is no fluid restriction unless indicated by the laboratory.
- The client may be requested to eat a high-fat diet (100 g of fat per day) for 3 days before the test. Procedure may be different; consult with the laboratory.
- Collect a random or 24–72-hour stool specimen and send the specimen immediately to the laboratory. Use a tongue blade to move stool to specimen container.
- Watery stools (diarrhea) can be used for fecal fat analysis.
- Stools collected at home or a medical facility should be refrigerated before sending to the laboratory. Once it is removed from the refrigerator, it should be sent immediately.
- Record client's name, date, and duration of collection time on the specimen container and/or laboratory slip.

Factors Affecting Laboratory Results

- Drugs: Ingestion of mineral oil, psyllium-based (fiber) laxatives such as Metamucil, rectal suppositories, cascara.
- Ingestion of low-fat caloric food.
- Ingestion of a high-fiber diet.
- A recent barium GI study.

NURSING IMPLICATIONS WITH RATIONALE

- Obtain a history of GI problems. Record the type of diet (food) the client is eating.
- Obtain a list of the client's medication. Note those drugs that can affect the test results.
- Ask the client if he or she has had any previous diagnostic testing that requires barium intake.
- Review the procedure with the client. An ingestion of 50–100 g of fat for 3 days prior to the test may have been prescribed. Check with the laboratory.

Client Teaching

- Inform the client of how to collect the stools. The stools should be refrigerated unless they are to be taken immediately to the laboratory.
- Instruct the client not to urinate in the stool container. Toilet paper should not be put in the stool container.
- Instruct the client not to take an enema or laxative during stool collection because it can alter the test results.
- Inform the client if the test is for a random stool collection or a 1- to 3-day collection period.
- Be supportive of the client. Answer questions or refer him or her to other health professionals.

Ferritin (serum)

F

Reference Values

Adult: *Female:* 10–235 ng/mL, 10–235 mcg/L (SI units). *Male:* 15–445 ng/mL, 15–445 mcg/L (SI units). *Postmenopausal:* 10–310 ng/mL.

Child: *1–16 Years:* 8–140 ng/mL. *Infant:* 2–12 months: 30–200 ng/mL, 1 month: 200–550 ng/mL.

Newborn: 20–200 ng/mL.

Description

Ferritin, an iron-storage protein, is produced in the liver, spleen, and bone marrow. The ferritin levels are related to the amount of iron stored in the body tissues. The body will release iron from tissue reserve as needed and will store excess iron to prevent damaging effects from iron over-load. One nanogram per milliliter of serum ferritin corresponds to 8 mg of stored iron.

Serum ferritin level is useful in evaluating the total body storage of iron. It can detect early iron-deficiency anemia and anemias due to chronic disease that resemble iron deficiency. Serum ferritin is not affected by hemolysis and drugs.

Purposes

- To evaluate the amount of iron stored in the body.
- To detect early iron-deficiency anemia.

Clinical Problems

Decreased Level: Iron deficiency, pregnancy, inflamed bowel disease, gastric surgery.

Increased Level: Metastatic carcinomas, leukemias, lymphomas, hepatic diseases (cirrhosis, hepatitis, cancer of the liver), iron overload (hemochromatosis), hemosiderosis, anemias (hemo-lytic, pernicious, thalassemia), acute and chronic infection and inflammation (renal disease, neu-roblastoma), tissue damage. *Drug Influence:* Oral or injectable iron drugs.

Procedure

- There is no food or fluid restriction.
- Collect 3–5 mL of venous blood in a red-top tube.
- List on the laboratory slip if the client is taking iron preparations.

Factors Affecting Laboratory Results

- None known.

NURSING IMPLICATIONS WITH RATIONALE

- Compare serum ferritin level with serum iron and transferrin percent saturation. Serum ferritin levels tend to be more reliable in determining iron deficiencies than serum iron levels. Serum ferritin levels decrease before iron stores are depleted.

Fetal hemoglobin (Hb F) (blood)

Hemoglobin F

F

Reference Values

From Total Hemoglobin:

Adult: 0–2%.

Child: *Newborn:* 60–90%. *1–5 Months:* Less than 70%. *6–12 Months:* Less than 5%. *Greater than 1 Year:* Less than 2%.

Description

For newborns, an elevated Hb F is normally found in the red blood cells. By the time the infant is 6 months old, the Hb F should be less than 5%, and the remaining hemoglobin should be comprised of Hb A_1 and Hb A_2. If the Hb F remains elevated after 6 months, hemoglobinopathy should be considered, such as minor or major thalassemias.

Purpose

- To diagnose various hemoglobinopathies, such as minor or major thalassemia.

Clinical Problems

Increased Level: Thalassemias (minor or major), sickle-cell anemia, acquired aplastic anemia (from drugs, toxins, etc.), hyperthyroidism, acute or chronic leukemia (especially juvenile myeloid leukemia), multiple myeloma, hemoglobin H disease, hereditary presence of Hb F.

Procedure

- There is no food or fluid restriction.
- Collect 7–10 mL of venous blood in a lavender- or green-top tube. Fill the tube. Invert the tube gently. Avoid hemolysis (do *not* shake tube).
- Collect capillary blood from a young child in a microcollection tube.

Factors Affecting Laboratory Results

- Hemolysis of the blood sample.
- Blood specimen that is older than 3 hours may cause a false-positive result.

NURSING IMPLICATIONS WITH RATIONALE

Client Teaching

- Explain the test procedure to the client or parent. Blood specimen can be taken from a finger or earlobe.
- Listen to client's concerns. Refer questions to which the answers are unknown to other health care professionals.

F

Fibrin degradation fragments (FDF)

See D-Dimer Test

Fibrin degradation products (FDP) (serum)

Fibrin or Fibrinogen Split Products (FSP)

Reference Values

Adult: 2–10 mcg/mL.

Child: Not usually done.

Description

The fibrin degradation products (FDP) test is usually done in an emergency when the client is hemorrhaging as the result of severe injury, trauma, and/or shock. Thrombin, which initially accelerates coagulation, promotes the conversion of plasminogen into plasmin, which, in turn, breaks fibrinogen and fibrin into FDP. The fibrin degradation (split) products act as anticoagulants, causing continuous bleeding from many sites. A clinical condition resulting from this fibrinolytic (clot-dissolving) activity is DIC (disseminated intravascular coagulation).

Purpose

- To aid in the diagnosis of disseminated intravascular coagulation.

Clinical Problems

Decreased Level: Cerebral thrombosis.

Increased Level: DIC caused by severe injury, trauma, or shock; massive tissue damage; surgical complications; septicemia; obstetric complications (abruptio placentae, preeclampsia, intrauterine death, postcesarean birth); acute myocardial infarction; pulmonary embolism; acute necrosis of the liver; acute renal failure; burns; acute leukemia. *Drug Influence:* Streptokinase, urokinase.

Procedure

- There is no food or fluid restriction.
- Collect 5–7 mL of venous blood in a blue-top tube. Avoid hemolysis.
- Draw blood before administering heparin.

Factors Affecting Laboratory Results

- Hemolysis of the blood sample can cause inaccurate test results.

NURSING IMPLICATIONS WITH RATIONALE

Increased Level

- Monitor vital signs and report shocklike symptoms, such as tachycardia, hypotension, pallor, and cold, clammy skin.
- Observe and report bleeding sites from the chest, the nasogastric tube, incisional or injured areas, and others.
- Report progressive discoloration of the skin (petechial, ecchymoses).
- Monitor infusion rates of IV fluids—crystalloids, colloids, and blood.
- Check urine output hourly. Report decreased urine output (less than 25 mL/h) and blood-colored urine.
- Provide comfort and support to the client and family.

Fibrinogen (plasma)

Factor I

Reference Values

Adult: 200–400 mg/dL.

Child: *Newborn:* 150–300 mg/dL. *Child:* Same as adult.

Description

Fibrinogen, a plasma protein synthesized by the liver, is split by thrombin to produce fibrin strands necessary for clot formation. A deficiency of fibrinogen results in bleeding. Low fibrinogen levels may be due to DIC (disseminated intravascular coagulation), which usually results from severe trauma or obstetric complications. Markedly prolonged PT (prothrombin time), an APTT (activated partial thromboplastin time), and a low platelet count suggest a fibrinogen deficiency and signs of DIC. Fibrin degradation products (FDPs) are usually measured to confirm DIC.

Purposes

- To check for a deficiency of fibrinogen as a cause of bleeding.
- To compare test results with FDPs in diagnosing DIC.

Clinical Problems

Decreased Level: Severe liver disease, hypofibrinogenemia, DIC, leukemia, obstetric complications.

Increased Level: Acute infections, collagen diseases, inflammatory disease, hepatitis. *Drug Influence:* Oral contraceptives, heparin.

Procedure

- There is no food or fluid restriction.
- Collect 5–7 mL of venous blood in a blue-top tube. Mix blood well with the anticoagulant in the tube (invert tube several times). Avoid hemolysis by not shaking the tube.

Factors Affecting Laboratory Results

- Postoperative surgery and third trimester of pregnancy could cause a false-positive fibrinogen elevation.
- Hemolysis of the blood sample can cause inaccurate results.
- Oral contraceptives and heparin can elevate test results.

F

NURSING IMPLICATIONS WITH RATIONALE

- Report if client had a blood transfusion within 4 weeks.
- Check laboratory results of PT, APTT, and platelet count. If an FDP level is ordered, check the laboratory result, since it confirms DIC.
- Monitor for signs and symptoms of DIC (petechiae and ecchymoses, hemorrhage, tachycardia, hypotension).
- Notify the health care provider if active bleeding occurs.

Client Teaching

- Instruct the client to inform the health care provider of any current, acute infection or illness that might be contributing to the bleeding.

Finger stick blood sugar (FSBS)
See Glucose Self-Monitoring Devices

Fluorescent treponemal antibody absorption (FTA-ABS) (serum)

Reference Values

Adult: Nonreactive (negative).

Child: Nonreactive (negative).

Description

The fluorescent treponemal antibody absorption (FTA-ABS) test uses the treponemal organism to produce and detect these antibodies. This test is most sensitive, specific, and reliable for diagnosing all stages of syphilis. It is more sensitive than the venereal disease research laboratory (VDRL) and rapid plasma reagin (RPR) tests. The FTA-ABS test is useful for confirming or ruling out suspected false-positive serology tests for syphilis. The limitations of this test are that the stage and activity of the disease cannot be identified, the effectiveness of the therapy cannot be measured, and the test for syphilis remains positive even after treatment for a very long time, or could remain positive forever.

Purpose

- To aid in the diagnosis of syphilis.

Clinical Problems

Reactive: *Positive:* Primary and secondary syphilis. *False Positives (Rare):* Lupus erythematosus, pregnancy, acute genital herpes.

Procedure

- There is no food or fluid restriction.
- Collect 3–5 mL of venous blood in a red-top tube. Avoid hemolysis.
- A borderline FTA-ABS test should be repeated.

Factors Affecting Laboratory Results

- Medical treatment does not eliminate the treponemal antibodies. The test results may remain positive after treatment.

F

NURSING IMPLICATIONS WITH RATIONALE

- Be supportive of the client and family. Keep conversation and information confidential except for what is required by law.
- Encourage the client to have his or her sexual partner seek medical care if the test is positive.
- Check the results of other serology tests for syphilis. A positive VDRL could be false positive because of acute or chronic illness. The FTA-ABS test is reliable for syphilis, giving accurate results; however, many laboratories have to send the blood sample out for testing. Ask the client if he or she has received treatment for syphilis. Positive FTA-ABS results can occur after treatment (penicillin, erythromycin) for months or several years, or for the rest of the client's life.
- Assess for signs and symptoms of syphilis. The primary stage begins with a small papule filled with liquid, which ruptures, enlarges, and becomes a chancre. With secondary syphilis, a generalized rash (macular and papular) develops and is found mainly on the arms, palms, soles of the feet, and face.

Folic acid (folate) (serum)

Reference Values

Adult: 3–16 ng/mL (bioassay), greater than 2.5 ng/mL (radioimmunoassay [RIA]; serum), 200–700 ng/mL (RBCs).

Child: Same as adult.

Description

Folic acid, one of the B vitamins, is needed for normal red and white blood cell function. Folic acid is present in a variety of foods: milk, eggs, leafy vegetables, beans, liver, fruits (oranges, bananas), and whole wheat bread. Dietary deficiency is the most common cause of a serum folic acid deficit, especially in children, older adults, and persons with chronic alcoholism. With a decreased folic acid intake, it takes approximately 3–4 weeks for folic acid deficiency to develop and 18–24 weeks before folic acid anemia will occur.

Usually the serum folic acid or folate test is performed to detect folic acid anemia, which is a megaloblastic anemia (abnormally large RBCs). Other causes of serum folic acid deficit are pregnancy (because of dietary deficiency and because the fetal requirement for folic acid is so great), alcoholism, and aging.

Purposes

- To check for folic acid deficiency during early pregnancy.
- To detect folic acid anemia.

Clinical Problems

Decreased Level: Folic acid anemia (megaloblastic anemia); vitamin B_6 deficiency anemia; malnutrition; malabsorption syndrome (small intestine); pregnancy; malignancies; liver diseases; celiac sprue disease. *Drug Influence:* Anticonvulsants—phenytoin (Dilantin), primidone (Mysoline); antineoplastic agents—methotrexate (folic acid antagonists); antimalaria agents; oral contraceptives.

Increased Level: Pernicious anemia.

Procedure

- There is no food or fluid restriction. Avoid alcohol.
- Collect 7–10 mL of venous blood in a red-top tube. Avoid hemolysis. Send blood to the laboratory immediately.
- If an RBC folate determination is requested, collect 7 mL of venous blood in a lavender-top tube. Send this to the laboratory immediately. Ascorbic acid will be added in the laboratory.

Factors Affecting Laboratory Results

- Drugs (*see Clinical Problems*).
- Alcohol—persons who consume large quantities of alcohol usually have poor nutritional intake (folic acid deficiency).

NURSING IMPLICATIONS WITH RATIONALE

- Obtain a dietary history. Collaborate with the dietitian on formulating a diet high in folic acid, and have the dietitian plan the diet with the client.
- Observe for signs and symptoms of folic acid deficiency, such as fatigue, pallor, nausea, anorexia, dyspnea, palpitations, and tachycardia.

Client Teaching

- Encourage the client to eat foods rich in folic acid, such as liver, lean meats, milk, eggs, leafy vegetables, bananas, oranges, beans, and whole wheat bread.

Follicle-stimulating hormone (FSH) (serum and urine)

Reference Values

Serum: *Adult:* Female: Follicular phase: 4–30 milliunit/mL. Midcycle: 10–90 milliunit/mL. Luteal phase: 4–30 milliunit/mL. Menopause: 40–170 milliunit/mL. Male: 4–25 milliunit/mL. *Child (Prepubertal):* 5–12 milliunit/mL.

Urine: *Adult:* Female: Follicular phase: 2–15 international unit/24 h. Midcycle: 8–60 international unit/24 h. Luteal phase: 4–20 international unit/24 h. Menopause: 50–150 international unit/24 h. Male: 4–18 international unit/24 h. *Child (Prepubertal):* less than 10 international unit/mL.

Description

Follicle-stimulating hormone (FSH), a gonadotropic hormone produced and controlled by the pituitary gland, stimulates the growth and maturation of the ovarian follicle to produce estrogen in females and to promote spermatogenesis in males. Infertility disorders can be determined by a serum and urine FSH test. Increased and decreased FSH levels can indicate gonad failure due to pituitary dysfunction.

Purposes

- To check for a FSH-producing pituitary tumor.
- To compare serum and urine FSH levels for determining the cause of infertility.

Clinical Problems

Decreased Level: Neoplasms of the ovaries, testes, adrenals; polycystic ovarian disease; hypopituitarism; anorexia nervosa. *Drug Influence:* Estrogens, oral contraceptives, testosterone.

Increased Level: Gonadal failure such as menopause, precocious puberty, FSH-producing pituitary tumor, Turner syndrome, Klinefelter syndrome, orchiectomy, hysterectomy, primary testicular failure.

Procedure

- No food or fluid restriction is required.
- State phase of menstrual cycle or if menopausal on the laboratory slip.
- Note on the laboratory slip if the client is taking oral contraceptives or any type of hormones.

Serum

- Collect 5–7 mL of venous blood in a red-top tube. Avoid hemolysis.
- Rest 30 minutes to 1 hour before blood is drawn.

Urine

- Collect a 24-hour urine specimen in a large container with a preservative. The pH of the 24-hour urine specimen should be maintained between 5 and 6.5 (glacial acetic acid or boric acid may be added).
- Avoid feces and toilet paper in the urine.

Factors Affecting Laboratory Results

- Alkaline urine can give an inaccurate test result.

NURSING IMPLICATIONS WITH RATIONALE

- Associate a decreased or increased urine FSH level with clinical problems. The excess production of estrogen with most ovarian tumors will decrease the production of FSH. After menopause, more FSH will be secreted to stimulate estrogen production.

Urine

- Label container with the client's name, the dates, and the exact times of urine collection (e.g., 5/10/20, 8 AM to 5/11/20, 8:01 AM).

Client Teaching

- Answer client questions concerning the test. Be supportive of the client and family.
- Inform the client to rest prior to a serum test, because exercise can increase FSH release.

Fungal antibody tests (serum, cerebrospinal fluid [CF])

Antifungal Antibodies, Fungal Antibody Screen

Reference Values

Negative, no antibodies.

Cerebrospinal Fluid (CF): Less than 1:8.

Description

Fungal antibody testing detects antibodies present in fungal diseases, such as blastomycosis, coccidioidomycosis, and histoplasmosis, which occurs in approximately 70–80% of infected clients. There are numerous species of fungi that are either superficial or systemic (deep). Fungal antibody test is not for superficial fungal infections (mycosis) that appear on the skin, hair, or nails. The systemic (deep) fungal infection that comes from inhaled spores can occur from bird droppings, soil, and dust. The antibodies can be present soon after the fungi invades the client. This test can indicate if the client has an active or a recent fungal infection.

The fungal antibody test can be done on cerebrospinal fluid. Refer to the laboratory test on fungal organisms that is in this text.

Purpose

- To identify the presence of fungal antibodies.

Clinical Problems

Increased Level: Acute fungal infection, antibodies to systemic (deep) mycosis, such as *Blastomyces dermatitidis*, *Coccidioides immitis*, or *Histoplasma capsulatum*.

Procedure

- Collect 5 mL of venous blood in a red-top tube. Place blood specimen in a biohazard bag if required.
- Avoid shaking the blood specimen to prevent hemolysis.
- Test may be repeated in 2 weeks depending on the client's condition and previous test results.

Factors Affecting Laboratory Results

- Hemolysis of the blood specimen.

NURSING IMPLICATIONS WITH RATIONALE

- Obtain a history of the client's exposure to bird droppings or contaminated soil.
- Determine if the client previously had a fungal infection.
- Record vital signs that would be the baseline numbers.
- Obtain the blood specimen for testing for fungal antibodies.
- Monitor the effects of antifungal medication if prescribed.

Client Teaching

- Encourage the client to report symptoms and changes occurring as the result of the fungal infection.
- Listen to the client's concerns and answer questions, or refer questions to other health care providers.

Fungal organisms: fungal disease, mycotic infections (smear, serum, culture—sputum, bronchial, lesion)

Actinomyces, Histoplasma, Blastomyces, Coccidioides, Cryptococcus, Candida, Aspergillus

Reference Values

Adult: Negative, serum: less than 1:8.

Child: Same as adult.

Description

There are more than 45,000 species of fungi, but only 0.01%, or 45, are considered pathogenic to humans. Fungal infections are more common today and can be classified as (1) superficial and cutaneous mycoses (tinea pedis [athlete's foot], tinea capitis [ringworm of the scalp], tinea barbae [ringworm of the beard], and tinea cruris [jock itch]), (2) subcutaneous mycoses, and (3) systemic mycoses (histoplasmosis, actinomycosis, and blastomycosis).

Most fungus organisms live in the soil and can be transmitted to humans and animals by way of the lungs or a break in the skin. The persons most susceptible to fungal infections are those with debilitating or chronic diseases (e.g., diabetes) or who are receiving drug therapy, such as steroids, prolonged antibiotics, antineoplastic agents, and oral contraceptives.

Purpose

- To assist in the diagnosis of selected fungal organisms.

Clinical Problems

ORGANISM	DISEASE ENTITY	COMMENTS
Actinomyces israelii	Actinomycosis	A gram-positive, non-acid-fast, anaerobic organism that can produce an abscess.
Histoplasma capsulatum	Histoplasmosis	The most common systemic fungal infection. It is commonly found in the eastern part of the United States and in the Mississippi and Ohio valleys. Usually the organism is carried by birds (e.g., starlings and chickens). In most clients, histoplasmosis is a localized pulmonary disease and resembles pulmonary tuberculosis.
Blastomyces dermatitidis	Blastomycosis	It causes granulomatous lesions that involve the skin or visceral organs. Histologically, it is similar to tuberculosis.
Coccidioides immitis	Coccidioidomycosis	It is commonly found in the Southwest and in the San Joaquin Valley of California. Usually the client has respiratory symptoms and fever of unknown origin. If the infection is overwhelming, it resembles military tuberculosis.

F

ORGANISM	DISEASE ENTITY	COMMENTS
Cryptococcus neoformans	Cryptococcosis Meningitis	Fungal disease usually begins as a pulmonary infection but disseminates to the central nervous system (brain). The organism is usually carried by pigeons. Clients with decreased immunologic resistance (such as those with acute leukemia or Hodgkin disease or who are receiving steroids or immunosuppressive agents) are susceptible to the disease.
Candida albicans, fungemia	Candidiasis (Moniliasis) Thrush	Clients with debilitating diseases or who are taking steroids, antineoplastic agents, or oral contraceptives are susceptible to this fungus.
Aspergillus fumigatus	Aspergillosis	Aspergillus organisms can cause severe respiratory infection. Fungus balls (aspergilloma) develop in the lung tissue. The sputum is golden brown and contains *Aspergillus hyphae*.

Procedure

Serum

- No food or fluid restriction is required. Suggest NPO for 12 hours. Check with your laboratory.
- Collect 5–7 mL of venous blood in a red-top tube.
- Obtain serum antibody test 2–4 weeks after exposure to organism.

Culture

- Follow directions from the special laboratory on collection of the specimen.

ORGANISM	TESTS
Actinomyces israelii	Smear and culture of lesion Biopsy
Histoplasma capsulatum	Sputum culture Histoplasmin skin test Serum test: complement fixation or latex agglutination Culture
Blastomyces dermatitidis	Smear, wet-mount examination of the material from the lesion Biopsy—histologic examination Skin test Serum test: complement fixation
Coccidioides immitis	Culture Sputum smears Skin test Serum test: complement fixation (sensitive), latex agglutination (very sensitive)
Cryptococcus neoformans	Culture of cerebrospinal fluid Serum test: latex agglutination (sensitive)
Candida albicans	Smear and culture of the skin, mucous membrane, and vagina
Aspergillus fumigatus	Sputum culture Skin test Serum IgE level and complement fixation

Factors Affecting Laboratory Results

- Contamination of the specimen affects results.

NURSING IMPLICATIONS WITH RATIONALE

- Associate mycotic infections with high-risk clients (e.g., those clients having chronic illnesses [such as diabetes mellitus] or debilitating diseases [such as cancer], or who are receiving prolonged antibiotics, antineoplastic agents [anticancer chemotherapy], steroids, or oral contraceptives).
- Use aseptic technique when collecting a specimen for culture. Preventing the transmission of the organism is most important. Contamination of the specimen can give inaccurate results.
- Obtain a history from the client—where he or she lives and occupation. Fungus organisms (e.g., *Histoplasma*, *Coccidioides*) are more prevalent in certain parts of the country. Report if the client works with chickens or pigeons.
- Teach the client to wear a mask when exposed to chicken feces. Explain that the *H. capsulatum* spores are in the feces and can be inhaled.
- Monitor the client's temperature. With many of the fungal diseases, the temperature is elevated.
- Report clinical signs and symptoms of respiratory problems (e.g., coughing up sputum, dyspnea, and chest pain).
- Check the color of the sputum. Certain fungi can be identified by the color of their secretions. Golden brown sputum is characteristic of the *Aspergillus* organism.
- Assess the neurologic status when cryptococcosis is suspected. Report headaches and changes in sensorium, pupil size and reaction, and motor function.

Galactose-1-phosphate uridyl transferase (GPT or GPUT) (blood)

Galactokinase (An enzyme that aids in the metabolism of galactose)

Reference Values

Negative: Quantitative test: 18.5–28.5 unit/g in hemoglobin (Hb).

Deficiency of the Enzyme: Less than 5 unit/g in Hb; Carrier of the deficiency: 5–18 unit/g of Hb.

Description

The enzyme, galactose-1-phosphate uridyl transferase (GPT), is needed to convert galactose to glucose during lactose metabolism. The enzyme deficiency is inherited or can be an acquired disorder that can occur during intrauterine development. If inherited, it is an autosomal recessive transmitted disorder. A deficiency of this enzyme can lead to galactosemia (increase in galactose in the blood due to the inability to metabolize galactose). Screening tests to detect the enzyme deficiency are performed at birth in some institutions. If the deficiency exists and is not treated soon after birth, this condition can cause mental retardation, failure to thrive, severe liver disorder, and/or irreversible cataracts due to the lack of brain, liver, or eye development.

Purpose

- To detect galactosemia in infants and carriers of the GPT enzyme deficiency.

Clinical Problems

Decreased Enzyme Level: Galactosemia.

Procedure

- There is no food or fluid restriction.
- Collect 5–7 mL of venous blood in a green- or lavender-top tube. Chill the tube of blood by placing it on ice. Avoid hemolysis.
- Take blood sample from the umbilical cord at birth or from the heel (heel stick). From the heel, place three drops of blood on a galactosemia screening filter paper.

Factors Affecting Laboratory Results

- Hemolysis from rough handling of blood specimen.
- Not chilling or putting the tube on ice.

G

NURSING IMPLICATIONS WITH RATIONALE

- Ascertain if the parent(s) is/are carriers of galactosemia. If the institution does not check for GPT deficiency at birth, the health care provider should suggest that the test be performed, especially if a client is a carrier.
- Assess the infant for symptoms suggesting GPT enzyme deficiency, such as vomiting, diarrhea, abdominal distention, liver enlargement, and central nervous system changes. A positive indication of galactose is elevated blood and urine levels of galactose and galactose-1-phosphate.

Client Teaching

- Instruct the parent who has an infant lacking the enzyme to avoid giving milk to the infant. Dietary alternatives for a galactose- and lactose-free diet, such as substituting with soy-bean milk, are suggested. A lactose-free diet avoids galactose toxicity.
- Inform the parent(s) to report vomiting or diarrhea that continues after implementing a lactose-free diet.
- Encourage the parent(s) to seek genetic counseling for a positive test.

Gamma-glutamyl transferase (GGT) (serum)

Gamma-Glutamyl Transpeptidase (GGTP, or GTP; γ-Glutamyl Transpeptidase, γ GT)

Reference Values 0–45 unit/L (overall average)

Adult: *Male:* 4–23 international unit/L, 9–69 unit/L at 37°C (SI units). *Female:* 3–13 international unit/L, 4–33 unit/L at 37°C (SI units). Values differ among institutions and methods used.

Elderly: Slightly higher than adult.

Child: *Newborn:* 5 times higher than adult. *Premature:* 10 times higher than adult. *Child:* Similar to adult.

Description

The enzyme gamma-glutamyl transferase (GGT) is found primarily in the liver and kidney, with smaller amounts in the spleen, prostate gland, and heart muscle. GGT is sensitive for detecting a wide variety of hepatic (liver) parenchymal diseases. The serum level will rise early and will remain elevated as long as cellular damage persists.

High levels of GGT occur after 12–24 hours of heavy alcoholic drinking and may remain increased for 2–3 weeks after alcohol intake stops. Some alcoholic rehabilitation programs use the GGT level as a guide to planning care as they work with alcoholic individuals.

The GGT test is considered more sensitive for liver dysfunction than the alkaline phosphatase (ALP) test.

Purposes

- To detect the presence of a hepatic disorder.
- To monitor the liver enzyme GGT during the liver disorder and treatment.
- To compare with other liver enzymes to identify liver dysfunction.

Clinical Problems

Increased Level: Cirrhosis of the liver, acute and subacute necrosis of the liver, alcoholism, acute and chronic hepatitis, cancer (liver, pancreas, prostate, breast, kidney, lung, brain), infectious mononucleosis, hemochromatosis (iron deposits in the liver), diabetes mellitus, hyperlipoproteinemia (type IV), acute myocardial infarction (fourth day), heart failure, acute pancreatitis, acute cholecystitis, epilepsy, nephrotic syndrome. *Drug Influence:* Phenytoin (Dilantin), phenobarbital, aminoglycosides, warfarin (Coumadin).

Procedure

- There is no food or fluid restriction.
- Collect 3–5 mL of venous blood in a red-top tube. Avoid hemolysis.

Factors Affecting Laboratory Results

- Phenytoin and barbiturates can cause a false-positive GGT test.
- Excessive and prolonged alcohol intake will elevate the GGT level.

NURSING IMPLICATIONS WITH RATIONALE

Increased Level

- Compare GGT with ALP, leucine aminopeptidase (LAP), and alanine aminotransferase (SGPT or ALT). The GGT test tends to be more sensitive for detecting liver dysfunction than the others.
- Report to the health care provider if the client is receiving phenytoin or phenobarbital when the test is ordered. Usually these medications cannot be withheld. Note on the laboratory slip the names of the drugs (affecting GGT levels) and the dosages the client is receiving.
- Assess the client's diet.
- Observe for signs and symptoms of liver damage, such as restlessness, jaundice, twitching, flapping tremors, spider angiomas, bleeding tendencies (nose and rectal bleeding), purpura, ascites, and others.

Client Teaching

- Instruct the client to maintain a well-balanced diet (adequate protein and carbohydrate).
- Encourage clients with an alcohol problem to participate in Alcoholics Anonymous or a rehabilitation program.

Gastrin (serum or plasma)

G

Reference Values

Adult: *Fasting:* Less than 100 pg/mL. *Nonfasting:* 50–200 pg/mL.
Child: Not usually done.

Description

Gastrin is a hormone secreted by the G cells of the pyloric mucosa that stimulates the secretion of gastric juices, namely hydrochloric acid (HCl). A very small amount of gastrin is secreted by the islets of Langerhans in the pancreas. Gastrin values follow a circadian rhythm, with the highest values occurring during the day, especially during meals. Hypersecretion of HCl inhibits gastrin secretion.

This test is usually ordered to diagnose pernicious anemia, gastric ulcer (mildly increased serum levels), and Zollinger-Ellison syndrome (high serum levels). Zollinger-Ellison syndrome may be due to pancreatic gastrinoma.

Gastrin stimulation tests aid in differentiating between Zollinger-Ellison syndrome and hypergastrinemia due to other causes. Either calcium infusion or secretion is administered intravenously. A marked increase in serum gastrin values occurs with Zollinger-Ellison syndrome and not with other probable causes of hypergastrinemia.

Purposes

- To aid in the diagnosis of pernicious anemia.
- To aid in the diagnosis of gastric ulcer.
- To differentiate between Zollinger-Ellison syndrome and hypergastrinemia from other causes.

Clinical Problems

Decreased Level: Vagotomy, hypothyroidism. *Drug Influence:* Atropine sulfate.

Increased Level: Pernicious anemia, Zollinger-Ellison syndrome, malignant neoplasm of the stomach, peptic ulcer, chronic atrophic gastritis, cirrhosis of the liver, acute and chronic renal failure. *Drug Influence:* IV calcium gluconate, insulin, catecholamines, and caffeine.

Procedure

- Food and fluids (except water) are restricted for 12 hours before the test.
- Collect 5–7 mL of venous blood in a red- or lavender-top tube.

Factors Affecting Laboratory Results

- IV infusion of calcium elevates the serum gastrin level.

NURSING IMPLICATIONS WITH RATIONALE

- For the gastrin stimulation test, infuse calcium gluconate intravenously over a period of 3–4 hours. Blood sample is taken before the test and then drawn every 30 minutes to 1 hour during the infusion. For the secretin test, infuse secretin intravenously over 1 hour. Obtain a blood sample before the test and then every 15–30 minutes for 1 hour as prescribed by the health care provider.
- Check the serum gastrin value. In Zollinger-Ellison syndrome, the serum level may reach 2,800–300,000 pg/mL.
- Observe for signs and symptoms of pernicious anemia (weakness, sore tongue, pallor of the gums and lips, anorexia, loss of weight, and numbness and tingling in the extremities).

Client Teaching

- Instruct the client that food and beverages are restricted (with the exception of water) for 12 hours before the test. A fasting blood sample is usually ordered.

Glucagon (plasma)

Reference Values

Adult: 50–200 pg/mL, 50–200 mg/L (SI units).

Description

Glucagon is secreted by the alpha cells of the pancreas. It functions as a counterregulatory hormone to insulin in regulating glucose metabolism. It increases blood glucose by converting glycogen to glucose in response to hypoglycemia.

High glucagon levels (500–1,000 pg/mL) occur in glucagonoma, pancreatic alpha cell tumor.

Purpose

- To detect an increase or deficit in serum glucagon that aids in the regulation of glucose metabolism.

Clinical Problems

Decreased Level: Glucose tolerance test during first hour, idiopathic glucagon deficiency, loss of pancreatic tissue.

Increased Level: Glucagonoma, acute pancreatitis, severe diabetic ketoacidosis, infections, pheochromocytoma.

Procedure

- Food and fluids are restricted for 10–12 hours prior to the test.
- Collect 5–7 mL of venous blood in a lavender-top tube. Avoid hemolysis. Chill the tube and take to laboratory immediately.
- Withhold drugs such as insulin, cortisone, growth hormones, and epinephrine, with health care provider's permission, until the test is completed.

Factors Affecting Laboratory Results

- Vigorous exercise, undue stress, trauma, and severe hyperglycemia affect test results.
- Administer steroids and insulin after the test.

NURSING IMPLICATIONS WITH RATIONALE

- Compare serum glucose and insulin levels. Glucose and insulin influence plasma glucagon levels.
- Record on the laboratory slip and report if client has taken large doses of steroids in the last 24 hours.
- Observe for signs and symptoms of hyperglycemia.

Client Teaching

- Instruct the client to relax by lying down for 30 minutes to 1 hour prior to the test. Stress and activity could cause false-positive test results.

Glucose—fasting blood sugar (FBS) (blood)

Reference Values

Adult: *Serum and Plasma:* 70–110 mg/dL; 3.9–6.1 mmol/L (SI units).
   Whole Blood: 60–100 mg/dL; 3.3–5.5 mmol/L (SI units).
   Prediabetes: 100–125 mg/dL.
   Panic Values: Less than 40 mg/dL; less than 2.2 mmol/L (SI units). Greater than 700 mg/dL; greater than 38.5 mmol/L (SI units).

Gestational Diabetes: Greater than 140 mg/dL; greater than 7.9 mmol/L (SI units).

Elderly: *Serum:* 70–120 mg/dL; 3.9–6.7 mmol/L (SI units).

Newborn: 30–80 mg/dL; 1.7–4.4 mmol/L (SI units).

Child: 60–100 mg/dL; 3.3–5.5 mmol/L (SI units).

Description

Glucose is formed from dietary carbohydrates and is stored as glycogen in the liver and skeletal muscles. Insulin and glucagon, two hormones from the pancreas, affect the blood glucose level. Insulin is needed for cellular membrane permeability to glucose and for transportation of glucose into the cells. Without insulin, glucose cannot enter the cells. Glucagon stimulates glycogenolysis (conversion of stored glycogen to glucose) in the liver.

A decreased blood sugar level (hypoglycemia) results from inadequate food intake or too much insulin. When elevated blood sugar (hyperglycemia) occurs, there is not enough insulin; this condition is known as diabetes mellitus. A fasting blood sugar level greater than 125 mg/dL usually indicates diabetes, and to confirm the diagnosis when the blood sugar is borderline or slightly elevated, a feasting (postprandial) blood sugar and/or a glucose tolerance test may be ordered.

Today, there are various home glucose monitoring devices available to monitor blood sugar, such as Accu-Chek blood glucose meter, Glucometer, MediSense Optium, and others. These glucose monitoring devices can be used for fasting blood sugar and can be used throughout the day to check blood sugars.

Purposes

- To confirm a diagnosis of prediabetic state or diabetic mellitus.
- To monitor blood glucose levels for diabetic clients taking an antidiabetic agent (insulin or oral hypoglycemic drug).

Clinical Problems

Decreased Level: Hypoglycemic reaction (insulin excess), cancer (stomach, liver, lung), adrenal gland hypofunction, malnutrition, alcoholism, cirrhosis of the liver, strenuous exercise, erythroblastosis fetalis (hemolytic disease), hyperinsulinism. *Drug Influence:* Insulin excess, acetaminophen, alcohol, propranolol, oral hypoglycemic agents.

Increased Level: Diabetes mellitus, diabetic acidosis, adrenal gland hyperfunction (Cushing syndrome), acute myocardial infarction, stress, crushed injury, burns, infections, renal failure, hypothermia, exercise, acute pancreatitis, cancer of the pancreas, heart failure, acromegaly, postgastrectomy (dumping) syndrome, extensive surgery. *Drug Influence:* ACTH, cortisone preparations, growth hormone, diuretics (hydrochlorothiazide [hydroDIURIL], furosemide [Lasix], ethacrynic acid [Edecrin]), anesthesia drugs, levodopa, estrogen, lithium, epinephrine, phenytoin, high doses of salicylates.

Procedure

- NPO except water for 10–12 hours before the test.
- Withhold insulin and oral hypoglycemic agents.
- Collect 3–5 mL of venous blood in a gray- or red-top tube. Blood is drawn between 7 AM and 9 AM.
- Give insulin as ordered and after the blood sample is taken.

Factors Affecting Laboratory Results

- Drugs—cortisone, thiazide, and the "loop" diuretics can cause an increase in blood sugar.
- Trauma—stress can cause an increase in blood sugar.

- The Clinitest for determining urine glucose (glycosuria) may be falsely positive if the client is taking excessive amounts of aspirin, vitamin C, and certain antibiotics (cephalosporin), because the test is not specific for glucose but for all reducing substances.
- High doses of vitamin C could cause false-negative results when using urine glucose testing tapes (e.g., Tes-Tape).

NURSING IMPLICATIONS WITH RATIONALE

- Hold morning insulin and drugs until the blood specimen is taken.
- Record on the laboratory slip if the client has been taking daily cortisone preparations, thiazides, or loop diuretics.

Decreased Level

- Recognize clinical problems associated with a low blood sugar level. Excessive doses of insulin, skipped meals, and inadequate food intake are the common causes of hypoglycemia.
- Observe for signs and symptoms of hypoglycemia (nervousness, weakness, confusion, cold and clammy skin, diaphoresis, and increased pulse rate).

Client Teaching

- Instruct the client to carry lumps of sugar or candy at all times. Most diabetic persons have warnings when hypoglycemia occurs.
- Teach the client to adhere to the medical nutrition therapy (ADA diet), as prescribed. Explain the exchange lists for meal planning.
- Encourage the client to contact the American Diabetic Association for literature and information concerning their meeting dates.
- Explain to the client that strenuous exercise can lower the blood sugar. Carbohydrate or protein intake should be increased before exercise or immediately after exercise; the health care provider should be contacted for food instruction.
- Encourage the client to take insulin ½ hour before breakfast and to eat meals on time.
- Teach clients with a hypoglycemic problem (blood sugar less than 50 mg/dL) to eat food high in protein and fat and low in carbohydrate. Too much sugar stimulates insulin secretion.

Increased Level

- Recognize clinical problems associated with high blood sugar levels. Diabetes mellitus, Cushing syndrome, and stressful situations (trauma, burns, extensive surgery) are the common causes of hyperglycemia.
- Consider drugs (such as cortisone, thiazides, and "loop" diuretics) as the cause of a slightly elevated blood sugar level. If blood sugar becomes too high, notify the health care provider—drug dosages may need to be decreased or insulin may need to be ordered or increased.
- Observe for signs and symptoms of hyperglycemia (excessive thirst [polydipsia], excessive urination [polyuria], excessive hunger [polyphagia], and weight loss). If the blood sugar is greater than 500 mg/dL, Kussmaul breathing (rapid, deep, vigorous breathing) caused by acidosis may be observed.

G

Client Teaching

- Instruct the client to test his or her blood before meals. Demonstrate how to use a glucose self-monitoring meter such as Accu-Chek, Glucometer, or others.
- Explain to the client that infections can increase the blood sugar level and that medical advice should be sought.

Glucose–postprandial (feasting blood sugar) (blood)

Two-Hour Postprandial Blood Sugar (PPBS)

Reference Values

Adult: *Serum and Plasma:* Less than 140 mg/dL/2 h; less than 7.8 mmol/L (SI units).
  Whole Blood: Less than 120 mg/dL/2 h; less than 6.7 mmol/L (SI units).

Elderly: *Serum:* Less than 160 mg/dL/2 h; less than 8.9 mmol/L (SI units).
  Whole Blood: Less than 140 mg/dL/2 h; less than 7.8 mmol/L (SI units).

Child: *Serum:* Less than 140 mg/dL/2 h; less than 6.7 mmol/L (SI units).

Description

A 2-hour PPBS or feasting sugar test is usually done to determine the patient's response to a high carbohydrate intake 2 hours after a meal (breakfast or lunch). This test is a screening test for diabetes, normally ordered if the fasting blood sugar was high normal or slightly elevated. A serum glucose greater than 140 mg/dL or a blood glucose greater than 120 mg/dL is abnormal, and further tests may be needed.

A glucose tolerance test may be prescribed for a client who has a feasting blood sugar (PPBS) between 140 and 200 mg/dL, to confirm diabetes mellitus. If the feasting blood sugar is greater than 200 mg/dL, a glucose tolerance test is not suggested and diabetes mellitus is confirmed.

Purposes

(*See Glucose—Fasting Blood Sugar.*)

Clinical Problems

Decreased Level: (*See Glucose—Fasting Blood Sugar.*)

Increased Level: (*See Glucose—Fasting Blood Sugar.*)

Procedure

- Food is restricted for 2 hours after breakfast or lunch before the test, but water is not.
- A high-carbohydrate meal might be requested at breakfast or lunch.
- Collect 3–5 mL of venous blood in a gray- or red-top tube 2 hours after the client finishes eating breakfast or lunch. If the nurse does not draw the blood, the laboratory needs to be notified when the client finished breakfast or lunch.

Factors Affecting Laboratory Results

- Smoking may increase the serum glucose level.
- (*See Glucose—Fasting Blood Sugar.*)

NURSING IMPLICATIONS WITH RATIONALE

- Determine the breakfast foods that the client likes and dislikes and notify the dietary department.

Client Teaching

- If the client is not hospitalized, instruct the person to be at the laboratory ½–2 hours after breakfast or lunch.

Increased Level

- (*See Glucose—Fasting Blood Sugar.*)

Glucose self-monitoring (self-testing) devices
Finger-Stick Blood Sugar, Glucose Capillary Test

G

Reference Values
Adult: *Blood:* 60–110 mg/dL, 3.3–6.1 μmol/L (SI units).
Child: *Blood:* 50–85 mg/dL, 2.7–4.7 μmol/L (SI units).
Urine: Negative.

Description
To control blood glucose levels, glucose monitoring devices are available for checking blood glucose levels. The glucose monitoring devices can be used in institutions such as hospitals, and clients with type 1, insulin-dependent diabetes mellitus and type 2, noninsulin dependent diabetes mellitus can use them in their homes. The test takes about 2 minutes, and test results are considered reliable.

The new generation of meters have greatly improved accuracy and precision over earlier models. They are less dependent on operator skill, and most have eliminated the need for timing, blotting, and wiping the strip. Though the manufacturers may not agree, most of the newer meters still are not as reliable as a laboratory test when the glucose levels are less than 50 or 60, or greater than 450 or 500 mg/dL. It varies with the manufacturer.

Usually the client tests his or her blood, by finger stick, before breakfast, and if indicated by the health care provider, before meals and at bedtime. A drop of blood from the finger stick is dropped on a reagent strip and the strip is inserted into the meter.

The use of reagent strips and tablets for urine testing (e.g., Clinistix, Diastix, Tes-Tape, and Clinitest) are less desirable for glucose accuracy than the self-monitoring metered devices. Clients who are unable to perform a finger stick and use the meter machine should use the urine testing method to evaluate blood glucose levels.

Purpose

- To check the blood glucose level.

Clinical Problems

Decreased Level: Insulin overdose, hypoglycemia, hypothyroidism, starvation.

Increased Level: Hyperglycemia, Cushing syndrome, excessive stress. *Drug Influence:* Corticosteroids (steroids), beta blockers, thiazides, estrogen.

Procedure

- NPO prior to the test unless otherwise instructed.

Blood: *Finger-Stick Capillary Method*
- Check procedure on the specific glucose monitoring device.
- Cleanse the finger site with alcohol; wipe dry.
- Puncture the lateral side of the finger using a lancet. Wipe off first drop of blood. Do not "milk" the finger.
- Let a large drop of blood drop onto the reagent strip. The blood should cover the pad of the strip.
- Place the reagent strip into the meter for reading. Follow directions on the meter.
- Apply pressure to the site with a gauze until bleeding has stopped.

Heel stick: Use the same method for obtaining a finger stick; however, hold the heel in a dependent position to allow the blood drop to accumulate. The use of a capillary tube to obtain the blood specimen may be necessary for blood glucose testing.

Urine

Clinitest: Dip the reagent strip into the urine specimen, remove the strip, wait 10 seconds, read by comparing strip to the color blocks.

Diastix: Dip the reagent strip into the urine specimen, remove the strip, wait 30 seconds, read by comparing strip to the color chart.

Tes-Tape: Tear off 1½ inches of reagent tape, dip into the urine specimen, remove tape, wait 60 seconds, read tape by comparing the dark part of tape to color chart.

Factors Affecting Laboratory Results

Blood
- Insufficient blood drop for the test.
- Milking the finger can cause false-low results.
- Certain drugs could cause false readings (*see Drug Influence*).

Urine
- Stale urine interferes with test results.
- Drugs that may cause a false-negative result include levodopa, aspirin, ascorbic acid, tetracycline, and methyldopa.

NURSING IMPLICATIONS WITH RATIONALE

- Obtain a history regarding the client's glucose testing method, including the past glucose testing results.
- Demonstrate how to use the glucose meter. Have the client repeat the procedure if he or she is unfamiliar with it.

Client Teaching

- Discuss the procedure (blood and/or urine) with the client. Answer questions concerning the meter.
- Discuss the course of action the client should take if the test result is abnormal.
- Instruct the client to take insulin or the oral hypoglycemic agent at the prescribed time.
- Tell the client to report immediately signs and symptoms of hypoglycemia or hyperglycemia.
- Instruct the client to keep accurate records of the glucose tests.
- Give the signs and symptoms of hypoglycemia and hyperglycemia. Answer questions concerning these signs and symptoms.
- Encourage the client to keep all medical appointments.

Glucose tolerance test (oral) (OGTT) (serum) and IV (IV-GTT)

G

Reference Values

Adult:

ORAL GTT

Time	Serum (mg/dL)	mmol/L	Blood (mg/dL)	mmol/L
Fasting	70–110	3.9–6.1	60–100	3.3–5.5
0.5 hour	less than 160	less than 8.9	less than 150	less than 8.3
1 hour	less than 170	less than 9.4	less than 160	less than 8.9
2 hours	less than 125	less than 6.9	less than 115	less than 6.9
3 hours	Fasting levels		Fasting levels	

IV GLUCOSE TOLERANCE TEST

Time	Serum (mg/dL)	mmol/L
Fasting	70–110	3.9–6.1
5 minutes	less than 250	less than 13.8
½ hour	less than 155	less than 8.5
1 hour	less than 125	less than 6.9

Child: Depends on the child's age. Infants normally have lower blood sugar levels (*see Glucose— Fasting Blood Sugar*). A child aged 6 or older has results similar to those of the adult.

Description

A glucose tolerance test (GTT) is done to diagnose diabetes mellitus in persons having high-normal or slightly elevated blood sugar values. The test may be indicated when there is a familial history of diabetes, in women having babies weighing 10 pounds or more, in persons having extensive surgery or injury, and in persons with obesity problems. The test should *not* be performed if the fasting blood sugar (FBS) is greater than 200 mg/dL. After the age of 60 years, the blood glucose level is usually 10–30 mg/dL higher than the "normal range."

The peak glucose level for the oral GTT (OGTT) is ½–1 hour after the ingestion of 100 g of glucose, and the blood sugar should return to normal range in 3 hours. Blood samples will be collected at specified times.

The *intravenous glucose tolerance test (IV-GTT)* is considered by many to be more sensitive than the oral GTT, because absorption through the gastrointestinal tract is not involved. The IV-GTT is usually done if the person cannot eat or tolerate the oral glucose. The blood glucose returns to the normal range in 2 hours. However, the values for the OGTT and IV-GTT slightly differ, because IV glucose is absorbed faster.

Hyperinsulinism can be detected with the OGTT. After 1 hour, the blood glucose level is usually lower than in the FBS test. The person might develop severe hypoglycemic reactions—there is more insulin being secreted in response to the blood glucose.

Purpose

- To confirm the diagnosis of diabetes mellitus.

Clinical Problems

Decreased Level: Hyperinsulinism, adrenal gland insufficiency, malabsorption, protein malnutrition.

Increased Level: Diabetes mellitus, latent diabetes, adrenal gland hyperfunction (Cushing syndrome), hyperlipoproteinemia, stress, infections, extensive surgery or injury, alcoholism, acute myocardial infarction, cancer of the pancreas, insulin resistance conditions (eclampsia, cancer metastases, acidotic conditions), duodenal ulcers. *Drug Influence:* Corticosteroids (cortisone), oral contraceptives, estrogens, diuretics, thiazides, salicylates, ascorbic acid.

Procedure

OGTT

- A diet adequate in carbohydrates should be consumed for 2–3 days prior to testing.
- The client remains NPO for 12 hours before the test, except for water.
- No coffee, tea, or smoking is allowed during the test. No food should be eaten.
- Drugs that affect test results should not be taken for 3 days prior to the GTT, if possible.
- Collect 5 mL of venous blood in a red- or gray-top tube for FBS. Collect a fasting urine specimen.
- Give 100 g of glucose, either lemon-flavored solution or Glucola. Some physicians will give glucose according to body weight (1.75 g/kg), as in pediatrics.
- Obtain blood and urine specimens ½, 1, 2, and 3 hours after glucose intake.

IV-GTT

- NPO 12 hours before test.
- Administer infusion of 50% glucose over 3–4 minutes.
- Obtain blood specimens at fasting, 5 minutes (blood only), ½, 1, and 2 hours.

Factors Affecting Laboratory Results

- Drugs (*see Drug Influence*).
- Age—older adults have higher blood sugar levels. Insulin secretion is decreased because of the aging process.
- Emotional stress, fever, infections, trauma, being bedridden, and obesity can increase the blood sugar level.
- Strenuous exercise and vomiting might decrease the blood sugar level. Hypoglycemic agents will decrease the blood sugar level.

NURSING IMPLICATIONS WITH RATIONALE

- Notify the laboratory of when (the exact time) the client drank the glucose solution. Laboratory personnel will collect the blood samples at specified times.

Client Teaching

- Explain to the client the procedure for the test. Explain that food, alcohol, and medications are restricted for 12 hours prior to the test. Water is permitted.
- Explain to the client that coffee, tea, and smoking are restricted during the test. Drinking water is allowed and encouraged; however, in some institutions, only 240 mL is permitted.
- Explain to the client that he or she may perspire or feel weak and giddy during the 2–3 hours of the test. This is frequently transitory; however, the nurse should be notified, and these symptoms should be recorded. They could be signs of hyperinsulinism.
- Inform the client to minimize his or her activities during the test. Increased activities could affect the glucose results.

Decreased Level

- Observe for signs and symptoms of hypoglycemia, especially when hyperinsulinism is suspected. Symptoms include nervousness; irritability; confusion; weakness; pale, cold, clammy skin; diaphoresis (excessive perspiration); and tachycardia.
- Obtain a history from the client as to when hypoglycemic symptoms occur (e.g., before meals). There may be periods of nervousness, "shakiness," and weakness.
- Explain that eating candy to correct nervousness and weakness should be avoided with hyperinsulinism, because it will temporarily correct the problem (the need for glucose) but will stimulate insulin secretion. Sugar will temporarily correct an insulin reaction in a diabetic.

Increased Level

- Identify factors affecting glucose results (e.g., emotional stress, infection, vomiting, fever, exercise, inactivity, age, drugs, and body weight). Most of these should be reported to the health care provider.
- Check previous FBS results before the test. A known diabetic normally does not, and in some cases should not, have this test performed because diabetic coma may ensue.

G

Glucose-6-phosphate dehydrogenase (G6PD or G-6-PD) (blood)

Reference Values

Adult: *Screen Test:* Negative. *Quantitative Test:* 8–18 international unit/g Hb, 125–281 unit/dL packed RBCs, 251–511 unit/106 cells, 1,211–2,111 milli-international unit/mL packed RBCs (varies with methods used).

Child: Similar to adult.

Description

Glucose-6-phosphate dehydrogenase (G6PD) is an enzyme in the red blood cells, or erythrocytes. It normally assists in glucose use in the RBCs, uses oxidative substances, and protects the integrity of the RBCs from injury.

A G6PD deficit is a sex-linked genetic defect carried by the female (X) chromosome, which will, in conjunction with infection, disease, and drugs, make a person susceptible to developing hemolytic anemia. With a moderate deficiency of G6PD enzyme, there is no apparent detectable RBC abnormality except for a decrease in the life span of the RBCs. Metabolites from certain drugs possessing an oxidizing action in the RBCs will cause an increased need for G6PD for glucose metabolism. A lack of this enzyme results in hemolysis (destruction of the RBCs) and hemolytic anemia when augmented by an oxidative drug.

Purpose

- To screen for hemolytic anemia.

Clinical Problems

Decreased Level: Hemolytic anemia, diabetic acidosis, infections (bacterial and viral), septicemia. *Drug Influence:* Acetanilid (acetylaniline), aspirin, ascorbic acid, nitrofurantoin (Furadantin), phenacetin, primaquine, thiazide diuretics, probenecid (Benemid), quinidine, quinine, chloramphenicol (Chloromycetin), sulfonamides, vitamin K, tolbutamide (Orinase). *Food:* Fava beans.

Procedure

- There is no food or fluid restriction.
- The laboratory methods used will vary. Screening tests for G6PD deficiency are methemoglobin reduction (Brewer's test), glutathione stability, dye reduction, and ascorbate and fluorescent spot tests. Check with the laboratory on whether capillary or venous blood is needed.
- Collect 5 mL of venous blood in a lavender- or green-top tube. Avoid hemolysis.

Factors Affecting Laboratory Results

- Drugs can decrease the level (*see Drug Influence*).

NURSING IMPLICATIONS WITH RATIONALE

Decreased Level

- Obtain a familial history of RBC enzyme deficiency. Black people are more prone to G6PD deficiency than white people; however, the degree of anemia is not as severe in black people as it is in white people.
- Observe for symptoms of hemolysis, such as jaundice of the eyes and skin.
- Check for decreased urinary output. Urine should be voided at a rate of at least 25 mL/hour or 600 mL/day. Prolonged hemolysis (destruction of RBCs) can be toxic to the kidney cells, causing kidney impairment.
- Check the hemology results.
- Record oxidative drugs the client is taking on the laboratory slip (*see Drug Influence*). Report your findings to the health care provider. Hemolysis usually occurs 3 days after the susceptible person has taken an oxidative drug. Hemolytic symptoms will disappear 2–3 days after the drug has been stopped.

Client Teaching

- Instruct the susceptible person to read labels on patent medicines and not to take drugs that contain phenacetin and aspirin. Most of these drugs, if taken continuously, can cause hemolytic anemia.

Glycosylated hemoglobin

See Hemoglobin A_1c (Blood)

Growth hormone (GH), human growth hormone (hGH) (serum)

Somatotrophic Hormone (STH)

Reference Values

Adult: *Male:* Less than 5 ng/mL. *Female:* Less than 10 ng/mL.
Child: Less than 10 ng/mL.

Description

Human growth hormone (hGH), hormone from the anterior pituitary gland, regulates growth of bone and tissue. Growth hormone levels are elevated by protein-rich food, fasting, stress, exercise, and deep sleep.

A low serum hGH level might be the cause of dwarfism. Elevated hGH levels cause gigantism in children and acromegaly in adults. From a random growth hormone level, a positive diagnosis cannot be made; therefore, *a growth hormone stimulation or suppression challenge test* would be suggested. A glucose loading GH suppression test should suppress hGH secretion. Failure to suppress hGH levels confirms gigantism (children) or acromegaly (adults).

Purposes

- To determine the presence of human growth hormone deficit or excess.
- To aid in the diagnosis of dwarfism, gigantism, or acromegaly.

Clinical Problems

Decreased Level: Dwarfism in children, hypopituitarism. *Drug Influence:* Cortisone preparations, phenothiazines, glucose.

Increased Level: Gigantism (children), acromegaly (adults), major surgery, premature and newborn infants. *Drug Influence:* Insulin, estrogens, amphetamines, beta blockers, levodopa, methyldopa (Aldomet).

Procedure

- The client is NPO for 8–10 hours except for water.
- Collect 3–5 mL of venous blood in a red-top tube, preferably in the early morning. Avoid hemolysis. Deliver the blood specimen immediately to the laboratory, because hGH has a short half-life.
- Have the client rest for 30 minutes to 1 hour before taking a blood sample.

Factors Affecting Laboratory Results

- Stress, exercise, food (protein), and deep sleep could cause an elevated hGH level.
- Drugs listed in *Drug Influence* could decrease or elevate hGH levels.
- Hemolysis of the blood sample affects test results.

H

NURSING IMPLICATIONS WITH RATIONALE

- Maintain a quiet environment so that stress will not affect test results.
- Notify the health care provider and/or laboratory if the client is anxious, has eaten, or has exercised before the test.

Client Teaching

- Instruct the client not to eat 8–10 hours before the test. Encourage the client to rest and not to exercise prior to the test.
- Inform the client that if the serum hGH is elevated, follow-up testing may be necessary.

Haloperidol (Haldol) (serum)

Reference Values

Adult: *Therapeutic Range:* 3–20 ng/mL. *Peak Time:* PO: 2–6 hours. *Toxic Level:* greater than 50 ng/mL.

Description

Haloperidol is used in the treatment of acute and chronic psychosis, in the manic phase of manic-depressive psychosis (bipolar disorder), and in some cases of schizophrenia. It is a drug frequently used in psychiatry.

Purposes

- To determine if the therapeutic haloperidol dose is within therapeutic range.
- To check for haloperidol toxicity.

Clinical Problems

Decreased Level: *Drug Influence:* Anticholinergics (used for parkinsonism).

Increased Level: Overdose of haloperidol.

Procedure

- There is no food or fluid restriction.
- Collect 3–5 mL of venous blood in a red-top tube.

Factors Affecting Laboratory Results

- Anticholinergics used for the pseudoparkinsonism effect can decrease the effect of haloperidol.
- Phenothiazines, benzodiazepines, or alcohol taken with haloperidol cause an additive central nervous system depressive effect.

NURSING IMPLICATIONS WITH RATIONALE

- Observe for side effects of haloperidol (e.g., dizziness, syncope, drowsiness, hypotension, pseudoparkinsonism, dry mouth, jaundice [due to large doses over a period of time]).
- Check vital signs.

Client Teaching

- Instruct the client to avoid driving and activities that require alertness when taking haloperidol.
- Instruct the client to avoid alcohol and other depressants that might cause side effects of haloperidol.
- Explain to the client the importance of checking with the health care provider about taking OTC (over-the-counter) drugs. Some OTC drugs might cause side effects.

Haptoglobin (Hp) (serum)

Reference Values

Adult: 60–270 mg/dL, 0.6–2.7 g/L (SI units).

Child: *Newborn:* 0–10 mg/dL (absent in 90%). *Infant (1–6 months):* 0–30 mg/dL, then gradual increase.

Description

Haptoglobins are alpha$_2$ globulins in the plasma. These globulin molecules combine with free (released) hemoglobin during red blood cell destruction (hemolysis). A decreased level of serum haptoglobin indicates hemolysis. Haptoglobins are decreased in severe liver disease, hemolytic anemia, and infectious mononucleosis and are elevated in inflammatory diseases, steroid therapy, acute infections, and malignancies. A hemolytic process may be masked in persons taking steroids.

Purposes

- To identify the occurrence of hemolysis.
- To assist in the diagnosis of selected health problems (*see Clinical Problems*).

Clinical Problems

Decreased Level: Hemolysis, anemias (pernicious, vitamin B$_6$ deficiency, hemolytic, sickle cell), severe liver disease (hepatic failure, chronic hepatitis), thrombotic thrombocytopenic purpura, disseminated intravascular coagulation, malaria.

Increased Level: Inflammation, acute infections, cancer (lung, large intestine, stomach, breast, liver), Hodgkin disease, ulcerative colitis, chronic pyelonephritis (active stage), rheumatic fever, acute myocardial infarction. *Drug Influence:* Steroids (cortisone).

Procedure

- There is no food or fluid restriction.
- Collect 3–5 mL of venous blood in a red-top tube. Avoid hemolysis.
- Haptoglobin levels can be measured by electrophoresis, radioimmunodiffusion, or spectrophotometry.

Factors Affecting Laboratory Results

- Steroids and inflammation may cause false results. Hemolysis could occur but the serum haptoglobin level may not indicate this.

NURSING IMPLICATIONS WITH RATIONALE

Decreased Level

- Associate a decreased serum haptoglobin level with conditions causing hemolysis, such as hemolytic anemias, severe liver disease, and others.
- Assess the client's vital signs. Report abnormal vital signs, especially if the client is having breathing problems. The oxygen capacity of hemoglobin may be reduced, causing a change in breathing pattern.
- Assess the client's urinary output. Excessive amounts of free hemoglobin may cause renal damage.

Increased Level

- Associate an elevated serum haptoglobin level with clinical problems, such as infections, inflammation, cancer, steroid therapy, and others.
- Check the serum haptoglobin level. The haptoglobin level may be masked by steroid therapy and inflammation. If hemolysis is suspected, the serum level may be normal instead of low because of steroid therapy or inflammation. Notify the health care provider of the findings.

Heinz bodies (blood)

Reference Values

Negative: Absence of Heinz bodies; less than 30% Heinz bodies present.

Description

Heinz bodies are small, irregular, decomposed particles of hemoglobin that accumulate on the red blood cells' membrane. Normally these bodies are removed by the spleen; however, they can be a cause of hemolytic anemia (hemolysis of RBCs) or hemoglobinopathy (hematologic disorder). After a splenectomy, the Heinz bodies increase in the blood, and the reference value can be greater than 30%.

Purpose

- To aid in identifying the cause of hemolytic anemia.

Clinical Problems

Increased Levels: Hemolytic anemia, hemoglobinopathies, glucose-6-phosphate dehydrogenase (G-6-PD) deficiency, post-splenectomy. *Drug Influence:* Analgesics including acetaminophen, antimalarials, certain sulfonamides, phenothiazines, phenacetin, procarbazine, nitrofurantoin, and chlorates.

Procedure

- There is no food or fluid restriction.
- Collect 7 mL of venous blood in a lavender-top tube. Avoid hemolysis; gently invert tube.

Factors Affecting Laboratory Results

- Hemolysis because of rough handling of blood specimen.
- Drugs that could induce hemolysis (*see Clinical Problems*).
- Blood transfusion(s) within the last week before the test.

H

NURSING IMPLICATIONS WITH RATIONALE

- Obtain a history from the client with regard to past and present health problems, drugs the client is taking, and any recent blood transfusions.
- Assess vital signs; report abnormal findings.
- Report jaundice that could result from red blood cell hemolysis. Bilirubin may be elevated.

Helicobacter pylori (serum, culture, breath analysis)

Reference Values

Negative findings. A positive or elevated titer level using enzyme-linked immunosorbent assay (ELISA) serology testing or the urea breath test indicates the presence of *Helicobacter pylori*.

Description

The gram-negative bacillus *Helicobacter pylori* is found in the gastric mucus layer of the epithelium in about 50% of the population by age 55. The majority of persons with the infection remain asymptomatic. *H. pylori* was first identified in 1983 as a cause of peptic ulcer disease. It is recognized as a primary cause of chronic gastritis, and it may progress over years to gastric cancer or gastric lymphoma. *H. pylori* is associated with 70–85% of clients with gastric ulcers and with 90–95% of duodenal ulcers. Duodenal ulcers due to Zollinger-Ellison syndrome are not associated with *H. pylori*.

The incidence of *H. pylori* increases with age. Between the ages of 45 and 55, the incidence of *H. pylori* antibodies is approximately 20%. The incidence of *H. pylori* grows to 50% over the next 10 years, and for persons over 65 years of age, the incidence increases to 75%. This organism is common in black people.

Eradication of *H. pylori* for asymptomatic clients usually is not suggested or prescribed but is definitely indicated for perforated, bleeding, or refractory ulcers. Treatment to eradicate the infection involves a dual, triple, or quadruple drug therapy program using a variety of drug combinations. Dual-drug therapy (omeprazole and amoxicillin) for 14 days has fewer side effects but is not as effective in eradicating *H. pylori* as the use of triple or quadruple therapy. Quadruple therapy has a 7-day treatment course that eliminates some of the side effects. After the drug therapy program, a 6-week standard acid suppression drug (histamine-2 blocker) is usually recommended.

Purposes

- To detect the cause of gastrointestinal disorder.
- To determine the presence of *H. pylori*.

Clinical Problems

Increased Level or Positive Culture: Presence of *H. pylori* causing acute or chronic gastritis, peptic ulcer disease, gastric carcinoma, gastric lymphoma.

Procedure

Serum (ELISA)
- No food or fluid restriction is required.
- Collect 7 mL of venous blood in a red-top tube.
- Use of a variety of commercial diagnostic kits.

Culture or Biopsy (Endoscopy)
- Obtain a culture or biopsy using endoscopy for detection of urease produced by *H. pylori*.

Urea Breath Test
- Use the urea breath test to diagnose urease, which is given off by *H. pylori*. It has a sensitivity of 92–94%.
- The urea test dose is accompanied by radioactive carbon 13 or 14. The expired air is tested for radioactivity.

Factors Affecting Laboratory Results

- None known.

NURSING IMPLICATIONS

- Obtain a familial history of gastrointestinal disorders, such as gastritis or peptic ulcer disease.
- Record symptoms client has related to gastritis or peptic ulcer disease, such as pain, abdominal cramping, gastroesophageal reflux disease, dyspepsia (heartburn), anorexia, nausea, vomiting, gastrointestinal bleeding, and tarry stools.
- Encourage the client to avoid smoking (if the client smokes), because smoking reduces bicarbonate content in the GI tract, allows reflux of the duodenum into the stomach, and slows the healing process.
- Listen to the client's concerns. Answer the client's questions or refer unknown answers to other health care providers.

H

Hematocrit (Hct) (blood)

Reference Values

Adult: *Male:* 40–54%, 0.40–0.54 (SI units). *Female:* 36–46%, 0.36–0.46 (SI units). *Panic Value:* Less than 15% and greater than 60%.

Child: *Newborn:* 44–65%. *1–3 Years Old:* 29–40%. *4–10 Years Old:* 31–43%.

Description

The hematocrit (Hct) is the volume (in milliliters) of packed red blood cells (RBCs) found in 100 mL (1 dL) of blood, expressed as a percentage. For example, a 36% hematocrit would indicate that 36 mL of RBCs were found in 100 mL of blood, or 36 vol/dL. The purpose of the test is to measure the concentration of RBCs (erythrocytes) in the blood.

Low hematocrits are found frequently in anemias and leukemias, and elevated levels are found in dehydration (a relative increase) and polycythemia vera. The hematocrit can be an indicator of the hydration status of the client. As with hemoglobin, an elevated hematocrit could indicate hemoconcentration because of a decrease in fluid volume and an increase in RBCs.

Purposes

- To check the volume of RBCs in the blood.
- To monitor the volume of RBCs in blood during a debilitating illness.

Clinical Problems

Decreased Level: Acute blood loss, anemias (aplastic, hemolytic, folic acid deficiency, pernicious, sideroblastic, sickle cell), leukemias (lymphocytic, myelocytic, monocytic), Hodgkin disease, lymphosarcoma, malignancy of organs, multiple myeloma, cirrhosis of the liver, protein malnutrition, vitamin deficiencies (thiamine, vitamin C), fistula of the stomach or duodenum, peptic ulcer, chronic renal failure, pregnancy, systemic lupus erythematosus, rheumatoid arthritis (especially juvenile). *Drug Influence:* Antineoplastic agents, antibiotics (chloramphenicol, penicillin), radioactive agents.

Increased Level: Dehydration/hypovolemia, severe diarrhea, polycythemia vera, erythrocytosis, diabetic acidosis, pulmonary emphysema (later stage), transient cerebral ischemia, eclampsia, surgery, burns.

Procedure

- No food or fluid restriction.

Venous Blood

- Collect 3–5 mL of venous blood in a lavender-top tube. Mix well. The tourniquet should be on for less than 2 minutes.
- Do not take the blood specimen from an arm in which there is an IV line.

Capillary Blood

- Collect capillary blood using the microhematocrit method. Blood is obtained from a finger prick, using a heparinized capillary tube.

Factors Affecting Laboratory Results

- If blood is collected from an extremity that has an IV line, the hematocrit will most likely be low. Avoid using such an extremity.
- If blood is taken to check the hematocrit immediately after moderate to severe blood loss and transfusions, the hematocrit could be normal.
- Age of the client—newborns normally have higher hematocrits because of hemoconcentration.

NURSING IMPLICATIONS WITH RATIONALE

- Explain the procedure to the client. If the microhematocrit method is used, explain that the finger will be cleansed with an alcohol sponge and pricked with a lancet or needle to obtain capillary blood.

Decreased Level

- Relate a decreased hematocrit to clinical problems and drugs. Blood loss and anemias are the most common causes of a low hematocrit. A hematocrit of 30% or less with no known bleeding frequently indicates a moderate to severe anemic condition.
- Assess for signs and symptoms of anemia (fatigue, paleness, and tachycardia).
- Assess changes in vital signs to determine whether shock is present because of blood loss. Symptoms could include rapid pulse, rapid respirations, and normal or decreased blood pressure.
- Recommend a repeat hematocrit several days after moderate/severe bleeding or transfusions. A hematocrit taken immediately after blood loss and after transfusions may appear normal.

Increased Level

- Relate an increased hematocrit to clinical problems. Dehydration and hypovolemia are common causes of hematocrit elevation because they result in hemoconcentration.
- Assess for signs and symptoms of dehydration/hypovolemia. A history of vomiting, diarrhea, marked thirst, lack of skin turgor, and shocklike symptoms (rapid pulse and respiration rates) could be indicative of a body fluid deficit.
- Administer IV or oral fluids according to the health care provider's order to reestablish body fluid volume.
- Avoid rapid administration of IV fluids to the older adult, child, or debilitated person so as to prevent overhydration and pulmonary edema. Signs and symptoms of overhydration are constant, irritated cough; dyspnea; hand and/or neck vein engorgement; and chest rales.
- Check the hematocrit daily, if ordered, when reestablishing body fluid volume. If the elevated hematocrit returns to normal, the elevation was due to hemoconcentration.
- Assess changes in urinary output. A urine output of less than 25 mL/hour or 600 mL daily could be due to dehydration/hypovolemia. Once body fluids are restored, urine output should be normal.

Hemoglobin (Hb or Hgb) (blood)

Reference Values

Adult: *Male:* 13.5–18 g/dL; 8.4–11.2 mmol/L (SI units). *Female:* 12–15 g/dL; 7.45–9.31 mmol/L (SI units).

Child: *Newborn:* 14–24 g/dL. *Infant:* 10–17 g/dL. *Child:* 11–16 g/dL.

Description

Hemoglobin (Hb or Hgb), a protein substance found in red blood cells, gives blood its red color. Hemoglobin is composed of iron, which is an oxygen carrier. Abnormally high hemoglobin levels may be due to hemoconcentration resulting from dehydration (fluid loss). Low hemoglobin values are related to various clinical problems.

The RBC count and hemoglobin level do not always increase or decrease equally. For instance, a decreased RBC count and a normal or slightly decreased hemoglobin level occur in pernicious anemia, and a normal or slightly decreased RBC and a decreased hemoglobin level occur in iron-deficiency (microcytic) anemia.

Purposes

- To monitor the hemoglobin value in RBCs.
- To assist in diagnosing anemia.
- To suggest the presence of body fluid deficit due to an increased hemoglobin level.

Clinical Problems

Decreased Level: Anemias (iron deficiency, aplastic, hemocytic), severe hemorrhage, cirrhosis of the liver, leukemias, Hodgkin disease, sarcoidosis, excess IV fluids, cancer (large and small intestine, rectum, liver, bone), thalassemia major, pregnancy, kidney diseases. *Drug Influence:* Antibiotics (chloramphenicol [Chloromycetin], penicillin, tetracycline), aspirin, antineoplastic drugs, doxapram (Dopram), hydantoin derivatives, hydralazine (Apresoline), indomethacin (Indocin), MAO inhibitors, primaquine, rifampin, sulfonamides, trimethadione (Tridione), vitamin A (large doses).

Increased Level: Dehydration/hemoconcentration, polycythemia, high altitudes, chronic obstructive pulmonary disease, heart failure, severe burns. *Drug Influence:* Gentamicin, methyldopa (Aldomet).

H

Procedure

- There is no food or fluid restriction.
- Do not take the blood sample from a hand or arm receiving IV fluid. The tourniquet should be on less than a minute.

Venous Blood: Collect 3–5 mL of venous blood in a lavender-top tube. Avoid hemolysis.

Capillary Blood: Puncture the cleansed earlobe, finger, or heel with a sterile lancet. Do not squeeze the puncture site tightly, for serous fluid and blood would thus be obtained. Wipe away the first drop of blood. Collect drops of blood quickly in micropipettes with small rubber tops or microhematocrit tubes. Expel blood into the tubes with diluents.

Factors Affecting Laboratory Results

- Drugs could increase or decrease hemoglobin (*see Drug Influence*).
- Taking blood from an arm or hand receiving IV fluids could dilute blood sample.
- Leaving the tourniquet on for more than a minute will cause hemostasis, which will result in a falsely elevated hemoglobin level.
- Living in high altitudes will increase hemoglobin levels.
- Decreased fluid intake or fluid loss will increase hemoglobin levels due to hemoconcentration, and excessive fluid intake will decrease hemoglobin levels due to hemodilution.

NURSING IMPLICATIONS WITH RATIONALE

- Explain the procedure to the client.

Decreased Level

- Recognize clinical problems and drugs that could cause a decreased hemoglobin level (*see Clinical Problems*). Anemia is a common cause, but usually the client is not considered anemic until the hemoglobin level is less than 10.5 g/dL. Hemorrhage could cause a low hemoglobin level if the blood is not replaced; however, the hemoglobin level does not decrease immediately. It may remain normal for hours or even several days.
- Observe the client for signs and symptoms of anemia (e.g., dizziness, tachycardia, weakness, dyspnea at rest). Symptoms depend on how low the hemoglobin level is (severe anemia).
- Check the hematocrit level if the hemoglobin level is low.

Increased Level

- Recognize clinical problems and drugs that can cause an increased hemoglobin level (*see Clinical Problems*). Dehydration is a major transient cause of an elevated level. Once the client is hydrated, the hemoglobin should return to the normal range.
- Observe for signs and symptoms of dehydration (e.g., marked thirst, poor skin turgor, dry mucous membranes, and shocklike symptoms [tachycardia, tachypnea, and, later, decreased blood pressure]).

Client Teaching

- Instruct the client to maintain an adequate fluid intake. Frequently, older adults tend to drink less fluid.

H

Hemoglobin A₁c (Hgb A₁c or Hb A₁c) (blood)

Glycosylated Hemoglobin (Hgb A₁a, Hgb A₁b, Hgb A₁c, Glycohemoglobin)

Reference Values

Total Glycosylated Hemoglobin: 5.5–9% of total Hgb (Hb).

Adult: *Hgb (Hb) A₁c:* Nondiabetic: 2–5%; Diabetic Control: 2.5–6%; high average; 6.1–7.5%; Diabetic Uncontrolled: greater than 8%.

Child: *Hgb (Hb) A₁c:* Nondiabetic: 1.5–4%.

Description

Hemoglobin A (Hgb or Hb A) comprises 91–95% of total hemoglobin. Glucose molecule is attached to Hb A₁, which is a portion of hemoglobin A. This process of attachment is called *glycosylation* or *glycosylated hemoglobin* or *hemoglobin A₁*. There is a bond between glucose and hemoglobin. Formation of Hb A₁ occurs slowly over 120 days, the life span of red blood cells. Hb A₁ is composed of three hemoglobin molecules—Hb A₁a, Hb A₁b, and Hb A₁c—of which 70% Hb

A_1c is 70% glycosylated (absorbs glucose). The amount of glycosylated hemoglobin depends on the amount of blood glucose available. When the blood glucose level is elevated over a prolonged period of time, the red blood cells become saturated with glucose; glycohemoglobin results.

A glycosylated hemoglobin represents an average blood glucose level during a 1- to 3-month period. This test is used mainly as a measurement of the effectiveness of diabetic therapy. Fasting blood sugar reflects the blood glucose level at a one-time fasting state, whereas the Hgb or Hb A_1c is a better indicator of diabetes mellitus control. However, a false decreased Hb A_1c level can be caused by a decrease in red blood cells.

An elevated Hb A_1c greater than 8% indicates uncontrolled diabetes mellitus, and the client is at a high risk of developing long-term complications, such as nephropathy, retinopathy, neuropathy, and/or cardiopathy. Total glycohemoglobin may be a better indicator of diabetes control for clients with anemias or blood loss.

Purposes

- To monitor the effectiveness of diabetic therapy.
- To manage diabetic therapy.
- To provide information regarding the presence of diabetes mellitus.
- To determine the client's compliance with diabetic therapy.

Clinical Problems

Decreased Level: Anemias (pernicious, hemolytic, sickle cell), thalassemia, long-term blood loss, chronic renal failure.

Increased Level: Uncontrolled diabetes mellitus, hyperglycemia, recently diagnosed diabetes mellitus, alcohol ingestion, pregnancy, hemodialysis. *Drug Influence:* Prolonged cortisone intake, ACTH.

Procedure

- Schedule the lab Hb A_1c test 6–12 weeks after diabetic treatment, unless otherwise indicated.
- Food restriction prior to the test is not required but is suggested.
- Collect 5 mL of venous blood in a lavender- or green-top tube. Avoid hemolysis; send specimen immediately to the laboratory.

Factors Affecting Laboratory Results

- Anemias may cause a low value result.
- Hemolysis of the blood specimen can cause an inaccurate test result.
- Heparin therapy may cause a false test result.

NURSING IMPLICATIONS WITH RATIONALE

- Monitor blood and/or urine glucose levels. Compare monthly fasting blood sugar with glycosylated hemoglobin (Hb A_1c) test result.
- Check previous fasting blood sugar results.
- Determine client's compliance to diabetic treatment regimen.
- Check the dose of daily insulin or oral hypoglycemic agent.

- Recognize clinical problems that can cause a false glycosylated hemoglobin result (*see Clinical Problems*).
- Observe for signs and symptoms of hyperglycemia.
- Report any complications the client has due to diabetes mellitus.

Client Teaching

- Inform the client that fasting prior to the test may or may not be prescribed. Tell the client to tell the laboratory person if he or she has not fasted prior to the test.
- Explain the purpose of the test—that is, it measures the effectiveness of the prescribed diabetic therapy.
- Instruct the client to comply with the diabetic treatment regimen, such as prescribed insulin, diet, and glucose monitoring.

Hemoglobin electrophoresis (blood)

Hemoglobins A_1, A_2, F, C, S

Reference Values

Adult: *Hemoglobin (Hb or Hgb) Electrophoresis:* A_1, 95–98% total Hb; A_2, 1.5%; F, less than 2%; C, 0%; D, 0%; S, 0%.

Child: *Newborn:* Hb, F, 50–80% total Hb. *Infant:* Hb F, 8% total Hb. *Child:* Hb F, 1–2% total Hb after 6 months.

Description

The normal types of hemoglobin are Hb A_1, comprising 95–98% of the total hemoglobin, Hb A_2, and Hb F (fetal). If Hb F makes up 5% or more of the total hemoglobin after the age of 6 months, thalassemia (Mediterranean anemia) could be a factor. There are three clinical types of thalassemia: thalassemia major (Hb F greater than 50%), thalassemia minor (increased Hb A_2 value), and thalassemia gene (combination of abnormal hemoglobins).

To identify normal hemoglobin types (A_1, A_2, and F) and abnormal hemoglobin types (Hb C, Hb M, Hb S, and others), a hemoglobin electrophoresis is usually ordered. It is not a routine test, but it is useful for identifying 150 or more types of hemoglobin. Many abnormal hemoglobin types do not produce harmful diseases; the common hemoglobinopathies are identified through electrophoresis.

Hemoglobin S: Hb S is the most common hemoglobin variant. If both genes have Hb S, sickle-cell anemia will occur; but if only one gene has Hb S, then the person simply carries the sickle trait. Approximately 1% of the black population in the United States has sickle-cell anemia, and 8–10% carry the sickle-cell trait. Sickle-cell anemia symptoms are usually not present until after the age of 6 months. In some cases, Hb S is combined with another abnormal hemoglobin type, Hb C or Hb D, Hb S/C or Hb S/D, to produce red blood cells (erythrocytes) that sickle. Those with sickle-cell anemia have low oxygen tension (*also see Sickle-Cell Test*).

Hemoglobin C: Hb C in the homozygous state (C/C) usually produces mild hemolytic anemia; in the heterozygous state (A/C), it produces the Hb C trait. This occurs more frequently in black people.

Purpose

- To detect abnormal hemoglobin types in the RBCs (e.g., sickle-cell anemia, which is characterized by the S-shaped hemoglobin).

Clinical Problems

HEMOGLOBIN TYPE	INCREASED LEVEL
Hemoglobin F	Thalassemia (after 6 months)
Hemoglobin C	Hemolytic anemia
Hemoglobin S	Sickle-cell anemia

Procedure

- There is no food or fluid restriction.
- Collect 3–5 mL of venous blood in a lavender-top tube. Send immediately to the laboratory. Abnormal hemoglobin is unstable.

Factors Affecting Laboratory Results

- Blood transfusions given 4 months before hemoglobin electrophoresis may cause inaccurate results.
- Collection of the blood sample in the wrong color tube can affect results.

H

NURSING IMPLICATIONS WITH RATIONALE

- Observe for signs and symptoms of sickle-cell anemia. Early symptoms are fatigue and weakness. Chronic symptoms are fatigue, dyspnea on exertion, swollen joints, bones that ache, and chest pains. Afflicted persons are susceptible to infection. Sickle-cell crisis is usually due to small infarcts to various organs. The crisis usually lasts 5–7 days, and immediate care is needed for the symptoms. Normally the hemoglobin level does not change.

Client Teaching

- Encourage the client to seek genetic counseling if he or she has sickle-cell anemia or is a carrier of the sickle-cell trait.
- Instruct the client with sickle-cell anemia to minimize strenuous activity and to avoid high altitudes and extreme cold. Encourage the client to take rest periods.
- Encourage the client to stay away from persons with infections.
- Suggest that the client carry a medical alert bracelet and/or card.

Hepatitis (profile)
Hepatitis A, B, C, D, E

Five major types of hepatitis virus can be identified through laboratory testing: hepatitis A virus (HAV), hepatitis B virus (HBV), hepatitis C virus (HCV), hepatitis D virus (HDV), and hepatitis E virus (HEV). These hepatitis viruses can be detected by testing serum antigens, antibodies, DNA, RNA, and/or the immunoglobins IgG and IgM. The following table differentiates between the hepatitis viruses according to method of transmission, incubation time, jaundice, acute and chronic phases of the disease, carrier status, immunity, and mortality rate.

Comparison of the Types of Viral Hepatitis

TYPES OF HEPATITIS					
Factors Associated with Hepatitis	HAV	HBV	HCV	HDV	HEV
Method of transmission	Enteral (oral–fecal) Water and food	Parenteral Intravenous Sexual Perinatal	Parenteral Sexual (possible) Perinatal	Parenteral Sexual (possible) Perinatal	Enteral (oral–fecal) Water and food
Incubation time	Abrupt onset; 2–12 weeks	Insidious onset; 6–24 weeks	Insidious onset; 2–26 weeks	Abrupt onset; 3–15 weeks	Abrupt onset; 2–8 weeks
Jaundice	Adult: 70–80% Child: 10%	20–40%	10–25%	Varies	25–60%
Hepatocellular carcinoma	None	Possible	Possible	Possible	None
Acute disease: serum markers	Anti-HAV-IgM	HBsAg, HBeAg, Anti-HBc-IgM	Anti-HCV	HDAg	Anti-HEV
Chronic disease: serum markers	None	HBsAg	Anti-HCV (50% of cases) Anti-HCV	Anti-HDV	None
Infective state: serum markers	None (HAV-RNA)	HBsAg, HBeAg, HBV-DNA	HCV-RNA	Anti-HDV HDV-RNA	None (HEV-RNA)
Fulminant hepatitis	Very low	Very low	Very low	High	Low
Chronic carrier	None	HbsAg (low incidence in adults; high incidence in children)	High incidence	Anti-HDV, HDAg low incidence (10–15%)	None
Immunity: serum markers	Anti-HAV total, Anti-HAV-IgG	Anti-HBs, Anti-HBc total	None	None	Anti-HEV
Mortality rate	less than 2%	less than 2%	less than 2%	less than or equal to 30%	less than 2%

H

Hepatitis A Virus (HAV): Hepatitis A virus is transmitted primarily by oral–fecal contact. Jaundice is an early sign of HAV, which can occur a few days after the viral infection and may last up to 12 weeks. The antibodies to hepatitis A, anti-HAV-IgM, and anti-HAV-IgG are used to confirm the phase of the hepatitis A infection. Anti-HAV-IgM denotes an acute phase of the infection, while anti-HAV-IgG indicates recovery, past infection, or immunity. Approximately 45–50% of clients having HAV may have a positive anti-HAV-IgG for life.

Hepatitis B Virus (HBV): The hepatitis B virus was once called serum hepatitis. There are numerous laboratory tests for diagnosing the acute or chronic phase of HBV. These include hepatitis B surface antigen (HBsAg), antibody to HBsAg (anti-HBs), hepatitis B e antigen (HBeAg), antibody to HBeAg (anti-HBe), and antibody to core antigen (anti-HBc-total).

HBsAg: The earliest indicator for diagnosing hepatitis B viral infection is the hepatitis B surface antigen. This serum marker can be present as early as 2 weeks after being infected, and it persists during the acute phase of the infection. If it persists after 6 months, the client could have chronic hepatitis and be a carrier. The hepatitis B vaccine will not cause a positive HBsAg. Clients who have a positive HBsAg should *never* donate blood.

Antibody to Hepatitis B Surface Antigen (Anti-HBs): With HBV, the acute phase of viral hepatitis B usually lasts for 12 weeks; therefore, HBsAg is absent and anti-HBs (antibodies to HBsAg) develop. This serum marker indicates recovery and immunity to the hepatitis B virus. An anti-HBs-IgM would determine if the client is still infectious. An anti-HBs titer of greater than 10 milli-international unit/mL and without HBsAg presence confirms that the client has recovered from HBV.

Hepatitis B e antigen (HBeAg): This serum marker occurs only with HBsAg. It usually appears 1 week after HBsAg and disappears before anti-HBs. If HBeAg is still present after 10 weeks, the client could be developing a chronic carrier state.

Antibody to HBeAg (Anti-HBe): The presence of anti-HBe indicates the recovery phase.

Antibody to Core Antigen (Anti-HBc): The anti-HBc occurs with a positive HBsAg within approximately 4–10 weeks of acute HBV. An elevated anti-HBc-IgM titer indicates the acute infection process. Anti-HBc can detect clients who have been infected with HBV. This serum marker may persist for years, and clients with a positive anti-HBc should not give blood.

Hepatitis C Virus (HCV): HCV is formerly non-A, non-B hepatitis. It is transmitted parenterally. It occurs more frequently with posttransfusion hepatitis, but also should be considered with drug addiction, needle sticks, hemodialysis, and hemophilias. Approximately half of the acute cases of HCV become chronic carriers.

Antibody to Hepatitis C Virus (Anti-HCV): HCV is confirmed by the anti-HCV test. Anti-HCV does not indicate immunity as it can with anti-HBs and anti-HBe.

Hepatitis D Virus (HDV): Hepatitis D (delta) virus is transmitted parenterally. HDV can be present only with HBV. It is coated by the HBsAg and depends on the HBV for replication. HDV is severe and usually occurs 7–14 days after an acute, severe HBV infection. It has a low occurrence rate except in IV drug abusers and clients receiving multiple transfusions. Its presence is in the acute phase of HBV or as a chronic carrier of HBV. Of all the types of hepatitis, it has the greatest incidence of fulminant hepatitis and death.

Hepatitis D Antigen (HDAg): Detection of HDAg and HDV-RNA indicates the acute phase of HBV and HDV infection. When HBsAg diminishes, so does HDAg. Anti-HDV appears later and may suggest chronic hepatitis D.

Hepatitis E Virus (HEV): HEV is transmitted by oral–fecal contact and not parenterally. It can result from drinking unsafe water as well as traveling in Mexico, Russia, India, or Africa. It is rare in the United States. Antibodies to hepatitis E (Anti-HEV) detect hepatitis E infection.

Hepatitis A virus (HAV) antibody (HAV ab, anti-HAV) (serum)

Reference Value

None detected.

Description

Hepatitis A virus (HAV), previously called infectious hepatitis, is usually transmitted by oral contact. The incubation period for HAV is 2–6 weeks, not like the 7–25 weeks for hepatitis B virus. HAV is not associated with chronic liver disease.

Antibodies to hepatitis A virus (IgM and IgG) indicate the presence of or past infection and possible immunity. Anti-HAV IgM (HAV ab IgM) appears early after exposure and is detectable for 4–12 weeks. Anti-HAV IgG appears postinfection (greater than 4 weeks) and usually remains present for life. Approximately 50% of the population in the United States have a positive anti-HAV IgG.

Purpose

- To determine the presence of or past infection of HAV.

Clinical Problems

Positive: Hepatitis A virus (HAV).

Procedure

- There is no food or fluid restriction.
- Collect 3–5 mL of venous blood in a red-top tube.

Factors Affecting Laboratory Results

- None known.

NURSING IMPLICATIONS WITH RATIONALE

- Obtain a history from the client of possible contact with a person having HAV. Record if the client has eaten shellfish that may have been obtained from contaminated water.

H

Client Teaching

- Explain to the client that HAV is normally transmitted by oral or fecal contact. A food handler with HAV could transmit the virus if the handler had poor personal hygiene (not washing hands after toileting).
- Alert the client that HAV can spread in institutions such as day care centers, prisons, and state mental institutions.

Positive Test

- Rest and nutritional dietary intake for several weeks according to the severity of the HAV are indicated. Fatigue is common. Rest periods are necessary as long as jaundice is present.
- Inform the client that effective personal hygiene is very important.

Hepatitis B surface antigen (HBsAg) (serum)

Hepatitis-Associated Antigen (HAA)

Reference Values

Adult: Negative.

Child: Negative.

H

Description

The hepatitis B surface antigen (HBsAg) test was originally called the Australia antigen test and later the hepatitis-associated antigen (HAA) test. This test is done to determine the presence of hepatitis B virus in the blood in either an active or a carrier state (as in a hepatitis B carrier). Approximately 5% of persons with diseases other than hepatitis B (serum hepatitis) will have a positive HBsAg test.

The HBsAg test is routinely performed on the donor's blood to identify the hepatitis B antigen. Transmission of hepatitis B in blood transfusions has greatly diminished through HBsAg screening of the donor's blood and excluding donors with a history of hepatitis. Though transfusion-related hepatitis B has decreased, the occurrence of hepatitis B is still on the increase.

In hepatitis B, the antigen in the serum can be detected 2–24 weeks (average 4–8 weeks) after exposure to the virus. The positive HBsAg may be present 2–6 weeks after onset of the clinical disease. Approximately 10% of clients with positive HBsAg are carriers, and their tests may remain positive for years.

In 75–90% of the clients, antibody to hepatitis B surface antigen (called anti-HBsAg or HBsAb) is found 2–12 weeks after HBsAg occurs. Anti-HBsAg can be detected for years after the acute viral infection, but it does not guarantee immunity against future hepatitis infection.

HBsAg test does not diagnose hepatitis A virus. Two tests for hepatitis A are anti-HAV-IgM (indicates an acute infection) and anti-HAV-IgG (indicates a past exposure).

Purposes

- To screen for the presence of hepatitis B in the client's blood.
- To detect the presence of hepatitis B in the donor's blood.

Clinical Problems

Increased Level (Positive): Hepatitis B, chronic hepatitis B. *Less Common:* Hemophilia, Down syndrome, Hodgkin disease, leukemia. *Drug Influence:* Drug addiction.

Procedure

- There is no food or fluid restriction.
- Collect 5–7 mL of venous blood in a red-top tube. Careful handling of the blood sample and washing the hands are most important to keep from contracting the viral hepatitis B.

Factors Affecting Laboratory Results

- None known.

NURSING IMPLICATIONS WITH RATIONALE

- Explain to the client the purpose of the test. If the person is a blood donor, the test is automatically done after the unit of blood is taken. Most of these persons do not know that the HBsAg test and other blood tests are done on donor blood.
- Obtain a history of any previous hepatitis infection and report it to the health care provider.

Increased Level (Positive Test)

- Handle blood obtained from the client with care, avoiding blood contact with your skin (especially if skin and nail cuts are present). If you accidentally stick yourself with the used needle, you should, in most cases, receive gamma globulin as a preventive measure to avoid the disease.
- Discard all needles and syringes used on clients having hepatitis B. Follow the hospital's isolation procedure.
- Observe for signs and symptoms of hepatitis, such as lethargy, anorexia, nausea and vomiting, fever, dark-colored urine, and jaundice.

Client Teaching

- Instruct the client to get plenty of rest; follow a nutritional diet, if tolerated; and drink fluids (juice and carbonated drinks).

H

Heroin (urine)

Reference Values

Normal: Negative.

Positive: >2 ng/mL.

Description

Heroin is an abuse drug made from morphine. It is metabolized back to morphine and is excreted in the urine as morphine or morphine glucuronides 8–24 hours later. About 50% of the heroin as morphine is excreted in 8 hours, 80–90% is excreted in 24 hours, and 100% in 48 hours. Street heroin is approximately 5–10% heroin, which is equivalent to 10–20 mg of morphine.

Purpose

- To detect the use of heroin or morphine from the urine sample.

Clinical Problems

Positive: Use of heroin or morphine.

Procedure

- A consent form may or may not be required. However, if the urine specimen is used for legal evidence, then a consent form would be needed and witnessed.
- Collect 50 mL of urine in a clean container. Write the client's name, date, and time of the urine collection. If it is for legal evidence, have a person witness the client's name, date, and time on the urine container and on the laboratory requisition slip.
- Serum and saliva may also be used to test for heroin.

Factors Affecting Laboratory Results

- False-positive result may occur if the client ingested cough medicine containing codeine or ate poppy seeds 1 day before the urine specimen was obtained.

NURSING IMPLICATIONS WITH RATIONALE

- Ask when the client had taken the drug substance and the name of the substance. The client may be unable to answer because of an unstable state of consciousness from an overdose of the drug substance.
- Obtain vital signs.
- Assess client for symptoms of heroin overdose: respiratory depression, pinpoint pupils of the eye, irritability, gastrointestinal hyperactivity, fatigue, and coma.
- Contact a professional employee in the health institution for crisis intervention assessment. Referrals to appropriate institutions or community programs may be necessary. Do not be judgmental of this acute or chronic situation.

Client Teaching

- Be available to the client and family and answer their questions and concerns. Give support as needed.
- Encourage the client and family to seek help for the addiction. A rehabilitation center or community group may be suggested. If unknown, refer them to professional personnel or counselors in the drug abuse programs.

Herpes simplex virus (HSV) antibody test (serum)
HSV-1 and HSV-2

Reference Values

Negative: Less than 1:10.

Positive: *Early Primary Herpes Simplex Infection:* 1:10–1:100. *Late Primary Herpes Simplex Infection:* 1:100–1:500. *Latent Herpes Simplex Infection:* Greater than 1:500. Fourfold titer increase between the acute and convalescent period.

Description

Herpes simplex is an infectious virus that can produce antibody titers. There are two types of herpes simplex: herpes simplex virus type 1 (HSV-1) and herpes simplex virus type 2 (HSV-2). HSV-1 infects the mouth, mostly the mucous membrane around the lip (cold sores), eyes, or upper respiratory tract. HSV-2 is frequently referred to as genital herpes, infecting the genitourinary tract. HSV-2 is transmitted primarily through sexual contact and can infect the newborn during vaginal delivery. Neonatal herpes may be mild, resulting in eye infection or skin rash, or it may result in a fatal systemic infection. Congenital herpes is not as common but may be acquired during early pregnancy, resulting in central nervous system disorders causing brain damage.

In addition to the serology blood test, a culture may be obtained to isolate the HSV. Herpchek from Du Pont Medical Products detects the herpes antigen from scrapings of suspected HSV genital vesicular lesions.

Antibodies for HSV-1 and HSV-2 begin to rise in 7 days and reach peak titers 4–6 weeks after infection. Usually recurrence or reinfection of HSV does not greatly change the titer level. Those infected may have an increased titer level for 6 months after infection or it may persist throughout their life. Genital herpes, HSV-2, tends to be more severe and needs appropriate medical care such as the topical antiviral drug acyclovir (Zovirax).

Purposes

- To detect the presence of HSV.
- To diagnose the convalescent phase of HSV.

Clinical Problems

Positive Titer: HSV-1, HSV-2, HSV-1 encephalitis, cervicitis, congenital herpes.

Procedure

- There is no food or fluid restriction.
- Collect 3–5 mL of venous blood in a red-top tube. Avoid hemolysis. Deliver the blood sample to the laboratory within 1 hour. Gloves should be worn when obtaining the blood specimen.
- The laboratory slip should indicate whether the test is for HSV-1 or HSV-2, or both.
- Cerebral spinal fluid may be obtained to determine the presence of HSV if HSV-1 encephalitis is suspected.

Factors Affecting Laboratory Results

- Hemolysis of the blood sample.
- Not delivering the blood sample to the laboratory within an hour.

NURSING IMPLICATIONS WITH RATIONALE

- Obtain a history from the client of a possible herpes infection of the mouth (HSV-1) or the genital area (HSV-2). Ascertain when the symptoms first occurred.
- Use gloves when inspecting the area because herpes simplex can be infectious.
- Listen to the client's concerns. If the herpes simplex is HSV-2, the client should be encouraged to have her or his sexual partner tested for HSV-2.

Client Teaching

- Inform the pregnant woman that it may be necessary to have a cesarean section if the virus is still present at the time of delivery. The health care provider will most likely culture the genital area near the time of birthing.
- Encourage the pregnant client to speak with appropriate health professionals. This helps in alleviating the client's fears and making the client well informed.

H

Heterophile antibody (serum, Monospot)

Reference Values

Adult: Normal, less than 1.28 titer; abnormal, greater than 1:56 titer.

Child: Same as adult.

Elderly: Normal, slightly higher titer than adult.

Description

This test is used primarily to check for infectious mononucleosis. Infectious mononucleosis is thought to be caused by the Epstein-Barr virus (EBV).

Heterophiles are a group of antibodies that react to sheep and horse red blood cells; if positive (titer), an agglutination occurs. Titers of 1:56–1:224 are highly suspicious of infectious mononucleosis; those of 1:224 or greater are positive for infectious mononucleosis. Elevated heterophile titers occur during the first 2 weeks, peak in 3 weeks, and remain elevated for 6 weeks. Sixty to 80% of persons with infectious mononucleosis have a positive heterophile antibody test.

There are several commercially prepared tests: Monospot by Ortho Diagnostics, Monoscreen by GlaxoSmithKline. A Monospot test is usually done first; if positive, then the titer test is performed.

Purposes

- To check for an elevated heterophile titer.
- To aid in the diagnosis of infectious mononucleosis.

Clinical Problems

Increased Level: Infectious mononucleosis, serum sickness, viral infections.

Procedure

Heterophile Antibody
- There is no food or fluid restriction.
- Collect 3–5 mL of venous blood in a red-top tube.

Monospot Screening Test: Collect 2 mL of venous blood in a red-top tube. Use a mono kit and follow directions. The client's serum is mixed with the guinea pig tissue on one spot of a glass slide, and at another spot on the slide it is mixed with beef red-cell stromata. Observe for 1 minute for agglutination. Results of the Monospot test are as follows:

1. If agglutination is stronger at the guinea-pig-kidney-tissue spot, the test is positive for infectious mononucleosis.
2. If agglutination is stronger at the beef red blood cells, the test is negative for infectious mononucleosis.
3. If agglutination is present at both spots, the test is negative for infectious mononucleosis.
4. If no agglutination is present at either spot, the test is negative.

There is no food or fluid restriction. Usually, in infectious mononucleosis, the white blood cell differential may show 10–25% atypical lymphocytes.

Factors Affecting Laboratory Results

- Serum sickness and Forssman antibodies can cause positive titers.

NURSING IMPLICATIONS WITH RATIONALE

- Explain to the client the procedure for the heterophile antibody test and the Monospot test.
- Obtain a history of the client's contact with any person or persons recently diagnosed as having infectious mononucleosis.
- Observe for signs and symptoms of infectious mononucleosis, such as fever, sore throat, fatigue, swollen glands.

H

- Determine when the symptoms (fever, fatigue, sore throat) first occurred. A repeat heterophile antibody or Monospot test may be needed if the first was done too early. Elevated titers take 4–8 weeks to return to normal.

Client Teaching

- Encourage the client to rest, drink fluids, and follow the health care provider's orders.

Hexosaminidase (total, A, and A and B) (serum, amniotic fluid)

Reference Values

Adult: *Total:* 5–20 unit/L. *Hexosaminidase A:* 55–80%.

Description

Hexosaminidase is a group of enzymes (isoenzymes A and B) responsible for the metabolism of gangliosides. It is found in brain tissue. Lack of hexosaminidase A causes accumulation of gangliosides in the brain, a condition known as Tay-Sachs disease. The total hexosaminidase may be normal or decreased. This test is used to confirm Tay-Sachs disease or to identify Tay-Sachs carriers.

Tay-Sachs disease is an autosomal-recessive disorder resulting in progressive destruction of the cells of the central nervous system. It is characterized by mental retardation, muscular weakness, and blindness. It primarily affects the Jewish population. Death usually occurs before the age of 5 years.

Sandhoff disease, a variant of Tay-Sachs, progresses more rapidly than Tay-Sachs disease. With this disorder, there is a deficiency of hexosaminidase A and B. It is not prevalent in any ethnic group.

Purposes

- To diagnose a deficit of hexosaminidase A (Tay-Sachs disease) or hexosaminidase A and B (Sandhoff disease).
- To identify carriers of Tay-Sachs disease or Sandhoff disease.

Clinical Problems

Decreased Level: *Hexosaminidase A:* Tay-Sachs disease. *Hexosaminidase A and B:* Sandhoff disease.

Procedure

- There is no food or fluid restriction.
- Collect 5–7 mL of venous blood in a red-top tube for serum value. Avoid hemolysis.
- Collect cord blood from newborn.

Factors Affecting Laboratory Results

- Hemolysis of the blood sample can cause an inaccurate test result.
- Pregnancy could increase total hexosaminidase values. *Note:* Most laboratories will not perform the test on pregnant women.

NURSING IMPLICATIONS WITH RATIONALE

- Talk with the health care provider and genetic counselor when both partners have a hexosaminidase A deficiency. It is important that correct information and answers be given to the couple.

Client Teaching

- Inform Jewish couples that the hexosaminidase screening test is to determine if they are Tay-Sachs carriers. Explain to the couple that it is a recessive trait and that both must carry the gene for their offspring to get Tay-Sachs disease.

HIV OraQuick test

OraSure Test, HIV Test, HIV Home Test

Reference Value

Negative.

Description

The OraQuick test (over-the-counter HIV test) to detect the presence of HIV in saliva is available for purchase in drugstores and online pharmacies. Approximately one-fifth (200,000) of the 1 million persons who are carriers of the HIV virus in the United States know that they are carriers of the virus. About 800,000 carriers are unaware that they have been infected. Those who are concerned if they are carriers can purchase the OraQuick test. FDA states that this home test is 92% correct in detecting HIV carriers. It is considered accurate in ruling out 99% of those who are not carrying the virus.

The cost of the OraQuick test (manufactured by OraSure) is about $40. Some stores, such as Walmart, may have a low price. The test may need to be repeated.

Purpose

- To determine if the person is an HIV carrier.

Clinical Problems

Positive HIV test result. A second test may be needed.

Procedure

- Purchase the HIV OraQuick test and follow directions.
- The mouth swab is used to collect the saliva. The results of the test are available in 20 minutes.

Factors Affecting Laboratory Results

- Inadequate saliva or not obtaining the saliva for the test.

NURSING IMPLICATIONS WITH RATIONALE

- Explain to the person who is concerned about being an HIV carrier about the OraQuick test. Inform him or her of where it can be purchased.
- Tell the person it is a kit. The person obtains his or her saliva by using a swab. The test result usually takes 20 minutes.

Client Teaching

- Advise the person to seek medical care when the test is positive. Retesting is suggested when it is positive.
- Suggest ways to prevent HIV, such as abstinence, condoms, or needle exchange as appropriate (*see Human Immunodeficiency Virus [HIV] test*).
- Be supportive and nonjudgmental.

Homocysteine (serum)

Reference Values

Adult: 4–17 µmol/L (fasting).

Description

Homocysteine is a by-product of protein. It is an amino acid found in the blood and is formed when protein-rich products, such as eggs, chicken, beef, or cheddar cheese, are eaten. A deficiency of certain B vitamins (e.g., B_6, B_{12}, and folate [folic acid]) can lead to an accumulation of homocysteine.

High levels of homocysteine have been linked to cardiovascular disease, stroke, and possibly Alzheimer disease. Also, homocysteine may promote blood clotting. Research has suggested that an increase in serum homocysteine can damage the inner lining of blood vessels and promote a thickening and loss of flexibility in the blood vessels. Persons who have undergone an angioplasty and have a high level of serum homocysteine generally have restenosis or repeated blockage of the coronary artery. Those who have a low serum homocysteine level usually have a lower rate of reblockage. It has been suggested that a person having an angioplasty take B vitamins following the procedure to decrease the homocysteine level and thus, hopefully, lower the incidence of restenosis.

Purposes

- To detect the risk of cardiovascular disease, including myocardial infarction and stroke.
- To detect a possible increased risk of Alzheimer disease.

Clinical Problems

Increased Level: Coronary artery disease, heart attack, thrombosis, stroke, possible Alzheimer disease, folic acid deficiency.

Decreased Level: Certain vitamin B drugs, folate.

Procedure

- Food and fluids are restricted for 12 hours before the test.
- Collect 3–5 mL of venous blood in a red-top tube.

Factors Affecting Laboratory Results

- Penicillamine reduces the serum homocysteine levels.

NURSING IMPLICATIONS WITH RATIONALE

- Obtain a dietary history of the client. Note if the client takes vitamins, especially B complex vitamins and folic acid.
- Report if the client is having symptoms of cardiovascular disease (e.g., pain).

Client Teaching

- Instruct the client with a high level of serum homocysteine to take vitamins B_6, B_{12}, and folate with the health care provider's consent. These vitamins help to lower the serum homocysteine level.
- Explain to the client that certain foods, such as cheddar cheese, eggs, and beef, can increase the serum homocysteine level when consumed in large quantities.
- Encourage the client to have repeated serum homocysteine tests when the level is elevated and measures are taken to lower the serum level.

H

Human chorionic gonadotropin (HCG) (serum and urine)
Pregnancy Test

Reference Values

Values may be expressed as international unit/mL or ng/mL. Check with your laboratory.

Adult: *Serum:* Nonpregnant female: Less than 0.01 international unit/mL (IU/mL).

PREGNANT (WEEKS)	VALUES
1	0.01–0.04 IU/mL
2	0.03–0.10 IU/mL
4	0.10–1 IU/mL
5–12	10–100 IU/mL
13–25	10–30 IU/mL
26–40	5–15 IU/mL

Urine: Nonpregnant: negative; pregnant: 1–12 weeks: 6,000–500,000 international unit/24 h. Many OTC pregnancy kits are available. The woman is usually tested 5–14 days after a missed menstrual period.

Description

Human chorionic gonadotropin (HCG) is a hormone produced by the placenta. In pregnancy HCG appears in the blood and urine 14–26 days after conception, and the HCG concentration peaks in approximately 8 weeks. After the first trimester of pregnancy, HCG production declines. HCG is not found in nonpregnant women, in death of the fetus, or after 3–4 days postpartum.

The immunologic test for pregnancy using anti-HCG serum is more sensitive, more accurate, less costly, and easier to perform than the older pregnancy test, which used live animals. The Aschheim-Zondek test and the Friedman test are no longer used.

Certain tumors (such as the hydatidiform mole, chorionepithelioma of the uterus, and choriocarcinoma of the testicle) can cause a positive HCG test. HCG levels may be requested on males for the determination of testicular tumor.

Purposes

- To determine if the client is pregnant.
- To detect a threatened abortion or dead fetus.

Clinical Problems

Decreased Level (Negative): Nonpregnant, dead fetus, postpartum (3–4 days), incomplete abortion, threatened abortion (decreased serum value).

Increased Level (Positive): Pregnancy, hydatidiform mole, chorionepithelioma, choriocarcinoma. *Drug Influence:* Anticonvulsants, hypnotics, tranquilizers (phenothiazines), antiparkinsonism drugs.

Procedure

- There is no food restriction.
- Perform the pregnancy test 2 weeks (no earlier than 5 days) after the first missed menstrual period. There are several commercially prepared kits for the immunologic pregnancy test.

Serum
- Perform the pregnancy test no earlier than 5 days after the first missed menstrual period.
- Collect 3–5 mL of venous blood in a red-top tube. Avoid hemolysis.

Urine
- The client should be NPO of fluid for 8–12 hours; no food is restricted.
- Take a morning urine specimen (60 mL) with specific gravity greater than 1.010 to the laboratory immediately. A 24-hour urine collection may be requested.
- Instruct the client to follow directions when using a commercial kit.
- Avoid blood in the urine, as false-positive results could occur.

Note: There are many commercial kits available. Follow the directions on the kit.

Factors Affecting Laboratory Results

- Diluted urine (specific gravity less than 1.010) could cause a false-negative test result.
- Certain drug groups can cause false-positive test results (*see Drug Influence*).

- Protein and blood in the urine could cause false-positive test results.
- During menopause, there may be an excess secretion of pituitary gonadotropin hormone, which could cause a false-positive result.

NURSING IMPLICATIONS WITH RATIONALE

- Ask the client when she had her last period. The test should be done 5 or more days after the missed period to avoid a false-negative result. Blood in the urine can cause a false-positive result.
- Listen to the client's concerns.

Client Teaching

- Inform the client who plans to use a commercially prepared pregnancy kit to follow the directions carefully.

Human immunodeficiency virus type-1 (HIV-1) or HIV* (serum)

Reference Values

Antibody Screening: *Adult and Child*: negative for antibodies, Enzyme-Linked Immunosorbent Assay (ELISA)

Antigen Screening: *Adult and Child*: Negative for p24 antigen, Polymerase Chain Reactions (PCR), bDNA

Description

HIV is a retrovirus that was discovered in 1983 and is identified as the cause of acquired immunodeficiency syndrome (AIDS). Retroviruses are composed of RNA instead of DNA. Retroviruses possess enzymes called reverse transcriptase and integrase that allow the conversion of the viral RNA into DNA, with integration and expression of the virus in the host cell's DNA. Although HIV infects multiple human cells, the predominant "host cell" for HIV is the CD4 +T lymphocyte since it possesses more receptor sites. The rate of HIV replication varies in infected individuals but is estimated at greater than a billion per day. The primary HIV syndrome is characterized by onset of symptoms in 2–4 weeks in 80–90% of clients. These are:

- Fever (96%), adenopathy (74%), pharyngitis (70%), rash (70%), and mouth ulcers (70%).
- Detectable virus in regional lymph nodes within 5 days.
- Seroconversion in 3 weeks but may take up to 3–6 months to produce enough detectable antibodies.

*Updated by Dr. Wesley Emmons, MD, FACP, Delaware.

The infected individual may be asymptomatic for up to 8–10 years. The CD4 is utilized as a marker of disease progression. A normal CD4 count is 800–1,200 cells/mm^3. With current medications, once CD4 cells increase above 200, the person is no longer considered to have AIDS. As HIV destroys CD4 cells, an individual may become AIDS defined. In 1993, the CDC identified 24 illnesses and conditions that are AIDS defining.

According to the CDC, as of 2014, 1.2 million people in the United States were HIV positive, and 36.7 million people were HIV positive worldwide. The incidence rate has remained stable as a result of prevention and testing efforts. Unfortunately, in the United States, over half a million HIV-positive individuals have died from AIDS-related illnesses since the first case was diagnosed.

Testing

Testing has changed significantly since the CDC released an update on June 27, 2014. Testing begins with a combination immunoassay that detects HIV-1 and HIV-2 antibodies and HIV-1, p24 antigen. All specimens reactive on this initial assay will undergo additional testing with an immunoassay that differentiates HIV-1 from HIV-2 antibodies. Specimens that are reactive on the initial assay and nonreactive or indeterminate on the differentiation assay proceed to HIV-1 nucleic acid testing for resolution.

The improved assay/algorithm, PCR, bDNA, allows for more accurate diagnosis of acute HIV-1 infection than previous immunoassays, which is important because this is when the client is most infectious. Also, it is more accurately used in the diagnosis of HIV-2 infection, having fewer indeterminate results, and it has a faster turnaround time.

No longer is Western blot part of the testing algorithm, as some false-negative results can be seen early in the course of HIV infection, and the majority of HIV-2 infections can be misclassified as HIV-1 by the Western blot. Rapid HIV-1/HIV-2 antigen/antibody combination testing was also not recommended, although FDA approved, as there was "insufficient evidence of performance." The new recommendation also includes tests for HIV antigen and HIV nucleic acid. bDNA is rarely used commercially.

Treatment

The goal of treatment is suppression of the virus to "undetectable" levels to restore and preserve immune function, prevent comorbidities such as opportunistic infections, and prevent transmission of the virus. The virus cannot be eradicated secondary to the long half-life of latently infected CD4 cells during the early stages of seroconversion.

There were six classes of ARV medication available as of 2011. Each class suppresses HIV viral replication of specific sites. To achieve "undetectable" viral suppression, a combination of at least three active drugs from two or more drug classes is required. The classes are (1) nucleoside reverse transcriptase inhibitors (NRTI), (2) non-nucleoside reverse transcriptase inhibitors (NNRTI), (3) protease inhibitors (PI), (4) integrase inhibitors (II), (5) fusion inhibitors, and (6) CCR5 antagonists. Three different assays are available to determine active ARVs. The genotype is used to determine specific mutations at the DNA level. Phenotype is used to determine the multiple indicator cluster (MIC) of each ARV. Trofile assay is used to determine if the HIV virus is susceptible to CCR5 antagonists.

Purposes

- To screen for the presence of HIV infections.
- To monitor HIV during drug therapy.

Clinical Problems

Seropositive Test: HIV infected

Procedure

- A signed consent form for the HIV antibody screen is usually required, however, oral consent may be acceptable.
- No food or fluid restriction is required.
- Collect 5–7 mL of venous blood in a red-top tube.

NURSING IMPLICATIONS WITH RATIONALE

- Develop an accurate understanding of HIV disease, including transmission, early infection, advanced disease, testing, treatment, and potential adverse illnesses.
- Learn to identify at-risk individuals by evaluating prevalence and incidence rate in their community. At-risk populations include IV drug users (IVDU), homosexuals, and individuals with recurrent STDs.
- Know state laws with respect to informed consent and opt-out testing.
- Understand what HIV test is being used and for what purpose: screening, confirmation, resistance testing, evaluation of disease progress, and evaluation of treatment.
- Document that the individual has signed an informed consent before testing is started.
- Understand that prenatal care includes HIV testing. Give the woman the option to decline.
- Offer opt-out rapid testing in the Labor and Delivery Department to all women with undocumented HIV status.
- Understand that infants born to mothers with HIV will have acquired maternal antibodies via the placenta. This does *not* diagnose the infant HIV positive. These antibodies can remain for up to 18 months after birth.
- Understand that infants younger than 18 months should not be HIV antibody tested.
- Know that HIV antigen testing, polymerase chain reactions, or bDNA is used to identify the presence of the HIV virus. The sensitivity of PCR at 3 months of age is 90% and almost 100% at 6 months of age.
- Know the intervals for testing. The test is performed at 1 day, 6 weeks, and 12 weeks. For infants at high risk, an additional test may be performed at 2 to 3 weeks. The sequence of tests is necessary because infection may take place during pregnancy, during delivery, or from breastfeeding. The majority of infections are picked up by 6 weeks. However, at 18 months an antibody test should be performed.
- Assess each HIV-positive individual for coinfections, such as hepatitis B and hepatitis C. That person is not immune to hepatitis A. The individual should receive the hepatitis A vaccine.
- Understand that if the individual is severely immune compromised, such as a CD4 of less than 200, the individual may not have a response to the TB skin test or the Interferon Gamma Release Assay. Testing should be repeated when the CD4 is greater than 200. Because HIV dramatically increases the risk of progression from latent to active disease, the individual should receive 9 months of isoniazid (INH) and vitamin B_6.

H

- Continue to employ universal body precautions with all blood and body fluids. Review OSHA and CDC guidelines for up-to-date information regarding bloodborne and body fluid–borne pathogen incidents, including needle sticks and splashes.

Client Teaching

- Teach the individual the meaning of HIV, a chronic viral infection that is treated with lifelong antiretroviral medication to preserve the immune system. Explain how the HIV virus infects the CD4 and the role of the medication to prevent this.
- Inform the client of the type of test being used. Explain that the ELISA and rapid tests are for detecting the presence of HIV antibodies. If the ELISA is positive, it must be repeated.
- Determine from the client when was the last possible exposure to HIV. For example, 90 days from the last known sexual encounter.
- Educate the client and community about routes of transmission. Explain that the HIV virus is present in blood and blood products, such as cerebrospinal fluid, semen, vaginal fluids, and breast milk. Transmission occurs when the HIV-infected fluids come in direct contact with damaged mucus membranes, tissue, and/or blood (needle stick, IVDU). HIV is not transmitted by talking, shaking hands, or hugging an HIV-positive individual. The HIV virus is *not* a foodborne or airborne virus. It cannot survive outside the body.
- Tell the client about primary and secondary prevention. Primary prevention is behavior and individual practices to prevent HIV infection, for example, abstinence, condom use, and needle exchange programs. Secondary prevention is behavior and individual practices to prevent transmitting the HIV virus: again, abstinence, condoms, needle exchanges, pregnant women engaging in HIV care, and taking antiretroviral drugs during pregnancy.
- Reinforce to each client that his or her care will be tailored to his or her needs and will be confidential. Know the impact the person's psychosocial and economic background will have on his or her willingness to participate in care.
- Be supportive to the client and family or partner and remain nonjudgmental.
- Encourage the client to participate in his or her own care and provide information regarding local HIV peer groups or HIV community case managers (www.aidsinfo.nih.gov; www.cdc.gov).

Human leukocyte antigen (HLA) (serum)

HLA Typing, Organ-Donor Tissue Typing

Reference Values

Histocompatibility match or nonmatch; no norms.

Description

Nucleated cells, including leukocytes, platelets, and many tissue cells, have antigens of the human leukocyte antigen (HLA) system on their surface membranes. The antigenic system is very complex as it relates to tissue compatibility for transplantation and immune response. The antigens are classified into five different series: A, B, C, D, and DR (D-related). There are many groups within these five series (20 A antigens, 40 B antigens, 8 C antigens, 12 D antigens, and 10 DR antigens) that can be HLA-phenotyped to determine histocompatibility.

The four main purposes for HLA testing are: (1) organ transplantation; (2) transfusion; (3) disease association, such as juvenile rheumatoid arthritis, ankylosing spondylitis, myasthenia gravis, Addison disease, and type 1 diabetes mellitus; and (4) paternity testing may be verified when the putative father has one haplotype (phenotyping) that is identical to the child. If the putative father does not have any antigen pair identical to one of the child's, he is excluded as the father. This test may be useful in genetic counseling when associated with susceptibility to certain disease.

Purposes

- To screen for histocompatibility in tissue typing.
- To determine paternity of a child.

Clinical Problems

Positive Histocompatibility: Tissue compatibility for grafts and organ transplants, father of child.

Procedure

- There is no food or fluid restriction.
- Collect 5–7 mL of venous blood in a green-top tube. Avoid hemolysis. Blood samples should be tested immediately.

Factors Affecting Laboratory Results

- Hemolysis of the blood sample.
- Blood transfusion in the last 3 days could affect test results.

NURSING IMPLICATIONS WITH RATIONALE

Client Teaching

- Encourage the client to express concerns related to health problems.
- Refer unknown questions to appropriate health professionals.

Human papilloma virus (HPV) (specimen)

Reference Values

Absence of human papilloma virus.

Description

The human papilloma virus (HPV) infection has been the primary cause of cervical cancer. There are more than 70 different types of HPV, and HPV types 16, 18, 33, 35, and 39 have been associated with invasive carcinoma of the cervix. HPV 16 and 18 are the most carcinogenic.

H

Some of the strains are low risk, for example, HPV 6, 11, 42, 43, and 44. These are associated with genital warts and mild dysplasia. However, some of the HPV types do not progress to cancer. Fifty percent of females do not know that a majority of cervical cancer is preventable. Some women believe that the HPV test isn't necessary if they aren't sexually active.

Frequently a specimen for HPV testing is obtained during the Papanicolaou (Pap) procedure. A HPV DNA detection of the virus is taken during the Pap procedure to determine the presence of the virus. Gardasil, an HPV vaccine, will guard against HPV 6, 11, 16, and 18. This vaccine is suggested by the Centers for Diseases (CDC) for clients in their teens or for young adults. The vaccine is also recommended for women 30 years old or older who have a positive test for low-risk HPV.

Purpose

- To detect the presence of HPV.

Clinical Problems

Increased Level: HPV infection, cancer in situ, infertility.

Procedure: DNA Probe

- No food or fluid restriction is required.
- Follow the directions on the HPV collection kit.
- Collect cervical cells using the HPV collection kit. Send the specimen to the laboratory. The test is usually performed during a Pap procedure.

Factors Affecting Laboratory Results

- Lubrication of the speculum.
- Inadequate amount of tissue.

H

NURSING IMPLICATIONS WITH RATIONALE

- Obtain a history of abnormal vaginal bleeding and previous abnormal Pap smear results.
- Determine if the client has had a test for human papilloma virus or has received the HPV vaccine.

Client Teaching

- Inform the female not to douche or have intercourse 24–48 hours before the HPV test. The health care provider should give the client the policy/information about the test and its preparation.
- Inform the client that usually he or she will not be notified of the results unless the test is positive for HPV. However, she may want to call the health care provider for the results.
- Answer the female's concerns or questions about HPV or refer questions to another health care provider.

Human placental lactogen (hPL) (serum)
Chorionic Somatomammotropin

Reference Values

Adult: *Nonpregnant Female:* Less than 0.5 mcg/mL.
Pregnant Female:

WEEKS OF GESTATION	REFERENCE VALUES
5–7	1 mcg/mL
8–27	greater than 4.6 mcg/mL
28–31	2.4–6 mcg/mL
32–35	3.7–7.7 mcg/mL
36–term	5–10 mcg/mL

Male: Less than 0.5 mcg/mL.

Description

Human placental lactogen (hPL), a hormone produced by the placenta, can be detected in the maternal blood after 5 weeks of gestation. The hPL increases slowly throughout the pregnancy. This test is useful for evaluating placental function and fetal well-being in high-risk pregnancies, especially from the 28th week to term. A marked decrease in the serum hPL level during the third trimester of pregnancy is indicative of fetal distress. Additional testing is recommended to determine fetal distress. A serum estriol and nonstress test are frequently ordered to verify the hPL test result.

Purposes

- To evaluate placental function.
- To determine fetal well-being after the 28th week to term.

Clinical Problems

Decreased Level: Fetal distress, toxemia of pregnancy, threatened-abortion, trophoblastic neoplastic disease (hydatidiform mole, choriocarcinoma).

Increased Level: Multiple pregnancy, diabetes mellitus, bronchogenic carcinoma, liver tumor, lymphoma.

Procedure

- There is no food or fluid restriction.
- Collect 5–7 mL of venous blood in a red- or green-top tube. Avoid hemolysis.
- The hPL level fluctuates; therefore, the test might need to be repeated.

Factors Affecting Laboratory Results

- Hemolysis of the blood sample.

NURSING IMPLICATIONS WITH RATIONALE

- Record the gestation week on the laboratory slip.
- Correlate the serum hPL result with the serum or urine estriol level. The human placental lactogen levels can fluctuate daily, so the hPL test is usually repeated. Other tests for detecting fetal distress are also ordered.

Client Teaching

- Inform the client that the test may be repeated because of frequent hPL fluctuations. Explain that other tests are usually ordered to monitor fetal well-being.

Hydroxybutyric dehydrogenase (HBD) (serum)

Hydroxybutyrate Dehydrogenase (HBDH), Alpha-Hydroxybutyric Dehydrogenase

Reference Values

140–350 international unit/L, 114–290 unit/L. *Ratio LD to HBD:* from 1.2:1 to 1.5:1.

Description

Hydroxybutyric dehydrogenase (HBD) enzyme is similar to the isoenzyme of lactate dehydrogenase, LD_1. HBD is found primarily in the heart muscle but can also be found in the brain and kidneys. This test is conducted to diagnose a myocardial infarction (MI). Frequently, it is used as a substitute for LD electrophoresis, which is a costlier test. Also, HBD levels are sustained longer than aspartate aminotransferase, creatine phosphokinase, and LD levels. HBD levels rise 8–10 hours following an MI, peak in 2–4 days, and can remain elevated for up to 18 days. Liver disease can complicate the use of HBD for diagnosing MI because an elevated LD_5 (liver) isoenzyme can cause an elevated HBD level. If there is a history of liver disease, then LD electrophoresis (identifying LD isoenzymes) should be used instead of HBD.

HBD is a useful test for aiding in the diagnosis of MI, mainly because other cardiac enzymes return to baseline sooner than HBD. However, HBD should not be the only test used for diagnosing MI, and it is usually not the first group of laboratory tests used for diagnosing an acute MI.

Purposes

- To aid in the diagnosis of an MI, especially a latent MI, when other cardiac enzymes do not show an increase.
- To monitor cardiac enzyme activity when LD electrophoresis is unavailable or too expensive to monitor.

Clinical Problems

Increased Level: Myocardial infarction, liver disease, nephrotic syndrome, leukemia, lymphomas, anemias (hemolytic or megaloblastic).

Procedure

- There is no food or fluid restriction.
- Collect 5–7 mL of venous blood in a red-top tube. A gray-top tube may also be used. Avoid hemolysis caused by rough handling. Send the specimen immediately to the laboratory.
- Do not freeze blood specimen; enzyme activity is lost during freezing. The specimen could be refrigerated, but the temperature should not be below 0°C, or 32°F.

Factors Affecting Laboratory Results

- Hemolysis of the blood specimen could cause a false elevation in the HBD level.
- Frozen blood specimen.
- Delay in taking the blood sample to the laboratory.

NURSING IMPLICATIONS WITH RATIONALE

- Obtain a history of the health problem.
- Monitor vital signs and electrocardiogram. Report abnormal findings to the health care provider.
- Monitor cardiac enzyme levels. Report abnormal levels to the health care provider.
- Provide comfort measures for the client.
- Encourage the client to immediately report chest discomfort/pain or shortness of breath.

17-hydroxycorticosteroids (17-OHCS) (urine)
Corticoids 17-OH, Porter-Silber Chromogens

H

Reference Values

Adult: *Male:* 3–12 mg/24 h. *Female:* 2–10 mg/24 h. Average 2–12 mg/24 h.

Elderly: Lower than adult.

Child: *Infant to 1 Year:* Less than 1 mg/24 h. *2–4 Years:* 1–2 mg/24 h. *5–12 Years:* 2–6 mg/24 h.

Description

17-OHCS are metabolites of adrenocortical steroid hormones, mostly of cortisol, and are excreted in the urine. Because the excretion of the metabolites is diurnal, a 24-hour urine specimen is necessary for accuracy of test results. This test is useful for assessing adrenocortical hormone function. An increased urinary concentration of 17-OHCS may indicate hyperadrenalism, and a decreased urinary concentration may indicate hypoadrenalism.

Purposes

- To assess adrenocortical hormone function.
- To detect disorders caused by deficit or excess of adrenocortical hormone.

Clinical Problems

Decreased Level: Addison disease, adrenogenital syndrome, hypopituitarism, myxedema (hypothyroidism). *Drug Influence:* Calcium gluconate, dexamethasone (Decadron), phenytoin (Dilantin), promethazine (Phenergan), reserpine (Serpasil).

Increased Level: Cushing syndrome, adrenal cancer, eclampsia, hyperpituitarism, hyperthyroidism, extreme stress. *Drug Influence:* Antibiotics (cloxacillin, erythromycin), acetazolamide (Diamox), ascorbic acid, chloral hydrate, chlordiazepoxide (Librium), chlorothiazide (Diuril), chlorpromazine (Thorazine), colchicine, cortisone, digoxin, digitoxin, estrogen, hydroxyzine (Atarax), iodides, oral contraceptives, meprobamate (Equanil or Miltown), methenamine (Urex), paraldehyde, quinine, quinidine, spironolactone (Aldactone).

Procedure

- No food or fluid is restricted, except for coffee and tea. Fluid intake should be encouraged.
- Collect urine in a large container/bottle, and add an acid preservative to prevent bacterial degradation of the steroids. The urine collection should be refrigerated if no preservative is added. No toilet paper or feces should be in the urine.
- Label container with client's name, date, and exact time of collection (e.g., 9/23/20, 7:20 AM to 9/24/20, 7:30 AM).
- Withhold drugs (with health care provider's approval) for 3 days before the test to prevent false results. Any drugs given should be listed on the laboratory slip.

Factors Affecting Laboratory Results

- Drugs (*see Drug Influence*). Cortisone can elevate the urinary levels of 17-OHCS, and dexamethasone (Decadron), a potent cortisone derivative, can decrease the 17-OHCS level. The potent cortisone drug inhibits ACTH production, which causes a decrease in adrenocortical hormone secretion.
- If the 24-hour urine sample is not refrigerated or does not contain a preservative, the results of the test could be inaccurate.

NURSING IMPLICATIONS WITH RATIONALE

- Encourage the client to drink 6–8 glasses of water or other fluid (except coffee) during the 24-hour test.
- Check the drugs the client is receiving, and withhold drugs (with the health care provider's permission) that may interfere with test results. Many times, medication cannot be withheld. In such cases, the drugs given should be listed on the laboratory slip and reported.
- Explain to the client and family that all urine should be saved during a 24-hour period and that there should be no toilet paper or feces in the urine.
- Label the urine bottle with the client's name and the date and exact time of the urine collection (e.g., 11/3/20, 7:20 AM to 11/4/20, 7:22 AM).
- Post a notice of urine collection on the client's door or bed and in the chart.
- Check the results of the plasma cortisol test.

Decreased Level

- Observe for signs and symptoms of hypoadrenalism (Addison disease). Symptoms include fatigue, weakness, weight loss, bronze coloration of the skin, postural hypotension, arrhythmia, craving for salty food, and fasting hypoglycemia. Report your findings to the health care provider.

Increased Level

- Observe for signs and symptoms of hyperadrenalism (Cushing syndrome). These symptoms include fluid retention, "moon face," hirsutism, "buffalo hump," hypertension, hyperglycemia, petechiae, and ecchymosis. Report your findings to the health care provider.

5-Hydroxyindoleacetic acid (5-HIAA) (urine)
5-OH-Indoleacetic Acid, Serotonin Metabolite

Reference Values

Adult: *Qualitative Random Samples:* Negative. *Quantitative 24 Hours:* 2–10 mg/24 h.

Child: Not usually done—results would be similar to adult results.

Description

5-Hydroxyindoleacetic acid (5-HIAA), a metabolite of serotonin, is excreted in the urine as the result of carcinoid tumors found in the appendix or in the intestinal wall. Serotonin is a vasoconstricting hormone secreted by the argentaffin cells of the gastrointestinal tract and is responsible for peristalsis. Carcinoid tumor cells, which secrete excess serotonin, are of low-grade malignancy. Early removal of this type of tumor ensures an 80–90% chance of cure. There have been reports of some noncarcinoid tumors producing high levels of 5-HIAA.

Certain foods may elevate the 5-HIAA urinary levels, and certain drugs may increase or decrease the 5-HIAA urinary levels. More than one random sample of urine for the 5-HIAA test may be needed to avoid false-positive or false-negative results. The 24-hour urine test usually follows the random urine screening test.

Purposes

- To confirm carcinoid tumor of the intestine.
- To compare with other laboratory tests for confirmation of carcinoid tumor.

Clinical Problems

Decreased Level: *Drug Influence* (depresses 5-HIAA): ACTH, heparin, imipramine (Tofranil), isoniazid (INH), MAO inhibitors, methyldopa (Aldomet), phenothiazines (chlorpromazine [Thorazine]), promethazine (Phenergan).

Increased Level: Carcinoid tumors of the appendix and intestine, carcinoid tumor with metastasis (greater than 100 mg/24 h), sciatica pain (severe), skeletal, and smooth muscle spasm. *Drug Influence:* Acetophenetidin (Phenacetin), glyceryl guaiacolate, methamphetamine (Methampex or Desoxyn), reserpine (Serpasil). *Foods:* Bananas, pineapple, avocados, plums, eggplant, and walnuts.

Procedure

- Foods (except for those listed) and fluids are not restricted.
- Eliminate the foods and drugs listed above for 3 days before the test, if possible.

Qualitative Random Urine Sample (for screening purposes): Collect a random urine sample and take it to the laboratory. If the urine sample is not tested immediately, it should be refrigerated. Collection of a random urine sample may need to be repeated to verify the results. The random urine screening test is usually done first, and if the test is positive, a 24-hour urine test for 5-HIAA is ordered.

Quantitative 24-Hour Urine Collection: Collect urine for 24 hours in a large container with a preservative. Some laboratories require no preservative, but the urine should be refrigerated during the 24-hour collection time. Label the bottle and laboratory slip with the client's name and the date and exact times of the urine collection (e.g., 6/24/20, 7:00 AM to 6/25/20, 7:00 AM).

Factors Affecting Laboratory Results

- Foods (*see Foods*).
- Drugs (*see Drug Influence*).
- A 24-hour urine sample that does not have a preservative and/or has not been refrigerated. (Check with the laboratory about the urine preservative and refrigeration.)

H

NURSING IMPLICATIONS WITH RATIONALE

- Instruct the client not to eat bananas, pineapple, avocados, plums, eggplant, or walnuts for 3 days before the test. Foods and fluid other than those mentioned are permitted before and during the test.
- Instruct the client and family not to throw away any urine during the 24-hour collection time. Instruct the client not to put toilet paper or feces in the urine.
- Inform the heath care provider of any drugs the client is taking that could cause a false-positive or false-negative result. These drugs should not be taken for 3 days before the test, if possible; if not, the names of the drugs should be listed on the laboratory slip and recorded in the client's chart.
- Check the 5-HIAA result of the random sample urine test and inform the health care provider if the result is unknown. A repeat test may be needed if the client has taken drugs that can depress the 5-HIAA or if the test is negative. If the urine test is positive, the health care provider may order the 5-HIAA 24-hour urine test.

Hydroxyproline (urine)

Reference Values

Adult: *18–39 Years:* 15–50 mg/24 h; *Greater than 40 Years Old:* 15–42 mg/24 h; 115–310 μmol/24 h; 0.4–4.5 mg/2 h; 3–38 μmol/2 h.

Child: *1–5 Years:* 20–65 mg/24 h; *6–10 Years:* 35–100 mg/24 h; *11–16 Years:* 65–180 mg/24 h.

Description

Hydroxyproline, an amino acid found in collagen, is increased during bone growth and bone disease. Collagen is a component of bone, cartilage, and skin. Urine hydroxyproline levels increase when there is collagen breakdown, as in bone destruction. Levels of hydroxyproline are higher during the night, in teenagers, and during the third trimester of pregnancy.

Urine excretion of hydroxyproline is an effective test for monitoring the progress of Paget disease (bone lesions, mainly of the long bones). Hydroxyproline levels decrease during treatment therapy for bone disorders.

Purposes

- To aid in the detection of bone disorders.
- To monitor the effect of treatment for bone disorders.

Clinical Problems

Decreased Level: Malnutrition, hypopituitarism, hypoparathyroidism. *Drug Influence:* Aspirin, ascorbic acid, glucocorticoids, calcitonin, plicamycin.

Increased Level: Paget disease, metastatic bone tumor, osteoporosis, bone growth, acromegaly.

Procedure

- Food and fluids are restricted for 8–12 hours before the 2-hour hydroxyproline test.
- The client should avoid meat, poultry, fish, jelly, and gelatin for 24–48 hours prior to the test.
- Collect a 2-hour or 24-hour urine specimen. A preservative is usually added to prevent degradation of hydroxyproline.
- Label the specimen with the client's gender and age and the exact time of urine collection.
- Keep the urine container refrigerated, and take it to the laboratory immediately following the specified urine collection time.

Factors Affecting Laboratory Results

- Drug influence (*see Clinical Problems*), decreased level.
- Meats and gelatin can cause false-positive test results.
- Faulty collection of urine specimen (e.g., not refrigerating the urine container).

NURSING IMPLICATIONS WITH RATIONALE

- Obtain a health and drug history. Record drugs the client is taking. If the client is receiving drugs to control bone disorder (e.g., Paget disease), the urine hydroxyproline level is expected to be lower.
- Provide comfort (e.g., position changes, pain medication) to alleviate pain.
- Be supportive of the client and family. Answer questions or refer questions to other health care providers.

Client Teaching

- Instruct the client to avoid meats and gelatin products for 24–48 hours prior to the test, because these foods can increase urine hydroxyproline levels. If the client consumes these foods prior to the test, it should be noted on the laboratory slip and the health care provider should be informed.
- Explain the procedure of urine collection to the client. Inform the client that the urine container should be refrigerated. If any of the urine is discarded accidently, the test should be restarted the next day.

Immunoglobulins (Ig) (serum)

IgG, IgA, IgM, IgD, IgE

Reference Values

	TOTAL Ig (99% mg/dL)	IgG (80% mg/dL)	IgA (15% mg/dL)	IgM (4% mg/dL)	IgD (0.2% mg/dL)	IgE (0.0002% U/mL)
Adult	900–2,200	650–1,700	70–400	40–350	0–8	less than 40
						(IgE 0–120 mg/Dl)
6–16 years		800–1,700	700–1,650	80–230	45–260	less than 62
4–6 years	700–1,700	550–1,500	50–175	22–100		less than 25
1–3 years	400–1,500	300–1,400	20–150	40–230		less than 10
6 months	225–1,200	200–1,100	10–90	10–80		
3 months	325–750	275–750	5–55	15–70		
Newborn	650–1,450	700–1,480	0–12	5–30		

Description

Immunoglobulins (Ig) are classes (groups) of proteins referred to as antibodies; they can be divided into five groups found in gamma globulin. Immunoglobulin is produced by the action of B lymphocytes and plasma cells, and, as is characteristic of all antibody actions, immunoglobulin responds to invading foreign antigens. As individuals are exposed to antigens, immunoglobulin (antibody) production occurs. With further exposure to the same antigen, immunity results.

The five classes of immunoglobulins—IgG, IgA, IgM, IgD, and IgE—are separated by the process of immunoelectrophoresis. Of these five classes, IgG, IgA, and IgM make up most of the total gamma globulin.

The immunologic functions of the immunoglobulins are as follows:

IgG: IgG is the major immunoglobulin. IgG results from secondary exposure to the foreign antigen and is responsible for antiviral and antibacterial activity. This antibody passes through the placental barrier and provides early immunity for the newborn. The IgG response is longer and stronger than that of the other immunoglobulins.

IgA: This immunoglobulin is found in the secretions of the respiratory, gastrointestinal, and genitourinary tracts; tears; and saliva. Its purpose is to protect mucous membranes from invading organisms (viruses, certain bacteria—*Escherichia coli* and *Clostridium tetani*). IgA does not pass the placental barrier. Those having congenital IgA deficiency are prone to autoimmune disease.

IgM: IgM antibodies are produced 48–72 hours after an antigen enters the body and are responsible for primary immunity. This immunoglobulin produces antibody activity against rheumatoid factors, gram-negative organisms, and the ABO blood group. IgM activates the complement system by destroying antigenic substances. Because it does not pass the placental barrier, the serum value is low in newborns; however, it is produced early in life and the level increases after 9 months of age.

IgD: Unknown.

IgE: This immunoglobulin increases during allergic reactions and anaphylaxis.

Purposes

- To identify the occurrence of total or a specific elevated immunoglobulin.
- To associate a specific immunoglobulin elevation with a health problem (*see Clinical Problems*).

Clinical Problems

Ig	DECREASED LEVEL	INCREASED LEVEL
IgG	Lymphocytic leukemia Agammaglobulinemia Preeclampsia Amyloidosis	Infections—all types Severe malnutrition Chronic granulomatous infection Hyperimmunization Liver disease Rheumatic fever Sarcoidosis
IgA	Lymphocytic leukemia Agammaglobulinemia Malignancies	Autoimmune disorders Rheumatic fever Chronic infections Liver disease
IgM	Lymphocytic leukemia Agammaglobulinemia Amyloidosis	Lymphosarcoma Brucellosis Trypanosomiasis Relapsing fever Infectious mononucleosis Rubella virus in newborns

(Continued)

Ig	DECREASED LEVEL	INCREASED LEVEL
IgE		Allergic reactions (asthma)
		Skin sensitivity
		Drug influence
		Tetanus toxoid
		Tetanus antitoxin
		Gamma globulin

Procedure

- There is usually no food or fluid restriction. Some laboratories request that the client refrain from eating and drinking 12 hours before the test. Check with your laboratory.
- Collect 5–7 mL of venous blood in a red-top tube.
- Record on the laboratory slip whether the client has received any vaccination or immunization, including toxoid, within the last 6 months, or any blood transfusion, gamma globulin, or tetanus antitoxin injections in the last 6 weeks.

Factors Affecting Laboratory Results

- Immunizations and toxoids received in the last 6 months, and blood transfusions, tetanus antitoxin, and gamma globulin received in the last 6 weeks can affect immunoglobulin results.

NURSING IMPLICATIONS WITH RATIONALE

- Obtain a history from the client concerning previous vaccination or immunization, including toxoids (tetanus), received in the last 6 months and blood transfusions or injections of gamma globulin or tetanus antitoxin received in the last 6 weeks.
- Report to the health care provider and record on the client's chart and the laboratory slip if the client has received recent blood transfusions, immunization or injections of toxoids, tetanus antitoxin, and gamma globulins.
- Check the client's temperature periodically.

Client Teaching

- Instruct the client to avoid infections by using preventive measures (e.g., avoiding persons with colds, getting adequate rest, eating balanced meals, and maintaining adequate fluid intake).

Infertility Screen (group of tests)

Reference Values

Female: Luteinizing hormone (LH). See LH values in text.
Follicle-stimulating hormone (FSH). See FSH values in text.

Male: Antisperm antibody. See antisperm antibody values in text.

Description

Infertility screening tests are a group of tests ordered by an infertility specialist, from either a private practice or clinic, to determine the cause of infertility. For the female, the reference values of her luteinizing hormone (LH) and follicle-stimulating hormone (FSH) are analyzed. For the male, the test determines whether antisperm antibodies are present.

Other causes of infertility are abnormal ovulation, tubal obstruction, endometrial polyps, low sperm count, sexual infections, and genetic causes. In some cases, clients with normal or abnormal test results may be referred to a psychologist or a psychiatrist.

Purposes

- To determine the cause of the infertility.
- To correct the cause of the infertility.

Clinical Problems

Causes of infertility may include a deficit in the LH or FSH, the presence of antisperm antibodies, sexual infections, female structural changes, low sperm count, or genetic causes.

Procedure

- Nothing by mouth 8 to 12 hours prior to LH, FSH, and antisperm antibody tests. Check with the person ordering the tests or the laboratory.
- Collect 5 to 7 mL of venous blood in a red-top tube.
- Semen collection may be used for the antisperm antibody test and the sperm count.
- Abstain from ejaculation for 24 to 48 hours before the test. Check with the physician.
- Follow procedure for other tests as ordered.

Factors Affecting Laboratory Results

- Hormones (estrogen, progesterone, and testosterone) and oral contraceptives could decrease serum LH values.
- Ejaculation occurring before semen collection.
- Heavy coffee consumption and smoking may decrease sperm motility.

NURSING IMPLICATIONS WITH RATIONALE

- Obtain a menstrual history from the female client.
- Obtain a history of drugs the clients are taking.
- Permit the clients to express their concerns about their infertility problem.
- Answer questions concerning the various tests that were ordered. If the answer is unknown, refer questions to the health care provider.

Influenza A and B titer (blood)

Reference Values

Normal: Negative titer; 1:8 titer influenza immunization.

Description

There are two main influenza viruses, A and B, that cause most major epidemics every 2 to 4 years. Influenza virus A has two subtypes: hemagglutinin (H) and neuraminidase (N). Hemagglutinin has three subtypes: H1, H2, and H3. Neuraminidase has two subtypes: N1 and N2. These types and subtypes are responsible for widespread epidemics of influenza. Virus B is associated with sporadic epidemics, mostly among children and young adults. Virus A spreads rapidly to many populations, whereas virus B is more local.

The incubation period of influenza is brief. The virus enters through the respiratory tract and spreads rapidly throughout the body. The symptoms include fever, chills, sore throat, cough, muscular pain and neuralgia, headache, and gastrointestinal upset. Antibiotics do not cure the virus, but they can prevent complications from secondary bacterial infections (acute bronchitis and pneumonia).

Annual influenza vaccination is suggested for the elderly, young children, health workers, and those with chronic health disorders, such as chronic heart, lung, and renal diseases and diabetes mellitus. The vaccine injection does not always provide immunity to all types of influenza viruses. Systemic reaction to the vaccine is rare, though it can occur.

Purposes

- To prevent at-risk populations from contracting the influenza virus.
- To be aware of the clients who are at higher risk of contracting influenza.
- To advise people to get a yearly influenza vaccine.

Clinical Problems

At Risk of Influenza: Elderly, young children, chronically ill persons, those with chronic health problems (heart, lungs, kidneys, diabetes mellitus), and health care personnel.

Procedure

- There is no food or fluid restriction.
- Obtain 7 mL of venous blood in a red-, gray-, or gold-top tube.
- A convalescent blood sample may be ordered 14 days later.

Factors Affecting Laboratory Results

- Not obtaining a convalescent blood sample to verify that the acute phase is finished.

NURSING IMPLICATIONS WITH RATIONALE

- Ask if the client has had a "flu shot," when, and how often. Advise the client that yearly flu vaccine injections are recommended.
- Inform the client that influenza is most prevalent from September to May.
- Advise the client to avoid crowded places when there is a local epidemic.
- Explain the importance of good hygiene to increase the body's resistance.
- Advise the client to avoid contact with a person with influenza.

Client Teaching

- Answer the client's questions and, if unknown, refer them to another health professional.

Insulin (serum), insulin antibody

Reference Values

Adult: *Serum Insulin:* 5–25 micro-unit/mL, 42–156 pmol/L (SI units). *Panic Value:* 7 unit/mL (7 µU/mL).

Insulin Antibody Test: No insulin antibodies detected.

Description

Insulin, a hormone from the beta cells of the pancreas, is essential in transporting glucose to the cells for metabolism. Increased glucose levels stimulate insulin secretion.

Serum insulin and blood glucose levels are compared to determine the glucose disorder. Serum insulin is valuable in diagnosing insulinoma (islet cell tumor), islet cell hyperplasia, and in evaluating insulin production in diabetes mellitus (DM). In insulinoma the serum insulin is high, and blood glucose is less than 30 mg/dL. Hyperinsulinemia can occur in obesity as well as in insulinoma.

Insulin values are more helpful during an OGTT (oral glucose tolerance test) for diagnosing an early pre-hyperglycemic DM. A normal fasting insulin level and a delayed rise in GTT curves occur frequently with mildly diabetic individuals.

An **insulin antibody test** is ordered when a diabetic requires a larger and larger insulin dosage. These antibodies are of immunoglobulin types, such as IgG (most common), IgM, and IgE. The IgG antibodies neutralize the insulin, thus preventing glucose metabolism. IgM antibodies can cause insulin resistance, and IgE could be responsible for allergic effects.

Years ago, the frequent cause of insulin antibodies were the use of beef and pork insulins. Pork insulin was closer in structure to human insulin. With an increase in the use of human insulin (Humulin insulin) in the United States and other countries, beef and pork insulins are not frequently given, thus fewer insulin antibodies occur.

Purposes

- To assist in the detection of an early pre-hyperglycemic diabetes mellitus state.
- To check for the presence of insulin antibodies that can affect insulin absorption and dosage.

Clinical Problems

Decreased Level: Diabetes mellitus, hypopituitarism. *Drug Influence:* Beta blockers, phenytoin, diuretics, calcium blockers.

Increased Level: Insulinoma, insulin-resistant diabetic state, Cushing syndrome, obesity. *Drug Influence:* Cortisone preparations, oral contraceptives, thyroid hormones, epinephrine, levodopa, terbutaline.

Procedure

- Food and fluids are restricted for 10–12 hours prior to the test. Insulin secretion reaches its peak in 30 minutes to 2 hours after meals.

- Collect 3–5 mL of venous blood in a red-top tube. Avoid hemolysis. The blood sample should be chilled. Serum must be separated within 30 minutes of collection. If blood glucose is needed, collect 3–5 mL in a gray- or red-top tube.
- Withhold medications that could affect test results, such as insulin and cortisone, until after the test.

Factors Affecting Laboratory Tests

- Drugs such as insulin, cortisone, oral contraceptives, and hormones could increase serum insulin levels.
- Hemolysis of the blood sample and not chilling the specimen could affect results.

NURSING IMPLICATIONS WITH RATIONALE

- Obtain a history of glucose disorders from the client or family. Report the client's complaints.
- Report if the client's insulin dosage has increased over a period of time.
- Be alert for signs and symptoms of hypoglycemia. If insulinoma is highly suspected, keep IV dextrose 50% available.

Client Teaching

- Explain to the client the importance of remaining NPO and resting (not exercising) before the test. Food and exercise increase blood glucose, thus increasing serum insulin level. Incorrect test results would occur.
- Instruct the client to report signs and symptoms of insulin reaction (e.g., nervousness, sweating, weakness, rapid pulse rate, confusion).

International normalized ratio (INR) (plasma)

Reference Values

Oral Anticoagulant Therapy: 2–3 INR.
Higher Value for Mechanical Heart Valve: 2.5–3.5 INR.

Description

The international normalized ratio (INR) was devised to monitor more correctly anticoagulant therapy for clients receiving warfarin (Coumadin) therapy. The World Health Organization recommends the use of INR for a more consistent reporting of PT (prothrombin time) results. The INR is calculated by the use of a nomogram demonstrating the relationship between the INR and the prothrombin time ratio. Usually both PT and INR values are reported for monitoring Coumadin therapy.

Refer to PT for the purposes, clinical problems, procedure, factors affecting laboratory results, nursing implications, and client teaching.

Inulin clearance

Reference Values

Adult: *Average Range for 21–69 Years:* 90–130 mL/min. *21–39 Years: Male:* 90–168 mL/min, *Female:* 84–150 mL/min. *40–49 Years: Male:* 78–162 mL/min, *Female:* 82–146 mL/min. *50–69 Years: Male:* 68–137 mL/min, *Female:* 66–130 mL/min. *70–79 Years: Male:* 42–122 mL/min, *Female:* 45–121 mL/min.

Child: *Less than 11 Years:* 82–122 mL/min. *11–20 Years:* 85–125 mL/min.

Description

The inulin clearance test is a reliable test used to assess the glomerular filtration rate (GFR) in relation to renal function. The substance given for the test is inulin, an inert sugar that is not metabolized nor absorbed from the renal tubules but is rapidly filtered through the glomeruli. If glomerular filtration is normal, the inulin clearance should be equivalent to the GFR. Decreased levels occur when greater than 50% of renal cells are nonfunctioning, thus indicating impaired glomerular filtration. Normal decreased glomerular filtration can occur during the aging process. Inulin clearance test is not suggested for a client who has a history of heart failure (HF).

Inulin clearance test is very time consuming and is not frequently performed. Blood urea nitrogen, serum creatinine, and creatinine clearance tests are normally ordered to determine renal function.

Purpose

- To assess renal function.

Clinical Problems

Decreased Level: Acute and chronic glomerulonephritis, acute tubular necrosis, nephrosclerosis, advanced chronic bilateral pyelonephritis, renal atherosclerosis, HF, renal malignancy, polycystic kidney disease, shock. *Drug Influence:* Aminoglycosides, penicillin preparations, amphotericin B, and phenacetin.

Procedure

Check your laboratory policy for consistency with this procedure.

- The client should not eat food for 4 hours prior to the test. Exercise should be avoided.
- The client is to drink a quart of water (4 full water glasses) in 30–60 minutes prior to the test.
- Collect 7 mL of venous blood in a green-top tube for use as a control blood sample.
- Insert a Foley catheter (indwelling urinary catheter) and save the urine for a baseline urine specimen.
- Start an IV line using 500 mL of 5% dextrose in water (D_5W) using a Y tubing set.
- Prepare 25 mL of 10% inulin for IV bolus. Inulin may be difficult to dilute; therefore, warming the vial may be necessary.

- Inject intravenously 25 mL of 10% inulin over 4 minutes.
- Wait 30 minutes and begin the infusion of 500 mL of 1.5% inulin solution using an IV pump at the rate of 4 mL/min or 240 mL/h.
- Obtain four urine samples: 30, 50, 70, and 90 minutes after the 1.5% inulin solution was started. Clamp the catheter between each collected urine specimen. Some institutions require three urine specimens, 20 minutes apart. Urine specimens should be refrigerated if not sent immediately to the laboratory.
- Collect four blood samples of 10 mL each in a green-top tube at 40, 60, 80, and 95 minutes after the 1.5% inulin solution was started. Some institutions require two blood samples, 20 minutes apart. Blood samples should be sent immediately to the laboratory.
- Label each specimen with the time of collection and the amount of inulin used.
- Remove the Foley catheter.

Factors Affecting Laboratory Results

- Hemolysis of the blood samples from rough handling can cause a false-negative result.
- Failure to infuse the inulin solution at the constant rate and prescribed rate of flow.
- Failure to collect the blood and urine specimens at the prescribed times and/or not labeling specimens correctly.
- Inadequate urine output due to inadequate water intake.

NURSING IMPLICATIONS WITH RATIONALE

- Assess vital signs. Auscultate the lungs to check for chest rales and peripheral edema. Excess fluid intake may increase the already overloaded vascular system. Report findings.
- Assess the urine output and fluid intake. Urine output of less than 600 mL/day can indicate renal dysfunction or inadequate fluid intake.
- Use the 25 mL of 10% inulin for IV bolus within 1 hour of preparation.
- One nurse should be assigned to monitor the test to maintain the correct procedure.

Client Teaching

- Explain the procedure for the inulin clearance test to the client (*see Procedure*). This may be written for the client so that he or she can follow the procedure.
- Inform the client that a catheter will be inserted in the bladder for the duration of the test. It will be removed following the test.
- Instruct the client not to eat for 4 hours before the test and not to exercise.
- Tell the client that the test usually takes about 2 hours. Explain that there will be 4–5 blood samples drawn and 4–5 urine samples collected according to the prescribed policy.
- Listen to the client's concerns. Answer questions.

Iron (Fe), total iron-binding capacity (TIBC), transferrin, transferrin saturation (serum)

Iron-Binding Capacity (IBC)

Reference Values

	SERUM IRON	TIBC	SERUM TRANSFERRIN	TRANSFERRIN SATURATION
Adult	50–150 mcg/dL 10–27 µmol/L (SI units) Males slightly higher	250–450 mcg/dL	200–430 mg/dL	30–50% (male) 20–35% (female)
Elderly	60–80 mcg/dL	less than 250 mcg/dL		
Child				
Newborn Infant	100–270 mcg/dL	60–175 mcg/dL 100–400 mcg/dL	125–275 mg/dL	
6 months– 2 years	40–100 mcg/dL	100–135 mcg/dL		
Greater than 2 years		40–100 mcg/dL		

Description

Iron (Fe) is absorbed from the duodenum and upper jejunum; the amount absorbed usually covers the amount of iron that has been lost. The average daily iron intake is 10–20 mg.

Iron is coupled with the iron-transporting protein transferrin. Transferrin is responsible for transporting iron to the bone marrow for the purpose of hemoglobin synthesis (*see Transferrin*). The storage compound for iron is ferritin (*see Ferritin*). Serum iron levels are elevated when there is excessive red blood cell destruction (hemolysis), and levels are decreased in iron-deficiency anemia.

Total iron-binding capacity (TIBC) measures the maximum amount of iron that can bind to the protein transferrin. The level of TIBC decreases with age. Usually, serum iron and TIBC are determined together.

Transferrin can be measured as serum and as a percentage of saturation (transferrin saturation). The transferrin saturation is the ratio between serum iron and TIBC relating to the availability of transferrin in binding with iron. Transferrin saturation is given in percent.

Serum iron, TIBC, transferrin, and transferrin saturation values are needed to adequately diagnose iron-deficiency anemia and other disorders. The table below gives the various tests used for diagnosing health problems related to iron and transferrin imbalances.

Serum Iron, TIBC, Transferrin, and Transferrin Saturation

SERUM IRON	TIBC	SERUM TRANSFERRIN	TRANSFERRIN SATURATION	HEALTH PROBLEMS
Low	High	High	Low	Iron-deficiency anemia
Low	Low	Low	Normal	Chronic illness: cancer, infection, cirrhosis
High	Normal or low	Low	Very high	Iron therapy overload

Purposes

- To determine a probable cause of iron excess (e.g., hemolysis) or deficit (e.g., iron-deficiency anemia).
- To compare serum iron and TIBC for diagnosing iron-deficiency anemia.

Clinical Problems

Decreased Level *Serum Iron:* Iron-deficiency anemia; cancer of the stomach, small and/or large intestines, rectum, and breast; rheumatoid arthritis; bleeding peptic ulcer; chronic renal failure; pregnancy; low-birth-weight infants; protein malnutrition; chronic blood loss (GI, uterine). *TIBC:* Hemochromatosis (excess iron deposits in organs and tissues), anemias (hemolytic, pernicious, sickle cell), renal failure, cirrhosis of the liver, rheumatoid arthritis, infections, cancer of the GI tract. *Drug Influence:* Cortisone preparations, dextran, testosterone. *Transferrin:* Anemia from chronic disease, hepatic damage, renal disease, cancer, acute or chronic infection. *Transferrin Saturation:* Chronic iron-deficiency anemia, anemia of chronic disease.

Increased Level *Serum Iron:* Hemochromatosis, anemias (hemolytic, pernicious, and folic acid deficiency), liver damage, thalassemia, lead toxicity. *TIBC:* Iron-deficiency anemia, acute chronic blood loss, polycythemia. *Drug Influence:* Oral contraceptives, iron preparations. *Transferrin:* Iron deficiency. *Transferrin Saturation:* Anemias (hemolytic, sideroblastic), hemochromatosis, iron overload.

Procedure

- NPO for 8 hours before the test. Serum iron levels are usually higher in the morning and following food intake.
- Collect 5–7 mL of venous blood in a red-top tube. Avoid hemolysis; false elevated readings can occur.

Factors Affecting Laboratory Results

- Oral iron medications and recent blood transfusion.
- Hemolysis of the blood sample.

NURSING IMPLICATIONS WITH RATIONALE

Decreased Level (Serum Iron)

- Observe for signs and symptoms of iron-deficiency anemia (e.g., pallor, fatigue, headache, tachycardia, dyspnea on exertion).

Client Teaching

- Instruct the client to eat foods rich in iron (e.g., liver, shellfish, lean meat, egg yolks, dried fruits, whole grain, wines, and cereals). Milk has little or no iron. Nutritional instruction is particularly important for preschool and adolescent children and for pregnant women.
- Recommend rest and avoidance of strenuous activity before test.

- Instruct the client on how to take iron supplements. Iron should be given following meals or snacks because it irritates the gastric mucosa. Orange juice and ascorbic acid promote iron absorption.
- Explain to the client that iron supplements can cause constipation and that the stools will have a tarry appearance.

Increased Level

- Observe for signs and symptoms of hemochromatosis (e.g., bronze pigmentation of the skin, dysrhythmias, and heart failure).

Ketone bodies, acetone (urine)

Reference Values

Adult: Negative test.
Child: Negative test.

Description

(*See Acetone, Ketone Bodies [serum].*)

Ketone bodies are produced to provide energy when carbohydrates (CHO) cannot be used, as in diabetic acidosis and starvation/malnutrition. When these excess ketones are produced, ketosis (in the blood) results, thus exhausting the alkaline reserve (e.g., bicarbonates) of the body, causing an acidotic state. Ketonuria (ketone bodies in the urine) occurs as a result of ketosis.

In testing for ketonuria, Acetest tablets are used to detect the two principal ketones (acetone and acetoacetic acid) in the urine. Ketostix can also be used, but this test method is more specific for acetoacetic acid.

Purpose

- To detect the presence of an acidotic state.

Clinical Problems

Positive Result: Diabetic acidosis (ketoacidosis), starvation/malnutrition, reducing diet ($\Downarrow$ CHO), fasting, severe vomiting, heat stroke, fetal death. *Drug Influence:* Ascorbic acid, levodopa compounds, insulin, isopropyl alcohol, paraldehyde, Pyridium, dyes used for the tests—bromsulfophthalein (BSP) and phenolsulfonphthalein (PSP).

Procedure

- There is no food or fluid restriction.
- Collect a random urine specimen. Two tests are usually performed, as follows.

Acetest: Place an Acetest tablet on a clean surface (preferably a white paper towel), and put a drop of fresh urine on the tablet. Wait 30 seconds; if the tablet changes color (lavender, medium purple, or dark purple), the result is positive for ketones.

K

The test is usually done on the same urine used for testing for glycosuria. The Clinitest is used for determining glycosuria and the Acetest for ketonuria.

Ketostix: Dip a reagent stick in fresh urine. Wait 15 seconds and compare it to the color chart. This test is more sensitive to acetoacetic acid than it is to acetone.

The urine should be fresh or refrigerated in a closed container. Waiting may cause false-negative results because of the instability of acetone.

Factors Affecting Laboratory Results

- A low-carbohydrate diet or a high-fat diet can cause false-positive results.
- Certain drugs can cause false-positive results (*see Drug Influence*).
- Urine kept at room temperature for 1 hour or more before testing may cause a false-negative result.
- Urinary tract infection—bacteria in the urine—will cause a loss of acetoacetic acid.
- Juvenile diabetics are more prone to ketonuria (ketosis) than adults.

NURSING IMPLICATIONS WITH RATIONALE

Positive Result

- Relate ketonuria to diabetic acidosis (ketoacidosis), starvation, fasting, or a low-carbohydrate diet. In severe diabetic acidosis, both ketonuria and glycosuria may be present. This would not be true in severe vomiting, starvation, reducing diets, and heat stroke, because in such cases only ketonuria would be present.
- Explain to the client that the urine should be freshly voided. Only 1 mL is needed. Acetone is lost in the urine if it stands at room temperature because it is volatile.
- Test and record the results of the Acetest and Clinitest on the client's chart. Notify the health care provider if results are abnormal.
- Assess for signs and symptoms of diabetic acidosis, such as rapid, vigorous breathing; restlessness; confusion; sweet-smelling breath; and a positive Clinitest and Acetest.

Client Teaching

- Instruct client on how to use the Acetest and Clinitest.
- Answer the client's questions concerning urine testing and diabetes mellitus.

K

17-Ketosteroids (17-KS) (urine)

Reference Values

Adult: *Male:* 5–25 mg/24 h. *Female:* 5–15 mg/24 h.

Elderly: 4–8 mg/24 h.

Child: *Infant:* Less than 1 mg/24 h. *1–3 Years Old:* Less than 2 mg/24 h. *3–6 Years Old:* Less than 3 mg/24 h. *7–10 Years Old:* Less than 4 mg/24 h. *10–12 Years Old:* 1–6 mg/24 h.

Adolescent: *Male:* 3–15 mg/24 h. *Female:* 3–12 mg/24 h.

Description

17-Ketosteroids (17-KS) are metabolites of male hormones that are secreted from the testes and adrenal cortex. 17-KS are excreted in the urine. In men, approximately one third of the hormone metabolites come from the testes, and two thirds come from the adrenal cortex. In women, nearly all of the excreted hormones (androgens) are derived from the adrenal cortex.

Because most of the 17-KS is derived from the adrenal cortex and not from the testes, the 17-KS level is more useful for diagnosing adrenal cortex dysfunction. This test is also useful for determining pituitary and gonadal hormone function. Usually plasma cortisol and 17-OHCS determinations are requested at the same time to further confirm adrenal dysfunctions.

Purpose

- To assist in the diagnosis of adrenal cortex dysfunction.

Clinical Problems

Decreased Level: Adrenal cortical hypofunction (Addison disease), hypogonadism, hypopituitarism, nephrosis, myxedema, severe debilitating diseases. *Drug Influence:* Thiazide diuretics, chlordiazepoxide (Librium), estrogen, oral contraceptives, paraldehyde, reserpine, probenecid (Benemid), promazine, meprobamate (Miltown),[*] quinidine, quinine.

Increased Level: Adrenocorticotropic hormone therapy, adrenal cortical hyperfunction (adrenocortical hyperplasia, Cushing syndrome, adrenocortical carcinoma), testicular neoplasm, ovarian neoplasm, hyperpituitarism, hirsutism, severe stress (burns, surgery, infectious diseases). *Drug Influence:* Acetazolamide (Diamox), antibiotics (chloramphenicol [Chloromycetin], cloxacillin, erythromycin), chlorpromazine (Thorazine), hydralazine, meprobamate (Miltown),[*] phenothiazines, spironolactone (Aldactone), phenazopyridine, dexamethasone (Decadron).

Procedure

- There is no food or fluid restriction.
- Drugs that interfere with test results should not be given for 48 hours before the test. Check with the health care provider first.
- Collect a 24-hour urine specimen in a large container, and keep the container on ice or refrigerated. An acid preservative is usually added to keep the urine at a pH less than 4.5, thus preventing steroid decomposition by bacterial growth.
- List on the laboratory slip the client's sex and age.
- Label container with the client's name, date, and exact time of collection, such as 9/23/20, 7:30 AM to 9/24/20, 7:32 AM.
- Postpone the test if the female has her menstrual period. Blood in the urine can cause false-positive results.

Factors Affecting Laboratory Results

- Drugs (*see Drug Influence above*).

---

[*] Meprobamate may increase or decrease the 17-KS value.

NURSING IMPLICATIONS WITH RATIONALE

- List on the laboratory slip the client's sex and age. If the client is a male, the laboratory results should be slightly higher than if the client is a female. In addition, if the client is over 65 years old, the test results should be low or low normal.
- Encourage the client to increase fluid intake.

Client Teaching

- Explain to the client and family that all urine will be collected for 24 hours in the large urine container/bottle, which is on ice or refrigerated. Inform the client that he or she should not put toilet paper or feces in the urine and should not urinate directly into the collection container. The container could contain an acid preservative, which could splash.

Decreased Level

- Observe for the signs and symptoms of adrenal gland insufficiency (Addison disease), such as weakness, weight loss, polyuria, hypotension, increased pulse rate, and shock (if severe).
- Record fluid intake and output. Report if the client's urine output is greater than normal (greater than 2,000 mL/24 h).
- Monitor weight loss. In Addison disease, sodium is not retained; therefore, both sodium and water are lost. Weight loss and dehydration usually occur.

Client Teaching

- Encourage the client to wear an identification bracelet containing emergency information.

Increased Level

- Observe for signs and symptoms of adrenal gland hyperfunction (Cushing syndrome), such as moon face, hirsutism, weight gain, a cervicodorsal fat pad (buffalo hump), a bleeding tendency, hyperglycemia, and edema in the extremities.
- Check serum potassium and blood glucose levels. Hypokalemia and hyperglycemia frequently occur; potassium supplements and insulin or a low-carbohydrate diet may be indicated.

Lactic acid (blood)

Reference Values

Adult: *Arterial Blood:* 0.5–2 mmol/L (SI units), less than 11.3 mg/dL. *Venous Blood:* 0.5–1.5 mmol/L, 8.1–15.3 mg/dL. *Panic Range:* Greater than 5 mEq/L, greater than 45 mg/dL.

Description

Blood lactic acid or lactate is an indicator of the presence of lactic acidosis. Increased secretion of lactic acid occurs following strenuous exercise and acute or prolonged hypoxemia (tissue hypoxia). A major cause of metabolic acidosis is excess circulating lactic acid. Shock and severe dehydration cause cell catabolism (cell breakdown) and an accumulation of acid metabolites, such as lactic acid.

Lactic acidosis is suspected if the anion gap is greater than 17 mEq/L and pH is decreased. Excess lactic acid decreases pH and causes lactic acidosis.

Purpose

- To detect the presence of acidosis related to shock, trauma, or severe illness (*see Anion Gap*).

Clinical Problems

Decreased Level: High lactic dehydrogenase (LDH) value.

Increased Level: Shock, severe dehydration, severe trauma, ketoacidosis, severe infections, neoplastic conditions, hepatic failure, renal disease, alcoholism, salicylate toxicity (severe), chronic alcoholism.

Procedure

- Collect 5–7 mL of blood in a green-top tube.
- Inform the client to avoid hand clenching, which can lead to a buildup of lactic acid caused by a release of lactic acid from muscle of the clenched hand.
- Avoid using a tourniquet if possible. It could increase the blood lactic acid level.
- Deliver blood specimen on ice to the laboratory immediately.

Factors Affecting Laboratory Results

- Delivery to the laboratory of an arterial blood specimen not on ice could cause an inaccurate result.
- Use of tourniquet could elevate lactic acid value.

NURSING IMPLICATIONS WITH RATIONALE

Increased Level

- Associate an elevated lactic acid value with shock, severe dehydration, severe trauma, severe infection, and other conditions.
- Observe for signs and symptoms of acidosis, dyspnea, or Kussmaul breathing, increased pulse rate, decreased pH, decreased serum carbon dioxide value, and decreased arterial bicarbonate value.
- Be supportive of the client and family. If shock is present, anxiety and fear are common.

L

Lactic (lactate) dehydrogenase (LD or LDH), LDH isoenzymes (serum)

Reference Values

Adult: *Total LDH:* 100–190 international unit/L, 70–250 unit/L. Values can differ according to the method used.

Isoenzymes: LDH_1, 14–26%; LDH_2, 27–37%; LDH_3, 13–26%; LDH_4, 8–16%; LDH_5, 6–16%. Differences of 2–4% are considered normal.

Child: *Newborn:* 300–1,500 international unit/L. *Child:* 50–150 international unit/L, 110–295 unit/L.

Description

Lactic dehydrogenase (LDH) is an intracellular enzyme present in nearly all metabolizing cells, with the highest concentrations in the heart, skeletal muscle, liver, kidney, brain, and red blood cells. LDH has two distinct subunits—M (muscle) and H (heart). These subunits are combined in different formations to make five isoenzymes.

- LDH_1: cardiac fraction; H, H, H, H; in heart, RBCs, kidneys, brain (some).
- LDH_2: cardiac fraction; H, H, H, M; in heart, RBCs, kidneys, brain (some).
- LDH_3: pulmonary fraction; H, H, M, M; in lungs and other tissues; spleen, pancreas, adrenal, thyroid, lymphatics.
- LDH_4: hepatic fraction; H, M, M, M; liver, skeletal muscle, kidneys, and brain (some).
- LDH_5: hepatic fraction; M, M, M, M; liver, skeletal muscle, kidneys (some).

Like other enzymatic tests, such as the creatine phosphokinase and aspartate aminotransferase tests, serum LDH and LDH_1 are used for diagnosing acute myocardial infarction. A high serum LDH (total) level occurs 12–24 hours after the infarction, reaches its peak in 2–5 days, and remains elevated for 6–12 days, making it a useful test for delayed diagnosis of MI. A flipped LDH_1/LDH_2 ratio, with LDH_1 the highest, indicates a myocardial infarction.

LDH_3 is linked to pulmonary diseases, and LDH_5 is linked to liver and skeletal muscle diseases. In acute hepatitis, total LDH rises, and the LDH_5 usually rises before jaundice develops.

Purposes

- To aid in the diagnosis of myocardial or skeletal muscle damage.
- To compare test results with other cardiac enzyme tests (e.g., CPK, AST).
- To check LDH isoenzyme results to determine organ involvement.

Clinical Problems

Increased Level: Acute MI, cerebrovascular accident, cancer (lung, bone, intestines, liver, breast, cervix, testes, kidney, stomach, melanoma of the skin), acute leukemia, acute pulmonary infarction, infectious mononucleosis, anemias (pernicious, folic acid deficiency, sickle cell, acquired hemolytic), acute hepatitis, shock, skeletal muscular disease, heat stroke. *Drug Influence:* Narcotics (codeine, morphine, meperidine [Demerol]).

L

Procedure

- There is no food or fluid restriction.
- Collect 5–7 mL of venous blood in a red-top tube. Avoid hemolysis.
- List on the laboratory slip any narcotics or intramuscular (IM) injections the client received within 8 hours before the test.

Factors Affecting Laboratory Results

- Narcotic drugs and IM injections can elevate serum LDH levels.
- Hemolysis of the blood sample can cause an elevated serum LDH level; the enzyme is plentiful in the RBCs.

NURSING IMPLICATIONS WITH RATIONALE

Increased Level

- Obtain a history of the client's discomfort. A complaint of severe indigestion several days before could be indicative of an acute MI. All information should be recorded and reported.
- Assess for signs and symptoms of an acute MI (e.g., pale or gray color, sharp stabbing pain or heavy pressure pain, shortness of breath, diaphoresis, nausea and vomiting, and indigestion).

Client Teaching

- Instruct the client to notify the nurse of any recurrence of chest discomfort or to seek medical care for indigestion lasting several days.

Lactose and lactose tolerance test (serum)

Reference Values

Serum/Plasma: Less than 0.5 mg/dL, less than 14.5 μmol/L (SI units).

Urine: 12–40 mg/dL.

Lactose Test: *Tolerance:* Fasting serum glucose plus 20–50 mg/dL. *Intolerance:* Fasting serum glucose plus less than 20 mg/dL.

Description

Lactose is a disaccharide sugar. Milk is rich in lactose. One glass of milk may contain 12 grams of lactose. For lactose to be absorbed, lactase (an intestinal enzyme) converts lactose to glucose and galactose. With a deficiency of the lactase enzyme, diarrhea, flatus, and abdominal cramping commonly occur due to excess lactose in the intestine.

When lactose intolerance is suspected, a lactose tolerance test is usually conducted. A large amount of lactose is ingested, and serum glucose levels are drawn at specified times. If the serum glucose level is more than 20 mg/dL greater than the fasting glucose level, lactose is tolerated and is being converted into glucose; if the increase in the serum glucose level is less than 20 mg/dL of the fasting glucose, lactose intolerance is occurring. Milk products should be avoided to decrease lactose intolerance.

Purposes

- To compare serum and urine lactose results for determining lactose deficiency.
- To diagnose lactose intolerance.

Clinical Problems

Decreased Glucose Level: Excess lactose in intestine, lactose intolerance.

Increased Glucose Level: Normal lactose tolerance.

Procedure

- The client should not eat or drink after midnight or at least 8 hours prior to the test.
- Collect 5–7 mL of a fasting venous blood specimen in a gray-top tube.
- The client drinks 50–100 g of lactose in 200–300 mL of water in 5–10 minutes. If severe lactase deficiency is suspected, the lactose dosage may be decreased.
- Collect blood samples following lactose ingestion in 30 minutes and in 1, 2, and 3 hours.
- Conduct test adjacent to a bathroom in the event that diarrhea because of lactose intolerance occurs.
- If the lactose tolerance test is abnormal, a glucose tolerance test may be ordered.

Factors Affecting Laboratory Results

- In the diabetic, an abnormal lactose tolerance can be due to abnormal carbohydrate metabolism.
- Twenty percent of individuals can have either a false-positive or false-negative test result.

NURSING IMPLICATIONS WITH RATIONALE

- Obtain a history from the client of abdominal cramps and diarrhea that occur following ingestion of milk. Notify the health care provider of finding because this usually indicates lactose intolerance. The test may be canceled.
- Assess the client during and following the procedure for symptoms of abdominal cramps, pain, nausea, and watery diarrhea. Report findings.

Client Teaching

- Instruct the client with a lactose intolerance to buy lactose-free milk. It can be purchased in most grocery stores. Calcium supplements may be necessary.
- Explain to the client the test procedure. Instruct the client to remain NPO for 8–12 hours (as determined by the institution's protocol) before the test. Tell the client that he or she will have four blood specimens collected within 2–2½ hours.
- Instruct the client not to exercise 8 hours before the test and not to smoke during the test because smoking can increase the blood glucose level.

Latex allergy testing (serum)

Latex-Specific IgE

Reference Values

Negative: Less than 0.35 international unit/mL by EIA.

Positive: Greater than 0.35 international unit/mL by EIA.

Description

Many persons, including health care professionals, are allergic to latex-containing medical products, such as gloves, catheters, condoms, and bandages. Allergic reactions can range from mild to severe. Clients, including health personnel, who have a questionable allergy to latex should be tested for latex allergy. Health professionals who are allergic to latex can use nonallergic gloves.

Since 1987, health care providers have been required to wear gloves as a standard precaution to protect self and others from organisms. It is predicted that 10–15% of health care providers are allergic to latex.

The latex allergy test measures IgE latex sensitivity. There are two types of allergic reactions to latex: type IV, which is allergic contact dermatitis caused by chemicals used in the process of manufacturing latex, and type I, which occurs from the proteins in the natural latex product. Latex actually comes from the rubber tree; it is collected from the tree before it hardens and becomes rubber.

Purpose

- To detect sensitivity to the use of latex products by clients or health professionals.

Clinical Problems

Increased Level: Allergy to latex products, industrial exposure to latex, use of latex catheter (retention latex catheters), multiple surgeries requiring latex products.

Procedure

- There is no food or fluid restriction.
- Collect 5–7 mL of venous blood in a red-top tube.

Factors Affecting Laboratory Results

- None known.

NURSING IMPLICATIONS WITH RATIONALE

- Obtain a history of allergy to latex products, such as gloves and retention catheters.
- Note if the client has swelling or itching from latex exposure to hands or body.
- Note if there is hand eczema present.
- Record the presence of latex allergy on the client's chart.

L

Client Teaching

- Instruct the client or health professional with an allergic reaction to latex to avoid contact with latex products. Inform him or her that there are nonallergic products available.
- Encourage the client to read labels before purchasing products that may contain latex.
- Instruct clients that when asked if they are allergic to drugs, they should include latex products if they have a latex allergy.

LDH isoenzymes

See Lactic Dehydrogenase

Lead (blood)

Reference Values

Adult: *Normal:* 10–20 mcg/dL. *Acceptable:* 20–40 mcg/dL. *Excessive:* 40–80 mcg/dL. *Toxic:* 80 mcg/dL.

Child: *Normal:* 10–20 mcg/dL. *Acceptable:* 20–30 mcg/dL. *Excessive:* 30–50 mcg/dL. *Toxic:* 50 mcg/dL.

Description

Excessive lead exposure due to occupational contact is a hazard to adults; however, most industries will accept a 40 mcg/dL blood lead level as a normal value. Lead toxicity can occur in children from ingesting chipped lead-based paint found in old houses. Sources of lead include leaded gasoline (fumes), lead-based paint, unglazed pottery, and "moonshine" whiskey prepared in lead containers.

Lead is usually excreted rapidly in the urine, but if excessive lead exposure persists, the lead will accumulate in the bones and soft tissues. Chronic lead poisoning is more common than acute poisoning. Lead colic (crampy abdominal pain) occurs in both acute and chronic lead poisoning.

Purpose

- To check for lead toxicity.

Clinical Problems

Increased Level: Leaded gasoline, including fumes; lead-based paint; unglazed pottery; batteries; lead containers used for storage; heat stroke (mobilizes lead stored in the body).

Procedure

- There is no food or fluid restriction.
- Collect 5–7 mL of venous blood in a brown- or royal-blue-top tube.
- Urine may be requested for a 24-hour quantitative test; a lead-free container must be used.

Factors Affecting Laboratory Results

- None reported.

NURSING IMPLICATIONS WITH RATIONALE

Increased Level

- Obtain a history from the client and/or parent concerning lead exposure. Record this history on the chart, and report the information to the health care provider.
- Observe for signs and symptoms of lead poisoning: lead colic (crampy abdominal pain), constipation, occasional bloody diarrhea, behavioral changes (from lethargy to hyperactivity, aggression, impulsiveness), tremors, and confusion.
- Monitor the urinary output, because lead toxicity can decrease kidney function. A urine output of less than 25 mL/h should be reported.
- Monitor the medical treatment for removing body lead, such as chelation therapy. The principal chelating agent is calcium disodium edetate, which combines metal with calcium substance.
- Provide adequate fluid intake. Adequate hydration prevents hemoconcentration.

Client Teaching

- Instruct those in high-risk groups to have their blood lead levels monitored.
- Instruct clients who are exposed to lead (in their occupations) that blood levels should be monitored. These persons should definitely keep medical appointments.
- Suggest to parents ways of satisfying children's hunger (e.g., attention) and a method of providing psychological satisfaction that may replace the child's desire to eat lead chips.

LE cell test; lupus erythematosus cell test (blood)
Lupus Test, LE Prep, LE Preparation, LE Slide Cell Test

Reference Values

Adult: Negative, no LE cells.

Child: Negative.

Description

The lupus erythematosus (LE) cell test, a screening test for SLE (systemic lupus erythematosus), is a nonspecific test. Positive results have been reported in those having rheumatoid arthritis, scleroderma, and lupus induced by drugs, such as penicillin, tetracycline, Dilantin, and oral contraceptives. The test is positive in 60–80% of those having SLE. Antinuclear antibodies or anti-deoxyribonucleic acid (anti-DNA) are more sensitive tests for lupus and should be used to confirm SLE. The LE cell test has been replaced by the ANA test.

Purposes

- To aid in the diagnosis of SLE.
- To compare with ANA and/or anti-DNA tests for diagnosing SLE.

Clinical Problems

Increased Level: Systemic lupus erythematosus, scleroderma, rheumatoid arthritis, chronic hepatitis. *Drug Influence:* Hydralazine (Apresoline), procainamide (Pronestyl), quinidine, anticonvulsants (phenytoin [Dilantin], Mesantoin, Tridione), oral contraceptives, methysergide, antibiotics (penicillin, tetracycline, streptomycin), sulfonamides, methyldopa (Aldomet), isoniazid (INH), clofibrate, reserpine, phenylbutazone.

Procedure

- There is no food or fluid restriction.
- Collect 3–5 mL of venous blood in a red-top tube.
- List on the laboratory slip drugs taken that might affect the test result.

Factors Affecting Laboratory Results

- Certain drugs can cause false-positive test results (*see Drug Influence*).
- Hemolysis of the blood sample could affect the test result.

NURSING IMPLICATIONS WITH RATIONALE

- Compare LE cell test results with those of serum ANA or anti-DNA, or both. The LE test should not be the only test used to diagnose SLE.
- Observe for signs and symptoms of SLE (e.g., fatigue, fever, rash [butterfly over the nose], leukopenia, thrombocytopenia).
- Be supportive of the client and family.

Client Teaching

- Encourage the client to have daily rest periods, which help to decrease symptoms.

Lecithin/sphingomyelin (L/S) ratio (amniotic fluid)

Reference Values

Before 35 Weeks of Gestation: 1:1. *Lecithin (L):* 6–9 mg/dL. *Sphingomyelin (S):* 4–6 mg/dL.
After 35 Weeks of Gestation: 4:1. *Lecithin (L):* 15–21 mg/dL. *Sphingomyelin (S):* 4–6 mg/dL.

Description

The lecithin/sphingomyelin (L/S) ratio can be used to predict neonatal respiratory distress syndrome (also called hyaline membrane disease) before delivery. Lecithin (L), a phospho-lipid, is responsible mostly for the formation of alveolar surfactant. Surfactant lubricates the alveolar lining and inhibits alveolar collapse, thus preventing atelectasis. Sphingomyelin (S) is another phospholipid, the value of which remains the same throughout pregnancy. A marked rise in amniotic lecithin after 35 weeks (to a level three or four times higher than that of sphingomyelin) is considered normal, and so chances for having hyaline membrane disease are small. The L/S ratio is also used to determine fetal maturity in the event that the gestation period is uncertain. In this situation, the L/S ratio is determined at intervals of a period of several weeks.

Purpose

- To check for possible neonatal respiratory distress syndrome (hyaline membrane disease) prior to delivery.

Clinical Problems

Decreased Ratio after 35 Weeks: Respiratory distress syndrome, hyaline membrane disease.

Procedure

- The client should sign a consent form.
- There is no food, fluid, or drug restriction.
- The physician obtains amniotic fluid by the method of amniocentesis. The specimen should be cooled immediately to prevent the destruction of lecithin by certain enzymes in the amniotic fluid. The specimen should be frozen if testing cannot be done at a specified time (check with the laboratory).
- Care should be taken to prevent puncture of the mother's bladder. If urine in the specimen is suspected, then the specimen should be tested for urea and potassium. If these two levels are higher than blood levels, the specimen could be urine and not amniotic fluid. Ultrasound is frequently used when obtaining amniotic fluid.

Factors Affecting Laboratory Results

- Maternal vaginal secretions or a bloody tap into the amniotic fluid may cause a falsely increased reading for lecithin.
- The amniotic fluid specimen should be tested immediately to prevent inaccurate results.

NURSING IMPLICATIONS WITH RATIONALE

- Check the procedures for amniocentesis. Explain the procedure to the client. Assist the health care provider in obtaining amniotic fluid.
- Obtain a fetal history of problems occurring during gestation. Also, ask for and report information on any previous children born with respiratory distress syndrome.
- Be supportive of the mother and her family before, during, and after the test. Remain with the client and answer her questions, if possible, or refer her questions to appropriate professional personnel.
- Assess the newborn at delivery for respiratory complications (substernal retractions, increased respiratory rate, labored breathing, and expiratory grunts).

L

Legionnaires antibody (serum)

Reference Value

Negative.

Description

Legionnaires disease, caused by a gram-negative bacillus, *Legionella pneumophila*, causes acute respiratory infections, such as severe, consolidated pneumonia. This organism is in the soil and water (lakes, streams, reservoirs) and is passed by inhalation of the bacillus in water aerosolized through plumbing fixtures (shower heads, whirlpool baths) and air-conditioning systems (cooling towers and condensers). The bacteria can be isolated from blood, sputum, pleural fluid, and lung-tissue specimen.

A fourfold rise in antibody titer greater than 1:128 during the acute and convalescent phase or a single titer greater than 1:256 is evidence of the disease. Several blood samples and a tissue specimen are useful in confirming Legionnaires disease.

Purpose

- To diagnose the presence of Legionnaires disease.

Clinical Problems

Increased Antibody Titer: Legionnaires disease.

Procedure

- There is no food or fluid restriction.
- Collect 3–5 mL of venous blood in a red-top tube. Tissue specimen from the lung or bronchiole site may be used.

Factors Affecting Laboratory Results

- None known.

NURSING IMPLICATIONS WITH RATIONALE

- Obtain a history from the client as to where he or she has been in the last week, such as hotel or other institutional site.
- Assess the client's respiratory status by inspection, palpation, percussion, and auscultation.
- Observe for signs and symptoms of Legionnaires disease, such as malaise, high fever, chills, cough, chest pain, and tachypnea. Fever rises rapidly to 39–41°C or to 102–105°F.

Client Teaching

- Inform the client that Legionnaires disease is not transmitted from person to person but through aerosol means, such as exhaust vents and fans.

Leucine aminopeptidase (LAP) (serum)

Reference Values

Adult: 8–22 microunit/mL, 12–33 international unit/L, 75–200 unit/mL, 20–50 unit/L at 37°C (SI units). Varies according to laboratory method.

Description

The leucine aminopeptidase (LAP) enzyme is produced by the liver and tends to parallel serum alkaline phosphatase (ALP), except that the LAP level is normal in bone disease or malabsorption syndrome. Alkaline phosphatase may be abnormal in liver and bone disease. LAP is not an indicator of pancreatic carcinoma as was once thought. It is an indicator for biliary obstruction caused by liver metastases and choledocholithiasis (calculi in the common bile duct).

This enzyme test is not frequently ordered, but it is useful as a supplement test in evaluating hepatobiliary disease.

Purpose

- To compare with other liver enzyme tests for diagnosing liver disease.

Clinical Problems

Increased Level: Cancer of the liver, extrahepatic biliary obstruction (stones), acute necrosis of the liver, viral hepatitis.

Procedure

- There is no food or fluid restriction.
- Collect 3–5 mL of venous blood in a red-top tube.

Factors Affecting Laboratory Results

- None reported.

L

NURSING IMPLICATIONS WITH RATIONALE

Increased Level

- Compare LAP with other tests for liver dysfunction, such as the alkaline phosphatase, alanine aminotransferase, and gamma glutamyl transpeptidase (GGT) tests. The LAP test is frequently used to verify the results of other laboratory tests. It is not considered as sensitive as the other tests, and therefore it is not as commonly used.

Leukoagglutinin test (blood, serum)

Reference Values

Negative: No dye uptake.

Positive: Dye uptake in the lymphocytes.

Description

Leukoagglutinins are antibodies that react with white blood cells and can cause a transfusion reaction. Fever may accompany the transfusion reaction. Usually the leukoagglutinin antibodies develop after the client has received white blood cells (WBCs) through transfusion or pregnancy. Normally the client has antibodies to the donor's WBCs; however, the donor could have antibodies to the client's WBCs. The transfusion reaction can occur even though compatible blood has been given. Severe transfusion reactions can lead to pulmonary infiltrates and multiorgan system failure.

To detect leukoagglutinins, the recipient's serum is tested with the donor's lymphocytes. The lymphocytes are examined under the microscope for cell damage. Agglutinating antibodies may be present in the donor or recipient's plasma.

Purpose

- To detect leukoagglutinin antibodies that may be a contributing factor to transfusion reaction.

Clinical Problems

Positive Test: Pregnancy, numerous transfusions.

Procedure

- No food or fluid restriction is required.
- Collect 7 mL of venous blood in a red- or lavender-top tube.

Factors Affecting Laboratory Results

- Blood transfusion dextran that has been previously administered.

NURSING IMPLICATIONS WITH RATIONALE

- Obtain a history of past blood transfusions and ascertain whether adverse effects occurred.
- Record baseline vital signs (VS). Vital signs can be compared with those taken during a transfusion or if a transfusion reaction occurs. Acetaminophen may be prescribed prior to a transfusion to avoid febrile state, as indicated.
- Administer leukocyte-poor blood that has been separated from the donor's blood when necessary to avoid a transfusion reaction.

Client Teaching

- Listen to the client's concerns. Answer questions or refer to other health professionals.

Lidocaine hydrochloride (blood, serum, plasma)
Xylocaine

Reference Values

Therapeutic Range: *Adult:* 1.5–5 mcg/mL, 6–22.5 µmol/L (SI units). *Child:* Similar to adult.
Toxic Level: *Adult:* 0.6 mg/mL. *Child:* Similar to adult.

Description

For treating acute ventricular arrhythmia, IV lidocaine is one of the drugs of choice. It obtains its antiarrhythmic effect by suppressing automaticity and increasing the electrical stimulation threshold of the ventricle. Lidocaine is also used as a local anesthetic.

Lidocaine is metabolized in the liver to active metabolites; about 70% of the metabolites are bound to plasma protein. An initial bolus of parenteral lidocaine (50–100 mg) has a half-life of 10 minutes; however, the half-life is lengthened to 2 hours with continuous IV administration. Steady state occurs 6–12 hours after IV lidocaine infusion. Ninety percent of the drug is excreted in the urine as metabolites and 10% is excreted unchanged.

Monitoring lidocaine levels is necessary to maintain therapeutic level and to avoid lidocaine toxicity. The maximum dose of lidocaine IV and bolus is 300 mg/h.

Purposes

- To monitor lidocaine levels for therapeutic effect.
- To check for lidocaine toxicity.

Clinical Problems

Decreased Level: *Drug Influence:* Barbiturates, phenytoin (Dilantin).
Increased Level: *Excess Dosage of Lidocaine:* Shock, liver and heart diseases. *Drug Influence:* Cimetidine (Tagamet), propranolol (Inderal).

Procedure

- There is no food or fluid restriction.
- Collect 3–5 mL in a red-top tube. Draw blood specimen 6–12 hours after starting lidocaine therapy for dysrhythmia prophylaxis. Then check serum levels daily as ordered.
- Record dose, time, and route (bolus or infusion) of lidocaine administration on the laboratory requisition slip.

Factors Affecting Laboratory Results

- Incorrect blood-collecting tube. Check with the laboratory for the type of collecting tube.

NURSING IMPLICATIONS WITH RATIONALE

- Monitor therapeutic drug level every 12 hours, especially when cardiac or liver insufficiency exists. The maximum dose is 300 mg/h.

L

- Regulate the IV rate using microchamber tubing and an infusion pump. Normally, no more than 4 mg/min should be infused.

Increased Level

- Observe for signs and symptoms of side effects of lidocaine and of lidocaine toxicity (drowsiness, dizziness, lightheadedness, confusion, disorientation, irritability, apprehension, double vision). High doses (greater than 9 mcg/mL, 38.4 µmol/L) may produce convulsions, hypotension, bradycardia, and shock.

Lipase (serum)

Reference Values

Adult: 20–180 international unit/L, 114–286 unit/L, 14–280 unit/L (SI units). Norms vary among laboratories.
Child: *Infant:* 9–105 international unit/L at 37°C. *Child:* 20–136 international unit/L at 37°C.

Description

Lipase, an enzyme secreted by the pancreas, aids in digesting fats. Lipase, like amylase, appears in the bloodstream following damage to the pancreas. Acute pancreatitis is the most common cause for an elevated serum lipase level. Lipase and amylase levels increase early in the disease, but serum lipase can be elevated for up to 14 days after an acute episode, whereas the serum amylase returns to normal after approximately 3 days. Serum lipase is useful for a late diagnosis of acute pancreatitis.

Purpose

- To suggest acute pancreatitis or other pancreatic disorders (*see Clinical Problems*).

Clinical Problems

Decreased Level: Late cancer of the pancreas, hepatitis.

Increased Level: Acute and chronic pancreatitis, cancer of the pancreas (early stage), perforated ulcer, obstruction of the pancreatic duct, acute cholecystitis (some cases), acute renal failure (early stage). *Drug Influence:* Codeine, morphine, meperidine (Demerol), bethanechol (Urecholine), steroids, guanethidine.

Procedure

- NPO except water for 8–12 hours.
- Collect 3–5 mL of venous blood in a red-top tube. Avoid hemolysis.
- Narcotics should be withheld for 24 hours prior to the test. If narcotics are administered within the 24 hours, the drug and the time administered should be written on the laboratory slip.

Factors Affecting Laboratory Results

- Most narcotic drugs elevate the serum lipase level.
- Food eaten within 8 hours prior to the test may interfere with serum lipase levels.
- The presence of hemoglobin and calcium ions may cause a decreased serum lipase level.

NURSING IMPLICATIONS WITH RATIONALE

Increased Level

- Relate elevated serum lipase and amylase levels to acute pancreatitis.
- Notify the health care provider when abdominal pain persists for several days. A serum lipase determination may be ordered because it is an effective test for latent diagnosis of acute pancreatitis. Lipase levels may remain elevated in the blood for 2 weeks.

Lipoproteins, lipoprotein electrophoresis, lipids (serum)

Reference Values

Adult: *Total:* 400–800 mg/dL, 4–8 g/L (SI units). *Cholesterol:* 150–240 mg/dL (*see test on Cholesterol*). *Triglycerides:* 10–190 mg/dL (*see test on Triglycerides*). *Phospholipids:* 150–380 mg/dL.

LDL: 60–160 mg/dL. *Risk for CHD:* High: Greater than 160 mg/dL. Moderate: 130–159 mg/dL. Low: Less than 130 mg/dL. Desirable: 100 mg/dL.

HDL: 29–77 mg/dL. *Risk for CHD:* High: Less than 35 mg/dL. Moderate: 35–45 mg/dL. Low: 46–59 mg/dL. Very low: Greater than 60 mg/dL.

Child: (*See tests on Cholesterol and Triglycerides.*)

Description

Lipoproteins are lipids bound to protein, and the three main lipoproteins are cholesterol, triglycerides, and phospholipids. The two fractions of lipoproteins—alpha (α), high-density lipoproteins (HDL), and beta (β), low-density lipoproteins (chylomicrons, VLDL, LDL)—can be separated by electrophoresis. The beta groups are the largest contributors of atherosclerosis and coronary artery disease. HDL, called "friendly lipids," are composed of 50% protein and aid in decreasing plaque deposits in blood vessels.

Increased lipoproteins (hyperlipidemia or hyperlipoproteinemia) can be phenotyped into five major types (I, IIA and IIB, III, IV, V). Cholesterol and triglycerides are the two lipids in each type found in varying amounts. With type II, the cholesterol is highly elevated, and the triglycerides are slightly increased. With type IV, the triglycerides are highly elevated, and the cholesterol is slightly increased. Types II and IV are the most common phenotypes and are the most prevalent in atherosclerosis and coronary artery disease.

Lipoprotein Phenotype: Hyperlipidemia

TYPE	LIPID COMPOSITION*
I	Increased chylomicrons, increased triglycerides; rare pattern of hyperlipidemia
IIA	Increased beta (low-density) lipoproteins (LDL); increased cholesterol, slightly increased triglycerides or normal; common pattern of hyperlipidemia
IIB	Increased beta and pre-beta lipoproteins, both cholesterol and triglycerides are elevated; common pattern of hyperlipidemia
III	Moderately increased cholesterol and triglycerides; uncommon pattern of hyperlipidemia
IV	Increase of pre-beta (very low-density) lipoproteins (VLDL); slightly increased cholesterol and markedly increased triglycerides; common pattern of hyperlipidemia
V	Increased chylomicrons, VLDL, and triglycerides, and slightly increased cholesterol; uncommon pattern of hyperlipidemia

*Types II and IV are increased in atherosclerosis and coronary artery diseases.

Purposes

- To identify clients with hyperlipoproteinemia.
- To distinguish between the phenotypes of lipidemias.
- To monitor lipid counts for clients with hyperlipidemia.

Clinical Problems

Decreased Level: Tangier disease, chronic obstructive lung disease. *Drug Influence: (See Cholesterol and Triglycerides.)*

Increased Level: Hyperlipoproteinemia, acute myocardial infarction, hypothyroidism, diabetes mellitus, nephrotic syndrome, eclampsia, Laënnec cirrhosis, multiple myeloma, diet (high in saturated fats). *Drug Influence: (See Cholesterol and Triglycerides.)*

Procedure

- NPO except for water for 12 hours before the test. The client should be on a regular diet for 3 days before the test. No alcohol intake for 24 hours.
- Collect 7 mL of venous blood in a red-top tube.

Factors Affecting Laboratory Results

- A diet high in saturated fats and sugar could elevate test results.
- Certain drugs can increase or decrease serum lipoproteins (*see Clinical Problems, Drug Influence for Cholesterol and Triglycerides*).

NURSING IMPLICATIONS WITH RATIONALE

- Check the client's serum cholesterol, serum triglyceride, LDL, and HDL levels. This information is helpful for teaching purposes and in answering the client's questions.

Client Teaching

- Instruct the client with hyperlipoproteinemia to avoid foods high in saturated fats and sugar (e.g., bacon, cream, butter, fatty meats, and candy).
- Answer client's questions concerning risk of coronary artery disease related to LDL and HDL.

Lithium (serum)

Eskalith, Lithobid, Eskalith CR, Lithotabs, Cibalith

Reference Values

Adult: *Normal:* Negative. *Therapeutic:* 0.8–1.2 mEq/L. *Toxic:* Greater than 1.5 mEq/L. *Lethal:* Greater than 4 mEq/L.

Child: Not usually given to children.

Description

Lithium, or lithium salt, is used to treat manic-depressive (bipolar) psychosis. This agent is used to correct the mania in manic-depression and to prevent depression. Because therapeutic and toxic lithium levels are narrow, serum lithium should be closely monitored.

Lithium salt was first used in the 1940s as a salt substitute; this practice was abandoned in the late 1940s because of its high toxicity. It was not used in the United States until after 1965, and then was used for treatment of manic-depression (bipolar).

Purposes

- To identify lithium toxicity.
- To monitor lithium levels for therapeutic effect and toxicity.

Clinical Problems

Increased Level: *Toxicity:* Lithium carbonate (Eskalith, Lithane, Lithonate), lithium bromide.

Procedure

- There is no food or fluid restriction.
- Collect 5–7 mL of venous blood in a red-top tube 8–12 hours after the last lithium dose.
- The lithium tolerance test may be ordered instead of the conventional blood sample. A base blood specimen is obtained, and then the lithium dose is given. Blood specimens are collected 1, 3, and 6 hours after the lithium dose.

Factors Affecting Laboratory Results

- None reported.

L

NURSING IMPLICATIONS WITH RATIONALE

- Observe for signs and symptoms of lithium overdose (slurred speech, muscle spasm, confusion, and nystagmus). Lithium dosage should be lower in the older adult (over 65 years) than in the middle-aged adult. Lithium test results should always be reported to the health care provider because of the narrow range of the "therapeutic" dosage.

Client Teaching

- Instruct the client to take the prescribed lithium dosage daily and to keep his or her medical appointments. Periodic blood specimens will need to be drawn to determine lithium levels.
- Suggest to the nursing mother taking lithium that the pediatrician should be notified before she breastfeeds the infant. Breast milk can contain high levels of lithium.
- Encourage adequate fluid and sodium intake while the client is maintained on lithium. Lithium inhibits antidiuretic hormone secretion, causing body water loss. Diuretics should be avoided.

Lupus erythematosus cell
See LE Cell Test

Luteinizing hormone (LH) (serum and urine)
Interstitial Cell-Stimulating Hormone (ICSH)

Reference Values

Ranges vary among laboratories.

Serum: *Adult:* Female: Follicular phase: 5–30 milli-international unit/mL (mIU/mL). Midcycle: 50–150 milli-international unit/mL. Luteal phase: 2–25 milli-international unit/mL. Postmenopausal: 40–100 milli-international unit/mL. Male: 5–25 milli-international unit/mL. *Child:* 6–12 years: Less than 10 milli-international unit/mL, 13–18 years: Less than 20 milli-international unit/mL.

Urine: *Adult:* Female: Follicular phase: 5–25 international unit/24 h. Midcycle: 30–90 international unit/24 h. Luteal phase: 2–24 international unit/24 h. Postmenopausal: greater than 40 international unit/24 h. Male: 7–25 international unit/mL.

Description

Luteinizing hormone (LH), a gonadotropic hormone secreted by the anterior pituitary gland, is needed (with follicle-stimulating hormone [FSH]) for ovulation to occur. After ovulation, LH aids in stimulating the corpus luteum in secreting progesterone. FSH values are frequently evaluated with LH values. In men, LH stimulates testosterone production, and with FSH, it influences the development and maturation of spermatozoa.

LH testing is usually ordered to evaluate infertility in women and men. High serum values are related to gonadal dysfunction, and low serum values are related to hypothalamus or pituitary failure. Women taking oral contraceptives have an absence of midcycle LH peak until the contraceptives are discontinued. This test might be used to evaluate hormonal therapy for inducing ovulation.

Purposes

- To evaluate the serum or urine LH level for determining the cause of hormonal dysfunction.
- To identify the gynecologic problem related to excess or deficit of LH.

Clinical Problems

Decreased Level: Hypogonadotropinism (defects in pituitary gland or hypothalamus), anovulation, amenorrhea (pituitary failure), hypophysectomy, testicular failure, hypothalamic dysfunction, adrenal hyperplasia or tumors. *Drug Influence:* Oral contraceptives, estrogen compounds, testosterone administration.

Increased Level: Amenorrhea (ovarian failure), tumors (pituitary, testicular), precocious puberty, testicular failure, Turner syndrome, Klinefelter syndrome, premature menopause, Stein-Leventhal syndrome, polycystic ovary syndrome, liver disease.

Procedure

Serum

- There is no food or fluid restriction.
- Collect 3–5 mL of venous blood in a red- or lavender-top tube. Avoid hemolysis. Daily blood samples must be taken at the same time each day to determine if ovulation occurs.
- Note on the laboratory slip the phase of the menstrual cycle, client's age, and if client is postmenopausal.
- Withhold, 24–48 hours before the test, medications that could interfere with test results (check with health care provider).

Urine

- Collect 24-hour urine specimen in a container with a preservative, or keep refrigerated if no preservative is added.
- Label the specimen with the client's name, date, and time.

Factors Affecting Laboratory Results

- Hormones (estrogen, progesterone, and testosterone) and oral contraceptives could decrease plasma LH value.
- Hemolysis of the blood sample could affect test result.
- Collection of the daily specimen at different times of the day may cause inaccurate result.

NURSING IMPLICATIONS WITH RATIONALE

- Obtain a menstrual history from the client. Record the menstrual phase on the laboratory slip.
- Check with the health care provider about withholding medications that could affect test results.
- Be supportive of client and family.

Client Teaching

- Instruct client to express concerns about infertility or other health problems.
- Explain to the client to keep an accurate account of her menstrual cycle.

Lyme disease (antibody)

Reference Value

Titer: Negative: Less than 1:256. Indirect fluorescent antibody (IFA) titer. ELISA or Western blot.

Description

Borrelia burgdorferi is the spirochete that causes Lyme disease. Several tick vectors, primarily the deer tick, carry the spirochete, which can be cultivated, with difficulty, from the blood, CSF, or skin biopsies. Lyme disease is most prevalent in the northeastern, upper midwestern, and western states.

A reddish, macular lesion usually occurs about 1 week after the tick bite. The infected tick bite can affect the central and peripheral nervous systems, causing a neuritis or aseptic meningitis. Also, it can affect the heart and joints, causing transient electrocardiographic abnormalities, carditis, and problems in one or more joints, mostly the knees, leading to arthritis (may take from a few weeks to 2 years to become symptomatic).

Immunoglobulins (IgM and IgG) aid in diagnosing early, late, or remission stage of Lyme disease. IgM titers occur approximately 2–4 weeks after the onset of disease, peaking at 6–8 weeks before levels decrease. IgG titers occur 1–3 months after onset of Lyme disease and peak at 4–6 months. IgG may remain elevated for months or years. Symptoms such as fever with flulike symptoms may begin 1 week after the spirochete infection. An erythematous, circular rash at the tick site frequently appears. The client may also suffer with malaise, headache, and muscle or joint aches and pain. Testing should be done 4–6 weeks after being infected. If the client has symptoms and the test is performed earlier with negative findings, a repeated test should be performed a week or two later. Antibiotic therapy is usually prescribed when symptoms are apparent even if the test result is negative.

Purpose

- To detect the occurrence of Lyme disease.

Clinical Problems

Positive Titer: Lyme disease.

Procedure

- There is no food or fluid restriction.
- Collect 3–5 mL of venous blood in a red-top tube.
- Repeat Lyme disease antibody test for symptomatic clients with early negative test result.

Factors Affecting Laboratory Results

- Persons with a high rheumatoid factor could have a false-positive test result.

NURSING IMPLICATIONS WITH RATIONALE

- Report a history of a tick bite.
- Assess for a macular lesion at the site of the tick bite and elsewhere.
- Check titer level. A fourfold rise in titer is indicative of a recent infection.

Client Teaching

- Instruct the client to wear clothing that completely covers the extremities when in the woods and areas infested by ticks and deer.
- Instruct the client to see his or her health care provider immediately if bitten by a tick or if a macular lesion results from a tick bite. Antibiotic therapy is frequently started.
- Inform the client that the most common complication of Lyme disease is arthritis. Others are cardiac dysrhythmias, carditis, and neuritis.

Lymphocytes (T and B) (blood)

T and B Lymphocytes; Lymphocyte Marker Studies; Lymphocyte Subset Typing

Reference Values

Adult: *T Cells:* 60–80%, 600–2,400 cells/µL. *B Cells:* 4–16%, 50–250 cells/µL.

Description

The two categories of lymphocytes are T lymphocytes and B lymphocytes. The T lymphocytes are associated with cell-mediated immune responses (cellular immunity), such as rejection of transplant and graft, tumor immunity, and microorganism (bacterial and viral) death. If the surface of the host's tissue cell is altered, the T cells might perceive that altered cell as foreign and attack it. This might be helpful if the altered surface is of tumor development; however, this T-cell attack might give rise to autoimmune disease.

The B lymphocytes, derived from bone marrow, are responsible for humoral immunity. The B cells synthesize immunoglobulins to react to specific antigens. An interaction between T and B lymphocytes is necessary for a satisfactory immune response.

Measurement of T and B lymphocytes is valuable for diagnosing autoimmune diseases (e.g., immunosuppressive diseases such as acquired immunodeficiency syndrome [AIDS], lymphoma, and lymphocytic leukemia). T and B cells can be used to monitor changes during the treatment of immunosuppressive diseases.

Purposes

- To detect selected autoimmune diseases, such as lymphoma and lymphocytic leukemia.
- To monitor the effects of treatment for immunosuppressive diseases, such as AIDS.

Clinical Problems

Decreased Level: *T Lymphocytes:* Lymphoma, systemic lupus erythematosus, thymic hypoplasia (DiGeorge syndrome), acute viral infections. *Drug Influence:* Immunosuppressive agents. *B Lymphocytes:* IgG, IgA, IgM deficiency, lymphomas, nephrotic syndrome, sex-linked agammaglobulinemia. *T and B Lymphocytes:* Immunodeficiency diseases. *Drug Influence:* Immunosuppressive agents.

Increased Level: *T Lymphocytes:* Autoimmune disorders such as Graves disease. *B Lymphocytes:* Acute and chronic lymphocytic leukemias, multiple myeloma, Waldenström macroglobulinemia.

Procedure

- There is no food or fluid restriction.
- Collect two 7 mL samples of venous blood in 2 lavender-top tubes. Refrigerate blood samples. *Check the laboratory procedures in your institution.*

Factors Affecting Laboratory Result

- An insufficient amount of blood drawn for the test could affect test result.

NURSING IMPLICATIONS WITH RATIONALE

- Keep the client free from exposure to infection.
- Observe for signs and symptoms of lymphocytic leukemias (e.g., fatigue, pallor, vesicular skin lesions, increased white blood cell count).

Client Teaching

- Instruct the client to stay away from persons with colds or communicable diseases.
- Listen to the client's concern.

Macular degeneration risk analysis (serum)

Reference Value

Absence of macular changes.

Description

Macular degeneration is a leading cause of blindness. Common symptoms include distorted, wavy lines or blurred vision and difficulty in adjusting to dim light. There are two types of macular degeneration: dry and wet. Wet macular degeneration is considered a more severe type. Two theories concerning the cause of this disease are genetic (Y402H and A695 variants) and environmental (such as smoking). Persons with an increase in either Y402H or A695 have a greater risk for developing macular degeneration. With clinical visual examination by an ophthalmologist, genetic type from blood sample, and environmental history, the diagnosis of macular degeneration can usually be made.

M

Purposes

- To assess the degree of macular degeneration.
- To obtain genetic information of macular degeneration and the degree of progression.

Clinical Problems

Increased Macular Changes: Dry or wet macular degeneration in variant degrees, environmental and genetic factors associated with macular degeneration.

Procedure

- There is no food or fluid restriction.
- Collect 5 mL of venous blood in a lavender-top tube to determine the genetic type if present.

NURSING IMPLICATIONS AND RATIONALE

- Obtain a familial history of macular degeneration.
- Report history of changes in vision.

Client Teaching

- Instruct the client to check his or her vision once a week using an Amsler grid. This is a home vision screening for macular degeneration. Check each eye by covering the opposite eye. Report blurred vision, wavy lines, and distorted vision of one or both eyes.
- Suggest taking an antioxidant (eye) vitamin such as PreserVision with lutein or Ocuvite with lutein, with the approval of the ophthalmologist or HCP.
- Answer questions or refer questions to the ophthalmologist.

Magnesium (Mg) (serum)

Reference Values

Adult: 1.5–2.5 mEq/L, 1.8–3 mg/dL.

Child: *Newborn:* 1.4–2.9 mEq/L. *Child:* 1.6–2.6 mEq/L.

Description

Magnesium is most plentiful in the cells (intracellular fluid). One third of the magnesium ingested is absorbed through the small intestine, and the remaining unabsorbed magnesium is excreted in the stools. The absorbed magnesium is eventually excreted through the kidneys.

As with potassium, sodium, and calcium, magnesium is needed for neuromuscular activity. Magnesium influences use of potassium, calcium, and protein, and when there is a magnesium deficit, there is frequently a potassium and calcium deficit. Magnesium is also responsible for the transport of sodium and potassium across the cell membranes. Another function of magnesium is its activation of enzymes for carbohydrate and protein metabolism.

Magnesium is found in most foods, so it would be difficult for a person who maintains a normal diet to have a magnesium deficiency. The daily required magnesium intake for an adult is 200–300 mg, or 0.2–0.3 g.

A serum magnesium deficit is known as hypomagnesemia, and a serum magnesium excess is called hypermagnesemia.

Purposes

- To detect hypomagnesemia or hypermagnesemia.
- To monitor magnesium levels when there is a probable magnesium loss.

Clinical Problems

Decreased Level: Protein malnutrition, malabsorption, cirrhosis of the liver, alcoholism, hypoparathyroidism, hyperaldosteronism, hypokalemia (decreased potassium), IV solutions without magnesium, chronic diarrhea, bowel resection complications, dehydration. *Drug Influence:* Diuretics (mercurial, ethacrynic acid [Edecrin]), calcium gluconate, amphotericin B, neomycin, insulin.

Increased Level: Severe dehydration, renal failure, leukemia (lymphocytic and myelocytic), diabetes mellitus (early phase). *Drug Influence:* Antacids (Maalox, Mylanta, Aludrox, Di-Gel), laxatives (Epsom salts [$MgSO_4$], milk of magnesia, magnesium citrate).

Procedure

- There is no food or fluid restriction.
- Collect 3–5 mL of venous blood in a red-top tube. Avoid hemolysis.

Factors Affecting Laboratory Results

- Hypokalemia and hypocalcemia will decrease the magnesium level.
- Drugs: Laxatives and antacids containing magnesium can cause hypermagnesemia, and diuretics, calcium gluconate, and insulin can cause hypomagnesemia. Insulin moves magnesium back into the cells, causing a serum magnesium deficit.

NURSING IMPLICATIONS WITH RATIONALE

Decreased Level

- Observe for signs and symptoms of hypomagnesemia, such as tetany symptoms (twitching and tremors, carpopedal spasm, generalized spasticity), restlessness, confusion, and arrhythmia. Neuromuscular irritability can be mistakenly attributed to hypocalcemia.
- Check serum potassium, sodium, calcium, and magnesium levels. Electrolyte deficits may accompany a magnesium deficit. If hypokalemia and hypomagnesemia are present, potassium supplements will not completely correct the potassium deficit until the magnesium deficit is corrected.
- Check for a positive Chvostek sign by tapping the facial nerve in front of the ear and observing for spasm of the cheek and twitching at the corner of the lip.

M

- Report to the health care provider if the client has been NPO and receiving IV fluids without magnesium salts for weeks. Hyperalimentation solutions should contain magnesium.
- Check clients receiving digitalis preparations for digitalis intoxication (anorexia, nausea, vomiting, bradycardia). A magnesium deficit enhances the action of digitalis, causing digitalis toxicity.
- Assess renal function when the client is receiving magnesium supplements. Excess magnesium is excreted by the kidneys.
- Assess electrocardiographic changes. A flat or inverted T-wave can be indicative of hypomagnesemia. It can also indicate hypokalemia.
- Administer IV magnesium sulfate in solution slowly to prevent a hot or flushed feeling.
- Have IV calcium gluconate available to reverse hypermagnesemia due to overcorrection. Calcium antagonizes the sedative effect of magnesium.

Client Teaching

- Instruct the client to eat foods rich in magnesium (fish, seafood, meats, green vegetables, whole grains, and nuts).

Increased Level

- Observe for signs and symptoms of hypermagnesemia, such as flushing, a feeling of warmth, increased perspiration (with the magnesium level at 3–4 mEq/L), muscular weakness, diminished reflex, respiratory distress, hypotension, a sedative effect (with the magnesium level at 9–10 mEq/L).
- Monitor urinary output. Effective urinary output (greater than 750 mL daily) will decrease the serum magnesium level.
- Assess the client's level of sensorium and muscle activity.
- Assess ECG changes. A peaked T-wave and wide QRS complex can indicate hyperkalemia (increased potassium) and hypermagnesemia, so the serum potassium and magnesium levels should be checked.
- Provide adequate fluids to improve kidney function and to restore body fluids. Dehydration can cause hemoconcentration and, as a result, magnesium excess.
- Check for digitalis intoxication if the client is receiving calcium gluconate for hypermagnesemia. Calcium excess enhances the action of digitalis.

Client Teaching

- Instruct clients to avoid constant use of laxatives and antacids containing magnesium. Suggest to clients that they check drug labels.

Malaria (blood)

M

Reference Values

Adult: Negative.

Child: Negative.

Description

Malaria is caused by malarial parasites transmitted by mosquitoes. The parasites rupture the red blood cells (hemolysis), causing the client to have chills and fever.

Malarial parasites can be detected by blood smears (venous or capillary blood). Blood samples are usually taken in the presence of chills and fever daily for 3 days or at specified times—every 6 or 12 hours.

Purpose

- To identify the presence of malarial parasites.

Clinical Problems

Positive: Malaria (*Plasmodium* species).

Procedure

- There is no food or fluid restriction.
- Venous or capillary blood can be used for the malarial smear.
- Collect 5 mL in a lavender-top tube.

Factors Affecting Laboratory Results

- None known.

NURSING IMPLICATIONS WITH RATIONALE

- Explain the procedure to the client. The client should inform the nurse when he or she is having chills and fever, because a blood sample is usually requested at that time. The blood sample may also be requested daily for 3 days or at specified times during the day.
- Monitor the client's temperature every 4 hours or as ordered. Record temperature changes.
- Report chills and fever to the health care provider.

Melanin (urine)

Reference Values

Negative for melanogen or melanin.

Description

The melanin urine test is prescribed to verify the presence or progression of a melanoma. Melanin, a pigment in the body, is highly elevated in malignant melanoma. With metastatic melanoma, melanin metabolites, melanogens, are usually found in high concentration in the urine. If the urine is exposed to air for many hours, melanogen is converted to melanin and the urine becomes deep brown and later black. Twenty-five percent of clients with malignant melanoma have melanogen in the urine (melanogenuria). Further testing is necessary to determine the extent of disease.

Purposes

- To detect melanogenuria.
- To aid in the detection of malignant melanoma.

Clinical Problems

Increased Level: Malignant melanoma. *Drug Influence:* Aspirin and aspirin compounds.

Procedure

- There is no food or fluid restriction.
- Collect a random urine specimen and send it immediately to the laboratory.

Factors Affecting Laboratory Results

- Aspirin can give a false-positive test result.
- When urine is left for hours at room temperature, the melanogen will convert to melanin and urine will become dark brown.

NURSING IMPLICATIONS WITH RATIONALE

- Obtain a history of health problems and drugs the client is currently taking. Drugs that contain aspirin can cause a false-positive test result.
- Listen to the client's concerns. Answer questions or refer the questions to other health professionals.

Client Teaching

- Instruct the client concerning urine collection. The urine container should be taken immediately to the laboratory.

Methemoglobin (blood)

Hemoglobin M, Hb M

M

Reference Values

Normal: Less than 1.5% of the total hemoglobin; 0.06–0.24 g/dL, 9.2–37 μmol/L (SI units).

Positive: 20–70%: Complaints of headache, dizziness, fatigue, tachycardia. Greater than 70%: Death.

Description

Methemoglobin (Hb M) occurs when the deoxygenated heme (iron portion of hemoglobin) is oxidized to a ferric state. In the ferric state, the heme cannot combine with oxygen; thus, cyanosis without dyspnea or other cardiovascular problems may result. Methemoglobinemia may be acquired from chemicals, radiation, and such drugs as nitrites, nitrates, certain sulfonamides, antimalarials, local anesthetics, or inherited enzyme deficiency. Poisoning from occupational or environmental contact could cause methemoglobinemia. A deficiency in the glucose-6-phosphate dehydrogenase (G-6-PD) enhances the production of Hb M.

If newborns are cyanotic after oxygen has been given, the methemoglobin level should be checked. Infants are more prone to develop methemoglobinemia.

Purposes

- To detect methemoglobin in the blood caused from an acquired chemical or drug condition.
- To detect congenital methemoglobinemia.

Clinical Problems

Increased Level: Acquired or hereditary methemoglobinemia, radiation, carbon monoxide poisoning, smoking. *Drug Influence:* Bromo-Seltzer, nitrates (include silver nitrate topical preparation), nitrites, nitrous oxide, nitroglycerin, antimalarials, analgesics, certain sulfonamides, fluoroquinolones, benzene derivatives such as chlorobenzene, phenacetin, isoniazid, lidocaine, chlorates. *Food Influence:* Sausage and other foods that contain nitrites.

Procedure

- There is no food or fluid restriction.
- Collect 7 mL of venous blood in a lavender- or green-top tube. Keep blood specimen on ice. Deliver blood specimen to the laboratory within 1 hour.

Factors Affecting Laboratory Results

- Certain drugs and foods can cause false results (*see Clinical Problems*).
- Not keeping the blood specimen chilled (on ice) and not delivering the specimen to the laboratory within 1 hour.

NURSING IMPLICATIONS WITH RATIONALE

- Obtain a history of the health complaints, drugs, and food the client is consuming. Certain drugs can enhance the production of Hb M (*see Clinical Problems*). Excessive use of Bromo-Seltzer can increase the Hb M level.
- Check vital signs. Continuously monitor heart rate with a pulse oximetry.
- Check O_2 saturation with the pulse oximetry or arterial blood gases.
- Administer oxygen. Blood transfusions may be prescribed.

Client Teaching

- Encourage client to rest if dizziness, fatigue, and headaches occur.
- Explain to the client that the health care provider may discontinue a drug that may be causing an increase in Hb M production.

Microalbumin (MA) (urine)

Reference Value
Microalbumin: 0.2–2 mg/dL.

Description
Microalbumin (MA) is a test for albumin accumulation in the urine that is greater than normal. Generally, the glomeruli filter albumin, and it is absorbed by the renal tubules. When the albumin level is not readily absorbed by the renal tubules, albumin spills into the urine. MA precedes nephropathy that is associated with diabetic nephropathy and renal disease. MA is elevated years before creatinine clearance shows abnormal levels.

With diabetics, presence of albumin in the urine as a result of the microalbumin test is an early indicator of diabetic nephropathy. It can also indicate hypertension and cardiovascular disease. MA can identify diabetic nephropathy 5–7 years before an abnormal protein urine level occurs.

It has been suggested that diabetics should have a yearly urine microalbumin test. Also, it is recommended that diabetic clients should keep their blood sugar levels in control. This would aid in decreasing the occurrence of diabetic nephropathy and CVD. For nondiabetics, an increase in urine microalbumin levels could indicate CVD.

Purposes
- To detect the presence of excess albumin in the urine.
- To diagnose the early signs of diabetic nephropathy.
- To identify early renal changes and pre-nephropathy.

Clinical Problems
Increased Level: Diabetic nephropathy, renal insufficiency/disease, hypertension, cardiovascular disease, urinary tract infections, preeclampsia.

Decreased Level: *Drug Influence:* Captopril, enalapril, perindopril, quinapril, ramipril, furosemide, dipyridamole.

Procedure
- There is no food or fluid restriction.
- Collect either a fresh urine specimen or a 24-hour urine specimen. The 24-hour urine specimen is refrigerated. If available, use the Micral Urine Test Strip and follow directions on the label.
- Label the urine specimen according to the time it was taken. Usually a single specimen is obtained in the morning and a 24-hour urine specimen begins in the morning. The first urine specimen is discarded. The urine specimen will be brought to room temperature when it is tested. Label for the 24-hour urine collection should indicate when the first urine specimen was discarded, for example, 6/2/20, at 7 AM to 6/3/20, 7:05 AM.
- The MA test may be repeated in a week if the test results were positive.

Factors Affecting Laboratory Results
- Feces or toilet paper in the urine collection.

NURSING IMPLICATIONS WITH RATIONALE

- Obtain a history of health problems, such as diabetes mellitus, hypertension, cardiovascular disease, renal disease, and urinary tract infections.
- Ascertain, if the client is a diabetic, whether his or her blood sugar is within controlled levels. Does the client have any diabetic complications, for example, eyes, circulation?
- Obtain vital signs. Compare vital signs to previous ones.

Client Teaching

- Explain the procedure for collecting the urine specimen. Normally, if it is a single fresh urine specimen, the client voids in the morning in the small container provided.
- If it is a 24-hour urine collection, instruct the client not to void in the large container but in a nonmetal urinal or container provided and to pour the urine from that container into the large refrigerated container. With a 24-hour urine specimen, the first urine specimen will be discarded. Fecal matter and toilet paper should *not* come in contact with any part of the urine specimens.
- Inform the client that he or she will be notified of the test results. A follow-up MA test may be requested.

Mumps antibody (serum)

Reference Values

Negative: Less than 1:8 titer.

Positive or Immunization: Greater than 1:8 (recent infection or immunization undetermined).

Description

Mumps, also called infectious parotitis, is an acute, contagious viral infection causing an inflammation of the parotid and salivary glands. The mumps virus can be spread by droplets or by direct contact with the saliva of an infected person. Complications of mumps include: (1) in adolescent or adult males, unilateral orchitis in approximately 20% of reported cases, (2) in adult women, oophoritis, and (3) in persons of all ages and genders, meningoencephalitis in 1–10% of infected cases.

Diagnosis may be made by blood specimen, culture of saliva, or mumps skin test. With a blood specimen, there should be two blood samples taken, one during the acute phase and one during the convalescent phase. For those persons who are at high risk or who have not had mumps, there is a vaccine to provide immunity.

M

Purpose

- To detect the presence of the mumps antibody in a person who may be at risk.

Clinical Problems

Positive: Mumps virus. *Complications:* Orchitis, oophoritis, meningoencephalitis.

Procedure

- There is no food or fluid restriction.
- Collect a total of two 3–5 mL samples of venous blood in a red-top tube, 1–2 weeks apart. The first specimen is drawn during the acute phase, and the second is taken 1–2 weeks later during the convalescent phase. Avoid hemolysis.
- Label the first specimen "acute."

Factors Affecting Laboratory Results

- Hemolysis of the blood sample.
- Obtaining one blood specimen only. A total of two blood samples should be obtained to determine not only the acute phase but also when the convalescent phase begins.

NURSING IMPLICATIONS WITH RATIONALE

- Assess the client for symptoms of mumps, which can include malaise, headache, chills, fever, pain below the ear, and swelling of the parotid glands.
- Assess if the client has been in contact with a person diagnosed as having mumps. Clients who are suspected of having mumps may be isolated up to 9 days after swelling occurs.
- Check if the client had received the mumps vaccine. Those who develop mumps normally have a lifetime immunity.

Client Teaching

- Explain to the client that he or she is to return for a second blood test. This is necessary to determine the convalescent phase of the mumps infection.
- Explain to the client that mumps is contagious and he or she should be isolated for approximately 9 days from persons who have never had mumps or the vaccine. The incubation period for mumps is 16 to 18 days.
- Inform the pregnant female that if mumps occurs during the first trimester of pregnancy, the fetus may have a higher risk of developing congenital anomalies. It is suggested to many young females that if they have not had mumps, they should be tested for mumps antibody; and if the result is negative, they should receive the mumps vaccine.

Myoglobin (serum)

M

Reference Values

Adult: 12–90 ng/mL, 12–90 mcg/L.

Female: 12–75 ng/mL, 12–75 mcg/L.

Male: 20–90 ng/mL, 20–90 mcg/L.

Description

Myoglobin is an oxygen-binding protein, similar to hemoglobin, that is found in skeletal and cardiac muscle cells. Myoglobin is released into circulation after an injury. Increased serum myoglobin occurs about 2–6 hours following muscle tissue damage. Serum myoglobin level reaches its peak approximately 8–12 hours following a myocardial infarction (MI). Elevated serum myoglobin (myoglobinemia) is short-lived; in 50% of persons having an MI, the serum level begins to return to normal range in 12–18 hours. Urine myoglobin may be detected for 3–7 days following muscle injury.

Because serum myoglobin is nonspecific concerning which muscle is damaged, myocardium or skeletal, cardiac enzymes should also be ordered. Creatine phosphokinase (CPK) and CPK isoenzyme (CPK-MB) should be checked because this enzyme rises early after an MI. Assessment of signs and symptoms of an acute MI need to be considered along with the blood tests. This test is not performed following cardioversion or after an angina attack.

Purpose

- To detect myoglobin protein, which is released in high amount during skeletal or cardiac muscle injury.

Clinical Problems

Increased Level: Acute MI, skeletal muscle injury, severe burns, polymyositis, trauma, surgical procedure, acute alcohol intoxication with delirium tremens, renal failure, metabolic stress.

Procedure

- There is no food or fluid restriction.
- Collect 3–5 mL of venous blood in a red-top tube. Avoid hemolysis. The blood sample should be drawn soon after an acute MI, following acute pain.

Factors Affecting Laboratory Results

- Blood sample taken for serum myoglobin a day or two after an acute injury, acute chest pain, or myocardial infarction.
- Hemolysis of the blood specimen.

M

NURSING IMPLICATIONS WITH RATIONALE

- Obtain a history of current discomfort. Differentiate, if possible, between heart and skeletal muscle discomfort. Record and inform the health care provider of your findings.
- Assess the client for signs and symptoms of an MI, such as sharp penetrating pain, intense chest pressure, diaphoresis, dyspnea, nausea and vomiting, and indigestion. Report findings immediately.
- Check vital signs. Compare with baseline vital signs. Report changes immediately.
- Compare serum myoglobin results with cardiac enzyme tests. Serum myoglobin usually increases before CPK; however, serum myoglobin elevation could indicate skeletal muscle injury. Various laboratory tests, history, and symptoms need to be considered.

Client Teaching

- Instruct the client to inform you when pain occurs or recurs. Have client describe the pain (type, intensity, duration).
- Allow the client and family member(s) time to express their concerns. As necessary, refer questions to other health care providers.

Myoglobin (urine)

Reference Values

Adult: None detected.

Description

Myoglobin is an oxygen-binding protein, similar to hemoglobin, that is found in skeletal and cardiac muscle cells. Myoglobin is released into circulation soon after a muscle tissue injury (skeletal or cardiac) occurs (*see Myoglobin [serum]*). Myoglobin passes rapidly from the blood through the glomeruli in the kidney and is excreted in the urine. Myoglobinuria can appear within 3 hours after a myocardial infarction (MI) and may be present in the urine up to 72 hours or longer. Usually, the serum myoglobin level returns to normal range within 18–36 hours.

Besides indicating myocardial damage due to a MI, myoglobinuria may occur following a traumatic muscle tissue injury, severe ischemia, diabetic ketoacidosis, delirium tremens, systemic infection with fever, severe burns, and muscular dystrophy. Client's symptoms and other tests should be considered to determine cause of urine myoglobin.

Purpose

(*See Myoglobin [serum].*)

Clinical Problems

Increased Level: Acute MI, skeletal muscle tissue injury, crush injuries from trauma, severe burns, surgical procedure, polymyositis, delirium tremens, metabolic stress.

Procedure

- There is no food or fluid restriction.
- Collect 5–10 mL of random urine specimen in a sterile plastic container. Deliver the urine specimen to the laboratory.

Factors Affecting the Laboratory Results

- Collecting the urine specimen within 3 hours of an acute injury. A repeat urine specimen should be collected 24 hours after the injury (skeletal or cardiac).

NURSING IMPLICATIONS WITH RATIONALE

- Obtain a history of the current muscle discomfort (skeletal or cardiac). Report your findings.
- Assess the client for signs and symptoms of an MI, such as sharp penetrating pain in the chest, radiating pain in the left arm, diaphoresis, dyspnea, nausea, and vomiting. Report your findings immediately.
- Check vital signs and report abnormal findings.
- Compare elevated serum myoglobin level with positive urine myoglobin. Cardiac enzymes should also be ordered.

Client Teaching

- Explain the procedure for urine collection to the client. Urine should be collected in a sterile plastic container. The client should clean the urinary orifice before urinating into the container.
- Instruct the client to give the urine specimen to the health care provider immediately so that the urine can be delivered to the laboratory. Urine should be tested soon after it is given.
- Answer client's and family's questions. Unknown answers should be referred to the appropriate health professional.

5' nucleotidase (5'N or 5'NT) (serum)

Reference Values

Adult: Less than 17 unit/L.

Pregnancy (Third Trimester): Slightly above normal value.

Child: Values lower than adults.

Description

This is a liver enzyme test that aids in the diagnosis of hepatobiliary disease. 5' nucleotidase (5'N) is not elevated in bone disorders as is alkaline phosphatase (ALP); therefore, it is useful in determining the origin of the problem. Elevated ALP and 5'N indicate liver disorder. Elevated ALP and normal 5'N indicate bone disorder. Usually several liver enzyme tests (e.g., ALP, leucine aminopeptidase [LAP], and gamma-glutamyl transferase [GGT]) are performed to evaluate liver function.

Purpose

- To compare test results with other liver enzyme tests for diagnosing a liver disorder.

Clinical Problems

Increased Level: Cirrhosis of the liver, biliary obstruction from calculi and tumor, and metastasis to the liver. *Drug Influence:* Phenothiazines, narcotics (codeine, morphine, meperidine [Demerol]).

Procedure

- There is no food or fluid restriction.
- Collect 3–5 mL of venous blood in a red-top tube. Avoid hemolysis.

Factors Affecting Laboratory Results

- Hemolysis of the blood specimen.

NURSING IMPLICATIONS WITH RATIONALE

- Check the venipuncture site; clients with liver disorders tend to have prolonged clotting times.

Elevated Level

- Compare 5′N levels with other liver enzyme levels. Elevated ALP, GGT, LAP, and 5′N values indicate that the problem is of liver origin.

Client Teaching

- Instruct the client that there could be a tendency toward bleeding. If bleeding occurs from the mouth, rectum, or elsewhere, the health care provider should be notified.
- Encourage the client to eat well-balanced meals, especially if the condition is cirrhosis of the liver or cancer of the liver.

N-telopeptide cross-links (NTx) (serum and urine)

Reference Values

Serum: *Female:* 6.2–19 nM BCE/L (bone collagen equivalents). *Male:* 5.4–24.2 nM BCE/L.
Urine: *Female:* 5–65 mM BCE/mmol creatinine. *Male:* 3–51 mM BCE/mmol creatinine.

Description

About 90% of the bone matrix consists of type I collagen that is cross-linked at the N-terminal and C-terminal ends. The N terminals of these proteins are cross-linked to give strength to the bones. The bone resorption by osteoclasts causes a production of cross-linked N-telopeptides of NTx type I collagen. This protein is found both in the serum and urine as an end product of bone degradation. The serum level of NTx correlates with bone resorption and bone density in older women with osteopenia or osteoporosis. It is also used to monitor the effects of the therapy for these conditions.

NTx serum levels correlate well with urine NTx normalized to creatinine.

Purposes

- To correlate with serum NTx and urine NTx to identify bone disease and osteoporosis.
- To monitor the effects of antiresorptive therapy with estrogen and/or calcium supplements.

N

O

Clinical Problems

Decreased Level: Hypoparathyroidism, hypothyroidism. *Drug Influence:* Cortisol therapy.

Increased Level: Osteoporosis, osteopenia, Paget disease, advanced bone tumors, acromegaly, hypoparathyroidism, hypothyroidism.

Procedure

Serum
- There is no food or fluid restriction.
- Collect 3–5 mL of venous blood in a red-top tube or serum separator tube.
- Take serum specimen to the laboratory immediately or refrigerate.

Urine
- Collect 20 mL of urine, the second void of the morning. A baseline urine specimen should be collected before correction therapy for the bone disease or osteoporosis has been started.
- Refrigerate specimen.

Factors Affecting Laboratory Results

- Hemolysis of the blood specimen.
- Unrefrigerated urine.

NURSING IMPLICATIONS WITH RATIONALE

- Obtain a health history related to symptoms of osteoporosis and bone disease.
- Compare serum levels with urine levels. Report findings.
- Ask the client when he or she had the last bone density scan. Record answer.
- Provide comfort measures to the client.

Client Teaching

- Explain to the client to collect the second urine sample in the morning.
- Tell the client to take the urine specimen to the laboratory or have it refrigerated. The specimen may be given in the laboratory.

Occult blood (feces)

Reference Values

Adult: Negative.

Child: Negative.

Note: A diet rich in meats, poultry, and fish, and certain drugs (cortisone, aspirin, potassium) could cause a false-positive occult blood test.

O

Description

Occult (nonvisible or hidden) blood in the feces usually indicates gastrointestinal bleeding. Bright red blood from the rectum can be indicative of bleeding from the lower large intestine (e.g., hemorrhoids), and tarry black stools indicate blood loss of greater than 50 mL from the upper GI tract.

Occult blood in the feces may be present days or several weeks after a single bleeding episode. False-positive occult blood test results may be due to ingestion of meats, poultry, fish, and certain drugs.

Purpose

- To detect blood in the feces.

Clinical Problems

Negative Results: *Drug Influence:* Ascorbic acid (large amounts of vitamin C).

Positive Results: Bleeding, peptic ulcer, gastritis, gastric carcinoma, bleeding esophageal varices, colitis, intestinal carcinoma, diverticulitis. *Drug Influence:* Aspirin, steroids (cortisone preparations), colchicine, iron preparations, iodine, indomethacin (Indocin), reserpine, potassium preparations, thiazide diuretics, bromides.

Procedure

- There are a variety of blood-test reagents that may be used to test for occult blood. Some are more sensitive than others. Orthotolidine (Occultest) is considered the most sensitive test, more sensitive than the guaiac (least sensitive).
- Meats, poultry, and fish should be avoided for 3 days prior to stool specimen, especially if orthotolidine or benzidine tests are used.
- Obtain a single, random stool specimen and send it to the laboratory. Only a small amount of fecal material is needed. Stool may be obtained from a rectal examination. Many times, the stool test is done on the nursing floor using a commercial kit.
- List on the laboratory slip any drugs the client is taking that could affect test results.
- The stool specimen does not need to be kept warm or examined immediately.

Factors Affecting Laboratory Results

- Drugs (*see Drug Influence*).
- Foods: meats; poultry; fish; and green, leafy vegetables can cause a false-positive test result.
- Urine and soap solution in the feces may affect the test result.

NURSING IMPLICATIONS WITH RATIONALE

Client Teaching

- Instruct the client not to eat meats, poultry, or fish for 3 days prior to the test. Green, leafy vegetables, if eaten in abundance, could cause a false-positive test result.
- Instruct the client not to take drugs, such as iron, that could cause false-positive results for 3 days prior to the test, if possible. Oral iron preparations can cause the stool to be black.

O

Positive Result for Occult Blood

- Obtain a history of recent or past bleeding episodes. Inform the health care provider of a history of GI bleeding. Only 2 mL or more blood can cause a positive test result.
- Inform the health care provider if the client is receiving medication that could cause a false-positive test result (*see Drug Influence*).
- Determine whether the client has had epigastric pain between meals. This type of pain could be indicative of a peptic ulcer.
- Be sure the stool is not contaminated with menstrual discharge.

Client Teaching

- Encourage the client to report abnormal-colored stools (e.g., tarry stools). Oral iron preparations can cause the stools to be black.

Opiates (urine and blood)

Reference Values

Negative.

Toxic Values: *Urine: Codeine:* Greater than 0.005 mg/dL (0.2 μmol/L). *Hydromorphone:* Greater than 0.1 mg/dL (5 μmol/L). *Meperidine:* Greater than 0.5 mg/dL (20 μmol/L). *Methadone:* Greater than 0.2 mg/dL (10 μmol/L). *Morphone:* Greater than 0.005 mg/dL (0.2 μmol/L). *Propoxyphene:* Greater than 0.5 mg/dL (20 μmol/L).

Blood: *Cocaine:* Greater than 1,000 ng/mL (greater than 3,300 μmol/L [SI units]).

Description

Testing for opiates is primarily done to screen for drug abuse or narcotic toxicity, or to check the progress of opiate detoxification. Specific opiates, such as codeine, morphine, methadone, hydromorphone, and meperidine, can be individually tested. Urine is the preferred specimen for checking for opiates; however, gastric secretions could be analyzed.

The liver detoxifies opiates and the urine excretes 90% of the opiates in 24 hours. The peak effect of opiates in the body occurs in approximately 1 hour.

Cocaine, a narcotic that is frequently abused, is a central nervous system stimulant. It increases blood pressure, respiratory rate, and heart rate and may lead to cardiopulmonary failure. Cocaine has many street names, such as coke, crack, gold dust, stardust, and happy dust.

Purposes

- To detect the presence of opiates.
- To check for opiate toxicity.
- To monitor the progress of opiate detoxification.

O

Clinical Problems

Increased Level: Specific opiate presence or toxicity: *Drug Influence:* Use of other opiates.

Procedure

- A signed consent may be necessary.
- There is no food or fluid restriction.

Urine
- Collect a random urine specimen and send the specimen immediately to the laboratory.
- List drugs taken by the client in the last 24 hours on the lab sheet, including over-the-counter drugs.
- Refrigerate the urine specimen if the test cannot be done immediately.

Blood
- Collect 5–7 mL of venous blood in a lavender- or green-top tube. Place tube on ice and send it to the laboratory immediately.
- If the test is for a legal purpose, have a witness present when obtaining the blood specimen. A signed consent form may be needed; check with hospital or state policy.
- If used for legal evidence, special handling and labeling of the specimen is essential; that is, it should be placed in a sealed container or bag and labeled with the date and time of the drawn blood specimen and the witness's name and signature.

Factors Affecting Laboratory Results

- Delay in testing the urine specimen without it being refrigerated.
- Blood specimen not tested within an hour after drawing and the tube not placed on ice.
- Blood specimen not drawn soon after cocaine use (cocaine has a short action).

NURSING IMPLICATIONS WITH RATIONALE

- Have the client sign a consent form if necessary.
- Explain the test procedure to the client.
- Obtain a drug history, including over-the-counter drugs. Explain that the drug information will be given to the health care provider.
- Send the random urine specimen immediately to the laboratory. If the opiate test is for methadone, a 24-hour urine specimen is needed. Inform the laboratory that the urine specimen should be tested immediately or refrigerated. Delay in testing could result in false-negative test result.

Client Teaching

- Explain to the client that addictive narcotic drugs can cause withdrawal symptoms when the drug is abruptly stopped.
- Inform the client of the adverse reactions to cocaine, such as lung and kidney problems, heart attacks, suicidal tendency, hallucinations, and others.
- Listen to the client's concerns. Be available to discuss drug problems or refer the discussion to an appropriate health care provider.

O Osmolality (serum)

Reference Values

Adult: 280–300 mOsm/kg.

Panic Values: Less than 240 mOsm/kg and greater than 320 mOsm/kg.

Child: 270–290 mOsm/kg.

Description

Serum osmolality is an indicator of serum concentration. It measures the number of dissolved particles (electrolytes, urea, sugar) in the serum and is helpful in the diagnosis of fluid and electrolyte imbalances. Sodium contributes 85–90% of the serum osmolality; changes in osmolality usually result from changes in the serum sodium concentration. Double the serum sodium can give a rough estimate of the serum osmolality.

The hydration status of the client is usually determined by the serum osmolality. An increased value (greater than 300 mOsm/kg) indicates hemoconcentration due to dehydration. A decreased value (less than 280 mOsm/kg) indicates hemodilution due to overhydration, or water excess. An osmometer is used in laboratories to determine serum osmolality; however, if the serum sodium, urea, and sugar levels are known, the serum osmolality can be calculated by the nurse as follows.

$$\text{Serum osmolality} = 2 \times \text{Serum sodium} + \frac{\text{BUN}}{3} + \frac{\text{Sugar}}{18}$$

Urine osmolality is more accurate than the specific gravity in determining the concentration, because it is influenced by the number of particles. The state of hydration affects the urine osmolality.

Purposes

- To monitor body fluid balance.
- To determine the occurrence of body fluid overload or dehydration.

Clinical Problems

Decreased Level: Excessive fluid intake, cancer of the bronchus and lung, adrenal cortical hypofunction, IV 5% dextrose in water (D_5W), syndrome of inappropriate diuretic hormone (SIADH) (serum only), diabetes insipidus (urine only).

Increased Level: Diabetes insipidus (serum only), dehydration, hypernatremia, hyperglycemia, uremia, SIADH (urine only), ethanol.

Procedure

Serum

- There is no food or fluid restriction.
- Collect 5–7 mL of venous blood in a red-top tube. Avoid hemolysis.

Factors Affecting Laboratory Results

- Hyperglycemia increases the serum osmolality.

O

NURSING IMPLICATIONS WITH RATIONALE

Decreased Level

- Associate a decreased serum osmolality with serum dilution caused by excessive fluid intake (overhydration).
- Observe for signs and symptoms of overhydration, such as a constant, irritated cough; dyspnea; neck- and hand-vein engorgement; and chest rales.
- Observe for signs and symptoms of water intoxication, such as headaches, confusion, and irritability. Excessive amounts of hypo-osmolar solutions can "superdilute" the intravascular fluid.

Client Teaching

- Instruct the client to decrease fluid intake.

Increased Level

- Assess for signs and symptoms of dehydration (thirst, dry mucous membranes, poor skin turgor, and shocklike symptoms).
- Check for glycosuria. Increased sugar in the urine could indicate the presence of hyperglycemia.
- Check the serum sodium, urea, and glucose for increased values. Calculate the serum osmolality by either doubling the serum sodium or using the formula given in the description.
- Compare the serum osmolality with the urine osmolality. If the serum is hypo-osmolar (hypo-osmolality), the problem could be due to the syndrome of inappropriate ADH (SIADH).

Client Teaching

- Encourage the client to increase fluid intake.

Osmolality (urine)

Reference Values

Adult: 50–1,200 mOsm/kg/H_2O, average 200–800 mOsm/kg H_2O.

Child: *Newborn:* 100–600 mOsm/kg/H_2O. *Child:* Same as adult.

Description

The urine osmolality test is more accurate than the specific gravity in determining the urine concentration, because its value reflects the number of particles, ions, and molecules and is not unduly influenced by large molecules. Specific gravity measures the quantity and nature of the particles, such as sugar, protein, and IV dyes (these elevate specific gravity but have little effect on osmolality).

The urine osmolality fluctuates in the same way that the urine-specific gravity does, and it can be low or high according to the client's state of hydration. A dehydrated client with normal kidney function could have a urine osmolality of 1,000 mOsm/kg H_2O or more. When hemoconcentration

O

occurs as a result of acidosis, shock, or hyperglycemia, the serum osmolality is elevated, and so should the urine osmolality be elevated.

If serum hypo-osmolality and hyponatremia occur with urine hyperosmolality, the problem is most likely the syndrome of inappropriate antidiuretic hormone secretion (SIADH). ADH causes water reabsorption from the kidney, thus diluting the serum.

Purposes

(*See Osmolality [serum].*)

Clinical Problems

Decreased Level: Excessive water intake, continuous IV 5% dextrose in water (D_5W), diabetes insipidus, glomerulonephritis, acute renal failure, sickle-cell anemia, multiple myeloma. *Drug Influence:* Diuretics.

Increased Level: High-protein diet, SIADH, Addison disease (adrenal gland insufficiency), dehydration, hyperglycemia with glycosuria.

Procedure

- Give a high-protein diet for 3 days prior to the urine osmolality test. Check with your laboratory.
- Restrict fluids for 8–12 hours before the test.
- Collect a random, morning urine specimen. The first urine specimen in the morning is discarded, and the second specimen, taken 2 hours later, is sent to the laboratory. Urine osmolality should be high in the morning.
- Send the urine specimen to the laboratory.

Factors Affecting Laboratory Results

- Diuretics can cause urine hyperosmolality.
- A high-protein diet can cause urine hyperosmolality.

NURSING IMPLICATIONS WITH RATIONALE

- Explain to the client that the purpose of the test is to determine the kidneys' ability to concentrate urine.
- Explain the procedure of the test if it requires more than a random urine sample for urine osmolality. A high-protein diet is taken for 3 days before the test, and oral fluids are restricted the night before. The first urine specimen of the morning is discarded, and the second specimen, taken 1–2 hours later, is sent to the laboratory.

Decreased Level

- Determine whether the decreased urine osmolality could be caused by excessive intake of water (greater than 2 quarts daily) or continuous IV administration of D_5W in water. A urine osmolality that remains less than 200 mOsm/kg after fluids are restricted could be indicative of early kidney impairment.

- Explain to the client the need to decrease excessive water intake.
- Report to the health care provider when the client is receiving D_5W continuously without any other solutes, such as saline (NaCl). The D_5W not only dilutes the urine; it can decrease the serum osmolality and cause water intoxication.
- Observe for signs and symptoms of water intoxication, such as headaches, confusion, irritability, weight gain, and, later, cerebral edema (if severe).

Increased Level

- Determine the hydration status of the client. Dehydration will cause an elevated urine osmolality as well as elevated serum osmolality. A urine osmolality of 1,000 mOsm/kg is not abnormal if the client has a decreased fluid intake.
- Check the serum osmolality. If the serum is hypo-osmolar and the urine is hyperosmolar, the problem could be due to SIADH. SIADH frequently occurs after surgery, trauma, or pain and will correct itself in a day or two. The function of ADH is to promote water reabsorption from the kidney tubules. The serum is diluted, and the decreased urine is concentrated.
- Keep an accurate intake and output record. The fluid intake should be comparable to the urine output.

Client Teaching

- Instruct clients on high-protein diets to increase water intake.

Osmotic fragility of erythrocytes (blood)

Erythrocyte Osmotic Fragility, Red Cell Fragility

Reference Values

Adult:

% SALINE (NaCl)	% HEMOLYSIS	
	FRESH BLOOD (LESS THAN 3 HOURS)	INCUBATED AT 37°C (24-HOUR BLOOD)
0.3	97–100	85–100
0.35	90–98	75–100
0.4	50–95	65–100
0.45	5–45	55–95
0.5	0–5	40–85
0.55	0	15–65
0.6	0	0–40

Child: Similar to adult.

O

Description

This is an infrequently performed test.

Water is normally exchanged between cells and extracellular fluid according to the osmolality (concentration) of fluid. Erythrocyte (red blood cell) fluid and plasma have similar ionic concentrations, iso-osmolar or isotonic. When there is an imbalance in one of the fluids, osmosis occurs. Fluid moves from the fluid with the lesser concentration to the fluid with the greater concentration. If erythrocytes are placed in a hypo-osmolar solution, fluid with less than the normal serum/plasma osmolality (less than 280 mOsm/kg) will move into the erythrocytes, causing them to swell and eventually to rupture.

The erythrocyte osmotic fragility test determines the erythrocytes' ability to resist hemolysis (RBC destruction) in a hypo-osmolar solution. Erythrocytes are placed in various concentrations of saline. If hemolysis occurs at a slightly hypo-osmolar concentration of saline (0.36–0.73% solution), there is increased osmotic fragility, and if hemolysis occurs at a severely hypo-osmolar concentration of saline, there is decreased osmotic fragility. With increased fragility, the erythrocytes are usually spherical, and with decreased fragility, the erythrocytes are thin and flat.

Purpose

- To determine erythrocyte osmotic fragility in a hypo-osmolar solution.

Clinical Problems

Decreased Level: Anemias (iron deficiency, folic acid deficiency, vitamin B_6 deficiency, sickle cell), thalassemia major and minor (Mediterranean anemia or Cooley anemia), hemoglobin C disease,[*] polycythemia vera, after splenectomy, acute and subacute necrosis of the liver, obstructive jaundice.

Increased Level: Hereditary spherocytosis, transfusion (incompatibility—ABO and Rh), acquired hemolytic anemia (autoimmune), hemoglobin C disease,[*] chemical or drug poisonings, chronic lymphocytic leukemia, burns (thermal).

Procedure

- There is no food or fluid restriction.
- The test is usually performed on fresh blood less than 3 hours old and/or on 24-hour-old blood incubated at 37°C.
- Collect 7 mL of venous blood in a lavender- or green-top tube. The tube should be filled to its capacity. A drop of blood is placed in tubes with decreasing saline concentration.
- Hemolysis is frequently determined by a colorimeter.

Factors Affecting Laboratory Results

- Plasma pH, temperature, glucose concentration, and oxygen saturation of the blood affect the osmotic fragility.
- Older erythrocytes have increased osmotic fragility.
- A blood sample more than 3 hours old may show an increase in osmotic fragility.

---

[*]Decreased or increased fragility may occur in hemoglobin C disease.

O

NURSING IMPLICATIONS WITH RATIONALE

Decreased Level

- Identify clinical problems related to a decreased erythrocyte osmotic fragility. Normally, complete hemolysis occurs with 0.3% saline. Thin, flat cells are usually resistant to hemolysis at 0.3%.
- Assess for signs and symptoms of anemias, such as fatigue, weakness, tachycardia, and dyspnea.

Increased Level

- Identify clinical problems related to an increased erythrocyte osmotic fragility (e.g., transfusion incompatibility, acquired hemolytic anemia, and chemical or drug poisoning [*see Clinical Problems*]).
- Monitor temperature when the client receives a blood transfusion. A slightly elevated temperature is an early sign of transfusion reaction.
- Observe for signs and symptoms of transfusion reactions other than changes in temperature (e.g., rash, difficulty breathing, and an increased pulse rate).

Osteocalcin (serum)

Bone G1a Protein (BGP); G1a Protein

Reference Values

Female: *Premenopausal:* 0.5–7.8 ng/mL, 0.5–7.8 mcg/L (SI units).
　　　 Postmenopausal: 1.2–11 ng/mL, 1.2–11 mcg/L (SI units).

Male: 1.5–11.5 ng/mL, 1.5–11.5 mcg/L (SI units).
　　　(Check reference values with your institution.)

Description

Osteocalcin or BGP, a biochemical marker, is useful in determining the effectiveness of treatment for bone disease and osteoporosis. This noncollagenous protein in the bone, produced by the osteoblasts, has a function in bone mineralization and bone formation. A small amount of osteocalcin enters the circulation. Osteocalcin synthesis is dependent on vitamin K. A reduced intake of vitamin K is associated with a decrease in the bone G1a protein.

It is an indicator for bone metabolism. Elevated levels occur during osteoporosis and bone disease.

Bone density scan can diagnose osteoporosis. The test cannot identify changes in bone metabolism. Bone density test is also more expensive than the laboratory tests for bone disease and osteoporosis.

Purposes

- To determine the effectiveness of bone therapy.
- To assess bone metabolism.
- To detect bone disease such as osteoporosis.

Clinical Problems

Decreased Level: Deficiency of growth hormone, hypoparathyroidism, multiple myeloma, cirrhosis of the liver. *Drug Influence:* Cortisone drugs, calcitonin, warfarin.

Increased Level: Fractures, osteoporosis, growth spurt (10–16 years old), acromegaly, bone cancer, Paget disease, hyperparathyroidism, hyperthyroidism, low estrogen production, low calcium intake, osteomalacia, renal failure with dialysis.

Procedure

- No food or fluid restriction is required.
- Collect 7 mL of venous blood in a red-, lavender-, or green-top tube. Check with your institution for the desired color-top tube.

Factors Affecting Laboratory Results

- None known.

NURSING IMPLICATIONS WITH RATIONALE

- Obtain a history of health problems, including symptoms of osteoporosis or bone disease.
- Determine if and when the client has had a bone density scan. The scan is useful to identify osteoporosis but is not effective for identifying changes in bone metabolism.
- Check the results of previous bone density and osteocalcin (BGP) tests. Compare other bone tests with the current BGP test.

Client Teaching

- Explain to the client that the BGP test is useful in determining the effects of the prescribed medication, for example, estrogen, raloxifene (Evista), alendronate (Fosamax).
- Answer client questions concerning the test and results or refer to other health professionals.

Ova and parasites (O and P) (feces)

Reference Values

Adult: Negative.

Child: Negative.

O

Description

Parasites may be present in various forms in the intestine, including the ova (eggs), larvae (immature form), cysts (inactive stage), and trophozoites (motile form) of protozoa. It is vitally important to detect parasites so that proper treatment can be ordered. Some of the organisms identified are amoeba, flagellates, tapeworms, hookworms, and roundworms. A history of recent travel outside the United States should be reported to the laboratory, because it may help in identifying the parasite.

Purpose

- To identify specific ova and parasites in fecal matter.

Clinical Problems

Positive Result: Protozoa—*Balantidium coli, Chilomastix mesnili, Entamoeba histolytica, Giardia lamblia, Trichomonas hominis*; helminths (adults)—*Ascaris lumbricoides* (roundworm), *Diphyllobothrium latum* (fish tapeworm), *Enterobius vermicularis* (pinworm), *Necator americanus* (American hookworm), *Strongyloides stercoralis* (threadworm), *Taenia saginata* (beef tapeworm), *Taenia solium* (pork tapeworm).

Procedure

- Collect stool specimens for 3 days or every other day. Stool specimens should be taken immediately to the laboratory.
- Mark on the laboratory slip the countries the client has visited outside the United States in the last 1–3 years.
- A loose or liquid stool is more likely to indicate that trophozoites are present. The stool must be kept warm and taken to the laboratory within 30 minutes. If the stool is semi-formed or well formed, it does not need to be kept warm but should be taken to the laboratory at once.
- If the stool is tested for tapeworm, the entire stool should be sent to the laboratory so that the head (scolex) of the tapeworm can be identified. The tapeworm will continue to grow as long as the head is lodged in the intestine.
- Anal swabs are used to check for pinworm eggs, and the swabbing should be done in the morning before defecation or the morning bath.
- No toilet paper or urine should be allowed in the fecal collection.
- Avoid taking mineral oil, castor oil, Metamucil, barium, antacids, or tetracycline for 1 week before the test.
- Laboratory results are available in 24–48 hours.

Factors Affecting Laboratory Results

- Urine, toilet paper, soap, disinfectants, antibiotics, antacids, barium, harsh laxatives, and hypertonic saline enemas (Fleet) may affect the result of the test.

NURSING IMPLICATIONS WITH RATIONALE

- Administer a mild laxative or normal saline enema, with the health care provider's approval, to obtain the stool specimen, if necessary.
- Take the fresh stool specimen to the laboratory immediately.
- Report if the client is taking antacids and/or antibiotics or has received barium in the last 7 days. These agents can alter the stool examination for parasites and ova.
- Obtain a history of the client's recent travel. Certain parasites are common to certain countries, and the health care provider and laboratory should be notified of this information.
- Handle the stool specimen with care to prevent parasitic contamination of yourself and other clients.
- Check for occult blood in the stool. The worm attaches itself to the bowel's lining.

Client Teaching

- Explain to the client the procedure for collecting the stool specimen. The stool should be collected in the morning, preferably before a bath. Explain to the client that he or she should not use soap or a Fleet enema, for this may destroy the parasite. The stool specimen should be obtained before treatment is initiated.
- Instruct the client not to put urine or toilet paper in the sterile bedpan. Disinfectants should not be used, because they can cause the ova to deteriorate.
- Instruct the client to wash hands thoroughly after urinating and defecating.

Parathyroid hormone (PTH) (serum)

Parathormone

Reference Values

Adult: *Intact PTH:* 11–54 pg/mL. *C-Terminal PTH:* 50–330 pg/mL. *N-Terminal PTH:* 8–24 pg/mL.

Description

Parathyroid hormone (PTH), secreted by the parathyroid glands, regulates the concentration of calcium and phosphorus in the extracellular fluid. The main function of PTH is to promote calcium reabsorption and phosphorus excretion. Serum calcium levels affect the secretion of PTH: low serum calcium levels stimulate the secretion of PTH; high serum calcium levels inhibit PTH secretion.

Two forms of PTH, inactive C-terminal PTH and active N-terminal PTH, are used in diagnosing parathyroid disorders. C-terminal assays (PTH-C) are an effective indicator of chronic hyperparathyroidism. N-terminal assays (PTH-N) detect acute changes in the PTH secretion, can differentiate between hypercalcemia due to malignancy or parathyroid disorder, and are useful for monitoring the client's response to PTH therapy. Both assays and serum calcium values are used in diagnosing early and borderline parathyroid disorders.

Purposes

- To identify hypo- or hyperparathyroidism (*see Clinical Problems*).
- To monitor the client's response to PTH therapy.

Clinical Problems

Decreased Level: *PTH-C Levels*: Hypoparathyroidism, nonparathyroid hypercalcemia. *PTH-N Levels*: Hypoparathyroidism, nonparathyroid hypercalcemia, certain tumors, pseudohyperparathyroidism. *PTH (Serum)*: Hypoparathyroidism, nonparathyroid hypercalcemia, Graves disease, sarcoidosis.

Increased Level: *PTH-C Levels*: Secondary hyperparathyroidism, tumors, hypercalcemia, pseudohypoparathyroidism. *PTH-N Levels*: Primary and secondary hyperparathyroidism, pseudohypoparathyroidism. *PTH (Serum)*: Primary and secondary hyperparathyroidism, hyper calcemia, chronic renal failure, pseudohyperparathyroidism (defect in renal tubular response).

Procedure

- NPO for 8 hours before the test.
- Collect 5–7 mL of venous blood in a red-top tube in the morning. Morning PTH is usually at its lowest point. Avoid hemolysis. Two tubes may be required (5 mL each). N-terminal PTH is unstable and needs to be chilled or frozen if test is not immediately run.
- N-terminal PTH levels decrease during hemodialysis. Collect blood specimens prior to dialysis.

Factors Affecting Laboratory Results

- Using a nonchilled tube for N-terminal PTH affects test result.
- Food, especially milk products, might lower the PTH level.
- Hemolysis of the blood sample could cause inaccurate results.

NURSING IMPLICATIONS WITH RATIONALE

- Check with the laboratory to verify the procedure for collecting blood sample(s).
- Assess for signs and symptoms of hypocalcemia (tetany [i.e., muscular twitching and tremors], paresthesia [tingling and numbness of fingers], spasmodic contractions).
- Assess for signs and symptoms of hypercalcemia (e.g., lethargy, muscle flaccidity, weakness, headaches, nausea, and vomiting).
- Recognize the relationship of serum calcium levels and PTH secretion and serum level.

Client Teaching

- Instruct the client not to eat until after the blood sample is taken. Explain to the client that foods high in calcium can affect test results.

Partial thromboplastin time (PTT), activated partial thromboplastin time (APTT) (plasma)

P

Reference Values

Adult: Results vary in accordance with equipment and laboratory values. *PTT:* 60–70 seconds. *APTT:* 20–35 seconds.

Child: Increased above adult level.

Anticoagulant Therapy: 1.5–2.5 times the control in seconds.
Note: Most laboratories do APTT only.

Description

The partial thromboplastin time (PTT) is a screening test used to detect deficiencies in all clotting factors except VII and XIII and to detect platelet variations. It is more sensitive than the prothrombin time in detecting minor deficiencies but is not as sensitive as the activated partial thromboplastin time (APTT).

The PTT is useful for monitoring heparin therapy. Heparin doses are adjusted according to the PTT test.

The APTT is more sensitive in detecting clotting factor defects than the PTT, because the activator added in vitro shortens the clotting time. By shortening the clotting time, minor clotting defects can be detected.

The APTT is similar to the PTT except that the thromboplastin reagent used in the APTT test contains an activator (kaolin, celite, or ellagic acid) for identification of deficient factors. This test is commonly used to monitor heparin therapy.

Purposes

- To monitor heparin therapy.
- To screen for clotting factor deficiencies.

Clinical Problems

Decreased Level: Extensive cancer.

Increased Level: Factor deficiency (factors V, VIII [hemophilia], IX [Christmas disease], X, XI, XII), cirrhosis of the liver, vitamin K deficiency, hypofibrinogenemia, prothrombin deficiency, von Willebrand disease (vascular hemophilia), disseminated intravascular coagulation, leukemias (myelocytic, monocytic), malaria. *Drug Influence:* Heparin, salicylates.

Procedure

- There is no food or fluid restriction.
- Collect 3–5 mL of venous blood in a blue-top tube. The tube should be filled to its capacity.
- An activated thromboplastin mixture (thromboplastin reagent and an activator, such as kaolin) is added to the client's plasma sample and the control sample. When a small amount of calcium solution is added, the stopwatch is started; it is stopped when fibrin strands are noted. The tests are usually duplicated and should agree to within 1–1.5 seconds. The test can also be done using a "fibrin meter."

Factors Affecting Laboratory Results

- A clotted blood sample.
- A test (collection) tube without an anticoagulant.

NURSING IMPLICATIONS WITH RATIONALE

- Check the APTT or PTT and report the results to the health care provider. The heparin dosage may need to be adjusted. The APTT range for heparin therapy is 1.5–2.5 times the normal value.
- Assess the client for signs and symptoms of bleeding (purpura [skin], hematuria, and nosebleeds).
- Administer heparin subcutaneously or intravenously through a heparin lock. Do not aspirate when giving heparin subcutaneously, because a hematoma (blood tumor) could occur at the injection site.

Parvovirus B 19 antibody (serum)

Reference Values

Negative: No IgG and IgM antibodies to parvovirus B 19.

Description

The parvovirus B 19, a human virus, destroys red blood cells (RBCs) and interferes with RBC production. This virus occurs more frequently in children. Erythema infectiosum causes a low-grade fever and rash, particularly in children; hydrops fetalis and aplastic anemia are associated with the parvovirus B 19.

The presence of IgM antibodies to parvovirus B 19 can indicate an acute infection, and the IgG antibodies can indicate a past infection or immunity. Joint inflammation and purpura are other clinical manifestations of the parvovirus B 19. A positive parvovirus B 19 has been associated with organ transplants; therefore, a serologic assessment should be made on organ donors.

Purposes

- To detect the presence of parvovirus B 19 antibody.
- To aid in the diagnosis of erythema infectiosum.

Clinical Problems

Positive Test: Erythema infectiosum (most common), transient aplastic anemia, joint arthritis, hydrops fetalis, fetal loss, bone marrow failure (aplastic anemia), chronic anemia in immuno-compromised clients.

Procedure

- There is no food or fluid restriction.

- Collect 5 mL of venous blood in a red-top tube. Avoid hemolysis (shaking tube or rough handling of the blood specimen). Keep blood specimen on ice.
- Take precaution with collection and delivery of the blood specimen to avoid spread of infection.

P

Factors Affecting Laboratory Results

- Hemolysis of the blood specimen.
- Blood specimen not kept cold or on ice.

NURSING IMPLICATIONS WITH RATIONALE

- Obtain a history of the health complaint from the child, parent, or family member. List symptoms.
- Record vital signs. Report abnormal findings.

Client Teaching

- Explain to the organ donors that a blood test may be prescribed to rule out the presence of a virus antibody (parvovirus B 19 antibody) that may affect organ donation. It is for preventive purposes.
- Answer the parent or family members' questions concerning the child or client condition or refer the person(s) to other health professionals for correct answers.

Pepsinogen I (PG-I) (serum)

Reference Values

Adult: 124–142 ng/mL, 124–142 mcg/L (SI units).

Child: *Premature Infant:* 20–24 ng/mL, 20–24 mcg/L (SI units). *Less than 1 Year:* 72–82 ng/mL, 72–82 mcg/L (SI units). *1–2 Years:* 90–106 ng/mL, 90–106 mcg/L (SI units). *3–6 Years:* 80–104 ng/mL, 80–104 mcg/L (SI units). *7–10 Years:* 77–103 ng/mL, 77–103 mcg/L (SI units). *11–14 Years:* 96–118 ng/mL, 96–118 mcg/L (SI units).

Description

There are seven fractions of pepsinogens in the blood. Five are classified as pepsinogen I (PG-I) and are secreted from the lumen of the stomach. The secretion of pepsinogen I is controlled by the hormone gastrin. Pepsinogen I is converted to pepsin when the stomach pH is acidic. Pepsin is needed in the process of digestion of proteins. Low gastrin and pepsinogen I levels are specific for atrophic gastritis. An elevated pepsinogen I level frequently occurs with duodenal ulcer. A high PG-I level can be inherited as an autosomal dominant trait.

Purpose

- To determine the cause of the gastric disorder.

Clinical Problems

Decreased Level: Atropic gastritis, gastric cancer, achlorhydria, pernicious anemia, Addison disease, myxedema, hypopituitarism.

Increased Level: Duodenal ulcer, acute gastritis, Zollinger-Ellison syndrome, hypergastrinemia.

Procedure

- NPO 8–12 hours before the test.
- Collect 5–7 mL of venous blood in a red-top tube.

Factors Affecting Laboratory Results

- Poor renal output can cause an elevated serum pepsinogen I level.

NURSING IMPLICATIONS WITH RATIONALE

- Assess the client's renal function, such as adequate urine output and blood urea nitrogen and serum creatinine levels. Poor renal function can cause a false-elevated serum PG-I level.
- Assess the client for complaints of gastric discomfort. Record findings.

Client Teaching

- Inform the client that the test requires a fasting blood specimen; therefore, the client should take nothing by mouth after midnight.
- Instruct the client to inform you of any abdominal discomfort. The time of gastric or intestinal discomfort should be recorded.

Phenothiazines (serum)

Reference Values

Adult

DRUG	THERAPEUTIC RANGE	PEAK TIME	TOXIC LEVEL
Chlorpromazine (Thorazine)	50–300 ng/mL	2–4 hours	greater than 750 ng/mL
Prochlorperazine (Compazine)	50–300 ng/mL	2–4 hours	greater than 1,000 ng/mL
Thioridazine (Mellaril)	100–600 ng/mL 0.2–2.6 mg/L	2–4 hours	greater than 2,000 ng/mL greater than 10 mg/L
Trifluoperazine (Stelazine)	50–300 ng/mL	2–4 hours	greater than 1,000 ng/mL

P

Description

Phenothiazines are major tranquilizers (neurolytics) used for the treatment of psychosis and emesis. They have many active metabolites that are excreted in the urine. Thus phenothiazines can be measured in the urine and also in gastric fluids. Because phenothiazines are metabolized to many metabolites, the serum value is difficult to measure.

The phenothiazines have a wide therapeutic index. Consequently, a large dosage or large overdoses are relatively safe. However, extremely large overdoses can cause drug toxicity.

Purposes

- To monitor a specific phenothiazine level for therapeutic effect.
- To check for specific phenothiazine toxicity.

Clinical Problems

Decreased Level: *Drug Influence:* Antacids, anticholinergics (for pseudoparkinsonism).

Increased Level: Phenothiazine overdose.

Procedure

- There is no food or fluid restriction.
- Collect 7 mL of venous blood in a red-top tube.

Factors Affecting Laboratory Results

- Barbiturates and other antipsychotic agents enhance the phenothiazine effect.
- Antacids slow down the phenothiazine absorption, and anticholinergics taken for the pseudoparkinsonism effect can decrease the phenothiazine effect.

NURSING IMPLICATIONS WITH RATIONALE

- Obtain a history from the client concerning drug dosage and frequency.
- Determine if the client smokes. Smoking increases metabolism of the drug, and the drug dosage might need to be increased.
- Check liver enzyme laboratory tests, especially if the client is taking chlorpromazine (Thorazine). Taking chlorpromazine for a long period of time could have an effect on the liver.
- Observe for side effects of phenothiazines, especially the common pseudoparkinsonism effect (e.g., muscle rigidity, tremors, bent-over position when walking).

Client Teaching

- Explain to the client the importance of taking the prescribed drug dosage. Desired effect from the drug cannot be obtained if the client is underdosed.
- Inform the client to use protective sunscreen, because photosensitivity is common with phenothiazines.
- Advise the client to check with the health care provider before taking over-the-counter drugs to avoid side effects.
- Inform the client that the urine may be pink or red-brown when taking chlorpromazine (Thorazine).

Phenylketonuria (PKU) (urine), Guthrie test for PKU (blood)

Reference Values

Adult: PKU and Guthrie test not usually done.

Child: *Phenylalanine:* 0.5–2 mg/dL. *PKU:* Negative, but positive when the serum phenylalanine is 12–15 mg/dL. *Guthrie:* Negative, but positive when the serum phenylalanine is 4 mg/dL.

Description

The urine phenylketonuria (PKU) and Guthrie (blood) tests are two screening tests used for detecting a hepatic enzyme deficiency, phenylalanine hydroxylase, that prevents the conversion of phenylalanine (amino acid) to tyrosine in the infant. Phenylalanine from milk and other protein products accumulates in the blood and tissues and can lead to brain damage and mental retardation.

At birth the newborn's serum phenylalanine level is less than 2 mg/dL because of the mother's enzyme activity. After the third day of life or after 48 hours of milk ingestion, the serum level increases if phenylalanine is not metabolized.

The Guthrie procedure is the test of choice because a positive test result occurs when the serum phenylalanine reaches 4 mg/dL at 3–5 days of life after milk ingestion. A positive Guthrie test does not always indicate PKU, but if it is positive, a specific blood phenylalanine test should be performed. The PKU urine test is done after the infant is 3–4 weeks old and should be repeated a week or two later. Significant brain damage usually occurs when the serum level is 15 mg/dL. If either the Guthrie test or the urine PKU is positive, the infant should be maintained on a low phenylalanine diet for 6–8 years.

Purposes

- To screen for phenylalanine hydroxylase deficiency.
- To repeat phenylketonuria test as indicated.

Clinical Problems

Increased Level: PKU, low-birth-weight infants, hepatic encephalopathy, septicemia, galactosemia. *Drug Influence:* Aspirin and salicylate compounds, chlorpromazine (Thorazine), ketone bodies.

Procedure

Guthrie Test (Guthrie Bacterial Inhibition Test): Phenylalanine promotes bacterial growth (*Bacillus subtilis*) when the serum level is greater than 4 mg/dL.

- Cleanse the infant's heel, and prick it with a sterile lancet. Obtain several drops of blood on the filter paper. The surface of the filter paper is streaked with *Bacillus subtilis*, and if the bacillus grows, the test is positive. Check the procedure outlined by your institution.
- The test should not be done before 2–4 days of milk intake, either cow's milk or breast milk, and is preferably done on or after the fourth day.
- Note on the laboratory slip the date of birth and the date the first milk was ingested.

Urine PKU*: There are several urine tests for detecting phenylpyruvic acid. All use the reagent ferric chloride, which causes the urine specimen to turn green when positive. The Phenistix is a dipstick with ferric salt in the filter paper; it is dipped in fresh urine or pressed against a wet diaper. The dipstick will turn green if positive.

- The urine PKU test should be done 3–6 weeks after birth, preferably at the fourth week. It is usually not positive for PKU until the serum phenylalanine levels are between 10 and 15 mg/dL.
- The infant should be receiving milk for accurate Guthrie and urine PKU test results.

Factors Affecting Laboratory Results

- Urine that is not fresh can cause an inaccurate result.
- Vomiting and/or decreased milk intake may cause a normal serum phenylalanine level in the infant with PKU.
- Aspirins and salicylate compounds can cause a false-positive result.
- Early PKU testing before the infant is 3 days old (Guthrie) or 2 weeks old (Phenistix) may cause a false-negative test result.

NURSING IMPLICATIONS WITH RATIONALE

Increased Level

- Relate positive Guthrie and urine PKU test results to the clinical problem phenylketonuria.
- Explain to the mother the screening tests used to detect PKU. The Guthrie test is normally done while the mother and infant are in the hospital. Many pediatricians want the urine PKU done at home by the parent or in the doctor's office 3–4 weeks after birth as a follow-up test.
- Determine whether the infant has been taking adequate feedings (cow's milk or breast milk) before performing the Guthrie test. Vomiting and/or refusing to eat are common problems of PKU infants. This may cause a normal serum phenylalanine level.
- Obtain history if mother was a "PKU baby." If so, the mother should be on a low-phenylalanine diet before and during pregnancy.

Client Teaching

- Instruct the mother on how to perform a urine PKU test accurately. A fresh wet diaper or a fresh urine specimen should be used.
- Instruct the mother that the baby should not receive aspirin or salicylate compounds for 24 hours before testing the urine. A false-positive test could result. Tylenol should be given instead of aspirin.
- Tell the mother which foods the baby should and should not have. The preferred milk substitute is Lofenalac (Mead Johnson and Co.), an enzymic casein hydrolysate with vitamins and minerals. It provides a balanced nutritional formula. Other low-phenylalanine foods are fruits, fruit juices, vegetables, cereals, and breads. High-protein foods should be avoided (e.g., milk shakes, ice cream, and cheese). It is thought that after the age of 6–8 years, 90% of the brain growth has occurred, and the diet does not need to be as restrictive.

---

*Most state laws require a repeat blood test instead of a urine test because it is more reliable.

Phenytoin sodium (serum)
Diphenylhydantoin (Dilantin)

P

Reference Values

Therapeutic Range: *Adult:* As an anticonvulsant, 10–20 mcg/mL, 39.6–79.3 µmol/L (SI units). As an antiarrhythmic, 10–18 mcg/mL, 39.6–71.4 µmol/L (SI units). *In Saliva:* 1–2 mcg/mL, 4–9 µmol/L.

Toxic Level: *Adult:* Greater than 20 mcg/mL, greater than 79.3 µmol/L (SI units). *Child:* Greater than 15–20 mcg/mL, 56–79 µmol/L (SI units).

Description

Phenytoin (Dilantin) reduces voltage, frequency, and transmission of electrical discharges within the motor cortex. It is used to prevent and control grand mal seizures. Phenytoin is also used as an antiarrhythmic drug for decreasing force of myocardial contraction, improving atrioventricular conduction depressed by a digitalis preparation, and prolonging the refractory period of the heart contraction.

Phenytoin sodium is absorbed from the gastrointestinal tract within 3–12 hours. Foods and antacids can decrease its absorption rate. Neonates and infants during their first 2–3 months of age cannot absorb phenytoin, so other anticonvulsants should be used during that period of time.

Approximately 90–95% of phenytoin is bound to plasma proteins, and the remainder is free. About 5–10% of the drug is excreted unchanged in the urine. Half-life in adults is an average of 24 hours and in children is an average of 15 hours. Frequent monitoring of serum phenytoin levels is indicated for checking the therapeutic level and for avoiding toxic level. It takes about 5–10 days to obtain steady state. With a change in phenytoin dosage, resampling is suggested in 48 hours.

General signs and symptoms of phenytoin toxicity include nystagmus (rapid movement of the eyeball), slurred speech, gingival hyperplasia, ataxia, drowsiness, lethargy, and confusion. IM injection might cause a slow and erratic absorption. Oral and IV routes (not to exceed 50 mg/min push) are preferred.

Purpose

- To monitor phenytoin (Dilantin) levels.

Clinical Problems

Decreased Level: Pregnancy, infectious mononucleosis. *Drug Influence:* Alcohol, carbamazepine (Tegretol), folate.

Increased Level: Phenytoin overdose, uremia, liver disease. *Drug Influence:* Aspirin, phenylbutazone (Butazolidin), dicumarol, chloramphenicol (Chloromycetin), sulfisoxazole (Gantrisin), chlorothiazide (Diuril), tranquilizers (chlordiazepoxide [Librium], chlorpromazine [Thorazine], prochlorperazine [Compazine], diazepam [Valium]), isoniazid (INH), phenobarbital, propoxyphene (Darvon).

Procedure

- There is no food or fluid restriction.
- Collect 5–7 mL of venous blood in a red-top tube. Avoid hemolysis.
- Record the dose, route, and last dose administered on the laboratory requisition slip. List drugs the client is taking that could affect test results.

Factors Affecting Laboratory Results

- Hemolysis of the blood specimen.
- Drugs that increase serum phenytoin level (*see Drug Influence*).

NURSING IMPLICATIONS WITH RATIONALE

- Check serum phenytoin result and immediately report nontherapeutic levels to the health care provider.
- Record dose, route, and last time the drug was given on the requisition slip.
- Note the method of drug administration. The oral and IV routes are commonly chosen methods for administration. The IM route might cause a slow and erratic absorption.

Increased Level

- Observe for signs and symptoms of phenytoin toxicity, such as nystagmus, slurred speech, ataxia, drowsiness, lethargy, confusion, and rash.

Phosphorus (P)—inorganic (serum)

Phosphate (PO_4)

Reference Values

Adult: 1.7–2.6 mEq/L or 2.5–4.5 mg/dL, 0.78–1.52 mmol/L (SI units).

Child: *Newborn:* 3.5–8.6 mg/dL. *Infant:* 4.5–6.7 mg/dL. *Child:* 4.5–5.5 mg/dL.

Elderly: Slightly lower than adult.

Description

Phosphorus is the principal intracellular anion; however, most of phosphorus exists in the blood as phosphate. From 80 to 85% of the total phosphates in the body are combined with calcium in the teeth and bones.

Phosphorus is the laboratory term used, because phosphates are converted into inorganic phosphorus for the test. Functions of phosphorus include metabolism of carbohydrates and fats, maintenance of the acid–base balance, use of B vitamins, promotion of nerve and muscle activity, and transmission of hereditary traits.

Phosphorus (P) metabolism is associated with calcium (Ca) metabolism. Both ions need vitamin D for their absorption from the gastrointestinal tract. Phosphorus and calcium concentrations are controlled by the parathyroid hormone. Usually there is a reciprocal relationship between calcium and phosphorus: when serum phosphorus levels increase, serum calcium levels decrease, and when serum phosphorus levels decrease, serum calcium levels increase. In certain neoplastic bone diseases, this relationship may be altered.

A high serum phosphorus level is called *hyperphosphatemia* and is usually associated with kidney dysfunction (poor urinary output). *Hypophosphatemia* means a low serum phosphorus level.

Purposes

- To check phosphorus level.
- To monitor phosphorus levels during renal insufficiency or failure.
- To compare the phosphorus level with those of other electrolytes (e.g., potassium, calcium).

Clinical Problems

Decreased Level: Starvation, malabsorption syndrome, hyperparathyroidism, hypercalcemia, hypomagnesemia, chronic alcoholism, vitamin D deficiency, diabetic acidosis, myxedema, continuous IV fluids with glucose. *Drug Influence:* Antacids such as aluminum hydroxide (Amphojel), epinephrine (adrenalin), insulin, mannitol.

Increased Level: Renal insufficiency, renal failure, hypoparathyroidism, hypocalcemia, hypervitaminosis D, bone tumors, acromegaly, fractures (healing). *Drug Influence:* Antibiotics (methicillin, tetracyclines), phenytoin (Dilantin), heparin, Lipomul, laxatives with phosphate.

Procedure

- The client should be NPO except for water for 8 hours before the test. Some laboratories will require NPO for 4 hours. Carbohydrates lower serum phosphorus levels because phosphate goes into the cells with glucose.
- Collect 3–5 mL of venous blood in a red-top tube. Avoid hemolysis.
- The blood sample should be taken to the laboratory within 30 minutes. The serum should be quickly separated from the red blood cells.

Factors Affecting Laboratory Results

- A high-carbohydrate diet and IV fluids with glucose can lower the serum phosphorus level; hence a fasting specimen is needed.
- Hemolysis of the blood sample can increase the serum phosphorus level. When RBCs rupture, they release intracellular phosphate into the serum.
- Late delivery of the blood sample (greater than 30 minutes) may cause the release of phosphorus from the blood cells into the serum. The serum should be separated from the blood clot within 30 minutes.
- Drugs (*see Drug Influence*). Amphojel can lower the serum phosphorus level.

NURSING IMPLICATIONS WITH RATIONALE

- Hold medications in the morning until the blood sample is taken.
- Hold IV fluid with glucose for 4–8 hours before the blood test, if possible. Glucose can lower the serum phosphorus level by promoting the shift of phosphate back into the cells.

P

Decreased Level

- Check the serum phosphorus, calcium, and magnesium levels, and report changes to the health care provider if the serum levels are unknown. An elevated calcium level causes a decreased phosphorus level.
- Monitor oral and IV phosphorus replacements. Some of the oral phosphate salts (Neutra-Phos) come in capsules and are indicated if nausea is present. Administer IV phosphate (KH_2PO_4) slowly to prevent hyperphosphatemia.
- Observe for signs and symptoms of hypophosphatemia, such as anorexia and pain in the muscles and bone.
- Observe for signs and symptoms of hypocalcemia (tetany) while the client is receiving phosphate supplements.

Client Teaching

- Instruct the client to eat foods rich in phosphorus (e.g., meats [beef, pork, turkey], milk, whole-grain cereals, and almonds) if the decrease is caused by malnutrition. Most carbonated drinks are high in phosphates.
- Instruct the client not to take antacids that contain aluminum hydroxide (Amphojel). Phosphorus binds with aluminum hydroxide; thus, a low serum phosphorus level results.

Increased Level

- Check the serum phosphorus, calcium, and magnesium levels. Observe for signs and symptoms of hypocalcemia (tetany). With an increased phosphorus level, calcium is usually low.
- Monitor urinary output. A decreased urine output (less than 25 mL/h or less than 600 mL/day) can increase the serum phosphorus level. Notify the health care provider of changes in urinary status.

Client Teaching

- Instruct the client to eat foods that are low in phosphorus (e.g., vegetables). Instruct the client to avoid drinking carbonated sodas that contain phosphates.

Placental Growth Factor (PGF) (serum)

Reference Values

Nonpregnant: Less than 50 pg/mL.

Pregnant female: 20 weeks: Greater than 200 pg/mL.

Description

When a pregnant female is prone to preeclampsia during pregnancy, various tests are performed to determine if she is likely to develop preeclampsia during this pregnancy. Normally the placental growth factor (PGF) rises throughout pregnancy to levels beyond 500 pg/mL. PGF is tested for pregnant clients prone to preeclampsia at 12 weeks of gestation and then monthly. If the PGF level is low or very low, she is at risk to develop preeclampsia during pregnancy.

Pregnancy associated plasma protein A (PAPP-A) aids in the diagnosis of preeclampsia. Other contributing factors of preeclampsia developing during pregnancy include a previous history of preeclampsia during other pregnancies, family history, increase in body weight, and African ancestry.

Purposes

- To determine the possibility of preeclampsia developing in regards to past and family history of preeclampsia.
- To monitor the PGF levels following 13 weeks of gestation.

Clinical Problems

Decreased Level: Risk for developing preeclampsia, hypertension.

Procedure

- There is no food or fluid restriction.
- Collect 3 to 5 mL of venous blood in a red-top tube.

NURSING IMPLICATIONS WITH RATIONALE

- Obtain a previous or family history of preeclampsia from the pregnant female.
- Record vital signs. Note if the blood pressure is elevated.

Client Teaching

- Explain the purpose for the PGF test and how often it may/will be taken. One test is not sufficient; monthly tests are needed, especially if there is a history of preeclampsia.
- Allow the client time to express her concerns about the test and/or possible preeclampsia.

Plasminogen (plasma)

Reference Values

Adult: 2.5–5.2 unit/mL, 7–16 mg/dL; 3.8–8.4 CTA (Council on Thrombolytic Agents).

Description

Plasminogen, inactive precursor of plasmin, is converted to plasmin, which activates the fibrinolytic process, a breakdown of fibrin clots in prevention of coagulation. Because plasmin cannot be measured in its active form in blood, plasminogen is measured to evaluate fibrinolysis. A decrease in plasminogen concentrate can indicate a tendency for thrombosis and also a serious secondary disease process (disseminated intravascular coagulation [DIC]).

Plasminogen is frequently monitored during administration of thrombolytic agents, such as streptokinase and urokinase, that are used to dissolve blood clots following an acute myocardial infarction. This test is also helpful in evaluating DIC.

P

Purposes
- To monitor the effect of thrombolytic therapy.
- To evaluate DIC.

Clinical Problems
Decreased Level: DIC liver disease (cirrhosis), thrombolytic therapy, tumors, preeclampsia. *Drug Influence:* Streptokinase.

Increased Level: Acute infection, MI, stress, surgery, trauma, malignant disease. *Drug Influence:* Oral contraceptives.

Procedure
- There is no food or fluid restriction.
- Collect 5 mL of venous blood in a blue-top tube. Avoid hemolysis. Avoid leaving the tourniquet on too long.

Factors Affecting Laboratory Results
- Hemolysis of the blood sample can affect results.
- Prolonged use of tourniquet could decrease plasma plasminogen level.
- Drugs (*see Drug Influence*).

NURSING IMPLICATIONS WITH RATIONALE

- Assess for bleeding tendencies, apprehension, petechiae, bleeding from orifices, tachycardia, and, later, hypotension.
- Check other laboratory findings (e.g., fibrin degradation products [FDPs]).
- Monitor vital signs.

Platelet aggregation and adhesions (blood)

Reference Values
Adult: Aggregation in 3–5 minutes.

Description
Platelet aggregation test measures the ability of platelets to adhere to each other when mixed with an aggregating agent, such as collagen, adenosine diphosphate (ADP), or ristocetin. This test is performed to detect abnormality in platelet function and to aid in diagnosing hereditary

and acquired platelet deficiencies, such as von Willebrand disease. Increased bleeding tendencies result from a decrease in platelet aggregation time.

The **platelet adhesion test**, like platelet aggregation, evaluates platelet function and helps to confirm hereditary diseases, such as von Willebrand disease. This test is also performed on clients taking large doses of aspirin for several weeks and on persons having a prolonged bleeding time. It is not performed in many laboratories because of the difficulty in standardizing the technique.

Clinical Problems

Decreased Platelet Aggregation: Von Willebrand disease, Bernard-Soulier syndrome, Glanzmann disease (thrombasthenia), leukemia, idiopathic thrombocytopenia, purpura, platelet release defects, afibrinogenemia, cirrhosis of the liver, uremia. *Drug Influence:* Aspirin and aspirin compounds, anti-inflammatory agents (ibuprofen [Motrin], indomethacin [Indocin], phenylbutazone [Butazolidin]), 5-fluorouracil, phenothiazines, tricyclic antidepressants, diazepam (Valium), antihistamines, dipyridamole (Persantine), clopidogrel (Plavix), cortisone preparations, theophylline, cocaine, marijuana.

Increased Platelet Aggregation: Diabetes mellitus, hyperlipemia, hypercoagulability.

Procedure

- The client should be NPO, including no medications, after midnight, except for water.
- Collect 5–7 mL of venous blood in a blue-top tube. Avoid hemolysis.
- Allow no aspirin or aspirin compounds for 7–10 days prior to the test. List drugs the client is taking on the laboratory slip.

Factors Affecting Laboratory Results

- Foods high in fat content eaten before the test; hyperlipemia increases platelet aggregation.
- Drugs that inhibit platelet aggregation (*see Drug Influence*).

NURSING IMPLICATIONS WITH RATIONALE

- Obtain a drug history from the client. Record and underline names of drugs the client is taking that could prolong platelet aggregation.
- List names of drugs that the client is taking that could affect test results on the laboratory slip.
- Check for bleeding tendencies, petechiae, purpura.

Client Teaching

- Inform the client of the importance of not taking aspirin and aspirin compounds 7–10 days before the test (check with the health care provider about the time period to avoid aspirin intake). Aspirin inhibits clotting time or prolongs bleeding time; thus the test could be invalidated.
- Inform the client that no medications, food, or fluids, except water, should be taken after midnight before the test (it may be necessary to take some medications before the test; check with health care provider).

Platelet antibody test (blood)

Platelet Antibody Detection Test, Antiplatelet Antibody Detection

P

Reference Values

Negative.

Description

When a client becomes sensitized to platelet antigens of transfused blood, platelet antibodies (autoantibodies) develop and thus cause thrombocytopenia because of destruction to the platelets. The platelet autoantibodies are IgG immunoglobulins of autoimmune origin. With idiopathic thrombocytopenic purpura (ITP), platelet autoantibodies are present.

Drug-induced thrombocytopenia is caused by platelet-associated IgG autoantibodies because of hypersensitivity to certain drugs. Some of the drugs that may cause drug-induced immunologic thrombocytopenia include salicylates, acetaminophen, antibiotics (sulfonamides, penicillin, cephalosporins), quinidine and quinidine-like drugs, gold compounds, cimetidine, oral hypoglycemic agents, heparin, digoxin.

Maternal–fetal platelet antigen incompatibility can occur if the mother has ITP autoantibodies that are passed to the fetus. Neonatal thrombocytopenia may result.

Purpose

- To detect the presence of platelet antibodies.

Clinical Problems

Positive Test: Thrombocytopenia because of platelet autoantibodies, idiopathic thrombocytopenic purpura, posttransfusion purpura, drug-induced thrombocytopenia.
Note: Drugs that may cause drug-induced thrombocytopenia (see Description).

Procedure

- No food or fluid restriction is required.
- Collect two 10 mL samples of venous blood in blue-top tubes. Deliver to the laboratory immediately with the time of collection written on the requisition form.

NURSING IMPLICATIONS WITH RATIONALE

- Obtain a drug history from the client.
- Check platelet count. If thrombocytopenia is present, a platelet antibody test may be ordered.
- Check for sites of petechiae and purpura. Report findings.

Client Teaching

- Instruct the client to report any abnormal bleeding.
- Listen to client's and family's concerns.

Platelet count (blood—thrombocytes)

Reference Values

Adult: 150,000–400,000 μL (mean, 250,000 μL), 0.15–0.4 $\times$ 10^{12}/L (SI units).

Child: *Premature:* 100,000–300,000 μL. *Newborn:* 150,000–300,000 μL. *Infant:* 200,000–475,000 μL (mm^3 or K/uL may be used for μl).

Description

Platelets (thrombocytes) are basic elements in the blood that promote coagulation. Platelets are much smaller than erythrocytes. They clump and stick to rough surfaces and injured sites when blood coagulation is needed. A decrease in circulating platelets of less than 50% of the normal value will cause bleeding; if the decrease is severe (less than 50,000 μL), hemorrhaging might occur.

Thrombocytopenia means platelet deficiency or a low platelet count. It is commonly associated with leukemias, aplastic anemia, and idiopathic thrombocytopenic purpura. Increased platelet counts (thrombocytosis) occur in polycythemia, in fractures, and after splenectomy.

Purposes

- To check the platelet count.
- To monitor the platelet count during cancer chemotherapy.

Clinical Problems

Decreased Level: Idiopathic thrombocytopenic purpura, multiple myeloma, cancer (bone, gastrointestinal tract, brain), leukemias (lymphocytic, myelocytic, monocytic), anemias (aplastic, iron deficiency, pernicious, folic acid deficiency, sickle cell), liver disease (cirrhosis, chronic active hepatitis), systemic lupus erythematosus, disseminated intravascular coagulopathy, kidney diseases, eclampsia, acute rheumatic fever. *Drug Influence:* Antibiotics (chloromycetin, streptomycin), sulfonamides, aspirin (salicylates), quinidine, quinine, acetazolamide (Diamox), amidopyrine, thiazide diuretics, meprobamate (Equanil), phenylbutazone (Butazolidin), tolbutamide (Orinase), vaccine injections, chemotherapeutic agents.

Increased Level: Polycythemia vera, trauma (surgery, fractures), postsplenectomy, acute blood loss (peaks in 7–10 days), metastatic carcinoma, pulmonary embolism, high altitudes, tuberculosis, reticulocytosis, severe exercise. *Drug Influence:* Epinephrine (adrenalin).

Procedure

- There is no food or fluid restriction.

Venous Blood: Collect 3–5 mL of venous blood in a lavender-top tube.

Capillary Blood: Discard the first few drips. Collect a drop of blood from a finger puncture, and dilute the blood immediately with the appropriate diluting solution.

Factors Affecting Laboratory Results

- Chemotherapy and x-ray therapy can cause a decreased platelet count.
- Drugs (*see Drug Influence*).

NURSING IMPLICATIONS WITH RATIONALE

- Explain to the client that the purpose of the blood test is to determine the platelet count.
- Check the platelet count, especially with bleeding episodes, and report abnormal levels.

Decreased Level

- Observe for signs and symptoms of bleeding (skin [purpura, petechiae] or gastrointestinal [hematemesis, rectal bleeding]). Record findings on the chart and report them to the health care provider.
- Monitor the platelet count, especially when the client is receiving chemotherapy or radiation therapy for cancer.

Client Teaching

- Instruct the client to avoid injury if possible. Mild injury could cause bleeding.

Porphobilinogen (urine)

Reference Values

Adult: *Random (qualitative)*: Negative. *24 Hour (quantitative)*: 0–2 mg/24 h.
Child: Same as adult.

Description

Porphobilinogen is one of the precursors of porphyrins, and large amounts are excreted during an acute attack of porphyria. Between attacks there may not be an appreciable amount of porphobilinogen present. The test should be conducted during the acute phase.

The urine porphobilinogen test is ordered to detect the presence of porphyrias. Porphyrias are inherent metabolic disorders that affect the synthesis of heme or hemoglobin. Congenital porphyria (erythropoietic porphyria) is characterized by pinkish brown-stained teeth, pinkish yellow to reddish black urine, and skin photosensitivity. Uroporphyrin and coproporphyrin I are excreted.

Hereditary hepatic porphyria can be divided into three types: acute intermittent porphyria, variegate porphyria, and hereditary coproporphyria. During an acute attack of porphyria, the urine becomes deep red and there are mental disturbances and severe abdominal pain. These attacks mimic various diseases, such as appendicitis and pancreatitis; the leukocyte (white blood cell) count becomes elevated. Barbiturates, alcohol, and estrogen can precipitate an acute attack of porphyria.

Purpose

- To detect the presence of porphyrias.

Clinical Problems

Increased Level: Acute intermittent porphyria, variegate porphyria, secondary malignant neoplasm, Hodgkin disease, cirrhosis of the liver (occasionally). *Drug Influence:* Antibiotics (penicillin, tetracyclines), antiseptics (phenol compounds, phenazopyridine [Pyridium]), barbiturates, hypnotics, phenothiazines (chlorpromazine [Thorazine]), procaine, sulfonamides.

Procedure

Qualitative (Screening Test)

- Collect a random sample of 30 mL or more of fresh urine during or immediately after an acute attack of porphyria, when the client has acute abdominal pain.
- Protect the specimen from light.

Quantitative (24 Hour)

- Collect the urine in a dark container. If it is collected in a clear container, protect it from light and refrigerate. The container should have an acidic preservative. Delta amino levulinic acid (ALA), which forms porphobilinogen, is not stable unless the urine is acidic. Urine should be collected immediately after the client has an acute attack.
- Have the client void, discard the urine, and then save all urine for 24 hours.
- Label the specimen with the date and the exact time the test started and ended.
- Encourage the client to take fluids. There is no food restriction.

Factors Affecting Laboratory Results

- Exposure of the urine sample to light.
- Drugs (*see Drug Influence*).
- Contamination of the urine with toilet paper or feces.

NURSING IMPLICATIONS WITH RATIONALE

Patient Teaching

- Explain the procedure to the client and family and tell them not to throw away any urine. Tell them that urine should not be exposed to light and should be refrigerated.
- Inform the client that he or she should not contaminate the urine with toilet paper or feces.

Increased Level

- Recognize that this test is usually done during an acute attack (acute abdominal pain) to detect porphyria.
- Observe and report urine color prior to an acute attack. The urine color should be amber to burgundy.
- Observe for signs and symptoms of an acute porphyria attack, such as severe abdominal pain (colicky), mental disturbances, and neuropathy. Respiratory distress could occur.

Client Teaching

- Instruct the client with porphyria to stay away from bright sunlight. Skin photosensitivity is a common problem, and skin lesions could result. Suggest that the client use sunscreen on exposed skin areas and wear protective clothing.
- Instruct the client not to take barbiturates, alcohol, or estrogens without permission. These agents can precipitate an acute attack of porphyria.

Porphyrins—coproporphyrins, uroporphyrins (urine)

Reference Values

Coproporphyrins: *Adult:* Random: 3–20 mcg/dL. Quantitative: 50–160 mcg/24 h. *Child:* 0–80 mcg/24 h.

Uroporphyrins: *Adult:* Random: Negative. Quantitative: Less than 30 mcg/24 h. *Child:* 10–30 mcg/24 h.

Description

Porphyrins are used in the synthesis of hemoglobin and of any hemoproteins that are carriers of oxygen. The porphyrins are eliminated from the body in feces and urine, mainly as coproporphyrins I and III and as uroporphyrins. Normal excretion of coproporphyrins is minimal, but the amount excreted rises during liver damage, lead poisoning, and congenital porphyria (an inherent error of metabolism).

There is an increase in urine porphobilinogen with disorders of porphyrin metabolism. Porphobilinogen is one of the precursors of porphyrins (formed in the liver).

Purposes

- To monitor porphyrin levels.
- To aid in the diagnosis of selected disease entities (*see Clinical Problems*).

Clinical Problems

Increased Level: Lead toxicity, cirrhosis of the liver, acute intermittent porphyria, viral hepatitis, infectious mononucleosis, porphyria variegata, porphyria cutanea tarda, acquired hemolytic anemia (autoimmune). *Drug Influence:* Antibiotics (tetracyclines, penicillin), antiseptics (ethoxazene [Diaphenyl], phenazopyridine [Pyridium]), sulfonamides (sulfamethoxazole [Gantanol], sulfisoxazole [Gantrisin]), barbiturates and hypnotics, phenothiazines such as chlorpromazine (Thorazine), procaine.

Procedure

- There is no food or fluid restriction.
- Collect urine in a dark container containing the preservative sodium carbonate. If a large, clear container is used, protect it from light and refrigerate it.
- Have the client void, discard the urine, and then save all urine for 24 hours.
- Label the specimen with the exact date and time the test started and ended (e.g., 7/24/20, 7:00 AM to 7/25/20, 7:01 AM).

Factors Affecting Laboratory Results

- Exposure of the urine to light.
- Drugs (*see Drug Influence*).
- Contamination of the urine with toilet paper and feces.

NURSING IMPLICATIONS WITH RATIONALE

Client Teaching

- Explain the procedure to the client. Inform the client and family that all urine must be saved for 24 hours. Emphasize that the urine should *not* be exposed to light.
- Inform the client not to contaminate the urine with toilet paper or feces.

Increased Level

- Recognize clinical problems and drugs related to elevated porphyrin levels. Liver disease and lead poisoning cause an excessive amount of coproporphyrin III to be excreted.
- Observe the color of a urine specimen exposed to light. A pinkish or red color should be reported.

Potassium (K) (serum)

Reference Values

Adult: 3.5–5.3 mEq/L, 3.5–5.3 mmol/L (SI units).
Panic Values: Less than 2.5 mEq/L and greater than 7 mEq/L.
Child: *Child:* 3.5–4.8 mEq/L. *Infant:* 3.5–5.5 mEq/L. *Newborn:* 3.8–5.8 mEq/L.

Description

Potassium is the electrolyte found most abundantly in intracellular fluids (cells). The serum potassium level has a narrow range, and cardiac arrest could occur if serum level is less than 2.5 mEq/L or greater than 7 mEq/L.

Eighty to 90% of the body potassium is excreted by the kidneys. When there is tissue breakdown, potassium leaves the cells and enters the extracellular fluid (interstitial and intravascular fluids). With adequate kidney functions, the potassium in the intravascular fluid (plasma/blood vessels) will be excreted, and with excessive potassium excretion, a serum potassium deficit (hypokalemia) occurs. However, if the kidneys are excreting less than 600 mL of urine daily, potassium will accumulate in the intravascular fluid and serum potassium excess (hyperkalemia) will occur.

The body does not conserve potassium, and the kidneys excrete an average of 40 mEq/L daily (the range is 25–120 mEq/L/24 h), even with a low dietary potassium intake. The daily potassium requirement is 3–4 g, or 40–60 mEq/L.

Purposes

- To check the potassium level.
- To detect the presence of hypo- or hyperkalemia.
- To monitor potassium levels during health problems (e.g., renal insufficiency, debilitating illness, cancer), and with certain drugs (e.g., thiazide diuretics).

P

Clinical Problems

Decreased Level: Vomiting/diarrhea, dehydration, malnutrition/starvation, crash diet, stress (trauma, injury, or surgery), gastric suction, intestinal fistulas, diabetic acidosis, burns, renal tubular disorders, hyperaldosteronism, excessive ingestion of licorice, excessive ingestion of glucose, alkalosis (metabolic). *Drug Influence:* Potassium-wasting diuretics (furosemide [Lasix], thiazides [Hydro-DIURIL], ethacrynic acid [Edecrin]), steroids (cortisone, estrogen), antibiotics (gentamicin, amphotericin, polymyxin B), bicarbonate, insulin, laxatives, lithium carbonate, sodium polystyrene sulfonate (Kayexalate), salicylates (aspirin).

Increased Level: Oliguria and anuria, acute renal failure, IV potassium in fluids, Addison disease (adrenocortical hormone), crushed injury and burns (with kidney shutdown), acidosis (metabolic or lactic). *Drug Influence:* Potassium-sparing diuretics, spironolactone (Aldactone), triamterene (Dyrenium), antibiotics (penicillin G potassium), cephaloridine (Loridin), heparin, epinephrine, histamine, isoniazid.

Procedure

- Food, fluid, and drug restrictions are not necessary.
- Collect 3–5 mL of venous blood in a red-top tube. Avoid hemolysis.
- Avoid leaving the tourniquet on for more than 2 minutes if possible.

Factors Affecting Laboratory Results

- The hydration status of the client can cause false potassium test values. Overhydration can cause a false serum potassium deficit through hemodilution. Dehydration can cause a serum potassium excess through hemoconcentration. After the client is hydrated, his or her serum potassium level may be normal or slightly low.
- The use of a tourniquet can cause an increase in the serum potassium level.
- Hemolysis of the specimen (blood) can result in a high serum potassium level.
- Drugs (*see Drug Influence*).
- Blood for transfusion that is 2 weeks or older has an elevated serum potassium level.

NURSING IMPLICATIONS WITH RATIONALE

- Compare serum potassium levels with urine potassium levels. When the serum potassium level is decreased, the urine potassium level is frequently increased, and vice versa.

Decreased Level

- Observe for signs and symptoms of hypokalemia, such as vertigo (dizziness), hypotension, cardiac dysrhythmias, nausea, vomiting, diarrhea, abdominal distention, decreased peristalsis, muscle weakness, and leg cramps.
- Record intake and output. Polyuria can cause an excessive loss of potassium. Potassium is not conserved well in the body, and the kidney excretes potassium regardless of potassium intake.
- Report serum potassium levels less than 3.5 mEq/L. If the potassium level is 3–3.5 mEq/L, it will take 100–200 mEq/L of potassium chloride (KCl) to raise the potassium level 1 mEq/L. If the potassium level is 2.9 mEq/L or less, it will take 200–400 mEq/L of KCl to raise the level 1 mEq/L.

- Determine the client's hydration status when hypokalemia is present. Overhydration can dilute the serum potassium level.
- Recognize behavioral changes as a sign of hypokalemia. Low potassium levels can cause confusion, irritability, and mental depression. The serum potassium level should be checked in the presence of any behavioral changes.
- Report electrocardiographic changes. A prolonged and depressed ST segment and a flat or inverted T-wave is indicative of hypokalemia.
- Dilute oral potassium supplements in at least 4 oz of water or juice. Potassium is a corrosive agent and is most irritating to the gastric mucosa.
- Monitor the serum potassium level in clients receiving potassium-wasting diuretics and steroids. Examples of potassium-wasting diuretics are HydroDIURIL, Lasix, and Edecrin. Cortisone steroids (such as prednisone) cause sodium retention and potassium excretion.
- Assess for signs and symptoms of digitalis toxicity when the client is receiving a digitalis preparation and a potassium-wasting diuretic or steroid. A lower serum potassium level enhances the action of digitalis. Signs and symptoms of digitalis toxicity are nausea and vomiting, anorexia, bradycardia, cardiac dysrhythmia, and visual disturbances.
- Monitor serum chloride, serum magnesium, and serum protein test results when hypokalemia is present. Correcting a potassium deficit with potassium only is not effective if chloride, magnesium, and protein levels are also low.
- Administer IV KCl in a liter of parenteral fluids. Never give an IV or bolus push of KCl, because cardiac arrest can occur. Parenteral KCl can only be administered intravenously when it is diluted (20–40 mEq per liter) and should never be given subcutaneously or intramuscularly. Concentrated IV KCl is irritating to the heart muscle and to the veins, causing phlebitis.
- Check the IV site when the client is receiving KCl in IV fluids. Infiltrated potassium is most irritating to the subcutaneous tissues (fatty tissues) and can cause tissue sloughing.
- Measure gastrointestinal fluid loss from suctioning, vomiting, or diarrhea for appropriate potassium and other electrolyte replacement. Potassium, sodium, hydrogen, and chloride are most plentiful in the gastrointestinal tract.
- Irrigate gastrointestinal tubes with normal saline solution to prevent electrolyte loss.

Client Teaching

- Instruct the client and family to eat foods high in potassium (fruits, dried fruits, vegetables, meats, nuts, coffee, tea, cocoa, and colas). The daily potassium requirement is 3–4 g, or 40–60 mEq/L.
- Teach clients to eat foods rich in potassium when they are taking drugs and foods that decrease body potassium (e.g., cortisone, potassium-wasting diuretics, laxatives, lithium carbonate, salicylates, insulin, glucose, and licorice).

Increased Level

- Observe for signs and symptoms of hyperkalemia, or serum potassium excess (slow pulse rate [bradycardia], abdominal cramps, oliguria or anuria, tingling, and twitching or numbness of the extremities).
- Assess urine output to determine renal function. Urine output should be at least 25 mL/h, or 600 mL daily, and a urine output of less than 600 mL/day could cause hyperkalemia.

P

- Report serum potassium levels greater than 5.3 mEq/L. High serum potassium levels can cause cardiac arrest.
- Regulate the rate of IV fluids so that no more than 10 mEq KCl are administered per hour. Rapid administration of KCl intravenously can result in hyperkalemia.
- Check the age of whole blood before administering it to a client with hyperkalemia. Blood 2 weeks old or older has an elevated serum potassium level.
- Assess the client's serum potassium level every 6 to 8 hours when it is elevated (greater than 6.5 mEq/L) and during treatment for hyperkalemia. The serum potassium level can change frequently during treatment.
- Monitor the electrocardiogram for QRS spread and peaked T-waves (signs of hyperkalemia). The pulse rate may be rapid, but if hyperkalemia persists, bradycardia or slow pulse can occur.
- Restrict potassium intake when the serum potassium level is greater than 6 mEq/L.
- Monitor clients receiving various medical treatments for hyperkalemia for signs and symptoms of continuous hyperkalemia or developing hypokalemia. The various medical treatments are as follows: (1) IV sodium bicarbonate increases the pH, causing potassium to shift back into the cells; (2) IV glucose and insulin can also cause potassium to shift back into the cells and are usually effective for 6 hours; (3) calcium gluconate decreases the myocardial irritability resulting from hyperkalemia but does not decrease the serum potassium level; (4) sodium polystyrene sulfonate (Kayexalate) is a drug used as ion exchange resin, sodium for potassium. It can be administered orally or rectally and is considered the most effective method for treating hyperkalemia.
- Notify the health care provider if the client is receiving a digitalis preparation when calcium gluconate is given. An elevated serum calcium level enhances the action of digitalis, causing digitalis toxicity.
- Observe for signs and symptoms of hypokalemia when administering Kayexalate for a prolonged period of time (2 or more days).

Potassium (K) (urine)

Reference Values

Adult: *Broad Range:* 25–120 mEq/24 h. *Average Range:* 40–80 mEq/24 h, 40–80 mmol/24 h (SI units).

Child: 17–57 mEq/24 h.

Description

Eighty to 90% of the body's potassium is excreted in the urine. A 24-hour urine potassium level is a valuable indicator of serum potassium status. A decrease in urinary potassium can indicate hyperkalemia (elevated serum potassium), and an increase in urinary potassium can indicate hypokalemia (low serum potassium) or may result from an increased potassium intake. If the kidneys are not functioning properly and there is decreased urine output (oliguria), the potassium excreted in the urine will be decreased and the serum potassium level will be elevated.

Purposes

(See Potassium [serum].)

P

Clinical Problems

Decreased Level: Elevated serum potassium level, acute renal failure, diarrhea. *Drug Influence:* Potassium-sparing diuretics (e.g., Aldactone).

Increased Level: Decreases serum potassium level, dehydration/starvation, chronic renal failure, diabetic acidosis, vomiting and gastric suction, increased adrenal cortical hormone or Cushing disease, salicylate toxicity. *Drug Influence:* Potassium-wasting diuretics (e.g., HydroDIURIL, Lasix), prednisone.

Procedure

- There is no food or fluid restriction.
- The 24-hour urine specimen should be kept on ice or refrigerated.
- Potassium supplements given as salt replacement should be eliminated for 48 hours.

Factors Affecting Laboratory Results

- Failure to refrigerate the urine container affects test results.
- Fecal material and toilet paper contaminate urine specimen.
- Vomiting or gastric suctioning can cause hypokalemia due to potassium loss from the gastrointestinal tract, and the accompanying metabolic alkalosis can cause an increase in urinary potassium loss. With a high urinary potassium excretion, the hypokalemic state could become more severe.

NURSING IMPLICATIONS WITH RATIONALE

Decreased Level

- Explain to the client that the purpose of the test is to determine whether the kidneys are excreting an adequate amount of potassium or whether the body is retaining it.
- Instruct the client to save all of his or her urine for 24 hours and to place it in the container, which should be on ice or refrigerated.
- Observe for signs and symptoms of hyperkalemia. When urinary potassium excretion is decreased, the serum potassium level may be increased. Signs and symptoms of hyperkalemia are oliguria, abdominal cramps, bradycardia, and tingling, twitching, or numbness in the extremities. Check the arterial pH or the serum carbon dioxide (CO_2) levels. If metabolic acidosis is present (decreased pH and serum CO_2), the serum potassium may be elevated and the urinary potassium may be decreased. Potassium is frequently retained in the body during metabolic acidosis.

Metabolic acidosis: $\downarrow$ pH, $\uparrow$ serum $CO_2 \rightarrow \downarrow$ serum K, $\downarrow$ urinary K

P

Increased Level

- Explain to the client that an increase in potassium intake or the use of diuretics (potassium wasting) will result in an excess urinary potassium excretion.
- Observe for signs and symptoms of hypokalemia. When urinary potassium excretion is increased, the serum potassium level is frequently decreased. Signs and symptoms of hypokalemia are vertigo (dizziness), hypotension, cardiac dysrhythmia, muscle weakness, and decreased peristalsis.
- Determine arterial pH or serum CO_2 levels. If metabolic alkalosis is present (elevated pH and serum CO_2), the serum potassium level may be low and the urine potassium may be increased. Hydrogen and potassium are excreted together in the urine and alkalosis results. Vomiting and gastric suction can cause metabolic alkalosis.

Metabolic Alkalosis: $\uparrow$ pH, $\uparrow$ serum $CO_2 \rightarrow \downarrow$ serum K, $\uparrow$ urinary K

Prealbumin (PA, PAB) antibody assay (serum)

Transthyretin (TTR), Thyroxin-Binding Prealbumin (TBPA)

Reference Values

Adult: 17–40 mg/dL, 170–400 mg/L (SI units). *Female (average):* 18 mg/dL, 180 mg/L (SI units). *Male (average):* 21.6 mg/dL, 216 mg/L (SI units).

Child: *Newborn:* 10–11.5 mg/dL, 100–115 mg/L (SI units). *2 to 3 Years:* 16–28 mg/dL, 160–280 mg/L (SI units).

Description

Prealbumin, also known as thyroxin-binding protein, thyroxin-binding prealbumin (TBPA), or transthyretin, is a test used primarily for nutritional assessment. Prealbumin has a shorter half-life (2–4 days) than albumin (20–24 days). This test is more sensitive for determining nutritional status and liver dysfunction than an albumin test.

It is also useful in monitoring the effectiveness of total parenteral nutrition (TPN) and evaluating the nutritional needs in critically ill clients. Prealbumin transports protein for triiodothyronine and thyroxine. It is also needed for the metabolism and transporting of vitamin A. Prealbumin is greatly reduced in hepatobiliary disease and chronic malignancy disease. This test is more sensitive for determining liver dysfunction than an albumin test. A prealbumin value of less than 5 mg/dL indicates severe protein depletion, and a value less than 10 mg/dL indicates severe nutritional deficiency.

Purposes

- To assess the client's nutritional status.
- To evaluate the client's nutritional needs postsurgery, and for the critically ill.

Clinical Problems

Decreased Level: Protein-wasting diseases, malnutrition, inflammation, malignancy, cirrhosis of the liver, zinc deficiency. *Drug Influence:* Estrogen, oral contraceptives.

Increased Level: Hodgkin disease, chronic kidney disease. *Drug Influence:* Steroids, nonsteroidal anti-inflammatory drugs (NSAIDs).

P

Procedure

- There is no food or fluid restriction.
- Collect 2–5 mL of venous blood in a red-top tube.
- Avoid hemolysis.

Factors Affecting Laboratory Results

- Hemolysis can cause a false test result.

NURSING IMPLICATIONS WITH RATIONALE

- Obtain a history of the client's nutritional intake. Record findings; relate findings to the health care providers (i.e., the physician or dietitian).
- Check vital signs and weight.
- Listen to the client's concerns; answer questions or refer them to other health care providers.

Client Teaching

- Inform the client of ways in which nutritional status can be improved.

Pregnancy-Associated Plasma Protein-A (PAPP-A) (serum)

Normal Values

Values differ with various laboratories.

Description

Pregnancy-associated plasma protein-A (PAPP-A) is useful in predicting preeclampsia and various fetal development disorders, such as Down syndrome, Trisomy 18 and 21, and Turner syndrome. A decreased value can also result in stillbirth. Normally the PAPP-A rises rapidly during the first trimester of pregnancy.

With Down syndrome, the PAPP-A level is half of the normal value. Amniocentesis may be suggested for a definitive diagnosis.

Purposes

- To check the PAPP-A level during the first trimester for fetal abnormalities.
- To determine if preeclampsia could occur during the pregnancy if the female has a history of past or familiar preeclampsia.

Clinical Problems

Decreased Level: Down syndrome, Trisomy 18 and 21, Turner syndrome, preeclampsia, stillbirth.

Procedure

- There is no food or fluid restriction.
- Collect 5 mL of venous blood in a red-top tube.

Factors Affecting Laboratory Results

- Maternal weight increase.

NURSING IMPLICATIONS WITH RATIONALE

- Record a past history of pregnancy problems, such as preeclampsia.
- Explain to the pregnant female that the purpose of the test is to check the status of the fetus. The test could be requested because of the late age of the client. Also this test can determine if the client is prone to preeclampsia.

Client Teaching

- Address the client's concerns regarding a possible unfavorable test result. Answer the client's questions or refer them to the health care provider.
- Inform the client that if the test is abnormal other tests and procedures may be requested for verification. For possible Down syndrome, an amniocentesis may be ordered.

Pregnanediol (urine)

Reference Values

Adult: *Male:* 0.1–1.5 mg/24 h. *Female:* 0.5–1.5 mg/24 h (proliferative phase), 2–7 mg/24 h (luteal phase), 0.1–1 mg/24 h (postmenopausal).

Pregnancy	
GESTATION WEEKS	**mg/24 h**
10–19	5–25
20–28	15–42
28–32	25–49

Child: 0.4–1 mg/24 h.

Description

Pregnanediol is the major metabolite of progesterone produced by the ovary during the secretory phase of the menstrual cycle (second half) and by the placenta. Progesterone is responsible for uterine changes after ovulation and for maintaining pregnancy after fertilization. A steady rise in urinary pregnanediol levels occurs during pregnancy, and a decrease in these levels indicates placental (not fetal) dysfunction and the possibility of an abortion. Progesterone therapy would be indicated when urine pregnanediol is decreased.

Urinary pregnanediol levels may be used to determine menstrual disturbances and are used to verify ovulation in those who have not been able to become pregnant. The pregnanediol levels rise rapidly after ovulation, and they can be used as an indicator of ovulation time. This test should not be mistaken for the pregnanetriol test.

Purposes

- To determine the occurrence of placental dysfunction.
- To compare test results with those of other laboratory tests for determining the cause of a menstrual disorder.

Clinical Problems

Decreased Level: Amenorrhea (menstrual disorder), ovarian hypofunction, threatened abortion, pregnancy complicated by intrauterine death, benign neoplasms of the ovary and breast, lutein cell tumor of the ovary, preeclampsia.

Increased Level: Pregnancy, ovarian cyst, choriocarcinoma of the ovary, adrenal cortex hyperplasia.

Procedure

- There is no food or fluid restriction.
- Collect urine over a 24-hour period in a large container or bottle with preservative and keep it refrigerated.
- Label the bottle with the client's name and the dates and exact times of collection (e.g., 4/10/20, 8:00 AM to 4/11/20, 8:00 AM).
- Record on the laboratory slip the date of the last menstrual period.
- Take the urine bottle to the laboratory immediately after the urine collection has been completed.
- The urine may also be used to determine estradiol (E3) levels in conjunction with the pregnanediol levels.

Factors Affecting Laboratory Results

- Toilet paper and feces in the urine.
- An unrefrigerated urine collection that has not been analyzed for several days.

NURSING IMPLICATIONS WITH RATIONALE

- Ask when the client had her last period; this should be recorded on the laboratory slip.

Client Teaching

- Explain to the client the procedure for collecting urine. Explain that all urine should be saved and placed in the labeled container in the refrigerator.
- Instruct the client not to put toilet paper or feces in the urine.

P

Decreased Level

- Recognize clinical problems that may cause a decreased pregnanediol level, such as menstrual disorder (amenorrhea), threatened abortion, and complicated pregnancy.
- Obtain a history of menstrual changes (menstruation patterns—frequency, length of period, flow, and discomfort).
- Obtain a history of pregnancy complications or problems. Record when the client had her last menstrual period and whether bleeding is present (how long has it occurred, how much bleeding, and is it continuous?).
- Give support to the client and family by listening, spending time with them, and answering questions, if possible. Supportive care can reduce anxiety.
- Monitor the urine pregnanediol levels if several tests have been ordered over a period of days or weeks. The levels can indicate progesterone production and whether progesterone therapy is needed.

Increased Level

- Recognize clinical problems that can cause an elevated pregnanediol level, such as pregnancy and an ovarian cyst. The pregnanediol level should increase during pregnancy. After 18–24 weeks, the level should be 13–22 mg/24 h, and after 28–32 weeks, the level should be 27–47 mg/24 h. In the last 2 weeks of pregnancy, the urine pregnanediol level decreases.

Pregnanetriol (urine)

Reference Values

Adult: *Male:* 0.4–2.4 mg/24 h. *Female:* 0.5–2 mg/24 h.

Child: *Infant:* 0–0.2 mg/24 h. *Child:* 0–1 mg/24 h.

Description

Pregnanetriol (17-hydroxyprogesterone) comes from adrenal corticoid synthesis. It should not be mistaken for pregnanediol because it is not a derivative of progesterone. The pregnanetriol test is useful in diagnosing congenital adrenocortical hyperplasia.

Purpose

- To detect anterior pituitary hypofunction or adrenocortical hyperfunction.

Clinical Problems

Decreased Level: Anterior pituitary hypofunction.

Increased Level: Adrenogenital syndrome, congenital adrenocortical hyperplasia, adrenocortical hyperfunction, malignant neoplasm of the adrenal gland.

Procedure

- There is no food or fluid restriction.

- Collect urine for 24 hours in a large, refrigerated container. No preservative is needed.
- Label the bottle with the client's name, date, and exact times of collection (e.g., 2/3/20, 8:00 AM to 2/4/20, 8:02 AM).

Factors Affecting Laboratory Results
- None known.

NURSING IMPLICATIONS WITH RATIONALE

- Monitor urine pregnanetriol levels with cortisone replacement.

Client Teaching
- Instruct the client and family to save all urine for 24 hours, to keep the urine refrigerated, and not to put toilet paper or feces in the urine.

Procainamide hydrochloride (serum)
Pronestyl, Procan, Procamide

Reference Values
Therapeutic Range: *Adult:* 4–10 mcg/mL, 5–30 mcg/mL, for sum of procainamide + NAPA. *Child:* Not done.

Toxic Level: *Adults:* Greater than 10 mcg/mL, greater than 30 mcg/mL, sum of procainamide + NAPA.

Description
Procainamide (Pronestyl, Procan), an antiarrhythmic agent, is used to treat cardiac arrhythmias. It acts by prolonging the refractory period of the heart, reducing conduction velocity, and decreasing myocardial excitability. This drug is absorbed readily from the gastrointestinal tract and is metabolized by the liver to active metabolites.

Procainamide can be administered orally, intramuscularly, and intravenously. The most common method is oral administration. The peak level occurs 1½ hours after oral administration. The steady state is about 24 hours after ingestion with good renal function. The half-life for procainamide is about 3–4 hours, and for the metabolite *N*-acetylprocainamide (NAPA) about 6–8 hours. Approximately 50% of the drug is excreted unchanged in the urine.

Common side effects of this drug are nausea, vomiting, bitter taste, hypotension, and bradycardia. Lupus erythematosus-like syndrome occurs in about 30–40% of clients on long-term procainamide therapy (1 year or more).

Purposes
- To monitor procainamide levels for therapeutic effect.
- To check for procainamide toxicity.

Clinical Problems

Increased Level: Overdose of procainamide, renal disease, liver disease. *Drug Influence:* Acetazolamide (Diamox), cimetidine (Tagamet), sodium bicarbonate. Increased hypotensive effect with methyldopa (Aldomet), reserpine (Serpasil).

Procedure

- There is no food or fluid restriction.
- Collect 3–5 mL of venous blood in a red-top tube.
- Record the dose, route, and last time the drug was administered on the laboratory requisition slip.
- Obtain blood samples during the peak level, 1–2 hours after oral administration, or ½ hour after IV administration.
- A trough level (before next dose) may be requested.

Factors Affecting Laboratory Results

- Drugs (*see Drug Influence*) could elevate the serum procainamide level.

NURSING IMPLICATIONS WITH RATIONALE

- Report the client with a history of renal disease to the health care provider. The procainamide dose might need to be adjusted.
- Monitor the serum procainamide level frequently, because one serum sample is not enough for evaluating therapy.
- Monitor IV procainamide; it should not exceed 25–50 mg/min.
- Administer oral dosage 1 hour before or 2 hours after meals with a glass of water to increase absorption.
- Assess vital signs frequently during oral and parenteral drug therapy. Report if the pulse rate and blood pressure decrease substantially from baseline levels. Fever may occur during the first few days of therapy. Report temperature elevation.

Increased Level

- Observe for signs and symptoms of side effects and procainamide overdose, such as anorexia, nausea, vomiting, bitter taste, dizziness, mental changes, muscle and joint pain, rash, hypotension, and bradycardia.
- Observe for signs and symptoms of lupus erythematosus-like syndrome (skin rash, erythema, fever, polyarthralgias, pleuritic pain). These symptoms are reversible.

Progesterone (serum)

Reference Values

Adult: *Female:* Follicular phase: 0.1–1.5 ng/mL, 20–150 ng/dL. Luteal phase: 2–28 ng/mL, 250–2800 ng/dL. Postmenopausal: Less than 1 ng/mL, less than 100 ng/dL. *Pregnancy:* First trimester: 9–50 ng/mL. Second trimester: 18–150 ng/mL. Third trimester: 60–260 ng/mL. *Male:* Less than 1 ng/mL, less than 10 ng/dL.

Description

Progesterone, a hormone produced primarily by the corpus luteum of the ovaries and in a small amount by the adrenal cortex, peaks during the luteal phase of the menstrual cycle for 4–5 days and during pregnancy. It prepares the endometrium for implantation of the fertilized egg. Only a small amount of progesterone is detected in the blood, because most is metabolized in the liver to pregnanediol, a progesterone metabolite.

Serum progesterone is useful in evaluating infertility problems, in confirming ovulation, and in assessing placental functions in pregnancy. A urine pregnanediol might be ordered to verify serum progesterone results.

Purposes

- To aid in the diagnosis of an ovarian or adrenal tumor.
- To assist in the diagnosis of placental failure.
- To evaluate infertility problems resulting from a decreased progesterone level.

Clinical Problems

Decreased Levels: Gonadal dysfunction, luteum deficiency, threatened abortion, toxemia of pregnancy, placental failure, fetal death. *Drug Influence:* Oral contraceptives.

Increased Levels: Ovulation, pregnancy, ovarian cysts, tumors of the ovary or adrenal gland. *Drug Influence:* ACTH, progesterone preparations.

Procedure

- There is no food or fluid restriction.
- Collect 5–7 mL of venous blood in a red-top (preferred) or green-top tube. Avoid hemolysis. Invert the green-top tube several times to mix with the anticoagulant in the tube.
- Note on the laboratory slip the phase of the client's menstrual cycle or weeks of gestation if pregnant.

Factors Affecting Laboratory Results

- Hemolysis from rough handling of the blood sample.
- Progesterone and estrogen therapy.

NURSING IMPLICATIONS WITH RATIONALE

- Obtain a history from the client of her menstrual phase or weeks or months of gestation. Record findings.

Client Teaching

- Inform the client that the blood test may be repeated or that a urine test may be ordered. Repeated tests at different times are usually performed to gather information concerning progesterone secretion.
- Listen to the client's concerns and fears. If unable to answer client's questions, direct to appropriate health professionals.

Prolactin (PRL) (serum)

Lactogenic Hormone, Lactogen

P

Reference Value

Female: *Nonpregnant:* Follicular phase: 0–23 ng/mL. Luteal phase: 0–40 ng/mL. Postmenopausal: Less than 12 ng/mL. *Pregnant:* First trimester: Less than 80 ng/mL. Second trimester: Less than 160 ng/mL. Third trimester: Less than 400 ng/mL.

Male: 0.1–20 ng/mL.

Pituitary Adenoma: Greater than 100–300 ng/mL.

Description

Prolactin, a hormone secreted by the anterior pituitary gland, is necessary in the development of the mammary glands for lactation and for stimulating and maintaining lactation postpartum. If the mother does not breastfeed, serum prolactin falls to normal range.

Serum prolactin levels 100–300 ng/mL in nonpregnant females and in males may indicate a pituitary adenoma (tumor). Bromocriptine (Parlodel) decreases the serum prolactin level and slows tumor growth until the pituitary tumor can be removed.

Prolactin levels may be monitored to determine the effects of surgery, chemotherapy, and/or radiation for treating prolactin-secreting tumors. Impotence in the male might be attributed to excess prolactin secretion that suppresses gonad function.

Purposes

- To detect various health problems related to an increased prolactin level (*see Clinical Problems*).
- To check drugs that the client is taking that influence increased prolactin levels.

Clinical Problems

Decreased Levels: Postpartum pituitary infarction. *Drug Influence:* Bromocriptine, levodopa, ergot derivatives, apomorphine.

Increased Levels: Pregnancy, breastfeeding, pituitary tumor, amenorrhea, ectopic prolactin-secreting tumors (such as of the lung), galactorrhea, hypothalamic disorder, primary hypothyroidism, endometriosis, chronic renal failure, polycystic ovary, Addison disease, stress, sleep, coitus, exercise. *Drug Influence:* Amphetamine, estrogens, antihistamines, oral contraceptives, phenothiazines, tricyclic antidepressants, monoamine oxidase inhibitors (MAO inhibitors), methyldopa (Aldomet), haloperidol (Haldol), cimetidine (Tagamet), procainamide derivatives, reserpine (Serpasil), isoniazid (INH), verapamil.

Procedure

- Withhold food, fluid, and medications for 12 hours prior to the test. If a medication needs to be taken within the 12 hours, the drug should be noted on the laboratory slip and recorded on the client's chart.
- Collect 3–5 mL of venous blood in a red- or lavender-top tube. Avoid hemolysis. The client should be awake for 1–2 hours before blood test. Sleep elevates the serum prolactin level.

Factors Affecting Laboratory Results

- Drugs can cause false-positive or negative laboratory test results (*see Drug Influence*).
- Exercise, stress, pain, surgical trauma, sleep.

NURSING IMPLICATIONS WITH RATIONALE

- Check with the health care provider to determine if drugs that could affect test results should be withheld for 12 hours before the test. Medication(s) that must be taken before the test should be recorded on the laboratory slip.

Client Teaching

- Inform the client that the blood sample will be drawn after the client is awake for at least 1 hour, preferably 2 hours. Sleep might cause false-positive results.
- Inform the client that test results might not be known for several days.
- Instruct the client to avoid stress and exercise before the test.

Propranolol hydrochloride (blood, serum, or plasma)

Inderal, Detensol, Novopranol

Reference Values

Therapeutic Range: *Adult:* 50–100 ng/mL, 193–386 nmol/L (SI units). *Child:* Not done.
Toxic Level: *Adult:* Greater than 150 ng/mL.

Description

Propranolol (Inderal) is a β-adrenergic blocking agent used in the treatment of angina pectoris, cardiac dysrhythmias, hypertension, and, in some cases, migraine headaches (prophylactically only). This drug blocks the cardiac effects of β_1-adrenergic stimulation, causing a decreased heart rate and force of heart contraction. Propranolol also blocks the bronchodilator effect of catecholamines, causing bronchoconstriction. In hypertensive clients, it will lower both supine and standing blood pressure by blocking sympathetic flow and suppressing renin activity.

Almost all of oral propranolol is absorbed through the gastrointestinal tract and is metabolized in the liver to a large number of metabolites. Ninety to 95% is bound to plasma protein and is excreted in urine as free and conjugated propranolol and as active metabolites. The half-life of plasma propranolol is 3–4 hours. Peak plasma level for the oral dosage form is 1–1½ hours and for an IV dose is 15 minutes. Propranolol crosses the placental and blood-brain barriers.

Careful monitoring for signs and symptoms of side effects of propranolol is necessary to prevent the three most common symptoms: bradycardia, hypotension, and bronchoconstriction. This drug is contraindicated for clients with asthma and low blood pressure.

Purposes

- To decrease blood pressure and irregular heart rate.
- To monitor propranolol levels for therapeutic effect.

Clinical Problems

Increased Level: Overdose of propranolol (Inderal), liver and renal diseases. *Drug Influence:* Quinidine, cimetidine (Tagamet).

Procedure

- There is no food or fluid restriction.
- Collect 5–7 mL of venous blood in a red-top tube.
- Record the dose, route, and last-administered dose on the laboratory requisition slip.

Factors Affecting Laboratory Results

- Spuriously low values have been reported with the use of certain blood collection tubes.

NURSING IMPLICATIONS WITH RATIONALE

- Record the dose, route, and last time the drug was given on the requisition slip.
- Check serum propranolol level, and report any nontherapeutic level to the health care provider.
- Take the apical pulse and blood pressure before administering propranolol. If the pulse rate and blood pressure are lower than the baseline levels, notify the health care provider before administering the drug.
- Check the daily intake and output and the client's weight. Propranolol can cause sodium retention.
- Recognize that digitalis glycoside (e.g., digoxin) taken with propranolol could cause bradycardia.

Increased Level

- Observe for signs and symptoms of drug side effects (e.g., decreased pulse rate or bradycardia, decreased blood pressure or hypotension, vertigo, syncope, dyspnea, bronchospasm, nausea, diarrhea, dry eyes, and dry skin).

Client Teaching

- Instruct the client on how to take a radial pulse. Inform the client to notify the health care provider if the pulse rate is lower than the baseline level or if the pulse becomes irregular.
- Explain to the client that propranolol should never be abruptly discontinued. Propranolol is tapered to lower doses over 1–2 weeks to prevent withdrawal syndrome (e.g., severe headaches, palpitation, and rebound hypertension).
- Inform the client that before general anesthesia for planned surgery is considered or given, the surgeon and anesthetist should be notified if the client is taking propranolol.

Prostate-specific antigen (PSA) (serum)

P

Reference Values

PSA: *Normal:* Less than 4 ng/mL. *Benign Prostatic Hypertrophy (BPH):* 4–10 ng/mL. *Prostate Cancer:* 10–120 ng/mL (depends on the stage of prostate cancer).

Total PSA: *Normal:* 2.5–4 ng/mL

Free PSA: *Normal:* Greater than 1 ng/mL.

% Free PSA: *Normal:* Greater than 25%.

% FREE PSA	PROBABILITY OF CANCER
0–10	56%
11–15	28%
16–20	20%
21–25	15%
greater than 26	8%

Description

Before the 1970s, prostate cancer was screened only by digital rectal examination and serum prostate acid phosphatase (PAP). By the time the PAP was elevated and the prostate gland was enlarged, metastasis had occurred. After the prostate-specific antigen (PSA) test was developed, fewer men were diagnosed with metastatic cancer.

Prostate-specific antigen, a glycoprotein from the prostatic tissues, is increased in both benign prostatic hypertrophy (BPH) and prostate cancer; however, it is markedly increased in prostate cancer. The PSA value may also be increased after a rectal examination and prostate surgery. An annual PSA test should be started at the age of 50. It should be started at the age of 40 if the male has a familial history of prostate cancer or is African American. A digital rectal exam (DRE) is usually done along with a PSA test. With an abnormal DRE, a biopsy of the prostate gland may be performed regardless of whether the PSA test is normal or elevated.

With serum PSA, there can be a false-positive or false-negative result. However, this test gives an indication of the risk of prostate cancer. If the PSA is less than 4 ng/mL, the chance of prostate cancer is very small, but not zero. If the PSA is over 10 ng/mL, there is a 70% chance the prostate gland is malignant. Doubling time of PSA results in 12 months is a concern, for example, 2–4 ng/mL. Also, an elevated PSA could be due to an enlarged prostate gland, such as benign prostatic hyperplasia or prostatitis, which is inflammation of the prostate gland from a bacterial infection or other causes.

The serum PSA may be used to monitor the effect of prostate cancer treatment with chemotherapy or radiation, determine disease process and prognosis, and detect a recurrence of the tumor. Repeating the PSA test may be necessary.

Today, the PSA assays are composed of three tests: serum PSA, total PSA, and % free PSA. If the serum PSA is slightly elevated or its previous result is doubled, the total PSA (tPSA) and % free PSA (%FPSA) are prescribed.

P

Total PSA (tPSA): The total PSA is comprised of a free portion and complexed (bound) PSA. The total PSA value is used for obtaining the % free PSA.

% Free PSA (%FPSA): If the percent of free PSA (%FPSA) is greater than 25%, the chance of having prostate cancer is very low, less than 8%. If the %FPSA is less than 25%, the chance of prostate cancer increases. The %FPSA can be determined from the total PSA and the free PSA by dividing the free PSA by the total PSA. If the total PSA is 2.4 ng/mL and the free PSA is 0.3 ng/mL, the percent of free PSA (%FPSA) would be 13%. This male would have a 28% chance of having prostate cancer (*see Reference Values*). A prostate gland biopsy would be suggested.

It has been suggested that the norm for serum PSA should be lower than 4 ng/mL. This may be true for men 50 years old or younger, but not for older men. If reference values need to be changed, then the normal serum PSA for men who are 50 years old or younger would be less than 2.5 ng/mL, and the serum PSA value for men 50 years old or older would remain as 4 ng/mL.

Purpose

- To aid in the diagnosis of prostate cancer.

Clinical Problems

Increased Level: Prostate cancer, benign prostatic hypertrophy, prostatitis, prostatic tissue biopsy, prostatic surgery.

Procedure

- No food or fluid restriction is required.
- Collect blood specimen before rectal and prostate examination.
- Collect 3–5 mL of venous blood in a red-top tube.

Factors Affecting Laboratory Results

- Rectal and prostate examinations can increase serum PSA levels.

NURSING IMPLICATIONS WITH RATIONALE

- Ascertain if there is a family history of prostate cancer.
- Obtain a history regarding changes in urinary pattern, such as interrupted urine flow; frequent urination, especially at night; difficulty in starting and stopping the urine flow; hematuria; and/or pain in the back during urination.
- Explain to the client that a blood sample will be obtained and the test results should be available within 24 hours.

Client Teaching

- Instruct the client that a manual rectal examination is usually part of the test regimen to determine prostatic changes. The prostatic palpation should be done *after* the blood sample is drawn.
- Be supportive of the client. Provide an atmosphere in which the client feels comfortable expressing his concerns.

Prostatic Acid Phosphatase (PAP)

See Acid Phosphatase (ACP)

Protein (total) (serum)

Reference Values

Adult: 6–8 g/dL.

Child: *Premature:* 4.2–7.6 g/dL. *Newborn:* 4.6–7.4 g/dL. *Infant:* 6–6.7 g/dL. *Child:* 6.2–8 g/dL.

Description

The total protein is composed mostly of albumin and globulins (*see Protein Electrophoresis*). The use of the total serum protein test is limited unless the serum albumin, A/G ratio, or protein electrophoresis test is also performed.

The protein level needs to be known to determine the significance of its components. With certain disease entities (e.g., collagen diseases, cancer, and infections), the total serum protein levels may be normal when the protein fractions are either decreased or elevated.

Purposes

- To differentiate between albumin and globulin.
- To monitor protein levels.
- To identify selected health problems associated with protein deficit.

Clinical Problems

Decreased Level: Prolonged malnutrition, starvation, low-protein diet, malabsorption syndrome, cancer of the gastrointestinal tract, ulcerative colitis, Hodgkin disease, severe liver disease, chronic renal failure, severe burns, water intoxication.

Increased Level: Dehydration (hemoconcentration), vomiting, diarrhea, multiple myeloma, respiratory distress syndrome, sarcoidosis.

Procedure

- There is no food or fluid restriction. High-fat foods should be avoided for 24 hours before the test. Check with your laboratory.
- Collect 5–7 mL of venous blood in a red-top tube. Avoid hemolysis.

Factors Affecting Laboratory Results

- A high-fat diet before the test.

P

NURSING IMPLICATIONS WITH RATIONALE

Client Teaching

- Instruct the client to avoid eating foods high in fat for 24 hours before the test.

Decreased Level

- Assess the client's dietary intake. If the deficit is due to poor nutrition, encourage the client to increase protein intake (e.g., eggs, cheese, meats, beans).
- Plan a well-balanced diet with the client. Collaborate with the dietitian and/or have the dietitian see the client.

Increased Level

- Recognize clinical problems associated with a serum protein excess. Hemoconcentration caused by dehydration is a frequent cause of total serum protein excess.
- Assess the client for signs and symptoms of dehydration, such as extreme thirst, poor skin turgor, dry mucous membranes, tachycardia, and increased respirations.
- Check urinary output. The serum protein level may be increased (it could also be decreased) with kidney dysfunction. If kidney dysfunction is due to dehydration, vomiting, or diarrhea, the serum protein level will most likely be elevated.
- Monitor fluid replacement (intravenously or orally). The serum protein level should return to normal when the client is adequately hydrated. Care should be taken to prevent overhydration when forcing fluids.

Protein (urine)

Reference Values

Random Specimen: *Negative:* 0–5 mg/dL. *Positive:* 6–2,000 mg/dL (trace to +2).

24-Hour Specimen: 25–150 mg/24 h.

Description

Proteinuria is usually caused by renal disease due to glomerular damage and/or impaired renal tubular reabsorption. With a random urine specimen, protein can be detected using a reagent strip or dipstick, such as Combistix. Normally albumin is measured with the dipstick, because it is sensitive to reagent strip. A positive urine specimen (proteinuria) suggests that a 24-hour urine specimen be obtained for quantitative analysis of protein.

The amount of proteinuria in 24 hours is an indicator of the severity of renal involvement. Minimal proteinuria (less than 500 mg or 0.5 g/24 h) may be associated with chronic pyelonephritis; moderate proteinuria (500–4,000 mg or 0.5–4 g/24 h) may be associated with acute or chronic glomerulonephritis or toxic nephropathies (e.g., use of aminoglycosides [gentamicin]); and marked proteinuria (greater than 4,000 mg or greater than 4 g/24 h) may be associated with nephrotic syndrome.

Emotions and physiologic stress may cause transient proteinuria. Newborns may have an increased proteinuria during the first 3 days of life.

Purposes

- To compare urine protein level with serum protein level in relation to health problems (*see Clinical Problems*).
- To identify renal dysfunction with increased protein level in the urine.

Clinical Problems

Decreased Level: Diluted urine. *Drug Influence:* Sulfosalicylic acid.

Increased Level: *Heavy Proteinuria:* Acute or chronic glomerulonephritis, nephrotic syndrome, lupus nephritis, amyloid disease. *Moderate Proteinuria:* Drug toxicities (aminoglycosides), cardiac disease, acute infectious disease, multiple myeloma, chemical toxicities. *Mild Proteinuria:* Chronic pyelonephritis, polycystic kidney disease, renal tubular disease. *Drug Influence:* Penicillin, gentamicin, sulfonamides, cephalosporins, contrast media, tolbutamide (Orinase), acetazolamide (Diamox), sodium bicarbonate.

Procedure

- There is no food or fluid restriction.
- List drugs client is taking that could affect test results.

Random Urine Specimen
- Collect clean-caught or midstream urine specimen.
- Place the reagent strip/dipstick (e.g., Combistix) in the urine specimen.
- Match the results from the dipstick with the color chart on the bottle.

24-Hour Specimen (Quantitative Analysis Test)
- Have client void prior to test and discard urine. Then save all urine for 24 hours in a urine collection container.
- Keep urine specimen bottle refrigerated or on ice.
- Label the urine bottle with the client's name, date, and exact time of collection (e.g., 7/12/20, 8:01 AM to 7/13/20, 8:02 AM).

Factors Affecting Laboratory Results

- Drugs (*see Drug Influence*).
- Diluted urine.
- Toilet paper or stool in the urine.

NURSING IMPLICATIONS WITH RATIONALE

- Explain the test procedure to the client (*see Procedure*). Emphasize the importance of following the test procedure for accurate results.
- Record on the laboratory slip all drugs that the client is taking and the date and time of last dose. The health care provider may withhold drugs for 24 hours prior to test.

P

- Assess for signs and symptoms of renal dysfunction, such as fatigue, decreased urine output, peripheral edema, increased serum creatinine.
- Answer the client's questions or refer the questions to the appropriate health professionals.

Protein electrophoresis (serum)

Reference Values

Adult

	WEIGHT (g/dL)	PERCENTAGE OF TOTAL PROTEIN
Albumin	3.5–5	52–68
Globulin	1.5–3.5	32–48
Alpha-1 (α_1)	0.1–0.4	2–5
Alpha-2 (α_2)	0.4–1	7–13
Beta (β)	0.5–1.1	8–14
Gamma (γ)	0.5–1.7	12–22

Child

	ALBUMIN (g/dL)	GLOBULINS (g/dL)			
		α_1	α_2	β	γ
Premature	3–4.2	0.1–0.5	0.3–0.7	0.3–1.2	0.3–1.4
Newborn	3.5–5.4	0.1–0.3	0.3–0.5	0.2–0.6	0.2–1.2
Infant	4.4–5.4	0.2–0.4	0.5–0.8	0.5–0.9	0.3–0.8
Child	4–5.8	0.1–0.4	0.4–1	0.5–1	0.3–1

Description

Serum proteins are made up of albumin and globulins. Albumin is the smallest of the protein molecules, but it makes up the largest percentage of the total protein value. Changes in the albumin level will affect the total protein value. Albumin plays an important role in maintaining serum colloid osmotic pressure. The globulin molecules are about 2.5 times as large as albumin molecules, but they are not as effective in maintaining osmotic pressure as albumin molecules are.

Serum protein electrophoresis is a process that separates various protein fractions into albumin: alpha-1 (α_1) globulin, alpha-2 (α_2) globulin, beta (β) globulin, and gamma (γ) globulin. The gamma globulins are the body's antibodies, which contribute to immunity.

Purposes

- To differentiate between the protein fractions.
- To determine disease entities among the protein fractions.

Clinical Problems

PROTEIN FRACTION	DECREASED LEVEL	INCREASED LEVEL
Albumin	Chronic liver disease Malnutrition Starvation Malabsorption syndrome Advanced malignancy Leukemia Heart failure Toxemia of pregnancy Nephrotic syndrome Chronic renal failure Burns (severe) Systemic lupus erythematosus (SLE)	Dehydration Exercise
Globulin		
α_1	Emphysema due to α-1-antitrypsin deficiency	Pregnancy Neoplasm Acute and chronic infection Tissue necrosis
α_2	Hemolytic anemia Severe liver disease	Acute infection Injury, trauma Burns (severe) Extensive neoplasms Obstructive jaundice Rheumatic fever Rheumatoid arthritis Acute myocardial infarction Nephrotic syndrome
β	Hypocholesterolemia	Hypothyroidism Biliary cirrhosis Kidney nephrosis Diabetes mellitus Malignant hypertension
γ	Nephrotic syndrome Lymphocytic leukemia Lymphosarcoma Hypogammaglobulinemia or agammaglobulinemia	Collagen disease Rheumatoid arthritis Lupus erythematosus Hodgkin disease Malignant lymphoma Chronic lymphocytic leukemia Multiple myeloma Liver disease
ELECTROPHORETIC PATTERNS		
Pattern I	$\downarrow$ albumin $\uparrow$ α_2-globulin	Acute stressful situation Acute infections Myocardial infarction Severe burns Surgery

(Continued)

ELECTROPHORETIC PATTERNS

Pattern II	↓ (slightly) albumin	Chronic infection and inflammation
	↑ (slightly) α_2-globulin	Cirrhosis
	↑ (slightly) γ globulin	Collagen disease (rheumatoid)
Pattern III	↓ (moderately) albumin	Collagen disease (lupus)
	↑ γ globulin	Subacute bacterial endocarditis
	↑ or normal β	Sarcoidosis

Procedure

- There is no food or fluid restriction.
- Collect 5–7 mL of venous blood in a red-top tube. Avoid hemolysis.

Factors Affecting Laboratory Results

- Hemolysis of the blood sample.

NURSING IMPLICATIONS WITH RATIONALE

- Check the albumin level from the protein electrophoresis results. Many clinical problems are the result of a serum albumin deficit.
- Assess for peripheral edema in the lower extremities when the albumin level is decreased. Albumin is the major protein compound responsible for plasma colloid osmotic pressure. With a decreased albumin level, fluid seeps out of the blood vessels into the tissue spaces. Cirrhosis of the liver and heart failure are clinical problems that can cause an albumin deficit and edema.
- Encourage the client to increase protein intake. Malnutrition and cirrhosis of the liver are associated with a poor-protein diet. Suggest foods high in protein (e.g., beans, eggs, meats, and milk).
- Assess urinary output. Renal and collagen (lupus) diseases occur with abnormal protein fractions. Urine output should be 25 mL/h or 600 mL/24 h.
- Check for albumin/protein in the urine.

Prothrombin time (PT) (plasma)

Pro-Time, International Normalized Ratio (INR)

Reference Values

Adult: 10–13 seconds (depending on the method and reagents used) or 70–100%. *For Anticoagulant Therapy:* 1.5–2 times the control in seconds or 20–30%. INR (international normalized ratio): 2–3.

Child: Same as adult.

P

Description

Prothrombin (factor II of the coagulation factors) is synthesized by the liver and is an inactive precursor in the clotting process (*see Factor Assay*). Prothrombin is converted to thrombin by the action of thromboplastin, which is needed to form a blood clot.

The prothrombin time (PT) measures the clotting ability of factors I (fibrinogen), II (prothrombin), V, VII, and X. Alterations of factors V and VII will prolong the PT for about 2 seconds, or 10% of normal. In liver disease, the PT is usually prolonged, because the liver cells cannot synthesize prothrombin.

The major use of the PT is to monitor oral anticoagulant therapy (i.e., with bishydroxycoumarin [dicumarol] and warfarin sodium [Coumadin]).

International Normalized Ratio: It has been recommended that the PT be reported as an International Normalized Ratio (INR). The INR was devised to improve the monitoring process for warfarin anticoagulant therapy. A client's response to the same dose of warfarin varies; thus the INR is used because it is an internationally standardized test for PT. The INR is designed for long-term warfarin therapy and should only be used after the client has been stabilized on warfarin. Stabilization takes at least 1 week. The INR should not be used when the client is beginning warfarin therapy in order to avoid misleading test results. The target INR range for a client taking warfarin is 2–3 and for a client having heart valve replacement is 2.5–3.5.

Purpose

- To monitor anticoagulant warfarin therapy.

Clinical Problems

Decreased Level: Thrombophlebitis, myocardial infarction, pulmonary embolism. *Drug Influence:* Barbiturates, digitalis preparations, diuretics, diphenhydramine (Benadryl), oral contraceptives, rifampin, metaproterenol (Alupent, Metaprel), vitamin K.

Increased Level: Liver diseases (cirrhosis of the liver, hepatitis, liver abscess, cancer of the liver), afibrinogenemia, factor II deficiency, factor V deficiency, factor VII deficiency, factor X deficiency, fibrin degradation products, leukemias, heart failure, erythroblastosis fetalis (hemolytic disease of the newborn). *Drug Influence:* Antibiotics (penicillin, streptomycin, carbenicillin, chloramphenicol [Chloromycetin], kanamycin [Kantrex], neomycin, tetracyclines), anticoagulants, oral (dicumarol, warfarin), chlorpromazine (Thorazine), chlordiazepoxide (Librium), diphenylhydantoin (Dilantin), heparin, methyldopa (Aldomet), mithramycin, reserpine (Serpasil), phenylbutazone (Butazolidin), quinidine, salicylates (aspirin), sulfonamides.

Procedure

- There is no food or fluid restriction.
- The INR may be checked with a CoaguChek test performed with finger prick.
- The collection tube for the PT test should contain an anticoagulant, either sodium oxalate or sodium citrate.
- Collect 3–5 mL of venous blood in a black-top tube (sodium oxalate). The blood must be tested within 1 hour after it has been drawn. The tube should be filled to its capacity. Some black-top tubes contain sodium citrate, so check with the laboratory.

OR

P

- Collect 3–5 mL of venous blood in a blue-top tube (sodium citrate). The blood should be tested within 2 hours to prevent inactivation of some of the factors. The tube should be filled to its capacity.
- Deliver the blood sample to the laboratory packed in ice. If the blood clots before testing, a new blood sample should be taken.
- Control values are given with the client's PT and/or INR. Control values may change from day to day; this is an indication of the minor variables in the testing conditions.
- List on the laboratory slip drugs the client is taking that could affect test results.

Factors Affecting Laboratory Results

- A clotted blood sample will cause an inaccurate result.
- A high-fat diet (decreased PT) and alcohol use (increased PT) may cause an endogenous change of PT production.
- Leaving a blood sample at room temperature for several hours (1–4 hours) may affect results.

NURSING IMPLICATIONS WITH RATIONALE

- Explain to the client that the purpose of the test is to determine how fast the blood clots. If the purpose of the test is to monitor anticoagulant therapy, inform the client that blood will be drawn daily or at specified times.
- Hold medications (if possible) that may affect the PT and/or INR until after the test. If such medications *are* given, list the names of the drugs on the laboratory slip and when the last dose was given.
- Take the blood sample immediately to the laboratory for testing. There should be an anticoagulant in the tube, and the blood should fill the tube.

Increased Level

- Monitor the PT and/or INR when the client is receiving anticoagulant therapy. The desired PT with anticoagulant therapy is 1.5–2 times the control PT in seconds. The desired INR is 2–3. The PT may be slightly lower when treating cardiac clients, 18–24 seconds. In clients with a thrombus, the desired PT range is 26–40 seconds. When the PT is above 40 seconds, bleeding may occur.
- Inform the health care provider of the client's PT and/or INR daily or as ordered. The health care provider may want the anticoagulant held (drug adjustment) until the current PT or INR has been received. The results are usually called to the floor by the laboratory personnel.
- Observe the client for signs and symptoms of bleeding (purpura [skin], hematuria [Hemastix test], hematemesis, nosebleeds). Report observations to the health care provider and record them in the client's chart.
- Administer vitamin K intramuscularly as ordered when the PT is over 40 seconds or when there is bleeding. IM injections can cause hematomas at the injection site when anticoagulants are used.

Client Teaching

- Instruct the client not to self-medicate when receiving anticoagulant therapy. Over-the-counter drugs may either increase or decrease the effects of the anticoagulants (drug interaction) and the results of the PT.
- Instruct the client to take the prescribed anticoagulants as ordered by the health care provider. Missed doses could affect the PT.
- Inform the client not to consume excess alcohol, because it can affect liver function and cause a prolonged PT. A high-fat diet may decrease the PT and INR.
- (*See Partial Thromboplastin Time, Activated Partial Thromboplastin Time.*)

Pyridinium (PYD) (urine)

Reference Values

Urine: *Female:* 15.3–33.6 nM/mm. *Male:* 10.3–33.6 nM/mm.

Description

Pyridinium (PYD) is another bone turnover biochemical marker that is used to monitor activity and effects of treatment for bone disease. PYD cross-links occur during the maturation of the type 1 collagen with bone formation. PYD cross-links are released into circulation during osteoclast (bone resorption). Bone is continuously being turned over, with bone resorption and bone formation.

In children, the bone biochemical markers are elevated because of growth of the long bones associated with bone resorption. At the age of 13, the child's levels gradually return to adult levels.

Purposes

- To monitor the activity of bone disease.
- To monitor the effects of the prescribed treatment for bone disease.

Clinical Problems

Decreased Level: Hypoparathyroidism, hypothyroidism. *Drug Influence:* Cortisol therapy, testosterone, estrogen drug.

Increased Level: Osteoporosis, Paget disease, cancer of the bone, child's growth of long bones, acromegaly, hyperparathyroidism, hyperthyroidism.

Procedure

- Discard the first morning urine specimen.
- Collect the second morning urine for specimen.
- Take urine to the laboratory immediately or refrigerate the urine specimen.
- Encourage the client to drink water, especially if the client has difficulty in providing a urine specimen.

Factors Affecting Laboratory Results

- Using the first morning urine sample.
- Contamination of the second urine sample.
- Not refrigerating the urine sample or not taking the specimen immediately to the laboratory.
- Testosterone can reduce N-telopeptide cross-links (NTx) levels.

R

NURSING IMPLICATIONS WITH RATIONALE

- Record the client's age and health problems, including osteoporosis and bone disease.
- Record which drug therapy the client is receiving.
- Compare the baseline PYD before drug therapy to the current PYD. Levels should be decreasing with use of antiresorption drugs, such as estrogen, raloxifene (Evista), and alendronate (Fosamax).

Client Teaching

- Instruct the client to save the second morning urine sample for the test.

Rabies antibody test (serum)
Fluorescent Rabies Antibody (FRA)

Reference Values

Indirect fluorescent antibody (IFA) less than 1:16.

Description

The rabies rhabdovirus affecting the central nervous system may be present in the saliva, brain, spinal cord, urine, and feces of rabid animals. This virus can be transmitted to the human by an infected dog, bat, skunk, squirrel, or other animal and is nearly 100% fatal if the person does not receive treatment before the symptoms occur.

   The rabies antibody test is performed to diagnose rabies in animals and humans that have been bitten by a rabid animal and to test the effects of rabies immunization on employees working in animal shelters. Brain tissue examined from the rabid animal can confirm the presence of the rabies virus. Both the rabies antibody test and the animal's brain tissue are preferred to positively diagnose rabies that was transmitted to the human. If the animal suspected of having rabies survives longer than 10 days, it is unlikely that the animal is rabid.

Purpose

- To aid in the diagnosis of rabies in animals and humans.

Clinical Problems

Increased (Positive) Titer Count: Rabies transmission.

Procedure

- There is no food or fluid restriction.
- Collect 5–7 mL of venous blood in a red-top tube. The animal brain should be sent along with the blood sample to the laboratory if possible.

Factors Affecting Laboratory Results

- None known.

R

NURSING IMPLICATIONS WITH RATIONALE

- Obtain a history of the animal bite. Rabies immunoglobulin (RIG) may be given soon after the exposure to neutralize the virus.
- The animal responsible for the animal bite should be captured. If the animal's rabies vaccination is not current, the animal is usually destroyed in order to test the brain tissue. A wait of 10 days to determine the survival of a "wild" animal is not suggested.

Client Teaching

- Suggest to persons working with animals, such as those working in veterinary practices, in kennels, in wildlife areas, and research laboratories, that they receive a preexposure rabies vaccine such as HDCV (human diploid cell rabies vaccine) to protect them from rabies exposure.
- Instruct the person who was bitten, or the family, to seek medical care immediately. Encourage the family to notify the humane society concerning the animal bite. The animal should be captured.
- Inform the client and/or family that if the animal is not located, the client should undertake a series of rabies vaccinations.
- Answer the client's questions. Refer questions to appropriate health professionals as needed.

Rapid plasma reagin (RPR) (serum)

Reference Values

Adult: Nonreactive.

Child: Nonreactive.

Description

(*See Description for VDRL.*)

The rapid plasma reagin (RPR) test is a rapid screening test for syphilis. A nontreponemal antibody test like the Venereal Disease Research Laboratory test (VDRL), the RPR test detects reagin antibodies in the serum and is more sensitive but less specific than the VDRL. Frequently, it is used on donor blood as a syphilis detection test. As with other nonspecific reagin tests, false positives can occur as the result of acute and chronic diseases. A positive RPR test should be verified by the VDRL and/or fluorescent treponemal antibody absorption (FTA-ABS) tests.

Purpose

- To compare test results with other laboratory tests for diagnosing syphilis.

Clinical Problems

Reactive (positive): Syphilis. *False Positive:* Tuberculosis, pneumonia, infectious mononucleosis, chicken pox, smallpox vaccination (recent), rheumatoid arthritis, lupus erythematosus, hepatitis, pregnancy.

Procedure

- There is no food or fluid restriction.
- Follow the directions on the RPR kit.

OR

- Collect 3–5 mL of venous blood in a red-top tube.

Factors Affecting Laboratory Results

- False-positive results caused by acute and chronic diseases (*see Clinical Problems for VDRL*).

NURSING IMPLICATIONS WITH RATIONALE

Reactive (Positive)

- Explain to the client that further testing will be done to verify test results.
- If the repeat result is positive, sexual contacts need to be notified to seek treatment.

Red blood cell indices (MCV, MCH, MCHC, RDW) (blood)

Erythrocyte Indices

Reference Values

	ADULT	NEWBORN	CHILD
RBC count (million/μL × 10^{12}/L [SI units])	Male: 4.6–6 Female: 4–5 4.6–6 × 10^{12} L	4.8–7.2 4.8–7.2 × 10^{12} L	3.8–5.5 3.8–5.5 × 10^{12} L
MCV (μm^3 [conventional]) or (fl [SI units])	80–98 μm^3	96–108 μm^3	82–92 μm^3
MCH (pg [conventional and SI units])	27–31 pg	32–34 pg	27–31 pg
MCHC (% or g/dL [conventional] or SI units)	32–36% 0.32–0.36	32–33% 0.32–0.33	32–36% 0.32–0.36
RDW (coulter S)	11.5–14.5%		

Description

Red blood cell (RBC) indices include the RBC count, RBC size (MCV: mean corpuscular volume), weight (MCH: mean corpuscular hemoglobin), hemoglobin concentration (MCHC: mean corpuscular hemoglobin concentration), and size differences (RDW: RBC distribution width). Other names for RBC indices are *erythrocyte indices* and *corpuscular indices*. To identify the types of anemias, the health care provider depends on the following RBC indices:

- *MCV:* MCV indicates the size of RBC: microcytic (small size), normocytic (normal size), and macrocytic (large size). A decreased MCV, or microcyte, might be indicative of iron-deficiency anemia and thalassemia. An example of an increased MCV, or macrocytosis, is pernicious anemia and folic acid anemia. MCV value can be calculated if the RBC count and hematocrit (Hct) are known.

$$MCV = \frac{Hct \times 10}{RBC\ count}$$

- *MCH:* MCH indicates the weight of hemoglobin in the RBC regardless of the size. In macrocytic anemias, the MCH is elevated, and it is decreased in hypochromic anemia. The MCH is derived by dividing the RBC count into 10 times the hemoglobin (Hb) value.

$$MCH = \frac{Hb \times 10}{RBC\ count}$$

- *MCHC:* MCHC indicates the hemoglobin concentration per unit volume of RBCs. A decreased MCHC can indicate a hypochromic anemia. The MCHC can be calculated from MCH and MCV, or from hemoglobin and hematocrit.

$$MCHC = \frac{MCH \times 100}{MCV} \quad OR \quad MCHC = \frac{Hb \times 100}{Hct}$$

- *RDW:* The RBC distribution width is the size (width) differences of RBCs. RDW is the measurement of the width of the size distribution curve on a histogram. It is useful in predicting anemias early, before MCV changes and before signs and symptoms occur. An elevated RDW indicates iron deficiency, folic acid deficiency, and vitamin B_{12} deficiency anemias. RDW and MCV are used to differentiate among various RBC disorders (*see Anemias: RDW and MCV Values*).

ANEMIAS: RDW AND MCV VALUES

RBC Disorder	RDW	MCV
Early factor deficiency (iron, folate, vitamin B_{12})	High	Normal
Iron-deficiency anemia	High	Low
Folic-acid-deficiency anemia	High	High
Vitamin B_{12} deficiency (pernicious anemia)	High	High
Hemolysis (RBC fragmentation)	High	Low
Hemolysis (autoimmune) anemia	High	High
Sickle-cell anemia	High	Normal
Sickle-cell trait	High	Normal

Purposes

- To monitor RBC count.
- To differentiate between the components of RBC indices to determine a health problem (*see Clinical Problems*).

Clinical Problems

INDICES	DECREASED LEVEL	INCREASED LEVEL
RBC count	Hemorrhage (blood loss) Anemias Chronic infections Leukemias Multiple myeloma Excessive intravenous fluids Chronic renal failure Pregnancy Overhydration	Polycythemia vera Hemoconcentration/dehydration High altitude Cor pulmonale Cardiovascular disease
MCV	Microcytic anemia: iron deficiency Malignancy Rheumatoid arthritis Hemoglobinopathies Thalassemia Sickle-cell anemia Hemoglobin C Lead poisoning Radiation	Macrocytic anemia: aplastic, hemolytic, pernicious Chronic liver disease Hypothyroidism (myxedema) Drug influence Vitamin B_{12} deficiency Anticonvulsants Antimetabolics
MCH	Microcytic, hypochromic anemia	Macrocytic anemias
MCHC	Hypochromic anemia Iron-deficiency anemia Thalassemia	
RDW		Iron-deficiency anemia Folic-acid-deficiency anemia Pernicious anemia Homozygous hemoglobinopathies (S, C, H)

Procedure

- There is no food or fluid restriction.
- Collect 3–5 mL of venous blood in a lavender-top tube. Avoid hemolysis. Avoid leaving the tourniquet on too long.
- Usually a particle counter is used that will provide all complete blood cell count results along with all the indices.

Factors Affecting Laboratory Results

- Drugs (*see Clinical Problems*).

NURSING IMPLICATIONS WITH RATIONALE

Decreased Level

- Relate a decreased RBC count, MCV, MCH, and MCHC to clinical problems.

- Assess for the cause(s) of a decreased RBC count. Check for blood loss, and obtain a history of anemias, renal insufficiency, chronic infection, or leukemia. Determine whether the client is overhydrated.
- Observe for signs and symptoms of advanced iron-deficiency anemia (fatigue, pallor, dyspnea on exertion, tachycardia, and headache). Chronic symptoms include cracked corners of the mouth, smooth tongue, dysphagia, and numbness and tingling of the extremities. With mild iron deficiency, the client is usually asymptomatic.

Client Teaching

- Instruct the client to follow the medical regimen, such as iron-supplement therapy and a diet rich in iron.
- Instruct the client to eat foods rich in iron (e.g., liver, red meats, green vegetables, and iron-fortified bread).
- Explain to the client who is taking iron supplements that the stools usually appear dark in color (tarry appearance). Tell the client to take an iron medication with meals. Milk and antacids can interfere with iron absorption.

Increased Level

- Relate an elevated RBC count, MCV, MCH, MCHC, and RDW to clinical problems and drugs.
- Assess for signs and symptoms of hemoconcentration. Dehydration, shock, and severe diarrhea are some of the causes of hemoconcentration that can elevate the RBC count.

Renin (plasma)

Reference Values

Adult: *Normal Sodium Diet: Supine:* 0.2–2.3 ng/mL. *Upright:* 1.6–4.3 ng/mL. *Restricted Sodium Diet: Upright:* 4.1–10.8 ng/mL.

Child: *1–3 Years:* 1.7–11 ng/mL. *3–5 Years:* 1–6.5 ng/mL. *5–10 Years:* 0.5–6 ng/mL.

Description

Renin is an enzyme secreted by the kidneys. This enzyme activates the renin-angiotensin system, which causes vasoconstriction and the release of aldosterone (a hormone from the adrenal medulla that causes sodium and water retention). Vasoconstriction and aldosterone can cause hypertension. Elevated plasma renin rarely occurs in essential hypertension, but its value is frequently elevated in renovascular and malignant hypertension.

Increased plasma renin levels can occur as a result of hypovolemia and kidney disorders. In addition, postural change (from a recumbent to an upright position) and a decreased sodium (salt) intake will stimulate renin secretion. Plasma renin levels are usually higher from 8:00 AM to noon and lower from noon to 6:00 PM.

Purpose

- To identify a possible cause of hypertension.

Clinical Problems

Decreased Level: Essential hypertension, Cushing syndrome, diabetes mellitus, hypothyroidism, high-sodium diet. *Drug Influence:* Antihypertensives (methyldopa [Aldomet], guanethidine [Ismelin]), propranolol (Inderal), levodopa.

Increased Level: Hypertension (malignant, renovascular), hyperaldosteronism, cancer of the kidney, acute renal failure, Addison disease, cirrhosis, chronic obstructive lung disease, manic-depressive disorder, pregnancy (first trimester), preeclampsia and eclampsia, hyperthyroidism, hypokalemia, low-sodium diet. *Drug Influence:* Estrogens, diuretics, antihypertensives (hydralazine [Apresoline], diazoxide [Hyperstat], nitroprusside), oral contraceptives.

Procedure

- Check with the laboratory and health care provider to determine whether the plasma renin test is to include urine aldosterone and/or urine sodium tests.

Plasma Renin

- Keep the tube and/or syringe cold in an ice bath before collection.
- The tourniquet should be released before the blood is drawn.
- Note on the laboratory slip if the client is in a supine or upright position.
- A normal or low-sodium diet may be indicated.
- Collect 5–7 mL of venous blood in a lavender-top tube.
- The blood sample should be placed in an ice bath; after centrifugation, the plasma is separated, frozen immediately to preserve renin activity, and sent to a special laboratory.

Factors Affecting Laboratory Results

- Drugs (*see Drug Influence*).

NURSING IMPLICATIONS WITH RATIONALE

- Check with the laboratory on procedural changes or modifications.

Increased Level

- Monitor the client's blood pressure every 4–6 hours or as ordered.
- Assess kidney function by recording urinary output. If urinary output is less than 25 mL/h or 600 mL/day, renal insufficiency should be suspected.

Reticulocyte count (blood)

Reference Values

Adult: 0.5–1.5% of all RBCs, 25,000–75,000 μL (microliter).

$$\text{Reticulocyte count} = \text{reticulocytes (\%) RBC count}$$

Child: *Newborn:* 2.5–6.5% of all RBCs. *Infant:* 0.5–3.5% of all RBCs. *Child:* 0.5–2% of all RBCs.

Description

The reticulocyte count is an indicator of bone marrow activity and is used for diagnosing anemias. Reticulocytes are immature, non-nucleated red blood cells that are formed in the bone marrow and passed into circulation. Normally, there is a small number of reticulocytes in circulation; however, an increased number (count) indicates RBC production acceleration. An increased count could be due to hemorrhage or hemolysis or the treatment of iron deficiency, vitamin B_{12} deficiency, or folic-acid-deficiency anemia. This test is also done to check on persons working with radioactive material or receiving radiotherapy. A persistently low count could be suggestive of bone marrow hypofunction or aplastic anemia.

Giving a percentage is not always the most accurate way of reporting the reticulocyte count, especially when the total RBC (erythrocyte) count is *not* within normal range. Both the RBC count and the reticulocyte count should be reported.

Purpose

- To aid in the diagnosis of anemias (pernicious, folic acid deficiency, hemolytic, sickle cell) (*see Clinical Problems*).

Clinical Problems

Decreased Level: Anemias (pernicious, folic acid deficiency, aplastic), radiation therapy, effects of x-ray irradiation, adrenocortical hypofunction, anterior pituitary hypofunction, cirrhosis of the liver (alcohol suppresses reticulocytes).

Increased Level: Anemias (hemolytic, sickle cell), thalassemia major, chronic hemorrhage, posthemorrhage (3–4 days), treatment for anemias (iron deficiency, vitamin B_{12}, folic acid), leukemias, erythroblastosis fetalis (hemolytic disease of the newborn), hemoglobin C and D diseases, pregnancy.

Procedure

- Venous or capillary blood could be used for the reticulocyte count test.

Venous Blood

- There is no food or fluid restriction.
- Collect 3–5 mL of venous blood in a lavender-top tube.

Capillary Blood

- There is no food or fluid restriction.
- Cleanse the finger and puncture the skin with a sterile lancet.
- Wipe the first drop of blood away. Collect the blood by using a micropipette. The blood is mixed in equal proportions with methylene blue solution. The reticulocytes stain blue.

Factors Affecting Laboratory Results

- The use of the wrong colored-top tube for venous blood. The tube should contain anticoagulant (EDTA).

R

NURSING IMPLICATIONS WITH RATIONALE

Decreased Level

- Recognize clinical problems related to a decreased reticulocyte count, such as pernicious and aplastic anemias.
- Obtain a history regarding radiation exposure—x-ray and others.

Increased Level

- Monitor the reticulocyte count when the client is being treated for pernicious anemia or folic acid anemia. There is usually an increase in reticulocytes.

Rheumatoid factor (RF), rheumatoid arthritis (RA) factor, RA latex fixation (serum)

Reference Values

Adult: Less than 1:20 titer; less than 1:40 chronic inflammatory disease; 1:20–1:80 positive for rheumatoid arthritis and other conditions; greater than 1:80 positive for rheumatoid arthritis.

Child: Not usually done.

Elderly: Slightly increased.

Description

The rheumatoid factor (RF) or rheumatoid arthritis (RA) factor test is a screening test used to detect antibodies (IgM, IgG, or IgA) found in the serum of clients with rheumatoid arthritis. RF occurs in 53–94% (average 76%) of clients with rheumatoid arthritis, and if the test is negative, it should be repeated.

The RF tests can be positive in many of the collagen diseases. The RF tests should not be used for monitoring follow-up or treatment stages of RA, because RF tests often remain positive when clinical remissions have been achieved. It also takes approximately 6 months for a significant elevation of titer. For diagnosing and evaluating RA, the ANA and the C-reactive protein agglutination tests are frequently used.

Purposes

- To screen for IgM, IgG, or IgA antibodies present in clients with possible RA.
- To aid in the diagnosis of RA.
- To compare test results in relation to other laboratory tests for diagnosing RA.

Clinical Problems

Increased Level: Rheumatoid arthritis, lupus erythematosus, dermatomyositis, scleroderma, infectious mononucleosis, tuberculosis, leukemia, sarcoidosis, cirrhosis of the liver, hepatitis, syphilis, chronic infections, old age.

Procedure

- There is no food or fluid restriction.
- Collect 3–5 mL of venous blood in a red-top tube.

Factors Affecting Laboratory Results

- A positive RF test result frequently remains positive regardless of clinical improvement.
- The RF test result can be positive in various clinical problems (e.g., collagen diseases, cancer, and liver cirrhosis).
- The older adult may have an increased RF titer without the disease.
- Due to the variability in the sensitivity and specificity of these screening tests, positive results must be interpreted in corroboration with the client's clinical status.

NURSING IMPLICATIONS WITH RATIONALE

Increased Level

- Relate an increased RF titer to clinical problems. A titer greater than 1:80 is most likely due to RA. Titers between 1:20 and 1:80 could be due to lupus, scleroderma, or liver cirrhosis.
- Consider the age of the client when the RF is slightly increased. There can be a slight titer increase in the older adult without clinical symptoms of RA. With juvenile rheumatoid arthritis, only 10% of the children have a positive RF titer.
- Assess for pain in the small joints of the hands and feet (especially the proximal interphalangeal joints), which could be indicative of an early stage of RA.

Rh typing (blood)

Reference Values

Adult: Rh + (positive), Rh – (negative).

Child: Same as adult.

Description

Rh typing is performed when typing donors'/recipients' blood and for crossmatching blood for transfusion. Rh factor (also known as Rh antigen) was first discovered by Landsteiner and Weiner in 1941; it was named Rh because of the use of rhesus monkeys in the research. Rh positive (most common Rh factor) indicates the presence of antigen on red blood cells; Rh negative indicates an absence of the antigen.

An Rh-negative woman carrying a fetus with an Rh-positive blood group can cause Rh-positive antigens from the fetus to seep into the mother's blood, causing Rh antibody formation. If the mother develops a high anti-Rh antibody titer, the child can be born with a condition called *erythroblastosis fetalis* (hemolysis of the RBCs). To prevent Rh antibodies, the Rh-negative woman is given Rho(D) immune globulin, such as RhoGAM, within 3 days after delivery with the first child or after a miscarriage to neutralize any anti-Rh antibodies.

Purpose

- To identify the client's Rh factor for pregnancy or for blood transfusion.

Clinical Problems

Increased (Positive) Anti-Rh Antibodies: *Infant:* Erythroblastosis fetalis.

Procedure

- There is no food or fluid restriction.
- Collect 5 mL of venous blood in a red-top tube. Do not use a serum separator tube.
- Blood testing for Rh factor (antigen) should be done with care to avoid false-positive and false-negative results.

Factors Affecting Laboratory Results

- None known.

NURSING IMPLICATIONS WITH RATIONALE

- Obtain a history of previous blood transfusions the client has received. If the client is a pregnant woman, determine whether she has been pregnant before and whether the child (children) was (were) born jaundiced.
- Ask the clients if they know their Rh factor. Compare the tested Rh factor with the client's stated Rh factor. This could prevent administering incorrect blood.

Client Teaching

- Inform the pregnant woman with Rh-negative factor that her blood will be tested at intervals during her pregnancy to find out whether antibodies are produced. The Rh-negative woman usually receives RhoGAM (Rh immune globulin) after delivery to prevent anti-Rh antibody production.

Rotavirus antigen (feces and blood)

Reference Values

Blood and Stool: Negative.

Description

Rotavirus is an RNA virus that frequently causes infectious diarrhea in infants and young children, usually between 2 months and 2 years. Rotavirus is a significant cause of enteritis in infants and gastroenteritis in very young children. It is more prevalent in the winter months in the United States; it is year-round in the tropical areas. Adults can also become infected with this virus. Clinical symptoms include vomiting (usually precedes diarrhea), diarrhea, fever, and abdominal pain. Symptoms in adults are normally mild.

The rotavirus is mainly transmitted by the fecal-oral route. It is frequently transmitted in infants and children in day care centers, group homes and preschools, and to the elderly in nursing homes. It can be detected in the stool using electron microscopy or preferably ELISA screening. Kits are available for testing the stool specimen.

Purpose

- To identify the rotavirus that is causing gastroenteritis in infants and young children.

Clinical Problems

Positive Test Result: Gastroenteritis caused by the rotavirus.

R

Procedure

- There is no food or fluid restriction.

Stool

- Obtain liquid stool and place the specimen in a closed container. The container should be placed on ice. A freshly soiled diaper may be used. Take immediately to the laboratory.
- A cotton-tip swab may be used to swab the rectum in a rotating motion. Leave the swab in the rectum for a few seconds for absorption. Place the swab in a tube or container, pack in ice, and send it immediately to the laboratory.
- No preservatives or metal container should be used. It interferes with ELISA testing.

Blood

- Collect 5 mL of venous blood in a red-top tube. Avoid hemolysis.

Factors Affecting Laboratory Results

- Not packing the stool specimen in ice can affect test results.
- Insufficient amount of stool specimen.
- Hemolysis of the blood sample.

NURSING IMPLICATIONS WITH RATIONALE

- Obtain a history of diarrhea, vomiting, and fever occurring in the child. Record frequency of the symptoms and color of the stool and vomitus.
- Take vital signs. Keep a chart of body temperatures.
- Collect stool according to the procedure. Have the specimen container iced and taken immediately to the laboratory.

Client Teaching

- Demonstrate to the parent how to collect the stool specimen. The stool specimen should be collected during the acute stage.
- Instruct the family member that the stool can be infectious and that the rotavirus could be transmitted to others if precautions are not taken. Hands should be thoroughly washed after changing soiled diapers. Dirty diapers should be carefully placed in a plastic bag and properly discarded.

- Answer the family's questions. Be supportive of the child and family members.
- Instruct the parent to check the child's body temperature at specified intervals.
- Encourage the parent to increase the child's fluid intake, particularly electrolyte-based fluids.
- Inform the parent that the rotavirus is easily transmitted and that there is a higher risk of transmission in nurseries, day care centers, group homes, and nursing homes.

R

Rubella antibody detection (serum)
Hemagglutination Inhibition Test (HI or HAI) for Rubella (German Measles)

Reference Values

Adult: *Susceptibility to Rubella:* Less than 1:8 titer. *Past Rubella Exposure:* 1:10–1:32 titer. *Immunity:* 1:32–1:64 titer. *Definite Immunity:* 1:64 titer and higher.

Description

Rubella (German measles) is a mild viral disease of short duration causing a fever and a transient rash. If it occurs in a woman in early pregnancy who is not immune from previous rubella infection and has not received rubella vaccination, the disease can produce serious deformities in her unborn child, especially if exposed during the first 2 months of gestation. Women should be immune to rubella (vaccinated) before marriage and definitely before pregnancy.

The rubella virus produces antibodies (natural immunity) against future rubella infections, but the exact antibody titer in the blood is unknown. Hemagglutination inhibition (HI or HAI) measures rubella antibody titers and is considered sensitive and reliable. If the antibody titer is 1:64 or higher, protection against rubella infection is assured.

Clinical indications for the HAI antibody (screening) test are as follows.

1. To determine the rubella antibody titer of a woman of child-bearing age if she has previously had the rubella infection. She will need the rubella vaccine if her titer is less than 1:8 (some state less than 1:20, others 1:32 or less).
2. To determine the rubella antibody titer at the first antepartum visit.
3. To check pregnant women (during their first trimester of pregnancy) at the time of rubella exposure and again in 3–4 weeks.
4. To check personnel who work in obstetrics in the hospital, clinic, or physician's office.
5. To diagnose a recent rubella infection in pregnant women (first trimester of pregnancy). The HAI test is done 3 days following the onset of the rash and is repeated 2–3 weeks later. A fourfold increase with the second HAI test usually indicates that the rash was due to rubella. A therapeutic abortion might be considered.

Purpose

- To identify clients who are susceptible to rubella or have immunity to the rubella virus.

Clinical Problems

Decreased Level (less than 1:8): Susceptible to rubella (German measles).

Increased Level (greater than 1:64): Definite immunity (resistance) to rubella.

Procedure

- There is no food or fluid restriction.
- Collect 3–5 mL of venous blood in a red-top tube.

Factors Affecting Laboratory Results

- None known.

R

NURSING IMPLICATIONS WITH RATIONALE

- Obtain a history of having rubella and recent exposure to rubella virus.

Client Teaching

- Explain to the client the HAI antibody titer for rubella susceptibility is less than 1:8 and for rubella immunity is 1:64 and greater. The antibody titer sufficient to protect the unborn child differs among experts. Some of them feel 1:20 gives adequate immunity, while others think it should be greater than 1:32. All agree that a 1:64 or higher dilution is a definite immunity titer.
- Teach young female adults and families about the need to have their blood checked for rubella immunity (against German measles). This test should be done before pregnancy, and if the titer is less than 1:8, they should receive the rubella vaccine. Some states require a rubella test before a marriage license is issued.
- Instruct pregnant women who are susceptible to German measles to avoid exposure to the disease if at all possible. If they have been exposed to German measles or develop a rash, they should notify the obstetrician immediately so that HAI antibody titer testing can be done. Exposure to German measles does not mean that the person will develop the disease, but it does mean that the antibody titer must be monitored. Emphasize the importance of calling the health care provider when exposed to German measles.
- Explain to interested persons some of the fetal abnormalities (congenital heart disease, deafness, mental retardation) that can occur if a woman develops German measles during the first 3 months of pregnancy.

Rubeola antibody detection (serum)

Reference Values

Negative: 0–4-fold titer.

Positive: Greater than 4-fold titer (current infection).

R

Description

Rubeola, "old-fashioned" measles (not German measles), is a contagious, viral communicable disease that is caused by the RNA paramyxovirus. It is transmitted via respiratory secretions. Since the 1970s, rubeola vaccine has been available to prevent the disease. Symptoms of rubeola include a rash that develops into a red color, maculopapular skin eruptions, fever, Koplik spots in the mouth, cough, conjunctivitis, and lymphadenopathy. An elevated immunoglobulin M (IgM) suggests an acute infection, and an elevated immunoglobulin G (IgG) suggests a current or past infection. IgM and IgG rubeola antibodies are tested to differentiate between an acute or a past infection. Immunity to rubeola can be obtained from past infection of the measle virus or from the vaccine.

Groups of people frequently tested are college students, women contemplating becoming pregnant, and pregnant women. If the woman has the measle infection during pregnancy, spontaneous abortion or preterm delivery might occur.

One or 2 weeks after the measle test, a retest may be suggested to determine the acute versus the convalescent period of the measle infection.

Purposes

- To determine the presence of the rubeola (measle) infection.
- To differentiate between the acute phase of the measle infection and the immunity phase according to IgM and IgG.

Clinical Problems

Increased Level: Measle infection, immunity to the measle virus.

Procedure

- No food or fluid restriction is required.
- Collect 5 mL of venous blood in a red-top tube.

Factors Affecting Test Result

- Hemolysis of the blood specimen.

NURSING IMPLICATIONS WITH RATIONALE

- Obtain a history of symptoms related to measle infection.
- Ask the client if she has been exposed to a person having measles.
- Determine if the client has had a previous measle vaccination or a previous measle infection.
- Ask if the client is pregnant.
- Explain to the client that test results are usually available in 24 hours.

Client Teaching

- Inform the client to return for a retest if indicated.
- Suggest to the woman of child-bearing age, who has not been infected during childhood years, to receive the rubeola (measle) vaccine before pregnancy.
- Be available to provide support to the client and family if the client has been infected with the measle virus.

Salicylate (serum)

Aspirin

Reference Values

Adult: *Normal:* Negative. *Therapeutic:* 5 mg (headache); 10–30 mg/dL (rheumatoid arthritis). *Mildly Toxic:* Greater than 30 mg/dL. *Severely Toxic:* Greater than 50 mg/dL. *Lethal:* Greater than 60 mg/dL.

Elderly: *Mildly Toxic:* Greater than 25 mg/dL.

Child: *Toxic:* Greater than 25 mg/dL.

Description

Salicylate levels are measured to check the therapeutic level, as in the treatment of rheumatic fever, and to check the levels caused by an accidental or deliberate overdose. Blood salicylate reaches its peak in 2–3 hours, and the blood level can be elevated for as long as 18 hours.

An overdose of aspirin will cause respiratory alkalosis, and if not corrected, metabolic acidosis will occur in response to cellular breakdown and the increase in organic acids. Prolonged use of salicylates (aspirins) can cause bleeding tendencies, because it inhibits platelet aggregation. It may be toxic in children because it increases the risk of Reye syndrome.

Purposes

- To monitor salicylate for daily therapeutic range.
- To check for salicylate toxicity.

Clinical Problems

Increased Level: Overdose or large, continuous doses of acetylsalicylic acid (aspirin), drugs containing aspirin.

Procedure

- Collect 5–7 mL of venous blood in a red- or green-top tube.
- There is no food or fluid restriction.
- A urine test may also be done as a screening test.

Factors Affecting Laboratory Results

- None reported.

NURSING IMPLICATIONS WITH RATIONALE

- Observe for signs and symptoms of early aspirin overdose (e.g., hyperventilation, flushed skin, and ringing in the ears).

- Obtain a history from the child or parent concerning the approximate number of aspirins taken. A toxic dose for a small child is 3.33 grains/kg, or 200 mg/kg. For a child weighing 15 kg (33 lb), the toxic dose would be 10 adult aspirins (5 grains each). Salicylates are not the choice agent for children with a virus because of the possibility of developing Reye syndrome.
- Recognize that acid–base imbalance is common with salicylate toxicity. Respiratory alkalosis usually occurs first, followed by metabolic acidosis. Symptoms of toxicity usually occur 6 hours following aspirin ingestion. Most of the aspirin has already been absorbed by that time.

Client Teaching

- Instruct the client who takes aspirins constantly that before any surgery the surgeon should be informed of the number of aspirins taken daily. Explain that aspirins will prolong bleeding time.

SARS (severe acute respiratory syndrome)

Reference Values

Normal WBC; no coronavirus antibodies.

Description

Severe acute respiratory syndrome, known as SARS, is an infectious disease believed to be caused by a coronavirus. SARS may have started in China in November 2002. By the first of June 2003, 6 months later, 31 countries had reported cases of SARS that had stricken 8,300 persons and caused 750 deaths.

Some people have mild cases of SARS, whereas others have become critically ill and died from SARS. The severity of the illness is unpredictable. The Centers for Disease Control (CDC) has developed recommendations and information regarding SARS. The CDC suggests for those persons caring for, or in contact with, SARS clients to use strict hand hygiene and to wear a surgical mask and, if available, an N–95 filtering disposable respirator. Isolation technique is essential.

The incubation period for SARS is 2–10 days. The symptoms of SARS include fever, chills, headache, malaise, myalgia that may progress to a dry cough, dyspnea, and hypoxemia. Abnormal laboratory findings include leukopenia, lymphopenia, thrombocytopenia, elevated LDH, CK, and AST levels. Antibodies to the virus may take more than 21 days after the illness to develop. During the acute stage of illness, the antibodies to the virus may not be isolated. In the early stage of the illness, the lungs can look normal; however, later the chest x-ray may show patchy infiltrates and even areas of consolidation. Some persons diagnosed as having SARS do not have the viral illness. It has been difficult to determine this illness.

Treatment includes supportive care, steroids, and antiviral agents such as oseltamivir and ribavirin. To identify and isolate suspected SARS cases, the CDC provides a website for case definition, http://www.cdc.gov/sars/guidance/B-surveillance/app1.html.

Purposes

- To prevent the spread of SARS.
- To provide effective care for patients with SARS.

Clinical Problems

Acute respiratory distress, severe acute respiratory syndrome.

Procedure

- Provide isolation for persons with acute respiratory distress symptoms if SARS is suspected, unless respiratory problem is known or until SARS is ruled out.
- Utilize mask and strict handwashing technique when in contact with SARS clients or if a client is suspected of having SARS.

NURSING IMPLICATIONS WITH RATIONALE

- Obtain a history of the client's travel to areas where SARS is prevalent, as well as fever, symptoms of respiratory problems, and contact with other persons having SARS.
- Obtain the blood specimens for tests such as white blood cells (WBC), creatine phosphokinase (CK), lactic dehydrogenase (LHD), aspartate aminotransferase (AST), or others as ordered.
- Monitor vital signs, especially the client's temperature.
- Use mask and strict isolation technique as indicated by the institution when caring for SARS clients or clients suspected of having SARS.

Client Teaching

- Give support to the client and family. Answer questions if known or have other health professionals answer questions.

Schilling test
See Diagnostic Tests

Sedimentation rate
See Erythrocyte Sedimentation Rate—ESR

Semen examination

Reference Values

Semen Examination: *Volume:* 1.5–5 mL. *Count:* 60–150 million/mL. *Mobility:* 3 hours greater than 60%. *Normal Forms:* Greater than 70%. *Appearance:* Translucent, turbid, viscous. *Viscosity:* Liquid after 30 minutes.

Antisperm Antibody Test: *Adult:* Negative to 1:32.

Description

Semen examination is used as one of the tests to determine the cause of infertility. The sperm count; volume of fluid; percentage of normal, mature spermatozoa (sperms); and percentage of actively mobile spermatozoa are studied when analyzing the semen content. Conception has been reported even when the sperm count has been as low as 10 million/mL.

Sperm count is frequently used to monitor the effectiveness of sterilization after a vasectomy (severing of the vas deferens). The sperm count is checked periodically. In cases of rape, a forensic or medicolegal analysis is done to detect semen in vaginal secretions or on clothes.

The three methods used to collect semen are masturbation, coitus interruptus, and intercourse using a condom. Sexual abstinence is usually required for 3 days before the test. Masturbation is the usual method for obtaining a semen specimen; however, for religious reasons intercourse with a condom is sometimes preferred. With coitus interruptus, only a partial semen specimen may be obtained. A semen specimen may be collected at home or in the health care provider's office.

The **antisperm antibody test** could be ordered to identify a possible cause of infertility. Autoantibodies to sperm might result from a blocking of the efferent ducts in the testes.

Purposes

- To check the sperm count.
- To determine if the decreased sperm count could be the cause of infertility.

Clinical Problems

Decreased Level: Vasectomy; infertility (0–2 million/mL). *Drug Influence:* Antineoplastic agents, estrogen.

Procedure

- Alcoholic beverages should be avoided for several days (at least 24 hours) before the test. There is no other fluid or food restriction.
- The client should abstain from intercourse for 3 days before semen collection.
- Collect semen by:
  1. Masturbation—collect in a clean container.
  2. Coitus interruptus—collect in a clean glass container.
  3. Intercourse with a clean, washed condom—place the condom in a clean container.
- Keep the semen specimen from chilling, and take it immediately to the laboratory. It should be tested within 2 hours after collection—the sooner, the better.

Factors Affecting Laboratory Results

- Recent intercourse (within 3 days) could have an effect on the sperm count.

NURSING IMPLICATIONS WITH RATIONALE

- Explain to the client the purpose of the test. He will most likely know the reason for semen collection and examination, which is either to determine the cause of infertility or to determine the effectiveness of sterilization following vasectomy.
- Be available to discuss methods of semen collection with the client and his spouse/partner (i.e., masturbation, coitus interruptus, and intercourse with a condom). This can be most embarrassing for the man and woman. Some persons prefer to discuss the test in detail with the nurse rather than with the health care provider. Religious beliefs need to be considered.
- Be supportive of the client and his spouse. Be a good listener and give them time to express their concerns.
- Answer their questions. If you are unable to respond, refer the question to the appropriate person (i.e., the health care provider, a clergyperson).
- Avoid giving your moral convictions about the test or the surgical procedure (vasectomy).

S

Serotonin (plasma)
5-Hydroxytryptamine

Reference Values

Adult: 50–175 ng/mL, 10–30 mcg/dL, 0.29–1.15 µmol/L (SI units).

Description

Serotonin is produced by the argentaffin cells of the intestinal mucosa. It is transmitted in the body by platelets and acts as a vasoconstrictor to small arterioles after tissue injury. It can also be found in the tissues of the central nervous system and has been classified as one of the neurotransmitters. Other functions of serotonin include contraction of smooth muscle such as in peristalsis, release of the growth hormone, and release of prolactin; it can cause hemocoagulation.

The primary purpose of this test is to confirm the diagnosis of carcinoid tumors of the argentaffin cells in the gastrointestinal tract. Most serotonin is excreted as the metabolite 5-hydroxyindole-acetic acid (5-HIAA) in the urine. The 5-HIAA urine test should be ordered with the plasma serotonin test. Ectopic production of serotonin can result from oat cell carcinoma of the lung, pancreatic tumors, and thyroid cancer.

Purpose

- To aid in the diagnosis of carcinoid tumors.

Clinical Problems

Decreased Level: Parkinson disease, Down syndrome, depression, renal insufficiency, phenylketonuria.

Increased Level: *Carcinoid Tumors:* Ectopic production due to oat cell carcinoma of the lung, pancreatic tumor, thyroid medullary cancer, myocardial infarction, endocarditis, chronic pain, cystic fibrosis. *Drug Influence:* Monoamine oxidase (MAO inhibitors), methyldopa, imipramine, reserpine.

Procedure

- There is no food or fluid restriction.
- Collect 7–10 mL of venous blood in a lavender-top tube. The blood specimen should be placed on ice immediately and sent promptly to the laboratory.
- Withhold MAO inhibitors for a week prior to the test with the health care provider's approval. MAO inhibitors taken prior to the test should be noted on the laboratory slip.

Factors Affecting Laboratory Results

- Blood specimen that has not been cooled and not taken immediately to the laboratory. Blood serotonin samples are unstable.
- Certain drugs can increase the plasma serotonin level, especially MAO inhibitors (*see Drug Influence*).
- The drug lithium may decrease or elevate the serotonin in the brain.
- A radioactive scan performed on the client 7 days before the serotonin blood sample is taken.

NURSING IMPLICATIONS WITH RATIONALE

- Obtain a list of drugs the client is taking. Notify the health care provider if the client is taking a drug that could elevate the plasma serotonin level, especially MAO inhibitors.
- Check if a urine 5-HIAA has been ordered. This urine test is usually ordered if a carcinoid tumor is suspected.
- Note if the client has chronic pain, which may increase the plasma serotonin level, or depression, which could decrease the plasma level.

Serum glutamic oxaloacetic transaminase (SGOT)

See Aspartate Aminotransferase

Serum glutamic pyruvic transaminase (SGPT)

See Alanine Aminotransferase

Severe combined immunodeficiency (SCID) (blood)

Reference Values

Normal: Presence of T cells.

Description

Severe combined immunodeficiency (SCID) is a screening blood test performed on infants 3 months or younger to determine the absence or deficiency of T cells in the body. The T cells are a type of white blood cells that are needed for immune system function. With a deficit or absence of T cells, the infant cannot fight off viruses, bacteria, or fungi. Death could occur as a result of severe infection.

The life expectancy for a child with a lack or absence of mature T cells without treatment is a year. SCID affects 1 in 40,000 to 1 in 100,000 infants each year. Early detection is imperative.

Duke University has a treatment program for infants with SCID. According to the program, the survival rate is 92% for infants diagnosed under 3 months. Delaware, Massachusetts, and Wisconsin have a routine SCID screening test on all newborns. The CDC and the federal government are pushing to make this screening test mandatory in all states.

At birth, the T cells and B cells of the white blood cells are immature stem cells and soon after become mature cells. The T cells promote immunity to infections resulting from bacteria, viruses, or fungi that enter the body. Treatment for SCID (lack or absence of T cells) is a bone marrow transplant from a parent, unaffected sibling, or a close relative. By replacing the marrow with healthy marrow, the child can be cured of SCID.

Purposes

- To detect the absence or a deficiency of T cells in the newborn.
- To prevent the presence of severe combined immunodeficiency.

Clinical Problems

Decreased Level: Absence of T cells, presence of SCID.

Procedure

- There is no food or fluid restriction.
- Obtain a drop of blood from the newborn's heel.

NURSING IMPLICATIONS WITH RATIONALE

- Determine if a SCID test is done on newborn infants in your state. The protocol for your state may include SCID test for all newborns.
- Obtain a history of any previous child's health problems, such as frequent severe infections or death of an infant/child before 1 year old.

Client Teaching

- Explain to the parent (s) that a routine blood sample is obtained to check for a lack of an important blood cell (T cell). A more detailed explanation may be needed.
- Explain that the blood test is usually performed a day or more after an infant's birth. However, it should be performed before the child is 3 months old.
- If the test is positive for SCID, be supportive to the family.

Sexual assault/attack
Rape Trauma, Rape Testing

Reference Values
Negative for physical sexual trauma.

Description
When a person has been physically and sexually assaulted/attacked, the person should have professional testing performed soon after the assault. If testing is performed several days after the assault, evidence would be diminished. The majority of health institutions (small and large) have a protocol for dealing with sexual assaults. The timing of the assault and a brief history from the person assaulted are essential. The emotional status of the person should be noted. The clothing of the person should be placed in a paper bag to preserve possible DNA (not a plastic bag). Photographs should be taken of any visual injury from the sexual attack.

Most health institutions have a kit, Sexual Assault Evidence Collection Kit (SAECK), with directions for testing persons who are sexually assaulted. A pelvic examination is usually performed to obtain sperm and other cells from the perpetrator.

Vaginal secretions may be taken to test for sexually transmitted diseases (STDs) such as for gonorrhea, syphilis, and trichomoniasis. Human immunodeficiency virus (HIV) and pregnancy tests may be performed at that time and repeated later. To prevent STDs, the health care provider may prescribe antibacterial agents. An antiretroviral drug to ward against HIV, such as zidovudine (Retrovir), may be prescribed. If pregnancy is a possibility, the health care provider may suggest and prescribe postcoital contraception if the rape occurred less than 3 days ago or an intrauterine contraceptive device if the rape happened more than a week ago.

Purposes
- To determine a possible sexual assault by using the SAEC kit.
- To obtain DNA evidence from vaginal secretions and clothing.

Clinical Problems
Positive Findings: Sexual assault vaginally and bodily harm, possible STD, possible HIV, and possible pregnancy.

Procedure
- Obtain a signed permission form from the client.
- There is no food or fluid restriction.
- Collect specimens according to the SAEC kit. This would include vaginal secretions and cells and blood samples for HIV and pregnancy tests.
- Refrigerate specimen(s) as needed to preserve DNA.

Factors Affecting Laboratory Results
- Not obtaining professional testing until several days following the assault.

NURSING IMPLICATIONS WITH RATIONALE

- Have the professional person who covers sexual assault or attack be responsible and in charge of the situation with the client and family.
- Obtain a signed consent form from the client.
- Place the clothing the client was wearing when she was attacked in a paper bag. Avoid using a plastic bag because it can promote bacteria growth and decrease the evidence of DNA. If the client has changed clothing, then special bagging would not be necessary.
- Photographs may be taken of any visual injury (pelvic and from the body).
- Assess the client's emotional status. Psychological counseling may be necessary.
- Notify the police if the police are not present.

Client Teaching

- Be supportive of the client and family. Professional counseling will most likely be necessary.

S

Sickle-cell (screening) test (blood)

Reference Values

Adult: 0.

Child: 0.

Description

(*See Hemoglobin Electrophoresis.*)

Hemoglobin S (sickle cell), an abnormal hemoglobin, causes red blood cells (erythrocytes) to form a crescent shape when deprived of oxygen. With adequate oxygen, the RBCs with hemoglobin S will maintain a normal shape.

If a sickle-cell screening test is positive for hemoglobin S, hemoglobin electrophoresis should be ordered to differentiate between sickle-cell anemia caused by hemoglobin S/S and sickle-cell trait caused by hemoglobin A/S. If the client's hemoglobin level is less than 10 g/dL or the hematocrit is less than 30%, test results could be falsely negative.

Purpose

- To screen for sickle-cell anemia.

Clinical Problems

Positive Results: Sickle-cell anemia, sickle-cell trait.

Procedure

- There is no food or fluid restriction.
- Collect 3–7 mL of venous blood in a lavender-top tube.

- If a commercial test kit (Sickledex) is used, follow the directions given on the kit.
- Note on the laboratory slip if blood transfusion was given 3–4 months before the screening test. If so, inaccurate results could occur.

Factors Affecting Laboratory Results

- A blood transfusion given within 3–4 months could cause inaccurate results.
- Hemoglobin less than 10 g/dL or hematocrit less than 30% could cause false-negative test results.
- Reagents from the test kit may deteriorate and may no longer be active test agents.
- The test result could be falsely negative in an infant less than 6 months old.

NURSING IMPLICATIONS WITH RATIONALE

- Explain to the client and/or family that the purpose of the test is to determine the presence of sickle cells (hemoglobin S).

Positive Test Results

- Observe for signs and symptoms of sickle-cell anemia. Early symptoms are fatigue and weakness. Chronic symptoms are dyspnea on exertion, swollen joints, "aching bones," and chest pains.

Client Teaching

- Instruct the client to avoid people with infections and colds. Persons with sickle-cell anemia are susceptible to infections.
- Encourage the client to seek genetic counseling if he or she has sickle-cell anemia or the sickle-cell trait.
- Instruct the client with sickle-cell anemia to minimize strenuous activity and to avoid high altitudes and extreme cold. Encourage the client to take rest periods.

Sodium (Na) (serum)

Reference Values

Adult: 135–145 mEq/L, 135–145 mmol/L (SI units). *Panic:* Less than 115 mEq/L.
Child: *Infant:* 134–150 mEq/L. *Child:* 135–145 mEq/L.

Description

Sodium (Na) is the major cation in the extracellular fluid (ECF), and it has a water-retaining effect. When there is excess sodium in the ECF, more water will be reabsorbed from the kidneys.

Sodium has many functions. It helps to maintain body fluids, is responsible for conduction of neuromuscular impulses via the sodium pump (sodium shifts into cells as potassium shifts out for cellular activity), is involved in enzyme activity, and it regulates acid–base balance by combining with chloride or bicarbonate ions.

The body needs approximately 2–4 g of sodium daily. Americans daily consume approximately 6–12 g (90–240 mEq/L) of sodium in the form of salt (NaCl). A teaspoon of salt contains 2.3 g of sodium.

Sodium imbalances are termed *hyponatremia* (serum sodium deficit) and *hypernatremia* (serum sodium excess). When the serum sodium level is 125 mEq/L, sodium replacement with normal saline (0.9% NaCl) should be considered, and if the serum sodium level is 115 mEq/L or lower, concentrated saline solutions (3% or 5% NaCl) might be ordered. When rapidly replacing sodium loss, assessment for overhydration is important.

Purposes

- To monitor the sodium level.
- To detect sodium imbalance (hypo- or hypernatremia).
- To compare the sodium level with that of other electrolytes (e.g., calcium, potassium, chloride).

Clinical Problems

Decreased Level: Vomiting, diarrhea, gastric suction, excessive perspiration, continuous intravenous 5% dextrose in water (D_5W), syndrome of inappropriate antidiuretic hormone (SIADH, due to surgery, trauma, pain, narcotics), low-sodium diet, burns, inflammatory reactions, tissue injury (fluid and sodium shift to the third space), psychogenic polydipsia, salt-wasting renal disease. *Drug Influence:* Potent diuretics (furosemide [Lasix], ethacrynic acid [Edecrin], thiazides, mannitol).

Increased Level: Dehydration, severe vomiting and diarrhea (water loss is greater than sodium loss), heart failure, Cushing disease, hepatic failure, high-sodium diet. *Drug Influence:* Cough medicines, cortisone preparations, antibiotics, laxatives, methyldopa (Aldomet), hydralazine (Apresoline), reserpine (Serpasil).

Procedure

- There are no restrictions on food and fluid. If the client has eaten large quantities of foods high in salt content in the last 24–48 hours, this should be noted on the laboratory slip and the health care provider should be notified. Sodium is rarely requested alone but is rather given as part of the serum electrolytes (i.e., sodium, potassium, chloride, carbon dioxide).
- Collect 3–5 mL of venous blood in a red- or green-top tube.

Factors Affecting Laboratory Results

- A diet high in sodium.
- Drugs—potent diuretics, cortisone preparations, various antihypertensive agents, cough medicines.

NURSING IMPLICATIONS WITH RATIONALE

Decreased Level

- Assess for signs and symptoms of hyponatremia (e.g., apprehension, anxiety, muscular twitching, muscular weakness, headaches, tachycardia, and hypotension).

- Recognize that hyponatremia after surgery is the result of SIADH. There is usually an excess secretion of antidiuretic hormone for a day or two after surgery, which causes water reabsorption from the kidneys and sodium dilution.
- Report if the client has received D_5W infusions for more than 2 days. Hyponatremia and water intoxication could occur. IV fluids with dextrose and one-third or one-half normal saline solution (0.33–0.45%) are frequently ordered.
- Monitor the medical regimen for correcting hyponatremia (i.e., water restriction, normal saline [0.9% percent] solution to correct a serum sodium level of 120–130 mEq/L, and 3% or 5% saline to correct a serum sodium level of less than 115 mEq/L).
- Observe for signs and symptoms of overhydration when the client is receiving 3% or 5% saline intravenously. Symptoms of overhydration are a constant, irritated cough; dyspnea; neck- and hand-vein engorgement; and chest rales.
- Check the specific gravity of urine. A specific gravity of less than 1.010 could indicate hyponatremia.
- Check serum sodium and other laboratory results and report serum electrolyte changes. An extremely low serum sodium level requires that the test be repeated.
- Irrigate nasogastric tubes and wound sites with normal saline instead of sterile water.
- Take vital signs to determine cardiac status during hyponatremia.
- Compare the serum sodium level with the urine sodium level. A low or normal serum sodium and a low urine sodium could indicate sodium retention or a decrease in sodium intake.

Client Teaching

- Encourage the client to avoid drinking only plain water. Suggest fluids with solutes (e.g., broth and juices).

Increased Level

- Observe for signs and symptoms of hypernatremia (e.g., restlessness; thirst; flushed skin; dry, sticky mucous membranes; a rough, dry tongue; and tachycardia).
- Check for body fluid loss by keeping an accurate intake and output record and weighing the client daily. A liter of fluid will add approximately 2.5 pounds of body weight.
- Check the specific gravity of the urine. A specific gravity greater than 1.030 could indicate hypernatremia.
- Report if the client is receiving IV fluids containing normal saline (0.9% NaCl). A liter of normal saline contains 155 mEq of sodium. The body needs 40–70 mEq/L of sodium daily, though the average daily intake for adults is 90–240 mEq/L. The maximum daily tolerance of sodium is 400 mEq/L, and if the client receives 3 liters of normal saline, he or she will receive 465 mEq/L.
- Observe for edema and overhydration resulting from an elevated serum sodium level. Signs and symptoms of overhydration are a constant, irritated cough; dyspnea; neck- and hand-vein engorgement; and chest rales.

Client Teaching

- Encourage the client to drink 8–10 glasses of water, unless this is contraindicated (for instance, with a history of heart failure).

- Instruct the client to avoid foods that are high in sodium (e.g., corned beef, bacon, ham, tuna fish, cheese, celery, catsup, pickles, olives, and potato chips). Avoid using salt when cooking or at mealtime.

Sodium (Na) (urine)

Reference Values

Adult: 40–220 mEq/L/24 h.

Child: Similar to adult.

Description

Sodium excretion varies according to the sodium intake, aldosterone secretion, urine volume, and disease entities, such as chronic renal failure, adrenal gland dysfunction (Addison disease and Cushing syndrome), cirrhosis of the liver, and heart failure.

When the urine sodium level is less than 40 mEq/24 h, the decreased sodium excretion could be due to sodium retention or decreased sodium intake. The body could be retaining sodium even with a low serum sodium level.

The urine sodium level should be monitored when edema is present and the serum sodium level is low or normal.

Purposes

(*See Sodium [serum].*)

Clinical Problems

Decreased Level: Cushing syndrome, heart failure, hepatic failure, renal failure, chronic obstructive pulmonary disease (COPD), low sodium (salt) intake. *Drug Influence:* Cortisone preparations.

Increased Level: Addison disease, dehydration, essential hypertension, diabetes mellitus, anterior pituitary hypofunction, high sodium intake. *Drug Influence:* Potent diuretics (furosemide [Lasix], ethacrynic acid [Edecrin]).

Procedure

- There is no food or fluid restriction.
- Collect a 24-hour urine sample and place it in a large specimen container. Label the container with the exact times the urine collection started and ended. First-voided specimen should be discarded.
- The urine specimen should be refrigerated or placed in a container of ice.

Factors Affecting Laboratory Results

- A diet high or low in sodium content.

- Drugs such as cortisone and potent diuretics.
- Renal dysfunction.
- Discarded urine.

NURSING IMPLICATIONS WITH RATIONALE

Client Teaching

- Explain the procedure for collecting the 24-hour urine. Inform the client that all voidings (urine) should be placed in the large container. Have clients inform their families of the procedure. Tell the client not to put toilet paper or feces in the urine.

Decreased Level

- Compare serum sodium level with the urine sodium level. A low or normal serum sodium and a low urine sodium could indicate sodium retention or a decrease in sodium intake.

Increased Level

- Report if the client is receiving several liters of normal saline solution intravenously (*see Sodium [serum]*).

Client Teaching

- Instruct the client to avoid eating foods high in sodium if the cause is due to high sodium intake.

Testosterone (serum or plasma)

Reference Values

Adult: *Male:* 0.3–1 mcg/dL, 300–1,000 ng/dL. *Female:* 0.03–0.1 mcg/dL, 30–100 ng/dL.

Child: *Male: 12–14 Years Old:* Greater than 0.1 mcg/dL, greater than 100 ng/dL.

Description

Testosterone, a male sex hormone, is produced by the testes and adrenal glands in the male and by the ovaries and adrenal glands in the female. It is useful in diagnosing male sexual precocity before the age of 10 years and male infertility.

In males, the highest serum testosterone levels occur in the morning. Serum testosterone is low in both primary and secondary hypogonadism.

Purposes

- To assess testosterone value.
- To detect testicular hypofunction.
- To aid in the diagnosis of male sexual precocity.

Clinical Problems

Decreased Level: Testicular hypofunction, Klinefelter syndrome (primary hypogonadism), alcoholism, anterior pituitary hypofunction, estrogen therapy, hypopituitarism.

Increased Level: Male sexual precocity, adrenal hyperplasia or tumor, neoplasm or hyperplasia of ovaries, adrenogenital syndrome in women, polycystic ovaries in females.

Procedure

- There is no food or fluid restriction.
- Collect 5–7 mL of venous blood in a red- or green-top tube. Avoid hemolysis.

Factors Affecting Laboratory Results

- None known.

NURSING IMPLICATIONS WITH RATIONALE

Decreased Level

- Determine whether the client is complying with medical treatment for testicular hypofunction or hypogonadism. Discuss the side effects of testosterone.
- Be supportive of the male client and his family concerning physical changes caused by hormonal deficiency.

Increased Level

- Observe for signs and symptoms of excess testosterone secretion (e.g., hirsutism, masculine voice, and increased muscle mass [especially in women]). Report abnormal findings.

Theophylline (serum)

Aminophylline, Theo-Dur, Theolair, Slo-Phyllin, Elixophyllin, Sustaire

Reference Values

Therapeutic Range: *Adult:* 5–20 mcg/mL, 28–112 μmol/L (SI units). *Elderly:* 5–18 mcg/mL. *Premature Infant:* 7–14 mcg/mL. *Neonate:* 3–12 mcg/mL. *Child:* Same as adult.

Toxic Level: *Adult:* Greater than 20 mcg/mL, greater than 112 μmol/L (SI units). *Elderly:* Same as adult. *Premature Infant:* Greater than 14 mcg/mL. *Neonate:* Greater than 13 mcg/mL. *Child:* Same as adult.

Description

Theophylline, a xanthine derivative, relaxes the smooth muscles of the bronchi and pulmonary blood vessels; reduces pulmonary hypertension; stimulates the central nervous system; stimulates myocardium, resulting in an increase in the force of contraction and cardiac output; increases renal blood flow, causing diuresis; and relaxes the smooth muscles of the gastrointestinal tract.

Usually theophylline products are given to control asthmatic attacks and to treat acute attacks. Oral theophylline preparations are well absorbed from the gastrointestinal tract.

Ninety percent of theophylline is metabolized in the liver, with about 60% bound to plasma protein and 40% free. Ten percent of the drug is excreted unchanged in the urine. The half-life of theophylline is 5–10 hours in a nonsmoker, 3½–5 hours in a smoker, and 3½ in children. Peak blood levels after an orally administered dose of theophylline occurs in 1–2 hours.

Persons with heart failure or liver disease or who are either very young or elderly could develop theophylline toxicity quickly. Serum theophylline levels in these persons should be monitored frequently.

Early signs and symptoms of theophylline toxicity are anorexia, nausea, vomiting, abdominal discomfort, nervousness, jitters, tachycardia, and cardiac arrhythmias. If severe theophylline toxicity occurs (greater than 30 mcg/mL), cardiac dysrhythmias, seizures, respiratory arrest, and/or cardiac arrest might result.

Purpose

- To monitor theophylline levels.

Clinical Problems

Decreased Level: Smoking. *Drug Influence:* Phenytoin (Dilantin).

Increased Level: Theophylline overdose, heart failure, liver disease, lung disease, renal disease. *Drug Influence:* Antibiotics (erythromycin, lincomycin), allopurinol, barbiturates, caffeine, cimetidine (Tagamet), furosemide (Lasix), ephedrine, propranolol (Inderal), sulfonamides, theobromine, other xanthines, flu vaccine.

Procedure

- The client should not drink coffee, tea, or colas, or eat chocolate 8 hours prior to the test.
- Collect 3–5 mL of venous blood in a red-top tube. Avoid hemolysis.
- Record the name of the drug, dose, route, and last dose administered on the laboratory requisition slip. Test might be ordered for peak levels or for trough levels (before next dose).
- Note on the laboratory requisition slip drugs the client is taking that could affect test results.
- Do not shake the collecting tube of blood specimen. This could decrease the serum theophylline level.

Factors Affecting Laboratory Results

- Drugs (*see Drug Influence*), food, and fluids, such as chocolate, coffee, tea, and colas, could increase serum theophylline level.
- Shaking the collecting tube vigorously could cause a false-negative test result.

NURSING IMPLICATIONS WITH RATIONALE

- Explain to the client that the purpose of the test is to monitor the therapeutic theophylline level.
- Check the theophylline level and report nontherapeutic levels to the health care provider immediately.

- Record name of the drug, dose, route, and last time drug was given on the requisition slip.
- Record the time the blood sample was drawn on the requisition slip. This informs the laboratory personnel and the health care provider of the theophylline level time (peak or trough before the next dose).

Decreased Level

- Recognize that smoking causes a short half-life and promotes a faster theophylline clearance. The drug phenytoin (Dilantin) has been reported to decrease the theophylline half-life.
- Report if the client is a smoker because a larger dose of theophylline might be needed.

Increased Level

- Recognize that liver, lung, and renal diseases and certain drugs might cause an elevated serum theophylline level (*see Drug Influence*).
- Observe for signs and symptoms of theophylline toxicity (e.g., anorexia, nausea, vomiting, abdominal discomfort, nervousness, irritability, tachycardia, and cardiac dysrhythmias).
- Monitor pulse rate and report signs of tachycardia and skipped beats.
- Monitor intake and output. Report if client's output has greatly increased because of diuresis.
- Check serum glucose level. Theophylline can cause hyperglycemia, also decreased clotting time.

Client Teaching

- Instruct the client not to drink coffee, teas, or colas, or eat chocolate within 8 hours of the test.
- Inform the client not to take other xanthines while taking theophylline to avoid theophylline toxicity.
- Suggest that the client avoid the herbal drug ephedra, which could cause theophylline toxicity.

Thyroid antibodies

See Thyroid Globulin Antibodies, Thyroid Peroxidase (TPO) Antibodies

Thyroid globulin antibodies (serum)

Thyroglobulin Antibodies, Thyroid Hemagglutination Test, Thyroid Autoantibodies, Antithyroglobulin Antibody, and Antimicrosomal Antibody

Reference Values

Adult: Negative to 1:20, antimicrosomal: negative to 100.

Child: Similar to adult but usually not done.

Description

A thyroid autoimmune disease usually produces thyroid antibodies (antithyroglobulin antibodies and antimicrosomal antibodies). These autoantibodies (against the body's own tissue) combine with thyroglobulin from the thyroid gland and cause inflammatory lesions of the gland.

If the thyroglobulin breaks away from thyroxine and enters the circulation, antithyroglobulin antibodies usually form. Antimicrosomal antibodies form if the microsomes of the thyroid epithelial cells are attacked. An increase in these thyroid antibodies damages the thyroid gland. Usually serum titers are ordered to detect the presence of one or both of the thyroid antibodies.

With thyrotoxicosis, a positive titer of 1:1,600 may occur, and with Hashimoto thyroiditis, the titer may be greater than 1:5,000. A positive thyroid antibodies (TA) test does not always confirm the diagnosis of Hashimoto thyroiditis, unless the titer is extremely high. The titer can also be elevated with carcinoma of the thyroid and rheumatoid-collagen diseases.

Antibodies to thyroglobulin may be detected in 40–70% of clients with chronic thyroiditis, 40% of clients with thyrotoxicosis (Graves disease), and 70% of clients with hypothyroidism (low to moderate titer elevation). Antibodies to thyroid microsomes occur in 70–90% of clients with chronic thyroiditis.

Purposes

- To aid in the diagnosis of Graves disease. Graves disease (hyperthyroidism) and Haskimoto's thyroiditis (hypothyroidism)
- To detect the presence of thyroid antibodies, which may cause a thyroid autoimmune disease.

Clinical Problems

Increased (Positive) Titer: Hashimoto thyroiditis, carcinoma of the thyroid gland, pernicious anemia, lupus erythematosus, rheumatoid arthritis, thyrotoxicosis (Graves disease).

Procedure

- There is no food or fluid restriction.
- Collect 5 mL of venous blood in a red-top tube. Avoid hemolysis.

Factors Affecting Laboratory Results

- Sex (thyroid disease is more common in women than in men).

NURSING IMPLICATIONS WITH RATIONALE

Increased Titer Level

- Check serum antithyroglobin antibody titer results and relate them to clinical problems. The test is usually ordered to diagnose Hashimoto thyroiditis; however, the titer level can be elevated in other clinical conditions (*see Clinical Problems*).
- Obtain a family history of thyroid disease. Determine whether the client has had a viral infection in the last few weeks or months. It is believed that viral infections can trigger autoimmune disease.

Thyroid peroxidase (TPO) antibody

TPO Antibodies, Antithyroid Peroxidase Antibodies, Antithyroperoxidase, Thyroperoxidase Antibodies

Reference Values

Negative for clients without TPO antibodies.

Description

Thyroid peroxidase (TPO) antibody test and thyroid globulin antibody test are frequently ordered at the same time. The thyroid antibodies are autoimmune antibodies that inhibit the synthesis of the thyroid hormone. TPO antibody test is the newer test for thyroid dysfunction. Thyroid peroxidase is essential for the synthesis of thyroid hormones, thyroxine (T_4), and triiodothyronine (T_3). Frequently, both tests are ordered to detect the cause of hypo- or hyperthyroidism. The most common thyroid diseases are Graves disease (hyperthyroidism) and Hashimoto thyroiditis (hypothyroidism). Thyroid antibodies can destroy thyroid function.

Hypothyroidism in a pregnant female can cause insufficient thyroxine levels in the brain, affecting the fetus's brain development. Hyperthyroidism during a female's child-bearing years can cause thyrotoxicosis, thus impairing fertility. In the pregnant female, hyperthyroidism could cause a miscarriage. It has been noted that TPO antibodies may cause mild depression in postpartum females.

Purposes

- To detect the presence of TPO antibodies.
- To determine the presence of hypo- or hyperthyroidism.

Clinical Problems

TPO antibodies: Graves disease (hyperthyroidism), Hashimoto thyroiditis, thyroid cancer, and others.

Procedure

- There is no food or fluid restriction.
- Collect 5 mL of venous blood in a red-top tube.

Factors Affecting Laboratory Results

- Hemolysis from rough handling of the blood sample.

NURSING IMPLICATIONS WITH RATIONALE

- Explain that the purpose of the test is to determine if thyroid antibodies (TPO antibodies) are present and causing the thyroid disease or dysfunction.
- Answer the client's questions or refer the questions to a health care provider.

Thyroid-stimulating hormone (TSH) (serum)

Reference Values

Values differ according to the laboratory method used.

Adult: 0.35–5.5 microinternational unit/mL (μIU/mL), less than 3 ng/mL.

Newborn: Less than 25 microinternational unit/mL by the third day.

Description

The anterior pituitary gland (anterior hypophysis) secretes thyroid-stimulating hormone (TSH) in response to thyroid-releasing hormone (TRH) from the hypothalamus. TSH stimulates the secretion of thyroxine (T_4) produced in the thyroid gland. The secretion of TSH is dependent on the negative-feedback system—a decreased T_4 level promotes the release of TRH, which stimulates TSH secretion. An elevated T_4 level suppresses TRH release, which suppresses TSH secretion.

TSH and T_4 levels are frequently measured to differentiate pituitary from thyroid dysfunctions. A decreased T_4 level and a normal or elevated TSH level can indicate a thyroid disorder. A decreased T_4 level with a decreased TSH level can indicate a pituitary disorder.

Purposes

- To suggest secondary hypothyroidism due to pituitary involvement.
- To compare test results with T_4 level to differentiate between pituitary and thyroid dysfunction.

Clinical Problems

Decreased Level: Secondary hypothyroidism (pituitary gland involvement), anterior pituitary hypofunction, Klinefelter syndrome. *Drug Influence:* Aspirin, steroid, dopamine, heparin.

Increased Level: Primary hypothyroidism (thyroid gland involvement with a decreased T_4); thyroiditis (Hashimoto disease, autoimmune disease); cirrhosis of the liver. *Drug Influence:* Antithyroid therapy for hyperthyroidism.

Procedure

- There is no fluid restriction. Shellfish should be avoided for several days prior to the test.
- Collect 5 mL of venous blood in a red- or green-top tube. Avoid hemolysis.

Factors Affecting Laboratory Results

- None known.

NURSING IMPLICATIONS WITH RATIONALE

- Recognize the cause of hypothyroidism by comparing the TSH level with the T_4 level. Decreased TSH and T_4 levels could be due to anterior pituitary dysfunction causing secondary hypothyroidism. A normal or elevated TSH level and a decreased T_4 level could be due to thyroid dysfunction.

- Observe for signs and symptoms of myxedema (hypothyroidism; e.g., anorexia; fatigue; weight gain; dry and flaky skin; puffy face, hands, and feet; abdominal distention; bradycardia; infertility; and ataxia).
- Monitor vital signs before and during treatment for hypothyroidism. Report immediately if tachycardia occurs.
- Refer to the client's triiodothyronine (T$_3$), T$_4$, and thyroglobulin results to observe correlations with the TSH result.

Thyroxine (T$_4$) (serum)

Reference Values

Adult: *Reported as Serum Thyroxine:* T$_4$ by column: 4.5–11.5 mcg/dL. T$_4$ (RIA): 5–12 mcg/dL. Free T$_4$: 1–2.3 ng/dL. *Reported as Thyroxine Iodine:* T$_4$ by column: 3.2–7.2 mcg/dL.

Child: *Newborn:* 11–23 mcg/dL. *1–4 Months Old:* 7.5–16.5 mcg/dL. *4–12 Months Old:* 5.5–14.5 mcg/dL. *1–6 Years Old:* 5.5–13.5 mcg/dL. *6–10 Years Old:* 5–12.5 mcg/dL.

Description

Thyroxine (T$_4$) is the major hormone secreted by the thyroid gland and is at least 25 times more concentrated than triiodothyronine (T$_3$). The serum T$_4$ levels are commonly used to measure thyroid hormone concentration and the function of the thyroid gland. The use of protein-bound iodine (PBI) is considered obsolete, and this test is seldom performed.

In some institutions, the T$_4$ test is required for all newborns (as is the phenylketonuria [PKU] test) to detect a decreased thyroxine secretion, which could lead to irreversible mental retardation.

Purposes

- To determine thyroid function.
- To aid in the diagnosis of hypo- or hyperthyroidism.
- To compare test results with other laboratory thyroid tests.

Clinical Problems

Decreased Level: Hypothyroidism (cretinism, myxedema), protein malnutrition, anterior pituitary hypofunction, strenuous exercise. *Drug Influence:* Cortisone, chlorpromazine (Thorazine), phenytoin (Dilantin), heparin, lithium, sulfonamides, reserpine (Serpasil), testosterone, tolbutamide (Orinase).

Increased Level: Hyperthyroidism, acute thyroiditis, viral hepatitis, myasthenia gravis, pregnancy, preeclampsia. *Drug Influence:* Oral contraceptives, estrogens, clofibrate.

Procedure

- There is no food or fluid restriction.
- Various methods are used for measuring T$_4$.

- Thyroid medication will interfere with the T$_4$ by column method. Check with your laboratory for an alternative procedure.
- Collect 5–7 mL of venous blood in a red-top tube. Avoid hemolysis.
- Note on the laboratory slip drugs the client is taking that could affect test results.

Factors Affecting Laboratory Results

- Drugs (*see Drug Influence*).

NURSING IMPLICATIONS WITH RATIONALE

Decreased Level

- Observe for signs and symptoms of hypothyroidism (e.g., fatigue, forgetfulness, weight gain, dry skin with poor turgor, dry and thin hair, bradycardia, decreased peripheral circulation, depressed libido, infertility, and constipation).

Increased Level

- Observe for signs and symptoms of hyperthyroidism (e.g., nervousness, tremors, emotional instability, increased appetite, weight loss, palpitations, tachycardia, diarrhea, decreased fertility, and exophthalmos).
- Monitor the pulse rate. Tachycardia is common and if severe could cause heart failure and cardiac arrest.

TORCH screen test
TORCH Battery, TORCH Titer

Reference Values

Maternal: *IgG Titer Antibodies:* Negative. *IgM Titer Antibodies:* Negative.

Infant: Same as maternal; infant should be under 2 months of age.

Description

TORCH stands for toxoplasmosis, rubella, cytomegalovirus (CMV), and herpes simplex. It is a screen test to detect the presence of these organisms in the mother and infant. During pregnancy, TORCH infections can cross the placenta and could result in mild or severe congenital malformation, abortion, or stillbirth. The severe effect from these organisms occurs during the first trimester of pregnancy. Prenatally the TORCH screening test is performed only when a TORCH infection is suspected, such as rubella infection.

TORCH screening test is more frequently performed when congenital infection in the infant is suspected. The IgG titers are compared with both mother's and infant's serum. If the IgG titer level is higher in the infant than mother and the IgM titer is present in the infant, congenital TORCH infection is likely. This test might be repeated in several weeks. Individual testing might be necessary along with clinical information to identify the TORCH infection. Rubella and CMV are the most common.

Purpose

- To detect TORCH infection in newborns and mothers.

Clinical Problems

Positive IgG, IgM Titers: Toxoplasmosis, rubella, CMV, herpes simplex.

Procedure

- There is no food or fluid restriction.
- Collect 7 mL of venous blood in a red-top tube.
- TORCH kits: Follow directions on the kit.

Factors Affecting Laboratory Results

- None known.

NURSING IMPLICATIONS WITH RATIONALE

- Obtain a history from the client about any previous infection.

Client Teaching

- Inform the client that if a positive test result occurs, more testing will be needed.

Toxoplasmosis antibody test (serum)

Reference Values

Titer: Less than 1:4, no previous infection from *T. gondii.*

Titer: 1:4–1:64, past exposure, may persist for life.

Titer: Greater than 1:256, recent infection.

Titer: Greater than 1:424, acute infection.

Description

Toxoplasma gondii (*T. gondii*) is a protozoan organism that causes the parasitic disease toxoplasmosis. Twenty-five to 40% of the population in the United States have antibodies to *T. gondii.* Half of these people are asymptomatic. This organism can remain in body muscle and be dormant for years or life. This organism is transmitted in raw or poorly cooked meat or by ingesting oocysts from feces of infected cats. Transmission from the latter may occur when changing the cat litter.

Congenital form of toxoplasmosis occurs to the fetus when the mother is acutely infected with the *T. gondii* during pregnancy and passes the organism via placenta to the unborn child. Most of these pregnant females having the *T. gondii* are asymptomatic. If the female is infected with *T. gondii* weeks or months before conception, the organism will not affect the fetus. Congenital toxoplasmosis may cause mental retardation, hydrocephalus, microcephalus, and chronic retinitis, and/or lead to fetal death. The Centers for Disease Control recommends a serological test for *T. gondii* antibody titer for all pregnant women before the 20th week (actually earlier is better). There usually is no risk for birth defects; if the titer is low-positive a repeat test may be suggested. However, if the pregnant woman acquires the organism (high titer level) during pregnancy, the fetus is at risk for birth defect. The fetus has been infected with the organism if the antibody titer of the infant persistently increases 2–3 months after birth. Toxoplasmosis is not communicable between individuals except for maternal–fetal transfer.

The IGM antibody titer begins to rise 1 week after infection and peaks in 1–3 weeks. The IgG antibody titer rises in approximately 4–7 days after the IgM antibody, peaks 1–3 weeks later, and falls slowly within 6 months. Sulfonamides may be used to treat toxoplasmosis.

Purposes

- To identify the *T. gondii* organism.
- To detect the *T. gondii* organism in pregnant woman before the 20th week.

Clinical Problems

Elevated Titers: Toxoplasmosis. *Low-Positive Titer:* Past infection of *T. gondii*. *High-Positive Titer:* Current active infection of *T. gondii*.

Procedure

- There is no food or fluid restriction.
- Collect 5–7 mL of venous blood in a red-top tube during early weeks of pregnancy or if suggestive symptoms are present. Test may be repeated in 2 weeks to determine if there is a rise in antibody titer.
- For cat owners, meticulous handwashing is essential after changing the cat litter. If possible, pregnant women should not change cat litter.

Factors Affecting Laboratory Results

- None known.

NURSING IMPLICATIONS WITH RATIONALE

- Obtain a history of meat ingested that was raw or poorly cooked or of contact with a cat and cat litter. Ask if the cat roams the street or is completely housebound.
- Check if the client is pregnant and has a cat. Ascertain if the pregnant woman handles the cat litter.
- Check if the client has ever been serologically tested for toxoplasmosis. Chronic toxoplasmosis has a low-positive titer.

Client Teaching

- Instruct the client to cook all meat thoroughly. Raw or poorly cooked meat may have the *T. gondii* organism.

- Instruct the pregnant woman not to handle the cat litter. Cat feces could be infected with the *T. gondii* organism, and if the pregnant woman is infected, the fetus could also be infected. Not all cats are infected with *T. gondii*; however, cats that roam the streets may have acquired the organism.
- Instruct the pregnant woman with an outdoor cat to inform her obstetrician so that a titer level can be taken and monitored.
- Answer client's questions or refer them to appropriate personnel.

Transferrin (serum)
Siderophilin

Reference Values
Adult: 200–430 mg/dL, 2–4.3 g/L (SI units).
Pregnancy (Full-Term): 300 mg/dL, 3 g/L (SI units).
Newborn: 125–275 mg/dL.
Transferrin Saturation: 20–50%.

Description
Transferrin is a β-globulin protein that is formed in the liver. Iron from the diet is absorbed from the intestinal mucosa and is transported by transferrin to the bone marrow for utilization in hemoglobin (hemoglobin synthesis), and to iron-storage sites, such as the muscle. When protein malnutrition is present, serum transferrin levels decrease quickly, even faster than serum albumin levels. Another purpose for transferrin is for stimulation of body growth.

The iron saturation of transferrin, called *transferrin saturation*, is calculated by percent using the following formula.

$$\% \text{ of transferrin saturation} = \frac{\text{serum iron level}}{\text{TIBC}} \times 100\%$$

A transferrin saturation of less than 15% can indicate chronic iron-deficiency anemia and other chronic illnesses. Additional information concerning iron, total iron-binding capacity (TIBC), and transferrin is discussed on page 415.

Purposes
- To detect a serum transferrin deficit.
- To aid in the diagnosis of chronic iron-deficiency anemia and iron overload.

Clinical Problems
Decreased Level: Chronic iron-deficiency anemia (% saturation), protein malnutrition, hepatic damage, renal disease, chronic infection or inflammation, cancer, rheumatoid arthritis, proteinuria, hemolytic states, iron overload.

Increased Level: Severe iron deficiency, pregnancy, polycythemia, acute hepatitis. *Drug Influence:* Oral contraceptives.

Procedure

- NPO for 12 hours before the test. Water is permitted.
- Collect 3–5 mL of venous blood in a red-top tube. Avoid hemolysis. The blood specimen should be taken in the morning if the transferrin saturation test is to be performed.

Factors Affecting Laboratory Test

- Hemolysis of the blood sample.
- Pregnancy or use of oral contraceptives may increase the serum transferrin level.

NURSING IMPLICATIONS WITH RATIONALE

- Compare serum transferrin level with serum iron level and the TIBC if these tests were ordered. To determine transferrin saturation (%), serum iron and TIBC values are needed.

Client Teaching

- Instruct the client to eat foods rich in protein, such as meats, beans, and fish.
- Answer the client's questions or refer the questions to other health professionals.

Transthyretin (TTR)

See Prealbumin Antibody Assay

Tricyclic antidepressants (TCA or TAD) serum

Reference Values

Adult:

DRUG	THERAPEUTIC RANGE	PEAK TIME	TOXIC LEVEL
Amitriptyline (Elavil)	125–200 ng/mL	2–12 hours	greater than 500 ng/mL
Desipramine (Norpramin)	125–300 ng/mL	4–6 hours	greater than 500 ng/mL
Doxepin (Sinequan)	150–250 ng/mL	2–4 hours	greater than 500 ng/mL
Imipramine (Tofranil)	150–300 ng/mL	1–2 hours (PO) 30 min (IM)	greater than 500 ng/mL
Nortriptyline (Aventyl)	50–150 ng/mL	8 hours	greater than 200 ng/mL
Protriptyline (Vivactil)	70–170 ng/mL	8–12 hours	greater than 200 ng/mL
Amoxapine (Asendin)	200–400 ng/mL	1½ hours	greater than 500 ng/mL
Maprotiline (Ludiomil)	200–300 ng/mL	12 hours	greater than 500 ng/mL

Description

Tricyclic antidepressants (TCAs) are useful in treating clinical depression and bipolar disorders. Laboratory measurements for TCAs are used to monitor the therapeutic range, to adjust drug dosages, and to detect toxic levels due to overdose (unintentional or intentional). Peak times should be noted when the client is obtaining maximum effects. The average time at which these drugs reach their steady state varies from days to 1–2 weeks. The serious toxic effect of these drugs is cardiotoxicity, which includes depressed myocardial contractility, decreased heart rate, and decreased coronary blood flow.

Purposes

- To monitor a specific TCA drug for therapeutic effect.
- To check for a specific TCA toxicity.

Clinical Problems

Decreased Level: *Drug Influence:* Barbiturates, alcohol.

Increased Level: Overdose of TCAs. *Drug Influence:* Steroids, antipsychotics (neuroleptics).

T

Procedure

- There is no food or fluid restriction.
- Collect 3–5 mL of venous blood in a red-top tube.

Factors Affecting Laboratory Results

- Drugs—barbiturates and alcohol can lower the serum TCAs, and steroids and antipsychotics can elevate the serum level.

NURSING IMPLICATIONS WITH RATIONALE

- Obtain a history from the client concerning daily drug dosing, having blood samples taken at regular intervals, and keeping doctor's appointments.
- Record and report noncompliance to drug regimen, if appropriate.

Client Teaching

- Instruct the client to follow the prescribed drug dosage. Explain to the client that if prescribed dose is not taken (undosing), therapeutic effects will not be obtained and depressed feelings might remain. Explain that with overdosing, serious cardiotoxicity might result.
- Encourage the client to express feelings about the drug regimen. Listen to the client's concerns.
- Explain to the client that when the dose is increased, it may take 7–10 days for a clinical change because the half-life is long with most of these agents.
- Explain to the client that when discontinuing the medication, the drug dosage should be tapered to avoid extrapyramidal side effects.

Triglycerides (serum)

Reference Values

Adult: *12–29 Years:* 10–140 mg/dL; *30–39 Years:* 20–150 mg/dL; *40–49 Years:* 30–160 mg/dL; *Greater than 50 Years:* 40–190 mg/dL, 0.44–2.09 mmol/L (SI units).

Child: *Infant:* 5–40 mg/dL. *Child:* 5–11 Years: 10–135 mg/dL.

Risk Values of Cardiovascular Disease: *Low Risk:* Less than 100 mg/dL. *Normal Risk:* 149 mg/dL. *Borderline High Risk:* 150–199 mg/dL. *High Risk:* 200–499 mg/dL. *Very High Risk:* Greater than 500 mg/dL.

Description

Triglycerides, blood lipids formed by esterification of glycerol and three fatty acids, are carried by the serum lipoproteins. The intestine processes the triglycerides from dietary fatty acids (exogenous), and they are transported in the bloodstream as chylomicrons (tiny fat droplets covered by protein), which gives the serum a milky or creamy appearance after a meal rich in fats. The liver is also responsible for manufacturing triglycerides, but these do not travel as chylomicrons. The majority of triglycerides are stored as lipids in the adipose tissue. A function of triglycerides is to provide energy to the heart and skeletal muscles.

Triglycerides are a major contributor to arterial diseases and are frequently compared with cholesterol by the lipoprotein electrophoresis. As the concentration of triglycerides increases, so will the very low-density lipoproteins (VLDL) increase, leading to hyperlipoproteinemia.

Persons who are at highest risk of elevated triglyceride levels are those who drink alcohol, are obese, consume foods high in simple sugars, take certain medications (thiazides, hormone therapy), have a familial history of high triglycerides, and medical conditions such as type 2 diabetes mellitus, hypothyroidism, and cardiac, kidney, and liver disease. The statins drugs for lowering cholesterol have less effect on lowering the triglycerides.

Purposes

- To monitor triglyceride levels.
- To compare test results with lipoprotein groups (VLDL) that indicate hyperlipemia.

Clinical Problems

Decreased Level: Congenital β-lipoproteinemia, hyperthyroidism, hyperparathyroidism, protein malnutrition, exercise. *Drug Influence:* Ascorbic acid, clofibrate (Atromid-S), phenformin, metformin.

Increased Level: Hyperlipoproteinemia, acute myocardial infarction, hypertension, cerebral thrombosis, hypothyroidism, nephrotic syndrome, arteriosclerosis, Laënnec or alcoholic cirrhosis, uncontrolled diabetes mellitus, pancreatitis, Down syndrome, stress, high-carbohydrate diet, pregnancy. *Drug Influence:* Estrogen, oral contraceptives.

Procedure

- Collect 3–5 mL of venous blood in a red-top tube.

- The client should be NPO (food, drink, or medications) after 6 PM the night before the test, except for water. Medications should be held until after blood is drawn. The client should be on a normal diet for several days before the test. No alcohol is allowed for 24 hours prior to the test.
- Note on the laboratory slip if the client's weight has increased or decreased in the last 2 weeks.

Factors Affecting Laboratory Results

- A high-carbohydrate diet and alcohol can elevate the serum triglyceride level.

NURSING IMPLICATIONS WITH RATIONALE

Increased Level

- Relate clinical problems and drugs to increased serum triglyceride levels. When triglycerides and/or cholesterol are elevated, a lipoprotein electrophoresis is frequently ordered.
- Check the serum cholesterol level. At times, only one of the body's lipids will be elevated. If the cholesterol level is elevated, suggest which foods should be avoided (*see Cholesterol*). Consult with the dietetics department.
- Check to determine if a lipoprotein electrophoresis has been ordered. This is frequently done when the triglycerides are elevated.

Client Teaching

- Instruct the client that he or she is not to eat food or to drink anything except water for 12–14 hours before the test. Client should avoid alcoholic intake for 24 hours. Medications may be withheld until after the test. Check with the health care provider and laboratory.
- Instruct the client with a high serum triglyceride level to avoid eating excessive amounts of sugars and carbohydrates as well as dietary fats. The client should be encouraged to eat fruit.

Triiodothyronine (T₃) (serum)

T₃ RIA

Reference Values

Adult: 80–200 ng/dL.

Child: *Newborn:* 40–215 ng/dL. *5–10 Years:* 95–240 ng/dL. *10–15 Years:* 80–210 ng/dL.

Description

Triiodothyronine (T₃), one of the thyroid hormones, is present in small amounts in blood and is more short acting and more potent than thyroxine (T₄). Both T₃ and T₄ have similar actions in the body. Serum T₃ is secreted in response to thyroid-stimulating hormone from the pituitary gland and thyroid-releasing hormone from the hypothalamus and is measured directly by radioimmunoassay (RIA).

Serum T_3 RIA measures both bound and free T_3. It is effective for diagnosing hyperthyroidism, especially T_3 thyrotoxicosis, in which T_3 is increased and T_4 is in the normal range. It is not as reliable for diagnosing hypothyroidism, because T_3 remains in the normal range. T_3 RIA and T_3 uptake are two different tests.

Purposes

- To aid in the diagnosis of hyperthyroidism.
- To compare T_3 with T_4 for determining a thyroid disorder.

Clinical Problems

Decreased Level: Malnutrition, severe acute illness and trauma. *Drug Influence:* Propylthiouracil, methylthiouracil, methimazole (Tapazole), lithium, phenytoin (Dilantin), propranolol (Inderal), reserpine (Serpasil), salicylates (aspirin), steroids, sulfonamides.

Increased Level: T_3 thyrotoxicosis, Hashimoto thyroiditis, toxic adenoma. *Drug Influence:* Estrogen, progestins, methadone, liothyronine (T_3).

Procedure

- Drugs that affect laboratory results should be withheld for 24 hours with the health care provider's approval. If the drugs are taken prior to the test, they should be listed on the laboratory slip.
- Collect 5–7 mL of venous blood in a red-top tube. Avoid hemolysis.
- Send the blood sample to the laboratory as soon as possible.

Factors Affecting Laboratory Results

- Drugs (*see Drug Influence*).
- Hemolysis of the blood specimen from rough handling.

NURSING IMPLICATIONS WITH RATIONALE

- List on the laboratory slip any drugs the client is taking that could cause false-negative or false-positive results.

Increased Level

- Observe for signs and symptoms of hyperthyroidism (e.g., nervousness, tremors, emotional instability, increased appetite, weight loss, palpitations, tachycardia, diarrhea, decreased fertility, and exophthalmos [protruding eyeballs]).
- Monitor pulse rate. Tachycardia is common and, if severe, could cause heart failure.

Triiodothyronine resin uptake (T_3 RU) (serum)

T_3 Uptake

Reference Values

Adult: 25–35 relative percentage uptake.

Description

Triiodothyronine (T$_3$) resin uptake is an indirect measure of free thyronine (T$_4$), whereas serum T$_3$ RIA is a direct measurement of T$_3$. This is an in vitro test in which the client's blood is mixed with radioactive T$_3$ and synthetic resin material in a test tube. The radioactive T$_3$ will bind at available thyroid-binding globulin (protein) sites. The unbound radioactive T$_3$ is added to resin for T$_3$ uptake. In hyperthyroidism there are few binding sites left, so more T$_3$ is taken up by the resin, thus causing a high T$_3$ resin uptake. In hypothyroidism there is less T$_3$ resin uptake.

This test can be performed when clients receive drugs, diagnostic agents (contrast media), and food containing iodine. Usually this test is not affected by inorganic or organic iodine, but it is affected by radioactive iodine, which interferes with the test reagents.

T$_3$ RU is one of the thyroid tests but should not be the only test used to determine thyroid dysfunction.

Purposes

- To differentiate between hypo- or hyperthyroidism.
- To compare test result with T$_3$ for determining thyroid disorder.

Clinical Problems

Decreased Level: Hypothyroidism (cretinism, myxedema), pregnancy, menstruation, thyroiditis (Hashimoto), acute hepatitis. *Drug Influence:* ACTH,[*] corticosteroids,[*] estrogen, oral contraceptives, antithyroid agents (methimazole, propylthiouracil), thiazides, chlordiazepoxide (Librium), sulfonylureas (e.g., tolbutamide [Orinase]).

Increased Level: Hyperthyroidism, protein malnutrition, malignancies (breast) and metastatic carcinoma, myasthenia gravis, nephrotic syndrome, uremia, threatened abortion. *Drug Influence:* ACTH,[*] corticosteroids,[*] anticoagulants (oral), heparin, phenytoin (Dilantin), phenylbutazone (Butazolidin), salicylates (high doses of aspirin compounds), thyroid agents.

Procedure

- There is no food or fluid restriction.
- Collect 5–7 mL of venous blood in a red-top tube. Avoid hemolysis.
- Note on the laboratory slip drugs the client is taking that could affect test results.

Factors Affecting Laboratory Results

- Drugs (*see Drug Influence*).
- Previous administration of radioactive iodine or other radioactive substances could cause inaccurate results.

NURSING IMPLICATIONS WITH RATIONALE

- List on the laboratory slip any drugs the client is taking that could cause a false-negative or false-positive result. Also note any radioactive substance the client has taken.
- Check results of the T$_4$ test.

[*]May cause decreased or elevated T$_3$ uptake levels.

Decreased Level

- Observe for signs and symptoms of hypothyroidism (e.g., fatigue, forgetfulness, weight gain, dry skin with poor turgor, dry and thin hair, bradycardia, decreased peripheral circulation, depressed libido, infertility, and constipation).

Increased Level

- Observe for signs and symptoms of hyperthyroidism (e.g., nervousness, tremors, emotional instability, increased appetite, weight loss, palpitations, tachycardia, diarrhea, decreased fertility, and exophthalmos [protruding eyeballs]).
- Monitor the pulse rate. Tachycardia is common and, if severe, could cause heart failure and cardiac arrest.

Troponins (serum, blood)

Cardiac-Specific Troponin 1 (cTn1), Cardiac-Specific Troponin T (cTnT)

Reference Values

Cardiac Troponin 1: 0.1–0.5 ng/mL; 0.1–0.5 mcg/L (SI units). Suspicious myocardium injury: 0.5–2 ng/mL. Positive myocardium injury: Greater than 2 ng/mL; greater than 2 mcg/L (SI units).

Cardiac Troponin T: Less than 0.2 ng/mL; less than 0.2 mcg/L (SI units).

Description

Troponins are biochemical markers for cardiac diseases especially for the diagnosis of acute myocardial infarction (AMI). The troponins are proteins, present in both the heart muscle and skeletal muscles; the enzyme-linked immunosorbent assay (ELISA) test can separate which muscle is involved. The cardiac-specific troponin 1 (cTn1) and the cardiac-specific troponin (cTnT) are released from the heart into the bloodstream 1–3 hours after the onset of symptoms of AMI. Thrombolytic treatment (clot busters) could be available for early onset of AMI. The troponins are also useful in detecting silent myocardial infarction and microinfarctions accompanied with chest pain. The electrocardiogram may not have changed.

Troponins are more specific for cardiac muscle injury than creatine phosphokinase MB (CPK-MB). CPK-MB can be elevated with severe skeletal muscle injury. The cardiac troponins are usually within normal range in noncardiac muscle diseases.

Following post infarction, the CTn1 remains elevated for 5–9 days and the cTnT remains elevated for 10–14 days. A new qualitative immunoassay testing for troponins may be performed at the bedside. The new test takes about 20 minutes and is read much like a glucometer.

Purposes

- To differentiate between cardiac and noncardiac chest pain.
- To evaluate clients with unstable angina pectoris with potential myocardial damage.
- To assist in the diagnosis of acute myocardial infarction.

Clinical Problems

Increased Level: Acute myocardial infarction, cardiac chest pain, myocardial damage.

Procedure

- No food or fluid restriction is required.
- Collect 5 mL of venous blood in a red-top tube or a heparinized green-top tube.
- Record on the laboratory slip the time the blood specimen was obtained.
- For qualitative immunoassay testing done at the bedside, a micropipette is used to obtain whole blood and is placed in the testing device.

Factors Affecting Laboratory Results

- Elevation of cTnT may occur with severe skeletal muscle injury.

NURSING IMPLICATIONS WITH RATIONALE

- Obtain a history of the chest pain and its severity.
- Check other cardiac enzyme levels (CPK-MB, etc.) with cardiac troponins.
- Record baseline vital signs. Keep a record of the vital signs taken periodically.
- Provide comfort measures for the client.

Client Teaching

- Instruct the client to notify the health professional immediately when chest pain occurs.
- Explain the bedside troponin test and how it will be done (if ordered).

Trypsin (stool)

Reference Values

Adult and Child: Positive in small amounts.

Cystic Fibrosis: Negative at dilutions greater than 1:10.

Description

Trypsin is an enzyme produced in the pancreas. Greater amounts of trypsin are found in stools of young children. Bacteria in the gastrointestinal tract destroys much of the trypsin in stool of older children and adults. With pancreatic insufficiency, the stool trypsin test is usually negative. A sample of stool specimens on 3 separate days should be sent for testing.

Purposes

- To determine if the stool specimen is negative for trypsin.
- To aid in the diagnosis of a pancreatic disorder or cystic fibrosis.

Clinical Problems

Lack of/Decreased Stool Trypsin: Pancreatic insufficiency, advanced cystic fibrosis, malabsorption (children), chronic pancreatitis.

Procedure

- There is no food or fluid restriction.
- Collect a morning stool specimen every morning for 3 consecutive days. Have client defecate in the bedpan. Stool collection from infants may be obtained from the diaper. Use a tongue blade and place the stool specimen in a clean, dry container.
- Deliver the container with the stool specimen immediately to the laboratory. The stool should be tested within 2 hours.

Factors Affecting Laboratory Results

- A stool specimen from a constipated stool could produce a false-negative result, which is due to the extended time the stool is in contact with intestinal bacteria.

NURSING IMPLICATIONS WITH RATIONALE

- Collect the stool specimen and place in a covered container. Send the specimen immediately to the laboratory.
- List on the laboratory slip the age of the client and the time the stool specimen was collected in addition to the client's name, identification number, room number, and the date.
- Note on the laboratory slip if the stool specimen was from a constipated stool.

Client Teaching

- Explain the stool collection procedure to the client and/or family member. Inform the client that 3 stool specimens are needed and that a stool specimen will be collected for the next 3 days.
- Instruct the client to have the bowel movement in a bedpan. The bedpan can be placed on a chair, on a bedside commode, or on the toilet seat area. Stool specimens from infants should be obtained from the diaper.
- Instruct the client not to urinate with the bowel movement and to inform you as soon as the stool is available.

Type and crossmatch
See Rh Typing and Cross Matching

Uric acid (serum)

Reference Values
Values may differ among laboratories.

Adult: *Male:* 3.5–8 mg/dL. *Female:* 2.8–6.8 mg/dL (normal range may differ slightly among laboratories). *Panic Values:* Greater than 12 mg/dL.

Child: 2.5–5.5 mg/dL.

Elderly: 3.5–8.5 mg/dL.

Description

Uric acid is a by-product of purine metabolism. Elevated urine and serum uric acid levels (hyper-uricemia) depend on renal function, purine metabolism rate, and dietary intake of purine foods. Excess quantities of uric acid are excreted in the urine. Uric acid can crystallize in the urinary tract in acidic urine; therefore, effective renal function and alkaline urine are necessary with hyperuricemia. The most common problem associated with hyperuricemia is gout. Uric acid levels frequently change from day to day; thus, several uric acid levels may be repeated over several days or weeks.

Clients with elevated serum uric acid should avoid foods high in purine.

Purposes

- To monitor serum uric acid during treatment for gout.
- To aid in the diagnosis of health problems (*see Clinical Problems*).

Clinical Problems

Decreased Level: Wilson disease, proximal renal tubular acidosis, folic-acid-deficiency anemia, burns, pregnancy. *Drug Influence:* Allopurinol, azathioprine (Imuran), Coumadin, probenecid (Benemid), sulfinpyrazone (Anturane).

Increased Level: Gout, alcoholism, leukemias (lymphocytic, myelocytic, monocytic), metastatic cancer, multiple myeloma, severe eclampsia, hyperlipoproteinemia, diabetic mellitus (severe), heart failure, glomerulonephritis, renal failure, stress, lead poisoning, x-ray exposure (excessive), strenuous exercise, high-protein weight-reduction diet, hemolytic anemia, lymphoma. *Drug Influence:* Ascorbic acid, diuretics (acetazolamide [Diamox], thiazides [chlorothiazide], furosemide [Lasix]), levodopa, methyldopa (Aldomet), 6-mercaptopurine, phenothiazines, salicylates (prolonged use), theophylline.

Procedure

- There is no food or drink restriction; however, in many cases, high-purine foods, such as meats (liver, kidney, brain, heart, and sweetbreads), scallops, and sardines, are restricted for 24 hours before the test.
- Collect 3–5 mL of venous blood in a red-top tube. Avoid hemolysis.
- List drugs the client is taking that could affect test results on the laboratory slip.

Factors Affecting Laboratory Results

- Excessive stress and fasting could cause an elevated serum uric acid level.
- Foods high in purine (*see Nursing Implications*).
- Drugs (*see Drug Influence*).

NURSING IMPLICATIONS WITH RATIONALE

- Check with the health care provider and/or laboratory to determine whether foods high in purine should be restricted.

Increased Level

- Recognize clinical problems and drugs related to hyperuricemia. Gout is a problem commonly associated with a high serum uric acid.
- Request the dietitian to visit the client to discuss food preference and to plan a low-purine diet.
- Observe for signs and symptoms of gout (e.g., tophi of the earlobe and joints, joint pain, and edema in the "big" toe). An elevated uric acid level leads to urate deposits in the tissues and in the synovial fluid of joints.
- Monitor the pH of the urine and the amount of the urinary output. The urine pH should be kept alkaline to prevent the formation of uric acid stones in the kidney. A decreased urine output (less than 600 mL/24 h) with an elevated serum uric acid could indicate kidney disease.
- Check serum urea and serum creatinine levels if the serum uric acid level is elevated and the urinary output is decreased. If the serum urea, creatinine, and uric acid are elevated and the urine output is decreased, kidney dysfunction should definitely be suspected. It could be secondary to another clinical problem.

Client Teaching

- Instruct the client to avoid eating foods that have moderate or high amounts of purines. Examples are as follows.

High (100–1,000 mg Purine Nitrogen/100 g Food)	Moderate (9–100 mg Purine Nitrogen/100 g Food)
Brains	Meat
Heart	Poultry
Kidney	Fish
Liver	Shellfish
Sweetbreads	Asparagus
Roe	Beans
Sardines	Mushrooms
Scallops	Peas
Mackerel	Spinach
Anchovies	
Broth	
Consommé	
Mincemeat	

- Instruct the client to decrease alcoholic intake. Ethanol causes renal retention of urate.

Uric acid (urine—24 hour)

Reference Values

Adult: 250–500 mg/24 h (low-purine diet), 250–750 mg/24 h (normal diet).
Child: Similar to adult.

Description

(*See Uric Acid [serum].*)

Uric acid is the end-product of purine metabolism, which takes place in the bone marrow, muscles, and liver. Excess quantities of uric acid are secreted in the urine unless there is renal dysfunction caused by obstruction of renal flow.

The main purpose of this 24-hour urine test is to detect and/or to confirm the diagnoses of gout or kidney disease.

Purpose

(*See Uric Acid [serum].*)

Clinical Problems

Decreased Level: Renal diseases (chronic glomerulonephritis, urinary obstruction, uremia), eclampsia (toxemia of pregnancy), lead toxicity. *Drug Influence:* Allopurinol, acetazolamide (Diamox), salicylates (prolonged low doses), triamterene.

Increased Level: Gout, high-purine diet, leukemias (lymphocytic, myelocytic), polycythemia vera, Fanconi syndrome, neurologic disorders (cerebral hemorrhage, cerebral thrombosis, brain infarction, cerebral embolism, encephalomyelitis), psychiatric disorders (manic-depressive [bipolar] disease, paranoid states, depressive neurosis), ulcerative colitis, viral hepatitis, x-ray therapy, febrile illnesses. *Drug Influence:* Bishydroxycoumarin, corticosteroids, cytotoxic agents (treatment for cancer), probenecid (Benemid), salicylates (high doses).

Procedure

- There is no drink restriction.
- A diet low or high in purines may be ordered before and/or during the time of urine collection.
- Collect a 24-hour sample in a large container and refrigerate. A preservative in the container may be necessary. Check with the laboratory on the need for preservative.
- Label the container with the client's name and the dates and times of urine collection (e.g., 9/23/20, 7:11 AM to 9/24/20, 7:11 AM).

Factors Affecting Laboratory Results

- Drugs (*see Drug Influence*).
- A high- or low-purine diet.
- Excessive x-ray exposure.
- Febrile illnesses.

NURSING IMPLICATIONS WITH RATIONALE

- Monitor urinary output. Poor urine output could indicate inadequate fluid intake or poor kidney function.
- Compare the serum uric acid level with the urine uric acid level. An elevated serum uric acid level (hyperuricemia) and a decreased urine uric acid level can indicate kidney dysfunction. Increased serum and urine uric acid levels are frequently seen in gout, so it is important to obtain both the urine and serum values.
- Check the urine pH, especially if hyperuricemia is present. Uric stones can occur when the urine pH is low (acidic). Alkaline urine helps to prevent stones in the urinary tract.

Client Teaching

- Explain to the client the purpose of and procedure for the test. Explain to the client and family that all urine should be saved for 24 hours. Tell the client not to put feces or toilet paper in the urine.
- Instruct the client as to which foods to avoid before and during the test, as ordered by the health care provider.

U

Urinalysis (routine)

Color, Appearance, Odor, pH, Specific Gravity, Protein, Glucose, Ketones, Blood, Nitrate, and Leukocyte Esterase (WBC)

Reference Values

	ADULT	NEWBORN	CHILD
Color	Light straw to dark amber		Light straw to dark yellow
Appearance	Clear	Clear	Clear
Odor	Aromatic		Aromatic
pH	4.5–8. Average is 6	5–7	4.5–8
Specific gravity (SG)	1.005–1.030 (1.015–1.024, normal fluid intake)	1.001–1.020	1.005–1.030
Protein	(2–8 mg/dL negative reagent strip test)		
Glucose	Negative		Negative
Ketones	Negative		Negative
Blood	Negative		Negative
Microscopic examination			
RBC	1–2 per low power field		Rare
WBC	3–4		0–4
Casts	Occasional hyaline		Rare

Description

Urinalysis is a physical, chemical, and microscopic analysis of the urine. Routine urine tests were performed as early as 1821. Until recently urine was manually tested for individual constituents, but now multiple-reagent strips are used for quick chemical screening.

Urinalysis is useful for diagnosing renal disease or urinary tract infection and for detecting metabolic disease not related to the kidneys. Many routine urinalyses are done in the health care provider's office as well as in the hospital or in a private laboratory. The color, appearance, and odor of the urine are examined, and the pH, protein, glucose, ketones, and bilirubin are tested with the reagent strips. Specific gravity is measured with a urinometer, and a microscopic examination of the urinary sediment is performed to detect red and white blood cells, casts, crystals, and bacteria.

Purposes

- To detect normal versus abnormal urine components.
- To detect glycosuria.
- To aid in the diagnosis of a renal disorder.

Clinical Problems

PROPERTY OR CONSTITUENT	CLINICAL CONDITIONS/ PROBLEMS	COMMENTS
Color		
Colorless (very pale)	Large fluid intake Diabetes insipidus Chronic kidney disease Alcohol ingestion Nervousness	A pale color usually indicates diluted urine, and dark yellow or amber indicates concentrated urine.
Red or red-brown	Hemoglobinuria Porphyrins Menstrual contamination Drug influence Sulfisoxazole with phenazopyridine (Azo-Gantrisin)	Drugs and foods will change the color of the urine.
Red or red-brown	Phenytoin (Dilantin) Cascara Chlorpromazine (Thorazine) Docusate Ca (Doxidan) Phenolphthalein (Ex-Lax) Foods Beets Rhubarb Food color	
Orange	Restricted fluid intake Concentrated urine Excess sweating Fever	

(*Continued*)

PROPERTY OR CONSTITUENT	CLINICAL CONDITIONS/ PROBLEMS	COMMENTS
	Drug influence	
	Amidopyrine	
	Furazolidone (Furoxone)	
	Nitrofurantoin	
	Phenazopyridine (Pyridium)	
	Sulfonamides	
	Foods and others	
	Carrots (carotene)	
	Rhubarb	
	Food color	
	Bilirubin	
Blue or green	*Pseudomonas* toxemia	
	Drug influence	
	Amitriptyline (Elavil)	
	Methylene blue	
	Methocarbamol (Robaxin)	
	Vitamin B complex	
	Yeast concentrate	
Brown or black	Lysol poisoning	
	Melanin	
	Bilirubin	
	Methemoglobin	
	Porphyrin	
	Drug influence	
	Cascara	
	Chloroquine (Aralen)	
	Iron injectable compounds	
Appearance		
Hazy, cloudy	Bacteria	
	Pus, tissue	
	RBCs	
	WBCs	
	Phosphates	
	Prostatic fluid	
	Spermatozoa	
	Urates, uric acid	
Milky	Fat	
	Pyuria	
Odor		
Ammonia	Urea breakdown by bacteria	
Foul or putrid	Bacteria (UTI)	
Mousey	Phenylketonuria	
Sweet or fruity	Diabetic acidosis (ketoacidosis)	
	Starvation	

PROPERTY OR CONSTITUENT	CLINICAL CONDITIONS/ PROBLEMS	COMMENTS
Foam		
Yellow— large amounts	Severe cirrhosis of the liver Bilirubin or bile pigment	
pH		
less than 4.5	Metabolic acidosis Respiratory acidosis Starvation Diarrhea Diet high in meat protein and/or cranberries Drug influence Ammonium chloride Methenamine mandelate (mandelic acid)	
greater than 8	Bacteriuria Urinary tract infection due to *Pseudomonas or Proteus* Drug influence Antibiotics Kanamycin Neomycin Streptomycin Sulfonamides Excess salicylates (aspirin) Sodium bicarbonate Acetazolamide (Diamox) Potassium citrate Diet High in citrus fruits High in vegetables	
Specific gravity (SG)		
less than 1.005	Diabetes insipidus Excess fluid intake Overhydration Renal disease Glomerulonephritis Pyelonephritis Polycystic disease Severe potassium deficit	Low, fixed SG can indicate kidney disease because of inability to concentrate urine.
greater than 1.026	Decreased fluid intake Fever Administration of IV dextran, albumin Diabetes mellitus Vomiting, diarrhea Dehydration X-ray contrast media	

(Continued)

PROPERTY OR CONSTITUENT	CLINICAL CONDITIONS/ PROBLEMS	COMMENTS

Protein

greater than 8 mg/dL or greater than 80 mg/24 h	Proteinuria
	Mild, transitory
	Protein
	Exercise
	Severe stress
	Cold baths
	Fever
	Acute infectious diseases
	Renal disease
	  Glomerulonephritis
	  Nephrotic syndrome
	  Polycystic kidney
	Lupus erythematosus
	Leukemia
	Multiple myeloma
	Cardiac disease
	Toxemia of pregnancy
	Septicemia
	Materials
	  Arsenic
	  Mercury
	  Lead
	  Carbon tetrachloride
	Drug influence
	  Barbiturates
	  Neomycin
	  Massive doses of penicillin
	  Sulfonamides
		Proteinuria is a sensitive indicator of kidney dysfunction.

less than 2 mg/dL	Very diluted urine	

Glucose

greater than 15 mg/dL (random) or +4	Diabetes mellitus CNS disorders Stroke (CVA) Meningitis Cushing syndrome Anesthesia Glucose infusions Severe stress Infections	The renal threshold for blood glucose is 160–180 mg/dL. Tes-Tape should be used in place of Clinitest when the client is receiving drugs.
greater than 15 mg/dL (random) or +4	Drug influence (false-positive results) Ascorbic acid Aspirin Cephalothin (Keflin) Streptomycin Epinephrine	

PROPERTY OR CONSTITUENT	CLINICAL CONDITIONS/ PROBLEMS	COMMENTS
Ketones	*(See Ketone Bodies, Acetone)*	Acetest or Ketostix should be tested when Clinitest or Tes-Tape is tested.
Positive +1 to +3	Ketoacidosis Starvation A diet high in protein and low in carbohydrates	
Microscopic Examination of Urinary Sediment RBCs		

RBCs and RBC casts greater than 2 per low power field	Trauma to the kidney
	Renal disease
	    Pyelonephritis
	    Glomerulonephritis
	    Hydronephrosis
	Renal calculi
	Cystitis
	Lupus nephritis (collagen disease)
	Aspirins (excess)
	Anticoagulants
	Sulfonamides
	Menstrual contamination	

WBCs		
WBC and WBC casts greater than 4 per low power field	Urinary tract infection Fever Strenuous exercise Lupus nephritis Renal diseases	If WBCs are present in the urine, a urine culture should be done.
Casts	Fever Renal disease Heart failure	

Procedure

- There is no food or fluid restriction unless the urinalysis is to be done in the early morning.
- Collect a freshly voided urine specimen, approximately 50 mL or more, in a clean, dry container and take it to the laboratory within 30 minutes. An early morning urine specimen collected before breakfast is preferred. The urine specimen could be refrigerated for 6–8 hours.
- A clean-caught or midstream urine specimen could be requested if WBCs are in the urine or if bacteria are suspected.

Factors Affecting Laboratory Results

- A urine specimen that has been sitting for an hour or longer without refrigeration.
- Drugs and foods (*see Clinical Problems*).
- Feces or toilet paper in the urine.

NURSING IMPLICATIONS WITH RATIONALE

- Assist the client with the urine collection as needed.
- Obtain a history of any drugs the client is currently taking. Such drugs as cascara, Azo-Gantrisin, nitrofurantoin, Thorazine, sulfonamides, Elavil, Ex-Lax, Pyridium, and others cause a discoloration of the urine. These should be noted on the laboratory slip.
- Assess the fluid status of the client. Urine should be concentrated if the urine specimen is obtained in the morning or if the client has a decreased fluid intake or is dehydrated. An increase in fluid intake will dilute the urine contents.
- Obtain a history of an excess amount of a certain food (e.g., carrots, rhubarb, beets) that can cause a change in the urine color or of foods (e.g., excess amounts of meat, cranberry juice) that could lower the urine pH (acidic).

Client Teaching

- Explain to the client the procedure for collecting the urine. Inform the hospitalized client that an early morning urine specimen taken before breakfast is needed. Instruct the client that approximately one third or one half of a small container of urine is needed. Have the client void in a clean, dry container or a clean urinal or bedpan that can be poured into the container. Inform the client not to put feces or toilet paper in the urine. The urine specimen should be taken to the laboratory within 30 minutes or refrigerated.
- Instruct the client at home to place the fresh morning urine specimen in the refrigerator. The urine specimen, however, should be taken to the laboratory within an hour. Urine is an excellent medium for the growth of bacteria, and the bacterial growth begins approximately a half hour after collection. Refrigeration may help to retard growth for a short period of time.
- Explain to the client the procedure for a clean-catch or midstream urine collection (see *Cultures*). This procedure may be requested when culture of the urine is needed as well as for urinalysis.

Urobilinogen (urine)

Reference Values

Adult: *Random:* Negative or less than 1 Ehrlich units. *2-Hour Specimen:* 0.3–1 Ehrlich units. *24-Hour Specimen:* 0.5–4 mg/24 h, 0.5–4 Ehrlich units/24 h, 0.09–4.23 μmol/24 h (SI units).
Child: Similar to adult.

Description

Bile, which is formed mostly from conjugated bilirubin, reaches the duodenum, where the intestinal bacteria change the bilirubin to urobilinogen. Most of the urobilinogen is lost in the feces. A large amount goes back to the liver through the bloodstream, where it is reprocessed to bile, and approximately 1% is excreted by the kidneys in the urine.

The urobilinogen test is one of the most sensitive tests for determining liver damage, hemolytic disease, and severe infections. In early hepatitis, mild liver cell damage, or mild toxic injury, the urine urobilinogen level will increase despite an unchanged serum bilirubin level. The urobilinogen level will frequently decrease with severe liver damage, because less bile will be produced. The urobilinogen test might be performed with the urinalysis.

Purpose

- To aid in determining liver damage.

Clinical Problems

Decreased Level: Biliary obstruction, severe liver disease, cancer of the pancreas, severe inflammatory disease, cholelithiasis, severe diarrhea. *Drug Influence:* Antibiotics (decreasing gut bacteria), ammonium chloride, ascorbic acid (vitamin C).

Increased Level: Infectious hepatitis, toxic hepatitis, cirrhosis of the liver (early and recovery stages), hemolytic anemia, pernicious anemia, erythroblastosis fetalis, sickle-cell anemia, infectious mononucleosis. *Drug Influence:* Sulfonamides, phenothiazines, acetazolamide (Diamox), cascara, phenazopyridine (Pyridium), methenamine mandelate (Mandelamine), procaine, sodium bicarbonate.

Procedure

- There is no food or fluid restriction.

Single Specimen

- The single urine specimen should be fresh and should be tested immediately. This may be done as part of the routine urinalysis. A reagent color dipstick is dipped in the urine and is compared with a color chart, in Ehrlich units.

2-Hour Urine Specimen

- Collect 2-hour specimen between 1 and 3 PM or between 2 and 4 PM, because urobilinogen peaks in the afternoon. Urine should be kept refrigerated or in a dark container. Urine should be tested within half an hour, because urine urobilinogen oxidizes to urobilin (orange substance).
- Label the container and laboratory slip with the exact time the urine was collected.

24-Hour Urine Specimen

- Discard the first urine specimen and then start urine collection.
- Collect 24-hour urine specimen, place in a large container, and keep refrigerated. A preservative may be added to the container. Keep urine collection from the light.
- Label the container with the client's name, the date, and the time of urine collection.
- Withhold client's medications that affect test results for 24 hours or until after the test, with the health care provider's permission. If drugs are given, list the drugs on the laboratory slip.

Factors Affecting Laboratory Results

- Antibiotics decrease the bacterial flora in the intestine.
- Certain drugs increase the urine urobilinogen level (*see Drug Influence*).

- pH changes (strongly acidic urine) could cause a decreased urobilinogen level, and strongly alkaline urine could cause an elevated level. Urine sitting for half an hour or longer may become alkaline.
- The urobilinogen level is highest in the afternoon and evening. The 2-hour urine specimen is frequently collected in the afternoon.

NURSING IMPLICATIONS WITH RATIONALE

- Explain to the client the procedure for collecting a 2-hour urine specimen or a 24-hour urine specimen. The bladder should be emptied before starting the 2-hour or 24-hour urine test. Inform the client that all urine must be saved during the specified time.
- Keep the collected urine from light in a urine container with a preservative. Refrigerate.
- Label the container and laboratory slip with the exact times urine collection begins and ends (after the last voiding).

Decreased Level

- Relate clinical problems and drugs to decreased urine urobilinogen. Most antibiotics will reduce the bacterial flora in the intestines, thus decreasing the formation of urobilinogen.

Increased Level

- Check for an increased urobilinogen level in freshly voided urine with a reagent color dipstick. Record the results of the single test. Note if the client is receiving drugs that could elevate the urobilinogen level.
- Assess for signs and symptoms of jaundice (yellow sclera, skin on the forearm is yellow).

Vancomycin (serum)

Reference Values

Therapeutic Range: *Peak:* 20–40 mcg/mL. *Trough:* 5–10 mcg/mL.
Toxic Level: Greater than 40 mcg/mL.

Description

Vancomycin is a potent antibiotic that is prescribed to treat serious gram-positive organisms by inhibiting cell-wall synthesis of the bacteria, thus causing its death. It may be ordered when the bacterium does not respond to penicillins or cephalosporins. Oral vancomycin is poorly absorbed; however, it may be ordered for treating some gastrointestinal infections such as that caused by *Clostridium difficile*. Intravenous vancomycin is the form most likely prescribed. Like aminoglycosides, vancomycin may cause ototoxicity and nephrotoxicity. Peak and trough levels should be closely monitored. The half-life for vancomycin in adults is 4–8 hours. In renal insufficiency, the half-life can be 4–8 days.

Purposes

- To monitor the vancomycin level.
- To check for vancomycin toxicity.

Clinical Problems

Uses: Methicillin-resistant *Staphylococcus aureus*, serious gram-positive organisms, staphylococcal septicemia in cancer.

Procedure

- There is no food or fluid restriction.
- Collect 3–5 mL of venous blood in a red-top tube. For peak level, draw a blood sample 30 minutes after administering intravenous vancomycin. For trough level, draw a blood sample prior to administering the next dose of IV vancomycin. Send blood samples immediately to the laboratory.

Factors Affecting Laboratory Results

- Inadequate renal function affects the peak and trough levels. The drug dose needs to be adjusted according to renal function.

NURSING IMPLICATIONS WITH RATIONALE

- Assess renal function. Urine output should be at least 600 mL/day. Vancomycin dose should be adjusted if renal function is inadequate. This drug may cause nephrotoxicity.
- Check hearing. High doses of vancomycin could damage the eighth cranial nerve. This drug may cause ototoxicity.
- Monitor intravenous flow rate for vancomycin. Rapid infusion could cause "red-man's syndrome." The skin becomes red (erythematous) and flushed. Itching may also occur.

Client Teaching

- Inform the client who is ambulatory to save urine so that it can be measured.
- Explain to the client that blood samples will be taken periodically 30 minutes after the drug has been infused and prior to the next drug dose.

Vanillylmandelic acid (VMA) (urine)

Reference Values

Adult: 1.5–7.5 mg/24 h, 35–45 µmol/24 h (SI units).

Child: Adolescent: 1–5 mg/24 h.

Description

Vanillylmandelic acid (VMA) is the major by-product of catecholamines (epinephrine and norepinephrine). An elevated level of VMA excretion might indicate severe hypertension or tumors of the adrenal medulla (pheochromocytoma in the adult and neuroblastoma and ganglioneuroblastoma in the child). Other methods should be used to verify positive VMA results, such as urine catecholamine.

The VMA test is a simple screening method. However, many foods (bananas, tea, coffee, chocolate, carbonated drinks, etc.) and drugs (aspirin, sulfonamides, some cough medicines, and others) produce false-positive results.

Purpose

- To screen for pheochromocytoma and other health problems (*see Clinical Problems*).

Clinical Problems

Decreased Level: Uremia. *Drug Influence:* clofibrate, antihypertensives (guanethidine [Ismelin], methyldopa [Aldomet], reserpine [Serpasil]), monoamine (MAO) inhibitors.

Increased Level: Pheochromocytoma, neuroblastoma, ganglioneuroblastoma, myasthenia gravis, muscular dystrophy (progressive), physical and mental stress. *Foods:* Fruits (bananas), fruit juices, chocolate, tea, coffee, carbonated drinks (except ginger ale), vanilla and vanilla products, candy, mints, jelly, cheese, gelatins, and cough drops. *Drug Influence:* Salicylates (aspirin), sulfonamides, penicillin, chlorpromazine (Thorazine), isoproterenol (Isuprel), levodopa, lithium carbonate, nitroglycerin, glyceryl guaiacolate, methenamine (Mandelamine), methocarbamol (Robaxin).

Procedure

- No drugs should be taken for 3 days before the test, *if possible*, especially those listed under Drug Influence.
- Those foods listed under Clinical Problems above should be omitted from the diet for 3 days before the test. Other foods and fluid are not restricted.
- Insert 10 mL of concentrated hydrochloric acid (HCl) into a large bottle. Some laboratories do not require that a preservative be added to the bottle.
- Label the bottle and laboratory slip with the client's name, dates, and times the urine collection started and ended. Keep the bottle refrigerated during the 24-hour collection time.

Factors Affecting Laboratory Results

- Drugs (*see Drug Influence*).
- Food (*see Clinical Problems*).
- Strenuous exercise will elevate VMA levels.
- Stress will elevate VMA levels.

NURSING IMPLICATIONS WITH RATIONALE

- Monitor vital signs, especially blood pressure. Maintain a blood pressure chart.

Client Teaching

- Explain to the client and family that all urine excreted over the 24-hour period must be saved and kept refrigerated. Inform the client not to put toilet paper or feces in the urine.
- Instruct the client not to eat the foods listed under Clinical Problems above for 3 days before the test. Write the restricted foods on a piece of paper for the client's reference.

- Explain to the client that he or she should eat well-balanced meals. Starvation or severe lack of food could increase the VMA levels.
- Encourage the client to avoid emotional stress and physical activity. Stress and activity increase VMA levels. Encourage the client to rest during the test.

VDRL (venereal disease research laboratory) (serum)
VDRL Screening Test

Reference Values

Adult: Nonreactive.

Child: Nonreactive.

Description

Syphilis, a venereal disease caused by the spirochete *Treponema pallidum*, is usually transmitted through sexual contact. There are stages of syphilis (primary, secondary, and tertiary) that, left untreated, could lead to death.

Primary Stage: *Duration After Contact:* 3–6 weeks. A chancre develops approximately 3 weeks after contact. Spirochetes in the exudate of the chancre lesion (sore) may be visualized with dark-field microscopy. Chancres are generally found in genital areas and in the mouth or on the lips.

Secondary Stage: *Duration After Contact:* 2 weeks to 6 months. Secondary lesions are highly contagious and at times may be visualized on dark-field microscopy. The lesions are usually red papular or "snail track" ulcers and may be seen anywhere on the body, especially in the palms of the hands and the soles of the feet. A relapse may occur in 2–4 years; this is called latent syphilis. The client may have a low fever.

Tertiary Stage: *Duration After Contact:* 4–20 years. This is referred to as late syphilis. Untreated syphilis (tertiary stage) normally does not have clinical signs. It does affect the person's cardio-vascular system and central nervous system. The person may develop cardiac valvular disease, aneurysms, general paresis, blindness, slurred speech, delusions, and delirium.

Two groups of blood tests are used to identify the spirochete *T. pallidum*: the nontreponemal antibody test (VDRL and rapid plasma reagin, RPR) and the fluorescent treponemal antibody absorption test (FTA-ABS, TPI).

The VDRL test is useful for detecting primary syphilis 1–3 weeks after the presence of a primary lesion and for detecting secondary syphilis

T. pallidum stimulates the development of nonspecific reaginic antibodies in the serum. If these antibodies are present and react with a lipid antigen (cardiolipin), the VDRL test is positive or reactive. A titer about 1:32 can indicate the secondary stage. With tertiary stage syphilis, the VDRL test is not sensitive and may fail to react or may produce variable titers.

The results of the VDRL test may be negative in the early infectious phase of syphilis or could produce biologic false positives (BFP) because of other acute or chronic diseases. If the VDRL test is negative, weekly VDRL tests may be indicated. The RPR test may be used first as a screening test for syphilis.

Purposes

- To detect the presence of *T. pallidum.*
- To screen for primary syphilis 1–3 weeks after the appearance of a primary lesion.

Clinical Problems

Nonreactive (Negative): *False Negatives:* Early primary stage of syphilis, tertiary stage of syphilis.

Reactive (Positive): Syphilis—*T. pallidum* organism. *False Positives (return to nonreactive within 6 months):* Tuberculosis, pneumonia, infectious mononucleosis, chicken pox, smallpox vaccination (recent), subacute bacterial endocarditis, leprosy. *False Positives (chronic; persist longer than 6 months):* Malaria, Hashimoto thyroiditis, rheumatoid arthritis, progressive systemic sclerosis, systemic lupus erythematosus, hepatitis.

Procedure

- There is no food or fluid restriction; however, some laboratories require that the client refrain from eating and drinking, so check with the laboratory. Alcohol should not be consumed for 24 hours before the VDRL test.
- Collect 3–5 mL of venous blood in a red-top tube. Avoid hemolysis.

Factors Affecting Laboratory Results

- Hemolysis of the blood sample could affect test result.
- Alcoholic intake decreases the test reaction.

NURSING IMPLICATIONS WITH RATIONALE

- Instruct the client not to drink alcohol for 24 hours prior to the test. If the client has consumed alcohol, the test may be postponed for 24 hours.
- Obtain a history of any acute or chronic disease. Related BFP may occur with certain diseases (*see Clinical Problems*).
- List present acute and/or chronic diseases in the client's chart and on the laboratory slip and notify the health care provider.
- Interpretation of tests for syphilis requires skill and experience.

Nonreactive (Negative)

- Relate a nonreactive VDRL test result to false-negative causes if the history and symptoms are suggestive of syphilis. Test should be repeated weekly for several weeks. Nonreactive (negative) results can occur in the early primary stage of syphilis.

Reactive (Positive)

- Relate a reactive VDRL test result to a positive indication of syphilis or a possible false positive due to acute or chronic diseases (*see Clinical Problems*). If the history is suggestive of syphilis but an acute or chronic disease is present, the FTA-ABS or TPI test may be performed.
- Check with the client about receiving treatment for syphilis. If primary syphilis persists for weeks before treatment, the VDRL test could remain positive for up to 6 months after

treatment. The test results after treatment for secondary syphilis could remain positive for 12–18 months. The history of treatment (where, when, how long, and what drugs) is extremely important. The health department should be notified when there is a positive test result.

- Be supportive of the client. Be willing to listen, and do not make a judgment concerning the client's lifestyle.
- Elicit from the client his or her sexual contacts so that they can be properly tested and treated. Explain the importance of preventing the transmission of the disease.
- Refer the client to a sexually transmitted disease (STD) clinic if one is available (with the health care provider's permission). Many clinics have case workers and a good follow-up care program.
- Emphasize the importance of follow-up care. Frequently clients are checked every 3 months for 2 years as a preventive measure for detecting a relapse (syphilis).
- Observe for signs and symptoms of tertiary (late) syphilis (*see Description*). These signs and symptoms should be documented and reported. The VDRL test is usually negative with tertiary syphilis.

Viral culture (blood, biopsy, cerebrospinal fluid, pharynx, rectum, sputum, stool, urine)

Reference Value

Negative culture result.

Description

The virus culture is performed to confirm a suspected viral infection. A blood sample, sputum, and pharyngeal swab are the most common specimens obtained for identifying a virus. The specimen is placed on a special viral culture media of growing cells. It will not grow on nonliving media.

Purpose

- To identify a viral infection.

Clinical Problems

Positive: Pneumonia (viral), meningitis (viral), rhinovirus, sinusitis, conjunctivitis, shingles, varicella-zoster virus, herpes simplex, enteroviruses, influenza, cytomegalovirus (CMV).

Procedure

- No food or fluid restriction is required.
- Collect 5 mL of venous blood in a green-top tube. Tube should be chilled. A repeated test is suggested in 14–28 days as a convalescent specimen.

- A culturette swab may be used to obtain a specimen from the conjunctiva, lesion, throat, and rectum. The swab should be placed in a chilled viral transport media.
- Obtain 5 mL of cerebrospinal fluid and place in a chilled sterile vial.
- Obtain a midstream, clean-caught urine specimen in a sterile container.
- Deliver the specimen immediately to the laboratory.

NURSING IMPLICATIONS WITH RATIONALE

- Obtain a history regarding the possibility of a viral infection. Note the severity of the infection.
- Record symptoms that the client is having in relation to the suspected virus.

Client Teaching

- Explain the procedure for collecting the specimen to the client.
- Inform the client that a second blood sample may be needed in 2–4 weeks. Check with the health care provider.
- Listen to the client's concerns

Vitamin A (serum)
Retinol

Reference Value

Adult: 30–95 mcg/dL, 1.05–3 µmol/L (SI units), 125–150 international unit/dL.

Child: *1–6 Years:* 20–43 mcg/dL, 0.7–1.5 µmol/L (SI units). *7–12 Years:* 26–50 mcg/dL, 0.91–1.75 µmol/L (SI units). *13–19 Years:* 26–72 mcg/dL, 0.91–2.5 µmol/L (SI units).

Description

Vitamin A is a fat-soluble vitamin that is absorbed from the intestine in the presence of lipase and bile. Vitamin A moves to the liver and is stored there as retinyl ester and in the body as retinol. It binds to the serum protein prealbumin.

The functions of vitamin A include mucous membrane epithelial cell integrity of the eyes, cornea, and the respiratory, gastrointestinal, and genito-urinary tracts; and skin integrity. Vitamin A has played a major role for years in treating acne; however, high doses of vitamin A can be toxic because it is a fat-soluble vitamin and accumulates in the body tissues. To determine if toxicity is present, a plasma retinyl ester level is obtained. During pregnancy, high doses of vitamin A may have a teratogenic effect on the fetus. Sufficient intake of vitamin A maintains cellular integrity, body growth, and night vision.

Purposes

- To detect a vitamin A deficit.
- To check for vitamin A toxicity.

Clinical Problems

Decreased Level: Night blindness; liver, intestinal, or pancreatic diseases; chronic infections; carcinoid syndrome; cystic fibrosis; protein malnutrition; malabsorption; celiac disease. *Drug Influence:* Mineral oil, neomycin, cholestyramine.

Increased Level: Hypervitaminosis, chronic kidney disease. *Drug Influence:* Glucocorticoids, oral contraceptives.

Procedure

- NPO for 8–12 hours before the test except for water.
- Collect 5–7 mL of venous blood in a red-top tube. Avoid hemolysis and protect the specimen from light. The blood specimen may be placed in a paper bag.

Factors Affecting Laboratory Results

- Selected drugs that can decrease or increase serum level.
- Hemolysis and prolonged exposure of the blood specimen to light.

NURSING IMPLICATIONS WITH RATIONALE

- Explain to the client that food and fluid, except for water, should be avoided until after the test.
- Obtain a history of the client's nutrient intake and supplementary vitamin intake. Note if the client avoids foods that are rich in vitamin A, such as green leafy and yellow vegetables; yellow fruits such as apricots and cantaloupe; eggs; whole milk; and liver. Individuals with a well-balanced dietary intake normally do not need vitamin supplements.

Decreased Level—Client Teaching

- Encourage the client to eat foods rich in vitamin A.
- Inform the client that vitamin supplements can be helpful in preventing vitamin deficiency. The client may wish to contact the health care provider concerning vitamin supplements.

Increased Level—Client Teaching

- Instruct the client that megadoses of vitamin A for treating acne can be toxic. Self-treating with vitamin A may be harmful because it is a fat-soluble vitamin and can have a cumulative effect. The health care provider should be contacted before taking megadoses of vitamin A.
- Instruct pregnant women that vitamins are usually prescribed during pregnancy; however, megadoses of vitamin A should be avoided because it may cause a birth defect in the newborn.

Vitamin B₁ (serum and urine)
Thiamine

Reference Values
Serum: 10–60 ng/mL, 5.3–8 mcg/dL.
Urine: 100–200 mcg/24 h.

Description
Vitamin B_1 is a water-soluble vitamin that is absorbed (effectively with the aid of folic acid) in the duodenum and is excreted in the urine. The functions of vitamin B_1 include the metabolism of carbohydrates, proteins, and fats, and maintaining nerve impulses. Thiamine is one of the B complex vitamins that is given to treat peripheral neuritis caused from alcoholism or beriberi. There are three types of beriberi: (1) wet beriberi, in which the myocardium dilates and becomes flabby, causing heart failure; (2) dry beriberi, characterized by nerve damage, causing peripheral neuritis and atrophy of muscles; and (3) cerebral beriberi (Wernicke-Korsakoff syndrome), which frequently occurs in chronic alcoholics and is characterized by ocular neuropathy and ataxia.

Foods rich in vitamin B_1 include enriched breads and cereals, yeast, fish, pork, liver, and milk. Asian clients whose diet consists of rice may develop a vitamin B_1 deficiency. Impaired absorption or utilization of vitamin B_1 due to intestinal or liver disease contributes to the vitamin B_1 deficiency.

Purpose
- To detect a vitamin B_1 deficit.

Clinical Problems
Decreased Level: Chronic alcoholism, beriberi, chronic diarrhea, pregnancy, severe liver disease, malabsorption. *Drug Influence:* Excessive and prolonged use of diuretics.

Procedure

Serum
- NPO for 8–12 hours except for water prior to the test.
- Collect 3–5 mL of venous blood in a red-top tube (serum) or green-top tube (plasma). Place blood specimen in a paper bag to protect the specimen from light.

Urine
- Discard the first urine specimen.
- Collect a 24-hour urine specimen in a large container (preferably a dark container to avoid light exposure), and keep the container refrigerated.
- Label the container with the client's name, the date, and the exact time of collection, such as 10/30/20, 7:00 AM to 10/31/20, 7:05 AM.

Factors Affecting Laboratory Results

- Prolonged light exposure of the specimens.
- Toilet paper or feces in the urine collection.
- High consumption of freshwater fish and tea may cause a decrease in vitamin B_1 levels.

NURSING IMPLICATIONS WITH RATIONALE

- Explain the test procedure to the client.

Client Teaching

- Instruct the client that food and fluids except water are prohibited for 12 hours or overnight (unless otherwise indicated by the health care provider).
- Instruct the client not to place toilet paper or feces in the urine specimen.

Decreased Level

- Obtain a history of the client's dietary intake. Note if the client consumes large quantities of alcoholic beverages.
- Note if the client is complaining of tingling and pain in the extremities. This could be an indication of peripheral neuritis.
- Administer oral or injectable thiamine drug (vitamin B_1) as prescribed.

Client Teaching

- Encourage the client to eat foods rich in vitamin B_1.
- Encourage the client to avoid alcohol consumption. Refer the client to Alcoholics Anonymous or counseling.

Vitamin B₆ (plasma)
Pyridoxine

Reference Values

Adult: 5–30 ng/mL, 20–120 nmol/L (SI units). Values depend on the method used.

Deficiency: Less than 5 ng/mL, or less than 20 nmol/L (SI units).

Description

Vitamin B_6, a water-soluble vitamin, is referred to as pyridoxine, pyridoxal, and pyridoxamine. Pyridoxine is converted to pyridoxal and pyridoxamine after absorption. The functions of vitamin B_6 include heme synthesis and as a coenzyme in amino acid metabolism. Vitamin B_6 may be partially destroyed by heat, so food processing can decrease the availability of vitamin B_6. Overheating of infant formulas may contribute to vitamin B_6 deficiency. Certain drugs block vitamin B_6, such as the long-term use of the antituberculin drug isoniazid (INH). Usually pyridoxine is given with isoniazid.

Foods rich in vitamin B_6 are whole grains, vegetables, eggs, bananas, fish, fowl, and lean meats. Very large doses of vitamin B_6 can cause peripheral neuropathy; however, this vitamin has a low toxic effect.

Purpose

- To detect a vitamin B_6 deficit.

Clinical Problems

Decreased Level: Malnutrition, malabsorption, chronic alcoholism, normocytic microcytic anemia, gestational diabetes, pregnancy, lactation, small bowel inflammatory disease, renal failure, asthma, heavy metal intoxication, carpal tunnel syndrome, pellagra. *Drug Influence:* Isoniazid, oral contraceptives, hydralazine, penicillamine, levodopa, anticonvulsants, cycloserine, pyrazinoic acid, tricyclic antidepressants, disulfiram.

Procedure

- NPO for 8–12 hours except for water. If the blood specimen was obtained from a nonfasting client, this should be noted on the laboratory slip.
- Collect 3–5 mL of venous blood in a lavender-top tube. Place the blood specimen in a paper bag to avoid light exposure. Time of specimen collection should be noted on the laboratory slip and the specimen should be delivered to the laboratory within 30 minutes.
- 24-hour urine specimen for vitamin B_6 has limited value.

Factors Affecting Laboratory Results

- Certain drugs can affect test results (*see Drug Influence*).
- Prolonged exposure of the blood specimen to light.
- Blood specimen not delivered to the laboratory within 30 minutes.

NURSING IMPLICATIONS WITH RATIONALE

- Explain test procedure to the client.

Decreased Level

- Report if the client is taking the antituberculin drug isoniazid and is not receiving pyridoxine.
- Observe infant suspected of vitamin B_6 deficiency for signs and symptoms of irritability, colic, startle reflex, and convulsion.
- Assess children and adults suspected of vitamin B_6 deficiency for irritability, dermatitis, glossitis, muscle weakness, polyneuritis, and a decrease in lymphocyte count.

Client Teaching

- Instruct the client to eat foods rich in vitamin B_6, such as whole grains, vegetables, eggs, fish, fowl, lean meats, and bananas. This is particularly necessary for clients with an alcoholic problem, during pregnancy and lactation, and those on strict diets. Vitamin supplements may be necessary.

Vitamin B$_{12}$ (serum)

Reference Values

Adult: 200–900 pg/mL.

Child: *Newborn:* 160–1,200 pg/mL.

Description

Vitamin B$_{12}$ is essential for red blood cell maturation and for gastrointestinal and neurologic function. The extrinsic factor of vitamin B$_{12}$ is obtained from foods and is absorbed in the small intestines when the intrinsic factor is present. The intrinsic factor is produced by the gastric mucosa, and when this factor is missing, pernicious anemia, a megaloblastic anemia, develops.

Purposes

- To detect pernicious anemia as determined by a decreased vitamin B$_{12}$ level.
- To suggest other health problems (*see Clinical Problems*).

Clinical Problems

Decreased Level: Pernicious anemia, malabsorption syndrome, liver diseases, hypothyroidism (myxedema), pancreatic insufficiency, sprue, Crohn disease, gastrectomy. *Drug Influence:* Neomycin, metformin, anticonvulsants, ethanol.

Increased Level: Acute hepatitis, acute and chronic myelocytic leukemia, polycythemia vera. *Drug Influence:* Oral contraceptives.

Procedure

- There is no food or fluid restriction.
- Collect 3–5 mL of venous blood in a red-top tube. Avoid hemolysis.

Factors Affecting Laboratory Results

- Drugs (*see Drug Influence*).
- Hemolysis of the blood specimen.

NURSING IMPLICATIONS WITH RATIONALE

- Assess for signs and symptoms of pernicious anemia, such as pallor; fatigue; dyspnea; sore mouth; smooth, beefy-red tongue; indigestion; tingling, numbness in the hands and feet; and behavioral changes.

Client Teaching

- Instruct the client to eat foods high in vitamin B$_{12}$, such as milk, eggs, meat, and liver. Contact the dietitian to assist the client in meal planning. Intramuscular vitamin B$_{12}$ may be ordered.

Vitamin C
See Ascorbic Acid

Vitamin D₃ (serum and plasma)
Cholecalciferol

Reference Values

Two Different Vitamin D₃s: Health care provider must specify which one: 1,25-dihydroxy (kidney) or 25-hydroxy (liver).

1,25-Dihydroxy: 20–76 pg/mL (serum). (Most potent. Stimulates calcium absorption by the small intestine and bone [along with PTH] and increases reabsorption of calcium by kidney.)

25-Hydroxy: 10–55 ng/mL (plasma). Reference values are usually higher in mid–late summer.

Description

Vitamin D is a fat-soluble vitamin occurring from exposure to the ultraviolet rays of sunlight and is absorbed in the presence of bile and stored in the liver. Most milk and milk products have been fortified with vitamin D. Vitamin D is needed for calcium absorption from the intestine and reabsorption from the bone.

A decrease in plasma vitamin D₃ occurs in aging and pregnancy. Rickets in children and osteomalacia in adults are caused by a vitamin D deficiency. Foods rich in vitamin D include vitamin D fortified milk, egg yolk, fish, liver, and butter.

Excess intake of vitamin D supplements could cause vitamin D toxicity. Hypercalcemia may occur with megadoses of vitamin D. Normally the serum calcium levels are checked with vitamin D₃ levels.

Purposes

- To detect a vitamin D deficit.
- To check for vitamin D toxicity when supplements are being taken.

Clinical Problems

Decreased Level: Malabsorption, cirrhosis of the liver, rickets, osteomalacia, steatorrhea, hypoparathyroidism, celiac disease, inflammatory bowel disease. *Drug Influence:* Anticonvulsants, isoniazid, mineral oil, glucocorticoids, aluminum hydroxide cholestyramine, colestipol.

Increased Level: Excessive intake of vitamin D supplements, excessive exposure to sunlight.

Procedure

- NPO for 8–12 hours prior to the test. If fasting is not required or if the client did not fast, this should be noted on the laboratory slip.
- Collect 3–5 mL of venous blood in a red-top tube (serum) or a green-top tube (plasma).

Factors Affecting Laboratory Results

- Certain drugs can decrease the vitamin D_3 level (*see Drug Influence*).
- Insufficient dietary intake of phosphorus can cause a decrease in vitamin D_3.
- Lack of exposure to sunlight can decrease the vitamin D_3 level.

NURSING IMPLICATIONS WITH RATIONALE

- Obtain a history of the client's exposure to sunlight. If the client has little to no sunlight exposure, the vitamin D_3 level will be decreased.
- Determine if the client is taking vitamin supplements and large doses of vitamin D. Hypervitaminosis D may occur, which can be toxic and could lead to nephrotoxicity.

Client Teaching

- Explain to the client that there should be nothing by mouth overnight prior to the test except for water unless otherwise indicated by the laboratory.

Decreased Level—Client Teaching

- Instruct the client to drink vitamin D fortified milk and/or take vitamin D supplements as indicated by the health care provider. Alert the client that massive doses of vitamin D can be toxic because it is a fat-soluble vitamin and can accumulate in the body.

Vitamin E (serum)

Tocopherol

Reference Values

Adult: 5–20 mcg/mL, 0.5–1.8 mg/dL, 12–42 μmol/L (SI units).

Child: 3–15 mcg/mL, 0.3–1 mg/dL, 7–23 μmol/L (SI units).

Description

Vitamin E is a fat-soluble vitamin that is plentiful in green, leafy vegetables, eggs, grains, oils, chicken, and fish. Vitamin E deficiency is not common unless it is due to malnutrition or malabsorption. Megadoses of vitamin E could impair absorption of vitamins D and K. Vitamin E is needed for muscle growth and development, adequate reproductive function, and neurologic function.

Purposes

- To detect a vitamin E deficit.
- To improve reproductive and neurologic functions.

Clinical Problems

Decreased Level: Malabsorption, malnutrition, neurologic abnormalities, platelet hyperaggregation, inadequate absorption of lipid, alcoholism, hemolytic anemia, cystic fibrosis. *Drug Influence:* Alcohol, phenytoin, cholestyramine, mineral oil.

Increased Level: Megadoses of vitamin E, hyperlipidemia.

Procedure

- There is no food or fluid restriction.
- Collect 3–5 mL of venous blood in a red-top tube. Place the blood sample in a paper bag to prevent light exposure. Send the blood specimen to the laboratory within 2 hours.

Factors Affecting Laboratory Results

- Exposure of the blood sample to light.

NURSING IMPLICATIONS WITH RATIONALE

- Obtain a history of dietary intake. Foods rich in vitamin E include green vegetables, grains, oils, eggs, fish, and chicken.
- Send the blood specimen to the laboratory in a paper bag to avoid light exposure.

Client Teaching

- Encourage the client to eat foods rich in vitamin E. Explain that vitamin E aids in muscle development, reproductive function, and neurologic function.
- Answer the client's questions concerning vitamin E intake. Excessively large doses should not be encouraged.

W

West Nile virus antibodies (serum and CSF)

Reference Values

Negative for IgM antibodies to flavivirus (10 days after flulike symptoms).

Description

West Nile virus is a flavivirus commonly found in Africa, West Asia, and the Middle East. West Nile virus first occurred in the United States in 1999. Since this time, almost every state has reported occurrences of the West Nile virus. It can infect humans, birds, mosquitoes, horses, and some other mammals. In people it is normally a mild disease, characterized by flulike symptoms (e.g., fever, headaches, lethargy, body aches, and possible skin rash), lasting only a few days. When it is severe, it may cause encephalitis, meningitis, or meningoencephalitis. This virus mainly occurs in late summer or early fall. The main route of infection is through the bite of an infected mosquito.

Purpose

- To aid in the diagnosis of West Nile virus infection.

Clinical Problems

Positive test: West Nile disease, flavivirus.

Procedure

- There is no food or fluid restriction.
- Collect 5 mL of venous blood in a red-top tube.
- Perform a spinal tap to obtain spinal fluid from the spinal cord. The CSF is evaluated for the flavivirus.

Factors Affecting Laboratory Results

- None known.

NURSING IMPLICATIONS WITH RATIONALE

- Ask the client if he or she has been bitten by a mosquito recently. Ascertain if the client has flulike symptoms.
- Check the vital signs. Continue to monitor vital signs.
- Note if the client has a severe headache, is confused, has difficulty in turning his or her head, or has any symptoms that may be due to meningitis or encephalitis.
- Provide comfort measures for the client.

Client Teaching

- Encourage the client to express to health professionals all symptoms that he or she is having.
- Tell the client to rest for several days after symptoms have ceased when flulike symptoms have occurred and have been severe. Temperature should be monitored.
- Inform the client that the test results for West Nile virus may take up to 2 weeks.

W

White blood cells (WBC) total (blood)

Leukocytes

Reference Values

Adult: Total WBC count: 4,500–10,000 μL (mm^3).

Child: *Newborn:* 9,000–30,000 μL. *2 Years:* 6,000–17,000 μL. *10 Years:* 4,500–13,500 μL.

Description

(*See White Blood Cell Differential [blood].*)

White blood cells, or leukocytes, are divided into two groups: the polymorphonuclear leukocytes (neutrophils, eosinophils, and basophils) and the mononuclear leukocytes (monocytes and lymphocytes). Leukocytes are a part of the body's defense system; they respond immediately to foreign invaders by going to the site of involvement. An increase in WBCs is called *leukocytosis*, and a decrease in WBCs is called *leukopenia*.

Purposes

- To assess WBCs as a part of a complete blood count (CBC).
- To determine the presence of an infection.
- To check WBC values for diagnosing health problems (*see Clinical Problems*).

Clinical Problems

Decreased Level: Hematopoietic diseases (aplastic anemia, pernicious anemia, hypersplenism, Gaucher disease), viral infections, malaria, agranulocytosis, alcoholism, systemic lupus erythematosus, rheumatoid arthritis. *Drug Influence:* Antibiotics (penicillins, cephalothins, chloramphenicol), acetaminophen (Tylenol), sulfonamides, propylthiouracil, barbiturates, cancer chemotherapy agents, diazepam (Valium), diuretics (furosemide [Lasix], ethacrynic acid [Edecrin]), chlordiazepoxide (Librium), oral hypoglycemic agents, indomethacin (Indocin), methyldopa (Aldomet), rifampin, phenothiazine.

Increased Level: Acute infection (pneumonia, meningitis, appendicitis, colitis, peritonitis, pancreatitis, pyelonephritis, tuberculosis, tonsillitis, diverticulitis, septicemia, rheumatic fever), tissue necrosis (myocardial infarction, cirrhosis of the liver, burns, cancer of the organs, emphysema, peptic ulcer), leukemias, collagen diseases, hemolytic and sickle-cell anemias, parasitic diseases, stress (surgery, fever, long-lasting emotional upset). *Drug Influence:* Aspirin, heparin, digitalis, epinephrine, lithium, histamine, antibiotics (ampicillin, erythromycin, kanamycin, methicillin, tetracyclines, vancomycin, streptomycin), gold compounds, procainamide (Pronestyl), triamterene (Dyrenium), allopurinol, potassium iodide, hydantoin derivatives, sulfonamides (long acting).

Procedure

Venous Blood
- There is no food or fluid restriction.
- Collect 3–5 mL of venous blood in a lavender-top tube. Avoid hemolysis.

Capillary Blood
- Collect blood from a finger puncture with a micropipette.
- Dilute immediately with the proper reagent.

Factors Affecting Laboratory Results

- Drugs that can increase and decrease the WBC count (*see Drug Influence*).
- The time the blood sample was taken. The WBC count is lower in the morning than in the afternoon.
- The age of the individual. Children can have a high WBC count, especially during the first 5 years of life.

NURSING IMPLICATIONS WITH RATIONALE

- Check the vital signs and note if the temperature and pulse rate are increased. Also check for signs and symptoms of inflammation and infection, such as redness, heat, swelling, and drainage at the tissue site.
- Note changes in the client's condition, such as fever, increased pulse and respiration rate, and leukocytosis.

Client Teaching

- Instruct the client to check the side effects of patent medicines, such as cold medications. These could cause severe leukopenia and agranulocytosis. With agranulocytosis, the major defense system is lost, and the client is susceptible to severe or long-lasting infection.
- Instruct clients with leukopenia to avoid persons with any contagious condition. Their body resistances are reduced, and they are prime candidates for severe colds or infections.

White blood cell differential (blood)

Differential WBC

Reference Values

DIFFERENTIAL WBC VALUES

WBC Type	Adult		Child
	%	μL (mm³)	Same as Adult Except
Neutrophils (total)	50–70	2,500–7,000	*Newborn:* 61%; *1 year old:* 32%
Segments	50–65	2,500–6,500	*1–12 years:* 4–9%.
Bands	0–5	0–500	*Newborn:* 34%. *1 year:* 60%.
Eosinophils	1–3	100–300	*6 years:* 42%. *12 years:* 38%.
Basophils	0.4–1	40–100	
Monocytes	4–6	200–600	
Lymphocytes	25–35	1,700–3,500	

Description

(*See White Blood Cells [WBC] Total.*)

The differential white blood cell count, part of the complete blood count, is composed of five types of WBCs (leukocytes): neutrophils, eosinophils, basophils, monocytes, and lymphocytes. The differential WBC count is expressed as cubic millimeters (mm³, μL) and percentage of the total number of WBCs. Neutrophils and lymphocytes make up 80–90% of the total WBCs. The differential WBC count provides more specific information related to infections and disease process.

Neutrophils: Neutrophils are the most numerous circulating WBCs, and they respond more rapidly to the inflammatory and tissue injury sites than other types of WBCs. During an *acute* infection, the neutrophils are the body's first line of defense. The segments are mature neutrophils, and the bands are immature ones that multiply quickly during an acute infection.

Eosinophils: Eosinophils increase during allergic and parasitic conditions. With an increase in steroids, either produced by the adrenal glands during stress or administered orally or by injection, eosinophils decrease in number.

Basophils: Basophils increase during the healing process. With an increase in steroids, the basophil count will decrease.

Monocytes: Monocytes are the second line of defense against bacterial infections and foreign substances. They are stronger than neutrophils and can ingest larger particles of debris. Monocytes respond late during the acute phase of infection and inflammatory process, and they continue to function during the chronic phase of phagocytes.

Lymphocytes: Increased lymphocytes (lymphocytosis) occur in chronic and viral infections. Severe lymphocytosis is commonly caused by chronic lymphocytic leukemia. Lymphocytes play a major role in the immune response system as B lymphocytes and T lymphocytes. Like eosinophils, lymphocytes decrease in number during excess adrenocortical hormone secretion or steroid therapy.

Purpose

- To differentiate between the various types of WBCs for diagnosing health problems (*see Description*).

Clinical Problems

Decreased Level *Neutrophils:* Viral diseases, leukemias (lymphocytic and monocytic), agranulocytosis, aplastic and iron-deficiency anemias. *Drug Influence:* Antibiotic therapy, immunosuppressive agents. *Eosinophils:* Stress, shock; adrenocortical hyperfunction. *Drug Influence:* Cortisone, ACTH. *Basophils:* Stress, hypersensitivity reaction, pregnancy, hyperthyroidism. *Monocytes:* Lymphocytic leukemia, aplastic anemia. *Lymphocytes:* Cancer, leukemia, adrenocortical hyperfunction, agranulocytosis, aplastic anemia, multiple sclerosis, renal failure, nephrotic syndrome, systemic lupus erythematosus.

Increased Level: *Neutrophils:* Acute infections (localized and systemic), inflammatory diseases (rheumatoid arthritis, gout, pneumonia), tissue damage (acute myocardial infarction, burns, crushed injury, surgery), Hodgkin disease, myelocytic leukemia, hemolytic disease of newborns, acute cholecystitis, acute appendicitis, acute pancreatitis. *Drug Influence:* Epinephrine, digitalis, heparin, sulfonamides, lithium, cortisone, ACTH. *Eosinophils:* Allergies, parasitic disease, cancer (bone, ovary, testes, brain), phlebitis, thrombophlebitis, asthma, emphysema, renal disease (renal failure, nephrotic syndrome). *Basophils:* Inflammatory process, leukemia, healing stage of infection or inflammation, acquired hemolytic anemia. *Monocytes:* Viral diseases (infectious mononucleosis, mumps, herpes zoster), parasitic diseases (Rocky Mountain spotted fever, toxoplasmosis, brucellosis), monocytic leukemia, cancer (esophagus, stomach, colon, liver, bone, prostate, uterus, brain, bladder), anemias (sickle cell, hemolytic), collagen diseases (SLE), rheumatoid arthritis, ulcerative colitis. *Lymphocytes:* Lymphocytic leukemia, viral infections (infectious mononucleosis, hepatitis, mumps, rubella, viral pneumonia, pertussis), chronic infections, Hodgkin disease, multiple myeloma, adrenocortical hypofunction.

Procedure

- There is no food or fluid restriction.
- Collect 7 mL of venous blood in a lavender-top tube. Avoid hemolysis.
- If eosinophils value is needed, record the time that the blood sample was drawn. If drawn in the afternoon or evening, the count could be slightly higher.

Factors Affecting Laboratory Results

- Steroids could decrease eosinophil and lymphocyte values.
- Certain drugs can increase or decrease blood values (*see Drug Influence*).

NURSING IMPLICATIONS WITH RATIONALE

- Check the WBC count and the differential WBC count. Elevated neutrophils may be indicative of an acute infection. Elevated eosinophils may be a sign of allergy. Increased basophils can be caused by the healing process. Increased monocytes occur during a bacterial infection, and increased lymphocytes occur in chronic or viral infections.
- Assess the client for signs and symptoms of an infection, such as elevated temperature, increased pulse rate, edema, redness, and exudate (wound drainage).
- Assess the client for signs and symptoms of allergies, such as tearing, runny nose, rash, and more severe reactions.
- Assess for signs and symptoms of healing, such as the ability to increase movement at the injured site and decreased edema and exudate.

Client Teaching

- Instruct the client to report any signs and symptoms of infection, such as the presence of a fever.
- Encourage the client to rest, take medications such as antibiotics as prescribed, increase fluid intake as appropriate, and monitor temperature.

Zika virus

Reference Values

Negative.

Description

Zika is a virus transmitted by the *Aedes aegypti* mosquito that was originally reported in Brazil in 2015; by 2016, the virus had been reported in 30 states of the United States, first in the Miami, Florida area. This mosquito virus is also in Puerto Rico, Virgin Islands, and American Samoa. Most of those who have contracted the Zika virus in the United States (except in Miami, Florida) have been persons visiting Brazil or countries affected by the mosquito virus. Approximately one out of five persons exposed to the Zika virus become ill. The most common symptoms are fever, rash, conjunctivitis, headaches, muscle aches, and joint pain.

The virus can affect the pregnant woman's fetus, causing various birth defects, such as premature birth, microcephaly (small brain size), and blindness. The Zika virus may also be sexually transmitted. To prevent sexual transmission, clients having contracted the Zika virus should use protection when having sex for the next 6 months.

The *Aedes aegypti* mosquito is more prevalent in warm weather, and this is especially true in warm/hot climates.

Purposes

- To identify clients who have been in contact with the mosquito carrying the Zika virus.
- To eradicate the *Aedes aegypti* mosquito population.

Clinical Problems

Clients who have been bitten by the *Aedes aegypti* mosquito that carries the Zika virus. Zika virus that has been sexually transmitted.

Procedure

- Obtain a blood sample from the affected person. Check with the laboratory in regards to method for obtaining the blood specimen.

NURSING IMPLICATIONS WITH RATIONALE

- Ask the client if he or she has been in any countries—such as Brazil, Puerto Rico, or Virgin Islands—where the *Aedes aegypti* mosquito is prevalent.
- Note if the client has any symptoms of Zika virus, such as a rash, fever, or joint pain.
- Report if the female client is pregnant. The Zika virus can be transmitted to the fetus. However, not all fetuses would contract the Zika virus.
- Inform all clients (female and male) with the Zika virus that the virus can be sexually transmitted, so they should use protection (e.g., a condom) for the next 6 months.
- Answer the client's questions and concerns about the Zika virus or refer questions to the health care provider.

Z

Zinc (plasma)

Reference Values

Plasma: *Adult:* 60–150 mcg/dL, 11–23 μmol/L (SI units).
Urine: 150–1,250 mcg/24 h.

Description

Zinc, a heavy metal, is an element found in the body and is required for body growth and metabolism. Approximately 80% of zinc is in the blood cells. About 30% of the zinc ingested is absorbed from the small intestine. Most of the body's excretion of zinc is in the stool, and a small amount is excreted in the urine.

Zinc is a component of many enzymes, such as carbonic anhydrase, DNA and RNA polymerases, lactic dehydrogenase, and alkaline phosphatase, and plays an important role in enzyme catalytic reactions. Plasma zinc levels are requested when a zinc deficiency or toxicity is suspected. Zinc deficiency is not apparent until it becomes severe and is manifested by growth retardation, delayed sexual development, severe dermatitis, alopecia, or poor wound healing. Zinc toxicity is rare, but it can be related to workers inhaling zinc oxide during industry exposure.

Purposes

- To detect a zinc deficiency.
- To determine the cause of diarrhea, growth retardation, delayed sexual development, alopecia, and poor healing.
- To detect zinc toxicity due to industry exposure (inhaling zinc oxide).

Clinical Problems

Decreased Level: Malnutrition, malabsorption, diarrhea, anemia, alcoholism, myocardial infarction, hereditary deficiency, cirrhosis, chronic renal failure, gallbladder disease. *Drug Influence:* Corticosteroids, estrogens, penicillamine, anti-cancer-antimetabolites, cisplatin, diuretics.

Increased Level: Ingestion of acidic food or beverages from galvanized containers, industrial exposure.

Procedure

- There is no food or fluid restriction.
- Collect 3–5 mL of venous blood in a metal-free, navy-blue-top tube. Avoid hemolysis.
- Send the blood specimen to the laboratory *immediately.*

Factors Affecting Laboratory Results

- Certain drugs decrease the plasma level (*see Drug Influence*).
- Hemolysis invalidates the test result.
- Use of a tube or needle containing metal.

Z

NURSING IMPLICATIONS WITH RATIONALE

- Obtain a history of the client's nutritional intake. Zinc is present in many foods. Malnutrition, cirrhosis of the liver, alcoholism, or severe diarrhea contributes to a zinc deficit.
- Monitor intravenous therapy including total parenteral nutrition (TPN). Continuous use can cause a zinc deficit.
- Check the history for anemia. With sickle-cell anemia, the zinc level is decreased because abnormal red blood cells cause excess loss of zinc.

Client Teaching

- Instruct the pregnant client that vitamins prescribed should contain zinc. Additional zinc is required during pregnancy and for lactation.
- Instruct the client who has poor nutrition to take vitamins. Tell the client to check the label on the vitamin container to determine that zinc is one of the elements.

Zinc protoporphyrin (ZPP) (blood)

Free Erythrocyte Protoporphyrin (FEP)

Reference Values

Adult and Child: 15–77 mcg/dL, 0.24–1.23 µmol/L (SI units). *Average:* Less than 35 mcg/dL, less than 0.56 µmol/L (SI units).

Description

Zinc protoporphyrin (ZPP) is a screening test to check for lead poisoning and iron deficiency. It can be checked by drawing a blood sample or by use of a hematofluorometer using several drops of blood. With iron deficiency, the ZPP level does not become elevated until a few weeks later. After iron therapy, the ZPP level returns to normal in 2–2½ months.

The use of the ZPP test for screening for increased blood lead levels has more than doubled within a year. ZPP is an effective indicator of the total body of lead. The blood lead level should also be checked.

Purpose

- To screen for lead poisoning or for iron deficiency.

Clinical Problems

Increased Level: Lead poisoning, iron deficiency, accelerated erythropoiesis, acute inflammatory processes. *Drug Influence:* Digitalis, riboflavin. *Laboratory Test:* Serum bilirubin can be elevated.

Procedure

- There is no food or fluid restriction.
- Collect 3–5 mL in a green- or lavender-top tube. Avoid hemolysis. A hematofluorometer with a few drops of blood may be used.

Factors Affecting Laboratory Results

- Hemolysis of the blood sample can increase the ZPP level.

NURSING IMPLICATIONS WITH RATIONALE

- Check with the laboratory concerning the type of blood specimen that should be obtained (drops of blood or use of a hematofluorometer with a few drops of blood).
- Obtain a history from the client or family concerning the child ingesting lead from paint. Older houses may still have lead paint.
- Obtain a history from the adult client concerning excessive lead exposure due to occupational contact. Other possible contact with lead includes use of unglazed pottery, "moonshine" whiskey prepared in lead containers, and lead gasoline fumes (not common today because of unleaded gasoline).
- Compare the blood lead level with the blood ZPP level. Report abnormal findings to the health care provider.
- Observe for signs and symptoms of lead poisoning, such as lead colic (crampy abdominal pain), constipation, occasional bloody diarrhea, behavioral changes (from lethargy to hyperactivity, aggression, impulsiveness), tremors, and confusion.
- Obtain a history of iron deficiency. Check the serum iron level, serum transferrin, and ferritin levels. Compare the above levels with the ZPP level.
- Check that blood ZPP levels are repeated after 2 months of iron therapy. ZPP levels should decrease after iron therapy for iron deficiency.

Z

Part I Situational Study Questions

Note: Answers are not given, and if the answers are unknown, the student should check the laboratory tests in the text (Part I).

SITUATION I: Hyperlipidemia

A.E., age 62, was ordered a serum lipoprotein test to check her cholesterol, LDL, and HDL values. Her findings were as follows: cholesterol 235 mg/dL; low-density lipoprotein (LDL) 130 mg/dL; and high-density lipoprotein (HDL) 40 mg/dL.

1. Were A.E.'s lipoproteins abnormal, and if so, which ones?
2. What are the normal reference values for triglycerides?
3. What is the purpose for lipoprotein phenotype in determining the lipid composition?
4. Should A.E.'s lipoprotein values be monitored, and if so, why?
5. Differentiate between atherosclerosis and coronary artery disease (CAD).

A.E. was ordered apolipoprotein (Apo) and apolipoprotein ratio tests.

6. What are apolipoproteins? Differentiate between the apolipoprotein A-1 (Apo A-1) and apolipoprotein B (Apo-B).
7. What are the major components of Apo B, and how do the two forms differ?
8. For what purpose was a ratio Apo A-1 and Apo B test ordered for A.E.?

An N-High Sensitivity CRP (hs CRP) test was ordered for A.E.

9. Why would an hs CRP test be ordered?
10. What is the reference value for hs CRP? What does a positive/increased CRP value indicate?

SITUATION 2: Possible Heart Attack (Possible MI)

T.F., age 58, complained of chest pain. Several laboratory tests were ordered: creatine phosphokinase (CPK, CK) and CPK isoenzymes, homocysteine, and troponins.

1. Where in the body are the creatine phosphokinase enzymes?
2. Why was the CPK isoenzyme test ordered for T.F.? Which CPK isoenzymes, if elevated, might be a cause of T.F.'s health problem?
3. T.F. was ordered a homocysteine test. How is an elevated homocysteine level associated with T.F.'s health problem?
4. What are troponins? What are the two types of troponins?
5. Why is the troponin level useful for determining the cause of T.F.'s complaint?
6. Why is the troponin level effective in determining the cause of chest/cardiac pain?
7. T.F. wants to know why these tests were ordered. What would your response be?

SITUATION 3: Heart Failure

G.H., age 72, has had some difficulty in breathing and her ankles were swollen in the morning. An atrial natriuretic peptide (ANP) and brain natriuretic peptide (BNP) levels were ordered.

1. What were the purposes for ordering ANP and BNP tests for G.H.?
2. What are the similarities and differences of ANP and BNP tests?

3. Explain how ANP values differ if G.H. has chronic or acute heart failure.
4. If G.H. has heart failure, would BNP be elevated, and if so, how high could the value be?
5. What other clinical problems might be associated with an elevated BNP?
6. What other tests might be ordered to rule out heart failure?

SITUATION 4: Breast Cancer

S.P., age 54, found a lump in her breast. A mammogram had been ordered along with several laboratory tests, such as breast cancer genetic testing, breast cancer tumor prognostic markers, and cancer tumor markers: CA 15-3, CA 27.29, CA 125, and CA 549.

1. What is the purpose for ordering a breast cancer genetic testing (BRCA-1 and BRCA-2 genes)?
2. Which of the breast cancer tumor prognostic markers might be indicative of breast cancer?
3. S.P. is postmenopausal. Would the estrogen receptor assay (ER assay) be more or less elevated compared to a premenopausal woman? Explain.
4. An increase in CA 15-3, CA 27.29, CA 125, and CA 549 could be an indicator of the presence of a tumor. Which one of the three cancer markers would be a more sensitive test for breast cancer?
5. Which cancer tumor marker would be a more sensitive test for ovarian cancer?
6. An elevated CA 50 marker might be present with what type of tumor?

SITUATION 5: Diabetes Mellitus

C.D., age 65, has been diagnosed with type 2 diabetes mellitus. C.D.'s fasting blood sugar is 225 mg/dL.

1. What is the "normal" range for a fasting glucose (sugar) level? What is the "normal" range for a postprandial (feasting) glucose level?
2. Should a glucose tolerance test be ordered for C.D.? Why or why not?

A hemoglobin A $_1$c test was ordered for C.D.

3. What was the purpose for ordering a hemoglobin A $_1$c test for C.D.?
4. Give another name for hemoglobin A $_1$c.
5. C.D.'s hemoglobin A $_1$c result was 7.6%. Is the result within the "normal" range for C.D.? What is the "normal" percentage for a diabetic and for a nondiabetic?
6. Why should C.D.'s hemoglobin A $_1$c be monitored? How often should it be monitored?
7. How does the hemoglobin A $_1$c compare with a glucose fasting blood sugar?

SITUATION 6: Older Adult: Laboratory tests were ordered before a biannual physical examination.

P.R., age 75, has an order for a complete blood count (CBC), basic metabolic panel test, INR, and lipid panel.

The results of her complete blood count are as follows: hemoglobin (Hgb) 13.2 g/dL; hematocrit (Hct) 35%; RBC count 5.5×10^{12}; WBC count 11,000 μL (mm^3); platelet count 300,000 μL.

1. What are the normal reference values for hemoglobin, hematocrit, red blood cell count, white blood cell count, and platelet count?
2. Are P.R.'s CBCs within normal reference values for a female? If not, which one(s) is/are not within normal range? Would there be additional testing done, and if so what?

3. What other CBC laboratory test could have been ordered? Check red blood cell indices.
4. The CBC can include the WBC differential count. This would include neutrophils, eosinophils, basophils, lymphocytes, and monocytes. What is the significance of each?
5. Is P.R.'s platelet count within normal range?

P.R.'s basic metabolic panel test results are as follows: sodium 148 mEq/L; potassium 4.5 mEq/L; calcium 4.9 mEq/L (9.8 mg/dL); chloride 100 mEq/L; carbon dioxide (CO_2) 24 mEq/L; glucose 142 mg/dL; blood urea nitrogen (BUN) 35 mg/dL; creatinine 1 mg/dL.

6. What are the normal reference values for each?

Sodium:	CO_2:
Potassium:	Glucose:
Calcium:	BUN:
Chloride:	Creatinine:

7. Which one(s) of the electrolytes is/are not in normal range? What could that indicate?
8. Is the glucose within normal range? If not, what could this indicate? What further laboratory studies might be suggested?
9. The BUN is elevated but not the creatinine. What could this indicate? Relate this to aging.
10. If the creatinine was elevated, what could this indicate?

P.R. is taking Coumadin 5 mg once a day. Her international normalized ratio or INR is 3.4.

11. What is the normal INR for a person taking warfarin (Coumadin)?
12. If the INR is elevated, does this mean that the blood is too thin or not thin enough?
13. Is P.R.'s INR within normal range? What could the health care provider suggest?

The lipid panel includes cholesterol, HDL, LDL, and triglycerides. P.R.'s lipid panel results are as follows: cholesterol 168 mg/dL; high-density lipoprotein (HDL) 58 mg/dL; low-density lipoprotein (LDL) 86 mg/dL; triglycerides 200 mg/dL. P.R. is taking Crestor 5 mg daily (statin drug).

14. What are the normal values for the lipid panel laboratory tests?

Cholesterol:_____	LDL: _____
HDL:_____	Triglycerides: _____

15. Are P.R.'s lipids within normal range? Explain.
16. P.R. is taking the statin drug Crestor. What effect does this drug have on the serum lipids? You may need to check with a drug reference book.

PART TWO

Diagnostic Tests

2

Acid perfusion
See Esophageal Studies

Amniotic fluid analysis
Amniocentesis, Amnioscopy

Normal Finding
Clear amniotic fluid, no chromosomal or neural tube abnormalities.

Description
Amniotic fluid analysis is useful for detecting chromosomal abnormalities, such as Down syndrome (Trisomy 21); neural tube defects (spina bifida); and sex-linked disorders, such as hemophilia; and for determining fetal maturity. The amniotic fluid is obtained by amniocentesis. This procedure involves the insertion of a needle into the suprapubic area after the fetus has been located and manually elevated and the aspiration of 5–15 mL of amniotic fluid. Ultrasound may be used to locate the placenta and to determine fetal position so that needle contact can be avoided. Amniocentesis is performed during the 14–16th weeks of pregnancy. It is usually not done before the 14th week because of the insufficient amount of amniotic fluid, or after the 16th week if a therapeutic abortion might be suggested.

Analyses of the amniotic fluid may also include color, bilirubin (present in the fluid until the 28th week but absent at full term), meconium (present during stress—e.g., in breech presentation), creatinine, lecithin/sphingomyelin (L/S) ratio (a decreased ratio can indicate respiratory distress syndrome), glucose, lipids, and alpha-fetoprotein (AFP).

Amnioscopy involves insertion of a fiberoptic lighted instrument (amnioscope) into the cervical canal to visualize the amniotic fluid. The color of the amniotic fluid can indicate fetal hypoxia. This test is normally performed close to full term, because it requires cervical dilation. Because there is a risk of rupturing the amniotic membrane and of intrauterine infection, the test is rarely performed.

Purposes
- To detect chromosomal abnormalities, neural tube defects, and sex-linked disorders.
- To determine fetal maturity.

Clinical Problems
Indications: Chromosomal disorders (e.g., Down syndrome), neural tube defects (e.g., spina bifida), and hemolytic disease due to Rh incompatibility; fetal sex (important for sex-linked disorders—e.g., hemophilia), fetal maturity, and pulmonary maturity of the fetus (L/S ratio).

Procedure
- The client should sign a consent form.
- Food and fluids are not restricted.

A

- Have the client void before the procedure to prevent puncturing the bladder and aspirating urine.
- Cleanse the suprapubic area with an antiseptic such as povidone-iodine (Betadine). A local anesthetic is injected at the site for the amniocentesis.
- The placenta and fetus should be located by ultrasound or manually (fetus only). A 22-gauge spinal needle with stylet is inserted through the skin to the amniotic cavity.
- An amount of 5–15 mL of amniotic fluid is aspirated. Apply a small dressing to the needle insertion site.
- The procedure takes approximately 30 minutes.

Foam Stability Test

This test determines if surfactant from mature fetal lungs is present in the amniotic fluid. When the test tube of amniotic fluid is shaken, bubbles appear around the surface if adequate amounts of surfactant are present.

Factors Affecting Diagnostic Results

A traumatic amniocentesis tap may produce blood in the amniotic fluid.

NURSING IMPLICATIONS WITH RATIONALE

Pretest

- Recognize when amniocentesis for amniotic fluid analysis is indicated (i.e., with a familial history of sex-linked, genetic, or chromosomal disorders; with a history of previous miscarriages; and in advanced maternal age [greater than 35 years old]). It is not a screening test.
- Obtain a list of medications the client is taking.
- Be sure that the client urinates before the test and that the consent form is signed.
- Review the procedure with the client. Encourage her to relax and control breathing during the procedure.
- Be supportive of the woman and her partner. Be a good listener. Allow them time to ask questions and to express any concerns. Refer questions you cannot answer to the appropriate health professionals.

Client Teaching

- Inform the client that normal results do not guarantee a normal infant, nor do they always predict sex correctly. The health care provider should tell the woman of potential risks, such as premature labor, spontaneous abortion, infection, and fetal or placental bleeding from the needle. These complications rarely occur, but the woman should be told of the risk factors.
- Instruct the client to notify the health care provider immediately of any of the following: bleeding or leaking fluid from the vagina, abdominal pain or cramping, chills and fever, or lack of fetal movement.
- Encourage the woman and her partner to seek genetic counseling, especially if a chromosomal abnormality has been determined. Usually the final decision about terminating a pregnancy rests with the pregnant woman and her partner.

Angiography (angiogram)

Arteriography: Cardiac (see Cardiac Catheterization), Cerebral Angiography, Pulmonary Angiography, and Renal Angiography

Normal Finding

Normal structure and potency of the blood vessels.

Description

In vivo angiography was first performed in the 1920s. The terms *angiography* (examination of the blood vessels) and *arteriography* (examination of the arteries) are used interchangeably. A catheter is inserted into the femoral, brachial, subclavian, or carotid artery, and a contrast dye is injected to allow visualization of the blood vessels. Normally the client feels a warm, flushed sensation as the dye is injected. Angiographies are useful for evaluating patency of blood vessels and for identifying abnormal vascularization resulting from neoplasms (tumors). This test may be indicated when computed tomography or radionuclide scanning suggests vascular abnormalities.

The new contrast media have a low osmolality. The older medias were hyperosmolar with a high content of iodine in relation to its solution. Examples of the low-osmolar contrast media include iopamidol, iohexol, and ioxaglate.

An embolus due to catheter clot formation is the most dangerous complication of angiography. Other complications include puncturing the site, causing hematoma and/or hemorrhage; contrast media reactions; and infection.

Cerebral Angiography: Any of the three arteries (femoral, brachial, or carotid) can be used for access. The dye will outline the carotid artery, vertebral artery, large blood vessels of the circle of Willis, and small cerebral arterial branches.

Pulmonary Angiography: The catheter is inserted into the brachial artery (in the arm) or the femoral artery and is threaded to the pulmonary artery. The dye is injected for visualizing pulmonary vessels. During the test, the client should be monitored for cardiac dysrhythmias.

Renal Angiography: The catheter is inserted into the femoral artery and is passed upward through the iliac artery and the aorta to the renal artery. This test permits visualization of the renal vessels and the parenchyma. An aortogram is sometimes made with real angiography to detect any vessel abnormality and to show the relationship of the renal arteries to the aorta.

Purposes

- To detect aneurysms, thrombosis, emboli, space-occupying lesions, stenosis, and plaques.
- To evaluate cerebral, pulmonary, and renal blood flow.

Clinical Problems

TYPE OF ANGIOGRAPHY	INDICATIONS/PURPOSES
Cerebral	To detect cerebrovascular aneurysm; cerebral thrombosis; hematomas; tumors from increased vascularization; cerebral plaques or spasm; cerebral fistula To determine cerebral blood flow, cause of increased intracranial pressure (↑ICP)
Pulmonary	To detect pulmonary embolism; tumors; aneurysms; congenital defects; vascular changes associated with emphysema, blebs, and bullae; heart abnormality To evaluate pulmonary circulation
Renal	To detect renal artery stenosis; renal thrombus or embolus; space-occupying lesions (i.e., tumors, cysts); aneurysms To determine the causative factor of hypertension, cause of renal failure To evaluate renal circulation

Procedure

All Angiographies

- A consent form should be understood and signed by the client or a designated family member.
- The client should have nothing by mouth (NPO) for 8–12 hours before the angiogram. Anticoagulants (heparin) are usually discontinued.
- Record vital signs (VS). Have client void before the test.
- Dentures and metallic objects should be removed before the test.
- The access site should be shaved.
- Premedications (i.e., a sedative or narcotic analgesic), if ordered, are administered an hour before the test. If the client has a history of severe allergic reactions to various substances or drugs, the health care provider may order steroids or antihistamines before and after the procedure as a prophylactic measure.
- Intravenous (IV) fluids may be started before the procedure so that emergency drugs, if needed, may be administered.
- The client lies in a supine position on an x-ray table. A local anesthetic is administered to the injection incisional site.
- The test takes approximately 1–2 hours.

Renal: A laxative or cleansing enema is usually ordered the evening before the test.

Pulmonary: Electrocardiography electrodes are attached to the client's chest for cardiac monitoring (tracings of heart activity) during the angiography. Pulmonary pressures are recorded, and blood samples are obtained before the contrast dye is injected.

Factors Affecting Diagnostic Results

- Feces and gas can distort or decrease the visualization of the kidneys.
- Barium sulfate from a recent barium study can interfere with the test results.
- Movement during the filming can distort the x-ray picture.

A

NURSING IMPLICATIONS WITH RATIONALE

Pretest

- Obtain a client history of hypersensitivity to iodine, seafood, or contrast dye from other x-ray procedures (e.g., intravenous pyelography [IVP]). The health care provider should also know if the client is highly sensitive to other substances. Skin testing could be done before the test, or prophylactic medications (i.e., steroids, antihistamines) may be given prior to and/or following the test.
- Record baseline vital signs.
- Give a laxative or cleansing enema, if ordered. Explain to the client that it will cleanse the lower intestinal tract, allowing better visualization.
- Have the client void, wear a gown, and remove dentures.
- Administer premedications (sedative and narcotic analgesic) as ordered. Check that the consent form has been signed before giving premedications. The client should be in bed with the bed sides up after the premedications are given.
- Encourage the client to ask questions. This test can be frightening to clients, and they will need time to express any concerns.
- Assess for vasovagal reaction (common complication; i.e., decreased pulse rate and blood pressure [BP], cold and clammy skin). Give IV fluids and atropine IV. This reaction lasts about 15–20 minutes.

Client Teaching

- Explain the procedure to the client (see *Description and Procedure*). Inform the client that the radiologist, surgeon, or health care provider will inject a contrast dye into an artery at the groin, elbow, or neck. The area will be numbed, and a catheter will be inserted and threaded with the guidance of fluoroscopy to the appropriate site.
- Inform the client that when the dye is injected, he or she will most likely feel a warm, flushed sensation that should last for a minute or two. Explain to the client that the test should not cause pain but can cause some periodic discomfort during the procedure.

Test

- Monitor vital signs: blood pressure, pulse, and respiration.
- Assess for vasovagal reaction (common complication, i.e., decreased pulse rate and blood pressure, cold and clammy skin). Give IV fluids and atropine IV (if indicated). This reaction lasts about 15–20 minutes.

Posttest

- Apply pressure on the injection site for 5–10 minutes or longer (venous access) or 30 minutes or longer (arterial access) until bleeding has stopped. Check the injection site for bleeding when taking vital signs.
- Monitor vital signs as ordered, such as every 15 minutes for the first hour, every 30 minutes for the next 2 hours, and then every hour for the next 4 hours, or until stable. The client's temperature should be taken every 4 hours for 24–48 hours or as ordered.

A

- Enforce bed rest for 5 hours for venous access or 6–8 hours for arterial access or as ordered. Activities should be restricted for a day.
- Assess the injection site for swelling and for hematoma.
- Check peripheral pulses in the extremities (i.e., dorsalis pedis, femoral, and radial). Absence or weakness in pulse volume should be reported immediately.
- Note the temperature and color of the extremity. Report changes (e.g., color—pale, pain in the extremity, especially distal to access site) to the health care provider immediately. Arterial occlusion to the extremity could occur.
- Apply cold compresses or an ice pack to the injection site for edema or pain, if ordered.
- Monitor electrocardiogram tracings, urine output, and IV fluids. IV fluids and cardiac monitoring may be discontinued after the angiography.
- Inform the client that coughing usually is not abnormal following a pulmonary angiography.
- Assess for dysphagia and for respiratory distress if the carotid artery was used for cerebral angiography.
- Assess for weakness or numbness in an extremity, confusion, slurred speech, or visual changes following a cerebral angiography. These could be symptoms of a transient ischemic attack (TIA), known as a "small stroke."
- Observe for a delayed allergic reaction to the contrast dye (i.e., tachycardia, dyspnea, skin rash, urticaria [hives], decreasing systolic BP, and decreased urine output).
- Inform the client to avoid heavy lifting for 24 hours or more as indicated by the health care provider.
- Be supportive of the client and his or her family. Answer questions, and explain your nursing implications.

Apnea test

Normal Findings

Positive test: *Presence of brain death.*

Negative test: *Absence of brain death.*

Description

The apnea test is primarily ordered to determine the absence or presence of spontaneous breathing when the client is taken off the ventilator. If the (adult) client does *not* have spontaneous breathing after 10 minutes (15 minutes for a child), the person is assumed brain dead. Arterial blood gases should be taken for the $PaCO_2$ level before and after the removal of the ventilator. A sign of respiratory distress is when the $PaCO_2$ is greater than 46 mmHg.

It should be noted if the client has a high-level spinal cord injury that has caused nonspontaneous breathing. Drug or alcohol poisoning can also cause a lack of spontaneous breathing. Usually the client is on a ventilator for a while before the apnea test is performed. It is mostly conducted when there is severe brain injury.

A

Brain death is when the entire brain including the brain stem has completely stopped functioning and breathing is only possible with the assistance of a ventilator. Brain death would not be considered if the client is on a ventilator to receive neuromuscular blocking agent(s) or has other physiological problems. This test is part of a neurologic examination for a client suspected to be brain dead.

Purpose

- To evaluate the presence of spontaneous breathing when client is taken off a ventilator.

Clinical Problems

Brain dead from an absence of spontaneous breathing after removal from a ventilator following 10–15 minutes. Other tests should be conducted to determine if a client is brain dead.

Procedure

- Obtain a signed consent form by the family or the appropriate person designated by the client's living will.
- Monitor arterial blood gases, before and after the ventilator is discontinued.
- Monitor a pulse oximeter, before and following the removal of the ventilator.
- Monitor vital signs before and during the test.
- Discontinue the ventilator. Give 6 L/min of oxygen when indicated by the health care provider.
- Observe chest for any spontaneous breathing or any effort to breathe.
- Restart ventilator if indicated.

Factors Affecting Diagnostic Tests

- Misinterpretation of brain death, such as from drug or alcohol intoxication, high-level spinal cord injury affecting respiration, myasthenia gravis, and other neurological causes.

NURSING IMPLICATIONS WITH RATIONALE

- Verify that the consent form is signed by the person(s) named in the living will or family members.
- Explain the test to the family members or the person(s) responsible for the client (see *Procedure*).
- Tell the client's family or the person(s) responsible for the client that the ventilator is usually restarted. The health care provider should explain the procedure to these individuals. If the test is positive that the client is brain dead, the health care provider may request that the family donate the client's tissue or organs, as appropriate.

Client Teaching

- Be available to answer the family and persons responsible for client care, or refer the questions to other health professionals.
- Be supportive to the family and others. Permit them time to express their concerns and grieve.

A

Arthrography

Normal Finding

Knee: Normal medial meniscus.

Shoulder: Bicipital tendon sheath, normal joint capsule, and intact subscapular bursa.

Description

Arthrography is an x-ray examination of a joint using air, contrast media, or both in the joint space. The purposes are to detect abnormalities of the cartilage and/or ligaments (e.g., tears) and to visualize structures of the joint capsule.

This procedure is performed when a client complains of persistent knee or shoulder pain or discomfort. Usually it is performed on an outpatient basis.

Arthrography is not indicated if the client is having an acute arthritic attack, has a joint infection, or is pregnant.

Purposes

- To visualize the structures of the joint capsule.
- To detect abnormalities of the cartilage and/or ligaments (tears).

Clinical Problems

Abnormal Findings: Osteochondritis dissecans, osteochondral fractures, cartilage abnormalities, synovial abnormalities, tears of the ligaments, and joint capsule abnormalities. *Shoulder:* Adhesive capsulitis, tears of rotator cuff, and bicipital tenosynovitis or tears.

Procedure

- Food and fluids are not restricted.
- Prepare the knee or shoulder area using aseptic technique.
- Local anesthetic is administered to puncture site.
- A needle is inserted into the joint space (e.g., knee), and synovial fluid is aspirated for synovial fluid analysis.
- Air and/or contrast medium is injected into the joint space, and x-rays are taken.
- The knee may be bandaged.

Factors Affecting Diagnostic Results

- None known.

NURSING IMPLICATIONS WITH RATIONALE

- Explain the procedure to the client to allay anxiety and fear and to increase the client's cooperation.

A

- Obtain a client history of allergies to seafood, iodine, and contrast dye. An antihistamine, diphenhydramine (Benadryl), may be given orally or intravenously if there is a history of iodine or seafood hypersensitivity.
- Provide ongoing assessment before, during, and after the procedure, including vital signs, discomfort, and others.

Client Teaching

- Inform the client that changes in body positions may be asked for during the procedure. At other times, the client is to remain still.
- Inform the client that he or she will not be asleep during the arthrography and may ask questions prior to, during, and after the test procedure.

Posttest

- Apply an Ace bandage to the leg, including the knee, if indicated, to decrease swelling and pain.

Client Teaching

- Instruct the client to rest the joint for the time specified, usually 12 hours.
- Inform the client that a crepitant noise may be heard with joint movement. This should stop in a few days; however, if the noise persists, the health care provider should be contacted.
- Instruct the client to apply an ice bag with a cover to the affected joint to decrease swelling if noted. An analgesic for pain and/or discomfort may be ordered or suggested.

Arthroscopy

Normal Finding

Normal lining of the synovial membrane. Cartilage is smooth and white, and ligaments and tendons are intact.

Description

Arthroscopy is an endoscopic examination of the interior aspect of a joint (usually the knee) using a fiberoptic endoscope. Normally an *arthrography* is performed prior to arthroscopy.

Arthroscopy may be used to diagnose meniscal, patellar, extrasynovial, and synovial diseases; to perform joint surgery; and to monitor disease processes or the effects of a medical or surgical therapeutic regimen. Frequently biopsy or surgery is performed during the test procedure. For a surgical procedure, spinal or general anesthesia is used, and for visualization of the interior joint space, a local anesthetic is used. Arthroscopy is contraindicated if a wound or severe skin infection is present or if the client has severe fibrous ankylosis.

A

Purposes

- To diagnose meniscal, patellar, extrasynovial, and synovial diseases.
- To perform joint surgery.

Clinical Problems

Abnormal Findings: Meniscal disease with torn lateral or medial meniscus, patellar disease, chondromalacia, patellar fracture, osteochondritis dissecans, osteochondromatosis, torn ligaments, Baker cysts, synovitis, and rheumatoid and degenerative arthritis.

Procedure

- A consent form should be signed by the client.
- There is no food or fluid restriction for local anesthetic. NPO after midnight for spinal and general anesthesia.
- Local, spinal, or general anesthesia is used, depending on the purpose and procedure for the test.
- Ace bandage and/or tourniquet may be applied to decrease blood volume in the leg.
- The arthroscope is inserted into the interior joint for visualization, for draining fluid from the joint, for biopsy, and/or for surgery.
- A dressing is applied to the incision site of the affected joint.

Factors Affecting Diagnostic Results

- Septic technique used during test procedure could cause pain and discomfort and could further complicate the joint disease.

NURSING IMPLICATIONS WITH RATIONALE

- Check on the type of anesthesia to be used. If general or spinal anesthesia is ordered, inform the client to remain NPO after midnight prior to the test.
- Assess the involved area for possible skin lesion or infection.
- Determine the client's anxiety level, and be available to answer questions. Be prepared to repeat information if the level of anxiety or fear is determined to be high.
- Use aseptic technique throughout the procedure. Sepsis can cause severe complications to the joint and tissues.

Posttest

- Assess the client before, during, and after procedure, including vital signs, bleeding, and swelling. Report abnormal findings to the health care provider.
- Apply an ice bag with cover to the area as indicated.
- Administer an analgesic for pain or discomfort as ordered.
- Answer the client's and family members' questions. If unable to supply answers, refer the questions to the appropriate health professionals.

Client Teaching

- Instruct the client to avoid excessive use of the joint for 2–3 days or as ordered. Walking should be minimized.

Barium enema
Lower Gastrointestinal Test, X-ray Examination of the Colon

Normal Finding

Adult: Normal filling, normal structure of the large colon.

Description

The barium enema test is an x-ray examination of the large intestine (colon) to detect the presence of polyps, an intestinal mass, diverticuli, an intestinal stricture/obstruction, or ulcerations. Barium sulfate (single contrast), barium sulfate or another prescribed contrast agent, and air (double contrast or air contrast) are administered slowly through a rectal tube into the large colon. The filling process is monitored by fluoroscopy, and then x-rays are taken. The colon must be free of fecal material so that the barium will outline the large intestine to detect any disorders. The double-contrast technique (barium and air) is useful for identifying polyps.

The barium enema test is indicated for clients complaining of lower abdominal pain and cramps; blood, mucus, or pus in the stool; changes in bowel habits; and changes in stool formation. The test can be performed in a hospital, in a clinic, or at a private laboratory.

Purpose

- To detect disorders of the large intestine.

Clinical Problems

Abnormal Findings: Carcinoma (tumor or lesion), inflammatory disease (ulcerative colitis, granulomatous colitis, diverticulitis), diverticuli, fistulas, polyps, and intussusception.

Procedure

In most institutions, the procedures for the barium enema are similar; however, they usually differ to some degree. Some institutions request that the client maintain a low-residue diet (tender meats, eggs, bread, clear soup, pureed bland vegetables and fruits, potatoes, and boiled milk) for 2–3 days before the test. Abdominal x-rays, ultrasound studies, radionuclide scans, and proctosigmoidoscopy should be done *before* the barium enema. It is important that the colon is free of fecal material.

Prepreparation

- Oral medications should not be given for 24 hours before the test, unless indicated by the health care provider. Narcotics and barbiturates could interfere with fecal elimination before and after the test.
- The client should be on a clear-liquid diet for 18–24 hours before the test. This would include broth, ginger ale, cola, black coffee or tea with sugar only, gelatin, and syrup from canned fruit. Some institutions permit a white chicken sandwich (*no* butter, lettuce, or mayonnaise) or hard-boiled eggs and gelatin for lunch and dinner, then NPO after dinner.
- Encourage the client to increase water and clear liquid intake 24 hours before the test to maintain adequate hydration.
- Prescribe laxatives (e.g., castor oil or magnesium citrate) to be taken the day before the test in the late afternoon or early evening (4 PM to 8 PM).

- A cleansing enema or laxative suppository such as bisacodyl (Dulcolax) may be given the evening before the test.
- Saline enemas (maximum three enemas) should be given early in the morning (6 AM) until the returned solution is clear. Some private laboratories have clients use bisacodyl suppositories in the morning instead of the enemas.
- Black coffee or tea is permitted 1 hour before the test. Some institutions permit dry toast.

Postpreparation

- The client should expel the barium in the bathroom or bedpan immediately after the test.
- Fluid intake should be increased for hydration and to prevent constipation due to retained barium.
- A laxative, such as milk of magnesia or magnesium citrate, or an oil retention enema should be given to remove the barium from the colon. A laxative may need to be repeated the day after the test.

Factors Affecting Diagnostic Results

- Inadequate bowel preparation with fecal material remaining in the colon could affect results.
- The use of barium sulfate in upper gastrointestinal and small bowel studies 2–3 days before the barium enema test could affect the results.

NURSING IMPLICATIONS WITH RATIONALE

Pretest (see also Procedure—Prepreparation)

- Review the written procedure for that institution. Explain the procedure to the client. Procedures do differ from one institution to another. Usually the preparations for a barium enema have similarities (clear liquids, increased fluid intake, laxatives, and cleansing enemas). Fecal material in the large intestine (bowel or colon) should be completely eliminated.
- List the procedure step by step for the client. Most private laboratories and hospitals have written preparation slips. The procedure may be sent to the client at home.
- Emphasize the importance of following dietary restrictions and of bowel preparation. Adequate prepreparation is essential or the test may need to be repeated.
- Notify the health care provider if the client has severe abdominal cramps and pain prior to the test. The barium enema test should not be performed if the client has severe ulcerative colitis, suspected perforation, or tachycardia.

Client Teaching

- Explain to the client that he or she will be lying on a tilting x-ray table for positioning purposes to increase the barium flow into the colon. Explain that a technician will be with him or her and will explain each step of the procedure.
- Inform the client that the test takes approximately ½–1 hour to complete. Tell the client to take deep breaths through the mouth, which helps to decrease tension and to promote relaxation.
- Administer a laxative or cleansing enema after the test. Instruct the client to check the color of the stools for 2–3 days. Stools may be light in color because of the barium sulfate. Absence of stool should be reported. Retention of barium sulfate after the test could cause obstruction and/or fecal impaction.

Biopsy (bone marrow, breast, endometrium, kidney, liver, lung, lymph nodes, prostate gland, and thyroid)

Normal Finding

Normal cells and tissue from the bone marrow, breast, endometrium of the uterus, kidney, liver, lymph nodes, prostate gland, and thyroid.

Description

Biopsy is the removal and examination of tissue from the body. Usually biopsies are performed to detect malignancy or to identify the presence of a disease process. Biopsies can be obtained by (1) aspiration by applying suction; (2) the brush method, using stiff bristles that scrape fragments of cells and tissue; (3) excision by surgical cutting at tissue site; (4) fine-needle or needle aspiration at tissue site with or without the guidance of ultrasound; (5) insertion of a needle through the skin; and (6) punch biopsy, using a punch-type instrument.

   Biopsies are performed on various organs and body structures, such as bone marrow, the breast, endometrium of the uterus, kidney, and liver. The methods used for the biopsy tissues of various organs may differ.

Bone Marrow: The bone marrow is composed of red and yellow marrow. The red marrow produces blood cells, and the yellow marrow has fat cells and connective tissue. The sternum and iliac crest are the most common sites for bone marrow aspiration.

Breast: Biopsy of the breast is mainly performed to determine if a breast lesion (nodule or mass) is a cyst or is cancerous. The majority of breast lumps are benign. The site of the breast lesion can be identified with the use of a fixed grid on the mammogram.

Endometrium of the Uterus: Endometrial biopsy can detect polyps, cancer, inflammatory condition, and defect in ovulation. The biopsy collection using a probe (blind technique) can be performed in the health care provider's office. Complications include perforation of the uterus, excessive bleeding, and aborting an early pregnancy. This procedure should not be performed if there is purulent discharge from the vagina. An endometrial biopsy differs from a D & C (dilation and curettage) in that dilation of the cervix is not needed. D & C requires general anesthesia because the entire endometrium is curettaged. With an endometrial biopsy, the affected tissue in the uterus could be missed with a sample biopsy; whereas with a D & C the total endometrium is obtained.

Kidney (Renal): A kidney biopsy is usually done with the guidance of ultrasound or fluoroscopy. The biopsy is performed to determine the cause of renal disease, to rule out metastatic malignancy of the kidney, or to determine if rejection of a kidney transplant is occurring. The biopsy can be obtained in three ways: (1) by use of a cystoscope, (2) by excision of the kidney, taking a wedge of tissue, and (3) percutaneously, using a needle.

Liver: Liver biopsy is not usually done unless the liver enzymes are greatly increased. It is performed to rule out metastatic malignancy or to detect a cyst or the presence of cirrhosis. Ultrasound is used to guide the biopsy needle to the pathologic site. Prior to a liver biopsy, the following laboratory levels should be checked: prothrombin time (PT), partial thromboplastin time (PTT), and platelet count. The liver is vascular, and if these laboratory results are abnormal, bleeding could occur following the test procedure.

Lung: Liver biopsy examines the lung tissue for pathological causes of lung disease. The causes could be due to cancer, granulomas, histoplasmosis, sarcoidosis, infection, and other lung diseases. The specimen from the lung could be obtained (1) by bronchial brushing at the affected area, (2) by a needle that is passed through a bronchoscope, or (3) by obtaining a specimen from an open lung biopsy that is performed by thoracotomy in a surgical area such as the operating room. Fluoroscopy is used to obtain the specimen.

Lymph nodes: Lymph node biopsy is usually ordered to detect abnormal tissue in the nodes, frequently the result of metastatic cancer. This is frequently done during the removal of breast tissue during surgery. It is also done to determine the presence of leukemia and lymphoma.

There are three usual sites for biopsies of the lymph nodes: (1) cervical nodes, (2) axillary nodes, and (3) inguinal nodes.

Prostate gland: The main reason for biopsy of the prostate gland is to diagnose whether cancer cells are present. When the prostate-specific antigen (PSA) is over 10 ng/mL or higher the prostate biopsy is usually done. The biopsy tissue also aids in the staging of the cancer tumor.

Though prostate cancer develops slowly, if the PSA is greater than 5 ng/mL, a biopsy of the prostate gland may be suggested.

Thyroid gland: A biopsy of the thyroid gland is the major diagnosis method for thyroid cancer. The biopsy of the thyroid can be performed by (1) needle aspiration or (2) surgical intervention. The biopsy is useful to determine if the mass is a cyst or tumor. The biopsy may also be performed to identify the cause of hyperthyroidism or the cause of an inflammatory thyroid disease.

Purposes

- To identify abnormal tissue from various body sites.
- To detect the presence of a disease process (e.g., cirrhosis).

Clinical Problems

Indications: Blood disorders, malignancies, cysts, polyps, infectious process, progressive disease entities (cirrhosis, nephrosis, lupus nephritis), ovulative defects, and rejection of an organ transplant.

Procedure

- A consent form should be signed by the client.
- Baseline vital signs are taken.
- Biopsy site is anesthetized.

Bone Marrow
- A local anesthetic is injected at the site (sternum or iliac spine).
- A needle with a stylet is inserted through a skin slit into the bone about 3 mm deep.
- The stylet is removed and a 10 mL syringe is attached to the needle. Bone marrow is aspirated; part is used for a blood smear and the remaining amount is placed in a green- or lavender-top tube.

Breast
- Needle aspiration or an excision of breast tissue can be performed.
- The skin is anesthetized; general anesthesia may be used if the biopsy tissue is difficult to obtain.

- A mammogram is usually needed to determine the placement of the needle or the excision site.
- Tissue obtained from biopsy is placed in formalin and sent immediately to the laboratory. The specimen from a needle aspiration is placed on a cytologic slide.

Endometrium of the Uterus

- The client is placed in the lithotomy position.
- A sound (probe) is inserted into the cavity of the uterus to determine its size. This is done as a precaution to prevent perforation of the uterus.
- A suction tube with curette is inserted into the cavity of the uterus, and sample specimens are obtained from the lateral, anterior, and/or posterior uterine wall.
- Specimen(s) is/are placed in formalin solution and sent to the laboratory for histologic testing.

Kidney (Renal) This test can be performed by use of a cystoscope with the brush method, excision of a wedge of renal tissue, or percutaneously with a special needle.

- The client is placed in the prone position.
- With the percutaneous method, the site is determined with the use of ultrasound or fluoroscopy.
- Anesthetic is given according to the procedure chosen.
- With needle insertion, the client is asked to take a breath and hold it. A small tissue specimen is obtained. Pressure is applied to the site for approximately 20 minutes to prevent bleeding, because the kidney tissue is very vascular.

Liver

- NPO for at least 6 hours prior to the test. The liver is less congested without food intake.
- Check that PT, APTT (PTT), and platelet count have been done and documented. Abnormal findings should be reported prior to the procedure to decrease/avoid excessive bleeding following the biopsy.
- A fine needle is inserted, usually with the guidance of ultrasound.
- The client is asked first to take a deep breath, then exhale and hold the breath. With expiration the diaphragm is motionless and remains high in the thorax.
- Apply a pressure dressing.
- The tissue specimen is placed in formalin solution or the specimen is swabbed on a slide and fixed in 95% alcohol.
- Place the client on his or her right side to decrease the chance of hemorrhage.

Lung

Bronchoscopy

- Client is placed in the supine position. A general anesthesia is given. However, the client may be given local anesthesia in which the tongue and the oropharynx are numbed.
- The bronchoscope or fiberoptic scope is passed through the mouth.
- A lung tissue sample is collected using either a biopsy forceps or bronchial brush.

Needle Biopsy

- Client is in a sitting position, bending over with hands on a table. A local anesthetic is injected.
- Client should not cough as the needle is inserted into the posterior chest wall in the intercostal space.
- Petroleum jelly gauze is applied to the injection site.

B

Surgical Biopsy
- General anesthesia is given. A thoracotomy is performed and a tissue specimen is collected from the suspicious area.
- A chest tube may be inserted following the procedure to avoid respiratory problems.

Lymph Nodes

Needle Biopsy
- Local anesthetic is injected.
- A needle attached to a syringe is inserted into the lymph node. The specimen is withdrawn.

Surgical Biopsy
- During surgery for cancer, lymph nodes near the site might be obtained to determine if the cancer has metastasized to the lymph nodes.

Prostate Gland

Transrectal Biopsy
- Client is in a Sim position.
- A rectal exam locates the site for the biopsy. A needle is guided to the site and cells are aspirated.

Transurethral Biopsy
- An endoscope is inserted into the urethra. Tissue from the prostate gland is excised.

Thyroid Gland

Needle Biopsy
- Local anesthetic is injected.
- A needle is inserted into the thyroid tissue. The client is instructed on breathing methods during the needle biopsy process.

Surgical Biopsy
- General anesthesia is administered.
- An incision is made at the site of the suspicious area, and tissue is collected.

Factors Affecting Diagnostic Results

- Blind biopsy can result in missing the diseased site (tissue).
- Improper care to the tissue specimen.

NURSING IMPLICATIONS WITH RATIONALE

- Check that the consent form has been signed.
- Check that the prescribed laboratory tests have been done.
- Explain the biopsy procedure to the client. Explanation can decrease client anxiety and increase cooperation with the procedure.
- Monitor vital signs as prescribed. Frequent vital signs will be taken during the test.
- Observe for bleeding and shortness of breath. If the client is taking warfarin (Coumadin) or any anticoagulant drug, it is advised not to take the drug four days before the test. Check with the health care provider.

Client Teaching

- Instruct the client to report excessive bleeding immediately to the health care provider.
- Instruct the client to report an elevated temperature.

- Instruct the client to take the prescribed pain medication. If pain intensifies, the health care provider should be notified.
- Advise the client to rest for 24 hours following the test procedure.
- Instruct the client to avoid heavy lifting for at least 24 hours, or longer if indicated (e.g., in liver, renal biopsy).
- Advise the client if an antibiotic drug is ordered following the test to take all the antibiotic as ordered. Some clients will stop taking the antibiotic if they feel better. Unless the client has an allergic reaction to the antibiotic, the prescribed amount of antibiotic pills should be taken.

Kidney

- Increase fluid intake following the biopsy.
- Check bowel sounds for several hours following the test. Abdominal intervention can cause a decrease in bowel sounds (decreased peristalsis).
- Instruct the client to report decreased urination or burning when urinating.

Liver

- Avoid heavy lifting.
- Check bowel sounds for several hours following the test. Report an absence of or decreased bowel sounds.

Bone densitometry

Bone Density (BD), Bone Mineral Density (BMD), Bone Absorptiometry

Normal Finding

Normal bone densitometry scan is determined according to the client's age, sex, and height.

Normal: 1 standard deviation below peak bone mass level.

Osteoporosis: Greater than 2.5 standard deviations below peak bone mass level (WHO standard).

Description

The bones are made up of minerals and protein. Bone mass peaks when the person is in the mid-30s. After that, bone is lost at a rate somewhat greater than new bone is made. When a woman reaches menopause, bone loss accelerates to about 1–3% a year. Osteopenia, which is a decrease in bone mass below the normal, is the first to occur. After age 60, bone loss in women slows, but it does not stop, and as she gets older, bone mass loss could be between 35 and 50%. The risk of bone fracture is greater in women than men. Men lose bone also; however, it is at a lower rate than women; 3–5% a decade. Usually, men develop osteoporosis about a decade later than women.

Bone density test is to detect early osteoporosis by determining the density of bone mineral content. Clients who have a loss of bone mineral are readily prone to have fractures. The bones that are usually examined are the lumbar spine and the proximal hip (neck of the femur). Another bone site, the heel bone, can be evaluated according to the client's symptoms.

The dual energy x-ray absorptiometry (DEXA) measures bone mineral density and only exposes the client to a minimal amount of radiation. Images from the detector/camera are computer analyzed to determine the bone mineral content. The computer can calculate the size and thickness of the bone.

Purposes

- To evaluate the bone mineral density.
- To identify early and progressive osteoporosis.

Clinical Problems

Abnormal Findings: Loss of bone mineral content, early and progressive osteoporosis.

Procedure

- A signed consent form may be required.
- No food or fluid restriction is required.
- Client is to remove all metal objects at the area to be scanned (e.g., keys, coins, zippers, belts).
- The client lies on an imaging table with a radiation source below and the detector above that measures the bone's radiation absorption.
- The bone density test takes approximately 30–60 minutes.

Factors Affecting Diagnostic Results

- Metallic objects in the bone scanning site.
- Previous fractures of the bone may increase the bone density.

NURSING IMPLICATIONS WITH RATIONALE

- Obtain family history of osteoporosis and client's skeletal problems, such as loss of height, fractures, and others.

Client Teaching

- Explain the procedure for bone density test.
- Inform the client that the test should not cause pain and the radiation is considered minimal.
- Instruct the client to remove all metal objects that would be within the scanning area.
- Tell the client that the test should take approximately 30–60 minutes.

Bronchography (bronchogram)

Normal Finding

Normal tracheobronchial structure.

Description

Bronchography is an x-ray test to visualize the trachea, bronchi, and entire bronchial tree after a radiopaque iodine contrast liquid is injected through a catheter into the tracheobronchial space. The bronchi are coated with the contrast dye, and a series of x-rays is then taken. Bronchography may be done in conjunction with bronchoscopy.

Bronchography is contraindicated during pregnancy. This test should also not be done if the client is hypersensitive to anesthetics, iodine, or x-ray dyes.

Purpose

- To detect bronchial obstruction, such as foreign bodies and tumors.

Clinical Problems

Indications: Bronchial obstruction (i.e., foreign bodies, tumors, cysts or cavities, bronchiectasis).

B

Procedure

- A consent form should be signed.
- The client should be NPO for 6–8 hours before the test.
- Oral hygiene should be given the night before the test and in the morning. This will decrease the number of bacteria that could be introduced into the lungs.
- Postural drainage is performed for 3 days before the test. This procedure aids in the removal of bronchial mucus and secretions. An expectorant (i.e., potassium iodide) may be ordered for 1–3 days before the test to loosen secretions and could detect an allergy to iodine.
- A sedative and atropine are usually given 1 hour before the test. The sedative/tranquilizer is to promote relaxation; atropine is to reduce secretions during the test.
- A topical anesthetic is sprayed into the pharynx and trachea. A catheter is passed through the nose into the trachea, and a local anesthetic and iodized contrast liquid are injected through the catheter.
- The client is usually asked to change body positions so that the contrast dye can reach most areas of the bronchial tree.
- Following the bronchography procedure, the client may receive nebulization and should perform postural drainage to remove contrast dye. Food and fluids are restricted until the gag (cough) reflex is present.

Factors Affecting Diagnostic Results

- Secretions in the tracheobronchial tree can prevent the contrast dye from coating the bronchial walls.

NURSING IMPLICATIONS WITH RATIONALE

Pretest

- Obtain a signed consent form. Check that the consent form is signed before premedication is given.
- Explain the procedure of the test. Generally, clients are extremely apprehensive about this test and are fearful that they may be unable to breathe. Reassure the client that the airway will not be blocked. Inform the client that he or she may have a sore throat after the test as the result of catheter irritation.
- Obtain a history of hypersensitivity to anesthetics, iodine, and x-ray dyes. Usually the client will receive an expectorant for several days before the test to loosen secretions.
- Record vital signs.

Client Teaching

- Instruct the client on how to perform postural drainage (over the side of the bed or in the Trendelenburg position for 15–20 minutes 3 times a day). It is important that chest secretions be removed prior to the test to ensure good visualization of the bronchial tree.

B

- Encourage the client to relax, and teach relaxation techniques.
- Instruct the client to practice good oral hygiene the night before and the morning of the test. Check the oral hygiene procedure. Dentures should be removed before the test.
- Answer the client's questions, and refer questions you cannot answer to other appropriate health professionals. Permit the client time to express his or her concerns.

Posttest

- Assess for signs and symptoms of laryngeal edema (e.g., dyspnea, hoarseness, apprehension). This could be caused by a traumatic insertion of the catheter.
- Assess for allergic reaction to the anesthetic and iodized contrast dye (i.e., apprehension, flushing, rash, urticaria [hives], dyspnea, tachycardia, and/or hypotension).
- Check the gag reflex to see that it has returned before offering food and fluids. Have the client swallow and cough, or tickle the posterior pharynx with a cotton swab; if gag reflex is present, offer ice chips or sips of water before food.
- Monitor vital signs. The temperature may be slightly elevated for 1 or 2 days after the test.
- Check breath signs. If rhonchi and fever are present, notify the health care provider and record on the client's chart.
- Have the client perform postural drainage posttest. This procedure helps with the removal of the contrast dye. Physiologic damage will not occur if some of the dye remains in the lung for a period of time.
- Offer throat lozenges or an ordered medication for sore throat.
- Be supportive of the client and family. Be available to answer their questions.

Bronchoscopy

Normal Finding

Normal structure and lining of the larynx, trachea, and bronchi.

Description

Bronchoscopy is the direct inspection of the larynx, trachea, and bronchi through a standard metal bronchoscope or a flexible fiberoptic bronchoscope called a bronchofiberscope. The flexible fiberoptic bronchoscope has a lens and light at its distal end, and because of its thinness and its flexibility, it allows for visualization of the segmental and subsegmental bronchi.

Through the bronchoscope, a catheter brush, biopsy forceps, or biopsy needle can be passed to obtain secretions and tissues for cytologic examination. A lung biopsy can be performed through the bronchoscope by the closed technique in which a transbronchial lung biopsy is obtained. When a transbronchial biopsy is performed using a bronchoscope, the specimen from the lesion is obtained using a forceps (with fluoroscopy). A transbronchial needle aspiration biopsy could be used for aspirating a specimen and fluid from the lesion. The open lung biopsy technique is by thoracotomy.

The two main purposes of bronchoscopy are visualization and specimen collection in the tracheobronchial tree. Other purposes include removal of the secretions and laser removal of the lesions.

B

Purposes

- To inspect the larynx, trachea, and bronchus for lesions.
- To remove foreign bodies and secretions from the tracheobronchial area.
- To improve tracheobronchial drainage.

Clinical Problems

Indications: Tracheobronchial lesion (i.e., a tumor), bleeding site, foreign bodies, secretions (liquid and tissue) for cytologic and bacteriologic examinations, mucus plugs, and tracheobronchial drainage.

Procedure

- A consent form for bronchoscopy should be signed by the client or an appropriate family member.
- The client should be NPO for 6 hours before the bronchoscopy and preferably for 8–12 hours.
- The client should remove dentures, contact lenses, and jewelry.
- Obtain a history of hypersensitivity to analgesics, anesthetics, and antibiotics.
- Check and record vital signs.
- Administer premedications.
- Record vital signs, premedications, and when the client voided on the preoperative checklist and the client's chart.
- The client will be lying on a table in the supine or semi-Fowler position with the head hyperextended, or he or she will be seated in a chair. Local anesthetic will be sprayed in the client's throat and nose, and the bronchoscope will be inserted through the client's nose or mouth by the health care provider. It is frequently inserted through the mouth when using the rigid scope and through the nose when using the fiberoptic scope.
- Specimen containers should be labeled, and specimens should be taken immediately to the laboratory. The procedure takes about 1 hour.

Factors Affecting Diagnostic Results

- Improper labeling of the specimen.
- Failure to take specimens immediately to the laboratory.

NURSING IMPLICATIONS WITH RATIONALE

Pretest

- Explain the procedure to the client. Explanation is important to help allay the client's anxiety.
- Check that the consent form is signed and that the client has voided before administering premedications. One of the drugs usually administered is atropine, which causes dryness of the mouth.
- Check that dentures, contact lenses, and jewelry have been removed.
- Obtain vital signs, and prepare a VS flow chart. Record admission and pretest vital signs, which will serve as baseline VS.
- Advise the client that the procedure takes about 1 hour.

Client Teaching

- Instruct the client to relax before and during the test. The premedications will aid in increasing relaxation and decreasing anxiety. Tell the client the health care provider will inform him or her of how the procedure is progressing. Bronchoscopy is usually performed under local anesthesia but could be performed under general anesthesia. The client should be told whether he or she will receive a local or a general anesthetic.
- Inform the client that the drugs will make him or her feel sleepy and the mouth feel dry. The client should remain in bed, and the bed sides should be up after premedications are given.
- Instruct the client to practice breathing in and out through the nose with the mouth opened. This is important if the bronchoscope is inserted through the mouth.
- Encourage the client to ask questions and give him or her time to express concerns. Inform the client that there may be some discomfort but that the spray will help to decrease it. Inform the client that he or she will receive adequate air exchange. Oxygen can be given through the side arm of the bronchoscope or rigid scope and by mask for fiberoptic scope.
- Inform the client that there may be hoarseness and/or a sore throat after the test.

Posttest

- Recognize the complications that can follow bronchoscopy (e.g., laryngeal edema, bronchospasm, pneumothorax, cardiac dysrhythmias, and bleeding from the biopsy site).
- Check VS until stable and as indicated.
- Elevate the head of the bed (semi-Fowler position). If the client is unconscious, turn him or her on the side with the head of the bed slightly elevated.
- Assess for signs and symptoms of respiratory difficulty (i.e., dyspnea, wheezing, apprehension, and decreased breath sounds). Notify the health care provider at once.
- Check for hemoptysis (coughing up excessive bloody secretions) and, if found, notify the health care provider. Inform the client that some blood-tinged mucus may be coughed up and that this is not abnormal. It usually occurs following a biopsy or after a traumatic insertion of the bronchoscope.
- Assess the gag (cough) reflex before giving food and liquids. Ask the client to swallow or cough. It normally takes 2–8 hours before the gag reflex returns. Offer ice chips and sips of water before offering food.
- Offer the client lozenges or prescribed medication for mild throat irritation after the gag reflex is present.
- Be supportive of the client. Touch the client's hand or arm for reassurance, as necessary.

Client Teaching

- Instruct the client not to smoke for 6–8 hours. Smoking may cause the client to cough and start bleeding, especially after a biopsy.
- Inform the client that collection of postbronchoscopic secretions may be required for cytologic testing.

Cardiac Calcium Scoring

Normal Findings

0–5% plaque in the coronary arteries.

Description

The amount of calcium in the coronary arteries can be scored using the multidetector CT (MDCT). Calcium in the coronary vessels is a significant cause of coronary atherosclerotic plaque and coronary disease. Earlier the calcified plaque in the coronary arteries was scored using the electron beam tomography (EBT), but heart motion affected the reading. The MDCT technique is newer and more accurate. The MDCT proves the early presence and severity of heart disease.

An Agatston (calcium) score indicates the amount and degree of calcium (plaque) in the coronary arteries. The following scale gives the Agatston score for the degree of coronary artery disease.

AGATSTON SCORE (CALCIUM)	DEGREE OF CORONARY ARTERY DISEASE
0–10	Minimal
11–100	Moderate
101–400	High
Greater than 400	Severe

Clients with an Agatston score over 400 have a greater occurrence of severe coronary problems, such as myocardial infarction (heart attack), heart failure, coronary bypass, and coronary stents. An extremely high score may indicate a high risk of cardiac death.

Purposes

- To assess the coronary arteries for calcium plaque buildup related to coronary artery disease and heart failure.
- To detect the amount of calcium buildup in the coronary arteries.
- To score the calcium buildup using the Agatston scoring scale.

Clinical Problems

Increased calcium buildup: Myocardial infarction, chest pain (angina), heart failure, shortness of breath, pulmonary emboli.

Procedure

- A signed consent form is usually required.
- Nothing by mouth for 4 to 6 hours before the procedure.
- Obtain baseline vital signs and scheduled VS during the test. If the client has a fast heart rate, a blocker or an ACE inhibitor may be given to slow the heart rate for better visualization of the calcium buildup in the vessel.

- IV dye may be administered intravenously if the calcium score is significantly lower than normal. If the client is on Metformin for diabetes mellitus, the Metformin should be withheld 1 day before the test; otherwise, lactic acidosis could occur due to the iodine contrast dye.

Factors Affecting Diagnostic Results

- Client could not remain still during the test.
- Client will not cooperate during the procedure. This could be due to age or mental status.
- Previous test (prior to 5 days) that used iodinated contrast medium could interfere with the test results.

NURSING IMPLICATIONS WITH RATIONALE

- Obtain a history of the client's complaints and cardiovascular symptoms.
- Ask the client if he or she has a history of allergy to iodinated dye or seafood.
- Explain the test procedure. ECG electrodes are applied to monitor the heart rate during the test. The client will lie in a supine position on a motorized table. The client will advance through a circular scanner and must remain still. At times the client will be told to hold his or her breath. An IV line may be inserted for IV fluids and for the use of IV iodinated dye, if needed. The procedure should take approximately 10 to 15 minutes.
- Observe the client following the test procedure for any adverse reactions to the test (i.e., changes in vital signs, chest pain, shortness of breath).

Client Teaching

- Advise the client to report any unusual symptoms that he or she may have later.
- Tell the client to increase the oral fluid intake especially if an iodine contrast agent was used during the procedure.
- Answer the client's questions or refer them to the health care provider.

Cardiac catheterization*
Cardiac Angiography (angiocardiography), Coronary Arteriography

Normal Finding

Patency of coronary arteries; normal heart size, structure, valves; normal heart and pulmonary pressures; normal left ventricular function; normal wall motion.

---

*Updated by Linda Dechant, APN, MSN, CCRN, CCNS, Clinical Nurse Specialist, Christiana Care Cardiology, Newark, Delaware.

Description

The first cardiac catheterization was performed in 1844 on a horse. It was not until 1929 that the first right-cardiac catheterization was performed on a human; the young Dr. Werner Forssmann catheterized himself. During the 1930s and 1940s there were a number of right-cardiac catheterizations done, but the first left-cardiac catheterization was not performed until the early 1950s. In the late 1960s and during the 1970s, the procedure and equipment for cardiac catheterization were greatly improved.

Cardiac catheterization is a procedure in which a long catheter is inserted into the femoral, brachial, or radial artery for left heart chamber (LHC), or femoral, jugular, or subclavian vein for right heart chamber (RHC). This catheter is threaded to the heart chambers and/or coronary arteries under the guidance of fluoroscopy. Contrast dye is injected for visualizing the heart structures. During injection of the dye, cineangiography is used for filming heart activity. The terms *angiocardiography* and *coronary arteriography* are used interchangeably with the term *cardiac catheterization*; however, with coronary arteriography, dye is injected directly into the coronary arteries, and with angiocardiography, dye is injected into heart, coronary, and/or pulmonary vessels.

With *right-cardiac catheterization*, the catheter is inserted into the femoral vein or an antecubital vein and threaded through the inferior vena cava into the right atrium to the pulmonary artery. Right atrium, right ventricle, and pulmonary artery pressures are measured, and blood samples from the right side of the heart can be obtained. While the dye is being injected, the functions of the tricuspid and pulmonary valves can be observed.

For *left-cardiac catheterization*, the catheter is inserted into the brachial or femoral artery and is advanced retrograde through the aorta to the coronary arteries and/or left ventricle. Dye is injected. The patency of the coronary arteries and/or functions of the aortic and mitral valves and the left ventricle can be observed. This procedure is indicated before heart surgery.

The frequency of complications arising from cardiac catheterizations is less than 2%. The complications that can occur, although rare, are myocardial infarction, cardiac dysrhythmias, cardiac tamponade, pulmonary embolism, cerebral vascular accident, dissection of the coronary arteries, cardiac arrest, and death.

Other rare complications include renal failure or anaphylactic reaction to contrast dye, blood clot at catheter site requiring anticoagulation, or significant internal bleeding near the insertion site, causing retroperitoneal hematomas. Complication to the vessel accessed may include pseudoaneurysm, arterial venous (AV) fistula formation, and artery occlusion.

Purposes

- To identify coronary artery disease (CAD).
- To evaluate cardiac valvular disease.
- To determine pressure in pulmonary vessels or heart chambers.
- To obtain a biopsy of myocardium.
- To evaluate artificial valves.
- To replace aortic valve via percutaneous approach.
- To perform percutaneous valvuloplasty.
- To angioplasty or stent an area resulting from coronary artery disease.
- To determine left ventricular injection fraction.
- To repair APFO, ASD percutaneously.

Clinical Problems

Abnormal Findings: *Right-Sided Cardiac Catheterization:* Tricuspid stenosis, tricuspid regurgitation, pulmonary stenosis, pulmonary hypertension, and septal defects. *Left-Sided Cardiac Catheterization:* Coronary artery disease, partial or complete coronary occlusion, mitral stenosis, mitral regurgitation, aortic regurgitation, aortic stenosis, left ventricular hypertrophy, ventricle aneurysm, and septal defect.

Procedure

- Obtain a signed consent form. Check that the health care provider has discussed possible risk factors before the consent form is signed.
- Food and fluids are restricted for 6–8 hours before the test, according to the hospital's policy. Some institutions permit clear liquids until 4 hours before the test.
- Antihistamines (e.g., diphenhydramine [Benadryl]) and steroids may be ordered the evening before and the morning of the test if the client has a history of allergic reactions.
- Medications should be given as ordered by the health care provider. Oral anticoagulants are discontinued to prevent excessive bleeding. Heparin may be ordered in an acute setting to prevent thrombi. Evaluate the INR (international normalized ratio) prior to procedure. Call the cardiologist if the INR is greater than 1.5.
- The injection site of the arm or groin is shaved and cleansed with antiseptics.
- Modified Allen test must be performed prior to utilizing the radial artery. This ensures collateral circulation to the hand during annulation of artery.
- The client's weight and height should be recorded. These are used to calculate the amount of dye needed (i.e., 1 mL/kg of body weight).
- The client should void before receiving the premedications. Dentures should be removed.
- Record baseline VS. Note the volume intensity of pulses. VS should be monitored during the test. Mark pulses with a pen if obtained via Doppler signal.
- Premedications may be given ½ to 1 hour before the cardiac catheterization.
- The client is positioned on a padded table. Skin anesthetic is given at the site of catheter insertion. Client lies still during insertion of the catheter and filming.
- A 5% dextrose in water (D_5W) infusion is started at a keep-vein-open (KVO) rate for administering emergency drugs, if needed. Occasionally, a higher rate of IV infusion of normal saline solution (NSS) or ½ NSS is administered prior to and during catheterization to prevent renal failure from contrast dye.
- Electrocardiography (ECG) leads are applied to the chest to monitor heart activity.
- A local skin anesthetic is injected at the catheter insertion site. A cutdown to locate the vessel may be needed. The client will feel a hot, flushing sensation for several seconds to a minute as the dye is injected.
- Vital signs and heart rhythm are monitored during the procedure.
- The health care provider may request that the client cough and breathe deeply. Coughing can decrease nausea and dizziness and possible dysrhythmia.
- The procedure takes 1–3 hours.

Factors Affecting Diagnostic Results

- Insufficient amount of contrast dye could affect results.
- Movement by the client could cause complications and interfere with the filming.
- Premature cessation of catheterization due to complications (e.g., anaphylaxis, coronary vasospasm, coronary artery dissection).

NURSING IMPLICATIONS WITH RATIONALE

Pretest

- Explain to the client that the purpose of the test is to check the coronary arteries for blockage, to check for heart valve defects, and/or to measure pressures in the pulmonary vessels, heart chambers, or obtain a biopsy of heart tissue. This test is often done before heart surgery to determine if bypass or valvular surgery is necessary.
- Explain the procedure to the client. The cardiologist or cardiac surgeon should explain the purposes, risk factors, and benefits of the catheterization.
- Obtain a client history of allergic reactions to seafood, iodine, or iodine contrast dye used in other x-ray tests (e.g., intravenous pyelography). A skin test may be performed to determine the severity of the allergy. An antihistamine (e.g., diphenhydramine [Benadryl]) and steroids may be given the day before and/or the day of the test as a prophylactic measure.
- Record baseline VS, and continuously monitor the VS during the procedure.
- Check that the catheter insertion site has been prepped (clipped and cleansed with an antiseptic). This will prevent infection.
- Assess the client with renal insufficiency. Premedication with acetylcysteine and/or sodium bicarbonate IV may be administered for renal protection from contrast dye 24 hours before and after the procedure. Alternatively, the client may receive IV hydration with a large volume of normal saline solution (NSS).
- If the client has diabetes and is on metformin, hold medication 2 days prior and 2 days postprocedure. Metformin and IV contrast may result in lactic acidosis.
- Encourage the client to ask questions, and allow the client and family time to express any concerns. Refer questions you cannot answer to the cardiologist or other health professionals.
- Administer premedications ½–1 hour before the test. Make sure that the client has voided and that the consent form has been signed before giving the premedications.

Client Teaching

- Inform the client that he or she will be in a special cardiac catheterization room. Give information about the padded table, the ECG leads to monitor heart activity, the IV fluids, the local skin anesthetic, and instructions that he or she may receive (such as to cough and to breathe deeply).
- Inform the client that there may be minimal discomfort at the catheter insertion site and from lying on the back. Instruct the client to ask any questions he or she may have during the test. Tell the client to tell the health care provider of any chest pain or difficulty in breathing during the procedure. The client's ECG and VS are monitored.
- Tell the client that a hot, flushing sensation may be felt for a minute or two because of the dye. The reason for this is a brief vasodilation caused by the dye.
- Tell the client that the test takes approximately ½–3 hours.

Posttest

- Monitor VS (blood pressure, pulse, respirations) every 15 minutes the first hour, every 30 minutes until stable, or as ordered. Temperatures are monitored for several days.
- Watch for cardiac rhythm and rate disturbances. Notify cardiologist of any changes from baseline.

C

- Assess client for complaints of chest heaviness, shortness of breath, and abdominal or groin pains. These may indicate complications.
- Observe the catheter insertion site for bleeding or hematoma. Change dressings as needed. If bleeding or hematoma develops at the site, hold pressure for 20 minutes and contact the cardiologist.
- Check peripheral pulses below the insertion site; if the femoral artery was used, then check the popliteal and dorsalis pedis pulses; if the brachial artery was used, then check the radial pulse. If the radial artery is utilized, check the ulnar pulse. Note the strength of the pulse beat. Perform neurovascular assessment of access limb with each vital sign check.
- Encourage client to increase fluid intake to flush dye from system.
- Assess the client's skin color and temperature.
- Be supportive of the client and family. Answer questions, or refer them to the appropriate health professionals. Communicate with the client about the nursing care being given.
- Administer analgesics as ordered for discomfort. Give antibiotics, if ordered.

Client Teaching

- Instruct the client that he or she is to remain on bed rest for 2–4 hours. This largely depends on the type of closure device used. The client can turn from side to side, and the bed may be elevated 30 degrees. The leg should be extended if the femoral artery was used. If the brachial artery was used, the head of the bed can be slightly elevated; however, the arm should be immobilized for 3 hours. If the radial artery is utilized, the compression device should be left on for 2 hours at a minimum. The client must keep the wrist immobilized but may be out of bed for 1 hour. Policy concerning positioning may differ among institutions. Some clients may be discharged on the same day depending on intervention and complications.
- Inform the client on discharge that if he or she experiences a small amount of bleeding, the client should lie down and apply pressure to the site. If there is a moderate to large amount of bleeding, call 911.
- Explain to the client that a small lump may form at the site of the incision. If the lump expands to the size of a golf ball or larger, the client should contact the cardiologist or go to the emergency room.
- The client should not do any heavy lifting or driving for 24–48 hours.
- Encourage fluid intake after the test, unless contraindicated (e.g., in the case of heart failure).

Cervicography (cervigram)

Normal Findings

Normal cervical tissue; no abnormal cells found.

Description

Cervicography is a photographic method to record an image of the cervix. This test may be done in conjunction with a Pap smear, colposcopy, and/or routine gynecologic examination. The Pap smear detects cellular changes, whereas the cervigram is a more sensitive means to detect cervical cancer. It can identify some cancerous lesions that were missed by the Pap smear.

Purpose

- To detect cervical cancer.

Clinical Problems

Abnormal Findings: Cancer of the cervix and invasive cervical cancer.

Procedure

- Food and fluids are not restricted.
- The client is placed in the lithotomy position.
- Acetic acid (5%) is swabbed on the cervical area.
- Pathographs are taken of the cervix.
- Aqueous iodine is then swabbed on the cervix; photos follow.
- An endocervical smear is taken; tissue obtained is applied to a slide(s).

Factors Affecting Diagnostic Results

- Cervical mucus that was not removed from the cervix prior to the application of acetic acid and the photography.

NURSING IMPLICATIONS WITH RATIONALE

- Obtain a signed consent form.
- Obtain a history of any gynecologic health problems (e.g., discharge, abnormal bleeding).
- Explain the procedure to the client. Explain that she may experience some discomfort due to the body position and the procedure; however, the discomfort should be mild and short term.
- Be supportive of the client. Allow the client time to express her fears and concerns.

Client Teaching

- Inform the client that she may experience a brown vaginal discharge following the procedure for a few days. The brown discharge is most likely due to the iodine swabbed on the cervix.
- Instruct the client that if great discomfort or heavy discharge occurs, the health care provider should be informed.

Cholangiography (intravenous, percutaneous, t-tube cholangiography)

Normal Finding

Patent biliary ducts (absence of stones and strictures).

Description

Intravenous (IV) cholangiography examines the biliary ducts (hepatic ducts within the liver, the common hepatic duct, the cystic duct, and the common bile duct) by radiographic and tomographic visualization. Often the gallbladder is not well visualized. The contrast substance, an iodine preparation such as iodipamide meglumine (Cholografin), is injected intravenously. Approximately

15 minutes later x-rays are taken. IV cholangiography is a tedious and time-consuming test, and reactions are more common with the IV contrast substance than with the oral agents.

Percutaneous cholangiography is indicated when biliary obstruction is suspected. The contrast substance is directly instilled into the biliary tree. The process is visualized by fluoroscopy, and spot films are taken.

T-tube cholangiography, also known as postoperative cholangiography, may be done 7–8 hours after a cholecystectomy to explore the common bile duct for patency of the duct and to see if any gallstones are left. During the operation, a T-shaped tube is placed in the common bile duct to promote drainage. The contrast substance is injected into the T-tube. A stone or two could be missed during a cholecystectomy, causing occlusion of the duct.

Clinical Problems

TEST	INDICATIONS/PURPOSES
IV cholangiography	To detect stricture, stones, or tumor in the biliary system
Percutaneous cholangiography	To detect obstruction of the biliary system caused from stones, cancer of the pancreas
T-tube cholangiography	To detect obstruction of the common bile duct from stones or stricture; fistula

Procedure

IV Cholangiography
- A consent form for IV cholangiography should be signed.
- The client should be NPO for 8 hours before the test. Some radiologists encourage fat-free liquids before the test to prevent renal toxicity caused by the injected dye.
- A laxative (i.e., citrate of magnesium or castor oil) may be given the night before the test, and a cleansing enema may be given in the morning. Keeping the gastrointestinal tract clear can prevent shadows in the x-ray films. Check with the radiology department for the exact preparation needed.
- A contrast agent, iodipamide meglumine (Cholografin) is injected intravenously while the client is lying on a tilting x-ray table. X-rays are taken every 15–30 minutes until the common bile duct is visualized.

Percutaneous Cholangiography
- A consent form for percutaneous cholangiography should be signed.
- The client should be NPO for 8 hours before the test.
- A laxative the night before and cleansing enema the morning of the test may be ordered.
- Preoperative medications usually include sedatives/tranquilizers. An antibiotic may be ordered for 24–72 hours before the test for prophylactic purposes.
- The client is placed on a tilting x-ray table that rotates. The upper right quadrant of the abdomen is cleansed and draped. A local (skin) anesthetic is given.
- The client should exhale and hold his or her breath while a needle is inserted with the guidance of fluoroscopy into the biliary tree. Bile is withdrawn, and the contrast substance is then injected. Spot films are taken.
- A sterile dressing is applied to the puncture site.

T-tube Cholangiography
- A consent form for T-tube cholangiography should be signed.
- The client should be NPO for 8 hours before the test.
- A cleansing enema may be ordered the morning before the test.

- The client lies on an x-ray table, a contrast agent such as sodium diatrizoate (Hypaque) is injected into the T-tube, and an x-ray is taken. The final x-ray is taken 15 minutes later.
- The T-tube may be removed after the procedure or it may be left in place.

Factors Affecting Diagnostic Results

- Obesity and gas or fecal material in the intestines can affect the clarity of the x-ray.

NURSING IMPLICATIONS WITH RATIONALE

Pretest

- Explain to the client the purpose and procedure for the IV cholangiography, percutaneous cholangiography, or T-tube cholangiography. Check with your institution to see if procedures differ, and make modifications in your explanation to the client. Explain the procedure step by step for the client, as requested. This can decrease high levels of anxiety.
- Obtain a client history of allergies to seafood, iodine, or x-ray dye. Report a history of allergies to these substances to the health care provider, and record in the client's chart.
- Permit the client to express his or her concerns. Answer questions, if possible. Refer questions you cannot answer to other health professionals.
- Check that the consent form has been signed by the client before giving a sedative and before the test.
- Administer the pretest orders (i.e., laxatives, sedatives, etc.).
- Inform the client having IV cholangiography that the test may take several hours (up to 4 hours).

Posttest

- Observe for signs and symptoms of allergic reaction to contrast agents (e.g., nausea; vomiting, flushing; rash; urticaria [hives]; hypotension; slurred, thick speech; and dyspnea).
- Check the infusion site for signs of phlebitis (i.e., pain, redness, swelling). Apply warm compresses to the infusion site if symptoms are present, as ordered.
- Check vital signs as ordered following the percutaneous cholangiography.

Client Teaching

- Instruct the client to remain in bed for 6 hours following percutaneous cholangiography.
- Advise the client to watch for symptoms of infections, such as fever, pain, and redness at the site.

Cholecystography (oral)
Gallbladder Radiography, Gallbladder (GB) Series

Normal Finding

Normal size and structure of gallbladder. No gallstones.

Description

Oral cholecystography is an x-ray test used to visualize gallstones in the gallbladder. There are two types of gallstones: radiopaque, usually composed of calcium carbonate, and radiolucent, composed of cholesterol or bile pigment. The radiolucent stones are the most common ones and can be visualized using contrast material (radiopaque dye) absorbed by the gallbladder. It takes 12–14 hours for the dye to be concentrated in the gallbladder. Nonfunctioning liver cells can hamper the excretion of the radiopaque dye.

Failure to visualize the gallbladder could be due to hypermotility of the bowel (diarrhea), liver disease, obstruction of the cystic duct, and inadequate client preparation (i.e., a high-fat diet the night before will cause the gallbladder to empty, thus losing the dye). If the gallbladder cannot be visualized using an oral-contrast substance, the IV cholangiography may be ordered.

Immediately after the oral cholecystography test, the client may be given a fat-stimulus meal. Fluoroscopic examination and x-rays are taken to observe the ability of the gallbladder to empty the dye. If x-rays of the gastrointestinal tract are ordered, the gallbladder x-ray should be obtained first, because barium could interfere with the test results.

Purposes

- To detect stones or tumor in the gallbladder.
- To check for obstruction of the cystic duct.

Clinical Problems

Abnormal Findings: Cholelithiasis (gallstones), neoplasms (tumors) of the gallbladder, cholecystitis (inflammation of the gallbladder, with or without stones), and obstruction of the cystic duct.

Procedure

- The client should have a fat-free diet 24 hours before the x-ray. Some x-ray departments suggest a high-fat meal at noon to empty the gallbladder and then a low-fat meal in the evening. After the dinner meal the night before the test, the client should be NPO except for sips of water.
- Two hours after the dinner meal, radiopaque tablets are administered according to the directions on the package. There are various commercial contrast agents (e.g., iopanoic acid [Telepaque], calcium or sodium ipodate [Oragrafin], iodoalphionic acid [Priodax], and iodipamide meglumine [Cholografin]). The client should take the tablets or capsules (six tablets of iopanoic acid) 5 minutes apart with a full glass of water (240 mL total).
- No laxatives should be taken until after the x-ray tests. Some x-ray departments request a saline enema the morning of the test to clear the gastrointestinal tract so that fecal material does not interfere with the gallbladder test.
- A high-fat meal (cream, butter, eggs) or synthetic fat-containing substances (Bilevac) may be given in the x-ray department after the fasting x-rays are taken. Post–fatty-meal films will be taken at intervals to determine how fast the gallbladder expels the dye.
- The fasting x-ray tests (stage I) takes from 45 minutes to 1 hour, and the post–fatty-meal tests (stage II) take another 1–2 hours.

Factors Affecting Diagnostic Results

- Inadequate patient preparation (i.e., a high-fat meal the night before, not taking all the tablets).
- Gastrointestinal series, barium enema, thyroid scan, I-131 uptake before the cholecystography test.
- Diarrhea or vomiting, which can inhibit absorption of the contrast substance.
- Liver disease.

NURSING IMPLICATIONS WITH RATIONALE

- Explain the test purpose and procedure to the client. Check your x-ray department's procedure for changes, and modify the procedure if needed. Some institutions send a written procedure to clients who are not hospitalized.
- Obtain a history of client allergies to seafood, iodine, or x-ray dye.
- Observe for signs and symptoms of jaundice (e.g., yellow sclera of the eyes, yellow skin, and a serum bilirubin level greater than 3 mg/dL).
- Administer the radiopaque tablets every 5 minutes with a full glass of water 2 hours after the dinner meal. Clients may take the tablets on their own, but they may need to be reminded.
- Observe for signs and symptoms of allergic reaction to the radiopaque tablets (e.g., elevated temperature, rash, urticaria [hives], hypotension, thick speech, and/or dyspnea).
- Report vomiting and diarrhea prior to the test to the health care provider. The tablets may not be absorbed because of hypermotility. The test is then canceled.
- Report to the health care provider and/or the x-ray department if the client is scheduled for a barium enema, gastrointestinal series, thyroid scan, or I-131 uptake before the GB series. These tests should be done after the GB series to prevent test interference.

Client Teaching

- Inform the client that the evening meal before the test should be fat free. If there are foods high in fat on the tray (e.g., whole milk, cream, butter, sauces, and fatty meats), the client should not eat them. In some institutions coffee or tea with sugar is given in the morning.
- Explain to the client that it is not uncommon for the test to be repeated and that he or she should not be alarmed. If the test is repeated, the client should remain on a low-fat diet, and the radiopaque tablets should be taken again as directed.
- Inform the client that the test does not hurt. Check to determine if there are two stages of the test; the first stage takes approximately 45 minutes to 1 hour. If the second stage is ordered, the client will receive a high-fat meal or fat-containing agent, and then more x-ray pictures will be taken.

Chorionic villi biopsy (CVB)

Normal Finding

Normal fetal cells.

C

Description

Chorionic villi sampling can detect early fetal abnormalities. Fetal cells are obtained by suction from fingerlike projections around the embryonic membrane, which eventually becomes the placenta. The test is performed between the 8th and 10th weeks of pregnancy. After the 10th week, maternal cells begin to grow over the villi.

The advantages of CVB over amniocentesis is that CVB may be performed earlier, and results can be obtained in a few days and not weeks. CVB can diagnose many chromosomal and biochemical fetal disorders. The disadvantage is that CVB cannot determine neural-tubal defects and pulmonary maturity.

Purpose

- To detect chromosomal disorders.

Clinical Problems

Indications: Chromosomal disorders, hemoglobinopathies such as sickle-cell anemia, and lyso-somal storage disorders such as Tay-Sachs disease.

Procedure

- A consent form should be signed by the client.
- There is no food or fluid restriction.
- Place the client in the lithotomy position.
- Ultrasound is used to verify the placement of the catheter at the villi. Suction is applied, and tissue is removed from the villi.
- Test takes approximately 30 minutes.

Factors Affecting Diagnostic Results

- Performing test after 10 weeks of gestation.

NURSING IMPLICATIONS WITH RATIONALE

- Obtain a history of last menstrual period (LMP) from the client and a history of family genetic disorders.
- Assess for signs of spontaneous abortion resulting from procedure, such as cramping, bleeding.
- Assess for infection resulting from procedure, such as chills, fever.
- Be supportive of client and family. Be a good listener.

Client Teaching

- Explain to the client that she will be in a lithotomy position and that ultrasound is used during the procedure.
- Instruct the client to report if excessive bleeding or severe cramping occurs after the procedure.

Colonoscopy*

Normal Finding
Normal mucosa of the large intestine; absence of pathology.

Description
Colonoscopy, an endoscopic procedure, is an inspection of the large intestine (colon) using a long, flexible fiberscope (colonoscope). The instrument is inserted anally and is advanced through the rectum, the sigmoid colon, and the large intestine to the cecum.

This test is useful for evaluating suspicious lesions in the large colon, such as polyps that could later develop into cancerous tumors, tumor mass, and inflammatory tissue. Biopsy of the tissue or polyp can be obtained. The biopsy forceps passes through the scope to obtain the tissue specimen. Polyps can be removed with the use of an electrocautery snare.

Colonoscopy should not be done on pregnant women near term, after recent abdominal surgery, or on a confused/uncooperative client. Caution should be taken in performing a colonoscopy following an acute myocardial infarction, in acute diverticulitis, or in severe (active) ulcerative colitis. Rarely colon perforation is caused by the fiberscope. Bleeding may occur after a biopsy or polypectomy.

Screening for polyps for the client over the age of 50 is important. However, if the client has a familial history of colon cancer, a colonoscopy may be recommended before the age of 50. Colon cancer is usually caused by adenomatous polyps, and if the polyps are removed early, cancer of the colon would be unlikely.

Virtual Colonography: A virtual colonography is an examination of the colon by computed tomography scanning of the entire large colon. It is currently not as accurate as the traditional colonoscopy, because it is difficult with this procedure to detect small polyps. In a major study, virtual colonography missed 45% of polyps that were 5 mm or smaller. Differentiation of stool from polyps can be difficult. The client still has to undergo the same "colon prep" before a virtual colonography as the person would with a traditional colonoscopy. Traditional colonoscopy is required to remove a polyp found on a CT scan of the colon. Virtual colonography has an advantage over traditional colonoscopy in that no sedatives are required. The procedure is less invasive. Additional information outside the colon may also be found, for example, incidental renal cell cancer.

Purposes
- To detect the origin of lower intestinal bleeding.
- To identify polyps in the large intestine.
- To screen for benign or malignant lesions (tumors) in the colon.

Clinical Problems
Indications: Intestinal bleeding, periodical screening for polyps or tumors, diverticular disease, benign or malignant lesions, and ulcerative colitis.

---

*Updated by Dr. Warren G. Butt, Gastroenterology-Stomach-Colon-Liver, Newark, Delaware.

Procedure

- A consent form should be signed by the client.
- Specific laboratory tests may be ordered, such as CBC and INR (if the client has taken Coumadin).
- Withhold medications that interfere with coagulation (Coumadin and Plavix), aspirin, NSAIDs (Advil, Motrin), iron medication, and alcohol 1 week prior to the test.
- Barium sulfate from other diagnostic studies can decrease visualization; therefore, the colonoscopy should not be attempted within 10 days to 2 weeks of a barium study.
- Avoid using soapsuds enemas. These can irritate the intestine.
- Emergency drugs and equipment should be available for hypersensitivity to medications (premedications and anesthetic).
- Specimen containers should be labeled with the client's name, date, and the type of tissue.
- Client should be accompanied by someone who can drive him or her home following the test.
- The procedure takes approximately 15 minutes to 1 hour.

Pretest Procedure

- The day before the procedure, the client may have "clear liquids" only, which include water, tea, coffee (without milk), strained fruit juices without pulp (apple, white grape, lemonade), plain gelatin (without added fruits or toppings), clear broths or bouillon (chicken or beef without noodles or solids), noncarbonated sports drinks (e.g., Gatorade), carbonated and noncarbonated soft drinks. All red fluids should be avoided due to the color of the dye, which can affect the visualization of the test.
- Two days prior to the exam, seeds, nuts, corn, and any other forms of roughage or fiber should be avoided. The client should *not* take Metamucil or Citrucel.
- One day before the test, the client should *not* eat any solid food.

Preparation: Use of Golytely/Colyte Solution or Magnesium Citrate Solution

Day Before the Test:

- Client taking Coumadin or Plavix should contact the physician's office. Discontinue iron supplements.
- Client should prepare GoLYTELY or Colyte solution according to instructions and refrigerate solution.
- Client should drink GoLYTELY/Colyte as instructed, usually 7 PM to 10 PM.
- If magnesium citrate is ordered, the client should purchase two 10-ounce bottles of magnesium citrate and follow the instructions given by the health care provider or physician.

Medication Procedure

- Intravenous fluids with propofol (Diprivan), midazolam (Versed), or meperidine (Demerol) for conscious sedation is given immediately prior to the test.

Factors Affecting Diagnostic Results

- A soapsuds enema can cause intestinal irritation.
- Barium sulfate from other diagnostic studies can decrease visualization; therefore, the study should not be attempted within 10 days to 2 weeks of a barium study.
- Inadequate bowel preparation with fecal material remaining in the colon will decrease visualization.

NURSING IMPLICATIONS WITH RATIONALE

Pretest

- The client should follow the pretest preparation procedure.
- Explain the test procedure. The client lies in the Sims position or left lateral position. A lubricated colonoscope is inserted. Air will be insufflated for better visualization. Photos are usually taken of any abnormal tissue or polyps.
- Record baseline vital signs and, if available, pertinent laboratory values.
- Report anxiety and fears to the physician or health professional prior to the test.

Client Teaching

- Instruct the client to bring someone to drive him or her home.
- Instruct the client to breathe deeply and slowly through the mouth during the insertion of the colonoscope.
- Inform the client that the procedure takes approximately 15 minutes to 1 hour.

Posttest

- Monitor vital signs and report abnormal changes.
- Assess for anal bleeding, abdominal distention, severe pain, severe abdominal cramps, and fever, and report any of the signs or symptoms immediately.

Colposcopy

Normal Finding

Normal appearance of the vagina and cervical structures.

Description

Colposcopy is the examination of the vagina and cervix using a binocular instrument (colposcope) that has a magnifying lens and a light. This test is for identifying precancerous lesions of the cervix and can be performed in the gynecologist's office or in the hospital. After a positive Papanicolaou (Pap) smear or a suspicious cervical lesion, colposcopy is indicated for examining the vagina and cervix more thoroughly. Atypical epithelium, leukoplakia vulvae, and irregular blood vessels can be identified with this procedure, and photographs and a biopsy specimen can be obtained.

Because this test has become more popular, there has been a decreased need for conization (surgical removal of a cone of tissue from the cervical os). Colposcopy is also useful for monitoring women whose mothers received diethylstilbestrol during pregnancy; these women are prone to develop precancerous and cancerous lesions of the vagina and cervix. Colposcopy is used to monitor female clients who have had cervical lesions removed.

Purposes

- To identify precancerous lesions of the cervix.
- To identify vaginal lesions.

Clinical Problems

Indications: Vaginal and cervical lesions, abnormal cervical tissue after a positive Pap smear, irregular blood vessels, leukoplakia vulvae, dysplasia and cervical lesions, and vaginal and cervical tissue changes for women whose mothers took diethylstilbestrol during pregnancy.

Procedure

- A consent form should be signed by the client.
- Food and fluids are not restricted.
- The client's clothes should be removed, and the client should wear a gown and be properly draped.
- The client assumes a lithotomy position (legs in stirrups). A speculum is inserted into the vagina, and a long, dry cotton swab applicator is used to clear away any cervical secretions. Another long cotton-swab applicator with saline may be used to swab the cervix for visualizing vascular patterns.
- Acetic acid (3%) is applied to the vagina and cervix. This produces color changes in the cervical epithelium and helps in detecting abnormal changes.
- A biopsy specimen of suspicious tissues and photographs may be taken. Pressure should be applied to control bleeding at the biopsy site, or cautery may be used.
- A vaginal tampon may be worn after the procedure.
- The test takes approximately 15–20 minutes.

Factors Affecting Diagnostic Results

- Mucus, cervical secretions, creams, and medications can decrease visualization.

NURSING IMPLICATIONS WITH RATIONALE

- Explain the purpose and procedure to the client.
- A consent form should be signed by the client.
- Encourage the client to ask questions and to express any concerns or fears. Reducing anxiety is important for the client and for the test. Remain with the client during the procedure.
- Place the biopsy tissue into a bottle containing a preservative and place the cells, if obtained, on a slide and spray them with a fixative solution.

Client Teaching

- Inform the client that she should not experience pain but there may be some discomfort with the insertion of the speculum or when the biopsy specimen is taken.
- Tell the client that the test takes 15–20 minutes.

Posttest Client Teaching

- Inform the client that she may have some bleeding for a few hours because of the biopsy. Tell the client that she can use tampons, and that if bleeding becomes heavy and it is not her menstrual period, she should call the gynecologist.
- Instruct the client not to have intercourse for a week until the biopsy site is healed or as ordered by the health care provider.
- Inform the client that she should be notified of the results, and tell her to call if she has not heard from the office in a week.

Computed tomography (CT) scan, computed axial tomography (CAT)*

CAT Scan, Computed Transaxial Tomography (CTT), EMI Scan

Normal Finding

Normal tissue; no pathologic findings.

Description

The computed tomography scan was developed in England in 1972 by Electric Music Industries Ltd., and was originally called the EMI scan. Other names for the CT scan are computed axial tomography, or CAT scan; computed transaxial (transverse) tomography, or CTT scan; and computer-assisted transaxial tomography, or CATT scan. The preferred term is "computed tomography," or CT scan.

The CT scanner produces a narrow x-ray beam that examines body sections from 360 degrees. The CT scanner's tube and detectors rotate around the client, who is lying on a table. It produces a series of cross-sectional images in sequence that build up a two-dimensional (2D) picture of the organ or structure. The traditional x-ray takes a flat or frontal picture, which also gives a two-dimensional view. The CT scanner is about 100 times more sensitive than the x-ray machine in separating different soft tissue densities. Although it is a costly diagnostic test, CT scanning is popular because it can diagnose at an earlier stage.

The CT scan can be performed with or without iodinated contrast media (dye). It is not an invasive test unless contrast dye is used. The contrast dye causes a greater tissue absorption and is referred to as *contrast enhancement*. This enhancement enables small abnormalities to be seen. Contraindications with using contrast would include clients having heart failure, pregnancy, renal insufficiency, and severe asthma.

CT is capable of scanning the head (internal auditory canal, brain, eye orbits, sinuses, and neck), abdomen (stomach, small and large intestines, liver, spleen, pancreas, bile duct, kidney, and adrenals), pelvis (bladder, reproductive organs, and small and large bowel within pelvis), chest (lung, heart, and mediastinal structure), and bones and joints. Magnetic resonance imaging (MRI), a noninvasive test, has *not* replaced CT scans; see discussion of MRI on pages 561–564.

Recent advances in helical (spiral) CT scanning techniques in combination with multirow solid-state detector arrays have allowed greater anatomic coverage with shorter scan times. This allows the imaging without blurring of moving organs such as the heart, including such small objects as the coronary arteries. Helical (spiral) CT imaging can take place in 30 seconds and can be performed with one breath held. This new technique is called multislice CT (MSCT).

Head and Brain CT: The CT of the brain/head provides two-dimensional views of the brain consisting of cross-sectional images of brain tissue layers. This procedure can differentiate between tumors, aneurysms, cerebral infarction, and intracranial hemorrhage and hematoma. Also, this CT scan can detect ventricular displacement or enlargement. Visualization of the pathology can be enhanced with IV iodinated contrast dye.

---

*Reviewed by Dr. Garth Koniver, Delaware; updated by Dr. Stephen Grahovac, Neurologist, Christiana Care, Newark, Delaware.

C

Chest (Thoracic) CT: CT of the chest gives a cross-sectional view of the chest to differentiate among various pathologic conditions: tumors, nodules, cysts, abscesses, hematomas, and aortic aneurysms. It can detect pleural effusion and enlarged lymph nodes in the chest area. The use of IV contrast media aids in highlighting blood vessels, thus identifying abnormalities of the vascular structures. CT of the chest can be useful in evaluating the effects of treatment therapy on the tumor and if metastasis has occurred. The helical or spiral CT imaging can readily detect pulmonary emboli over 90% of the time.

Abdominal CT: CT of the abdomen is useful for diagnosing tumors, obstructions, cysts, hematoma, abscesses, bleeding, perforation, calculi, fibroids, and other pathologic conditions that appear in the liver, biliary tract, pancreas, spleen, GI tract, gallbladder, kidneys, adrenals, uterus and ovaries, and prostate. IV contrast dye may be used to enhance visualization. The kidney and urinary flow is easily seen with the use of contrast dye. Oral contrast media may be used for scanning the GI tract. The CT scan is useful for staging tumors and monitoring the effects of treatment therapy on the tumor.

Spine CT: CT scan of the spine gives cross-sectional images that are displayed as two-dimensional views on a monitor. It can be reconstructed in the sagittal and coronal plane, or as a 3D surface rendering. It is mainly used to view the bony anatomy. Contrast dye may be injected into the spinal column via lumbar puncture, that is, CT myelography for clearer visualization of nerve roots and disc herniation. MRI is the preferred study of the spine; however, if MRI is contraindicated or unavailable, then contrast CT would likely be ordered. CT is better than MRI for spinal fractures and bony detail.

Long Bones and Joints CT: Skeletal CT provides cross-sectional images of the bone. This procedure is useful to detect bone and soft tissue tumors and bone metastases. Joint abnormalities can be identified with this CT. Contrast dye may be ordered.

Purposes

- To screen for coronary artery disease; head, liver, and renal lesions; tumors; edema; abscesses; infection; metastatic disease; vascular diseases; stroke; and bone destruction.
- To locate foreign objects in soft tissues, such as the eye.

Clinical Problems

CT TYPE	ABNORMAL FINDINGS
Head	Cerebral lesions: hematomas, tumors, cysts, abscess, infarction, edema, atrophy, hydrocephalus
Internal auditory canal	Acoustic neuroma, cholesteatoma, bone erosion
Eye orbits	Bone destruction, optic nerve tumors, muscle tumor, orbital tumor
Sinus	Bone destruction, sinusitis, polyps, tumors
Neck (soft tissue)	Tumors, abscess, stones in the salivary ducts, enlarged nodes
Abdomen	
Liver	Hepatic lesions: cysts, abscess, tumors, hematomas, cirrhosis with ascites
Biliary	Obstruction due to calculi
Pancreatic	Acute and chronic pancreatitis; pancreatic lesions: tumor, abscess, pseudocysts

CT TYPE	ABNORMAL FINDINGS
Kidney	Renal lesions: tumors, calculi, cysts, congenital anomalies; perirenal hematomas and abscesses
Adrenal	Adrenal tumors
Chest and thoracic	Chest lesions: tumors, cysts, abscesses; aortic aneurysm; enlarged lymph nodes in mediastinum; pleural effusion
Spine	Tumors, paraspinal cysts, vascular malformation, congenital spinal anomalies (e.g., spina bifida, herniated intervertebral disk)
Bony pelvis, long bones, joint	Bone destruction, fractures, tumors
Guided needle biopsy	For lung or liver masses, adrenal mass, kidney, spine, neck tumors

Procedure

General Preparation for All Scans

- A consent form should be signed by the client.
- There is no food or fluid restriction if contrast dye is *not* used.
- For IV contrast injection studies, usually there is NPO (nothing by mouth) 4 hours prior to the CT. Clients with diabetes may be given orange juice instead of water; check with the health care provider or CT supervisor. Oral hypoglycemic agents (Glucophage) are contraindicated to iodinated contrast. For PM scheduling: NPO after a liquid breakfast.
- Prescribed medications may be given with a small amount of water prior to the CT scan; check with the health care provider or CT supervisor.
- A mild sedative may be ordered for some clients to alleviate anxiety.
- Client should remain motionless during the procedure.
- If contrast media (dye) is ordered and the client is allergic to iodine products, steroids or antihistamines may be given before the scan or he or she may be given IV during the CT scan.

Suggested Prophylactic Premedication for Clients Allergic to Contrast Dye

TIME BEFORE CT	DRUG	DOSE
13 hours	Prednisone, PO	50 mg
7 hours	Prednisone, PO	50 mg
1 hour	Prednisone, PO	50 mg
	Benadryl, PO	50 mg
	Zantac, PO	150 mg

Veterans Affairs Medical Center, Wilmington, DE.

- IV infusion or heparin lock insertion may be required prior to test. Use a 19- or 20-gauge needle. Never insert the needle into the antecubital area (anterior bend of the elbow).
- CT scanning usually takes 15 minutes.

Head CT

- Remove hairpins, braids, clips, and jewelry (earrings) before the test.
- Remove dentures prior to the use of contrast dye.
- A mild sedative or analgesic may be ordered for restless clients or for those who have aches and pains of the neck or back.

- Head is positioned in a cradle, and a wide, rubberized strap is applied snugly around the head to keep it immobilized during the test.

Neck CT

- IV contrast media is usually used. Check general preparation for scan for IV contrast injection studies.

Abdominal and Pelvic CT

- Abdominal x-ray (including the kidneys, ureters, and bladder) may be requested before the CT scan.
- The gastrointestinal tract must be free from barium. An enema may be ordered.
- Current laboratory reports of serum creatinine and blood urea nitrogen should be available to determine if there is kidney dysfunction, and if so, to what degree. These tests should be done 7 days prior to the CT scan with contrast injection.
- For an AM abdominal/pelvic scan, give the oral contrast media (15 oz) between 8 PM and 10 PM the evening before the scan. NPO after 10 PM. One hour prior to the CT, give half the bottle of the oral contrast. Thirty minutes prior to the CT, give the remaining half bottle of oral contrast.
- For a PM abdominal/pelvic scan, give 1 bottle (15 oz) of oral contrast media at 7 AM the morning of the scan. NPO after 7 AM. One hour prior to the CT, give half a bottle of the oral contrast. Thirty minutes prior to the CT, give half a bottle of the oral contrast.

Chest CT

- A chest x-ray may be requested before a chest scan.
- IV contrast media is frequently given in the left arm.

Spine CT

- NPO is not indicated, because contrast media is usually not ordered.
- Spine x-rays taken prior to scan should be available. Spine CT should be done after myelography.

Bony Pelvis, Long Bone, and Joint CT

- The nuclear medicine study to locate "hot areas" should be done before the CT scan of the bones and joints.

Factors Affecting Diagnostic Results

- Barium sulfate can obscure visualization of the abdominal organs. Barium studies should be performed 4 days before the CT or after the CT.
- Excessive flatus can cause client discomfort and may cause an inaccurate reading.
- Movement can cause artifacts.
- Metal plates in skull and metal bridges.
- Dental fillings.

NURSING IMPLICATIONS WITH RATIONALE

Pretest

- Explain the procedure to the client. The CT scanner is circular, with a doughnut-like opening. The client is strapped to a special table, with the scanner revolving around the body area that is to be examined. Clicking noises will be heard from the scanner. The radiologist or specialized technician is stationed in a control room and can observe and communicate with the client at all times through an intercom system. The test is not painful.

- Inform the client that he or she may be asked to hold the breath several times during an abdominal or thoracic scan.
- Inform the client that the CT of the head takes 5 minutes without contrast media and 10 minutes with use of contrast. For body CT, the test takes 5–15 minutes.
- Obtain a history of allergies to seafood, iodine, and contrast dye from other x-ray tests. Contrast enhancement is not always done with CT.
- Advise the client that if contrast dye is injected by IV, a warm, flushed sensation may be felt in the face or body. A salty, "fishy," or metallic taste, and a sensation of urinating (does not occur) may be experienced. Nausea is not uncommon. These sensations usually last for 1 or 2 minutes.
- Observe for signs and symptoms of a severe allergic reaction to the dye (e.g., dyspnea, palpitations, tachycardia, hypotension, itching, and urticaria). Emergency drugs should be available.

Posttest

- Observe for delayed allergic reaction to the contrast dye (e.g., skin rash, urticaria, headache, vomiting, and/or renal dysfunction). Increased creatinine level can follow IV contrast use. An oral antihistamine may be ordered for mild reactions.
- If contrast dye has been used, instruct the client to increase fluid intake to enhance the excretion of the dye.
- Be supportive of the client and family. The CT scan can be frightening. The major risk involved is an allergic reaction to the dye (not common with nonionic contrast).

Client Teaching

- Instruct the client to resume his or her usual level of activity and diet, unless otherwise indicated.

Cordocentesis
See Fetoscopy

Corneal staining

Normal Finding
The cornea is free of injuries.

Description
Corneal staining with fluorescein dye enhances the visualization of corneal injuries, such as scratches and abrasions. The use of slit-lamp examination may be used along with the corneal staining to identify the type of injury to the cornea.

Purpose

- To detect a corneal injury.

Clinical Problems

Abnormal Findings: Corneal abrasions, scratches, and ulcerations.

Procedure

- A signed consent form may be required.
- Fluorescein strip deposits the dye by the strip touching the lower conjunctival sac.
- Client closes his or her eyes, and opens and closes the eyes again to spread the dye over the cornea.
- With the forehead placed against a bar, the client looks straight ahead, and the eye(s) are examined.
- For several hours after the procedure, blurring may occur.

Factors Affecting Diagnostic Results

- The inability of the client to remain still.

NURSING IMPLICATIONS WITH RATIONALE

- Obtain a history of the eye injury.
- Ask if the client is allergic to dye, particularly fluorescein dye.

Client Teaching

- Inform the client that this procedure should not cause pain but may cause some discomfort.

Cystometry (cystometrogram) (CMG)

Normal Findings

Adult: *Urine stream:* Strong and uninterrupted. Normal filling pattern and sensation of fullness. *Bladder capacity:* 300–600 mL; *Residual urine:* 0–30 mL; *Urge to void:* Greater than 150 mL; *Fullness felt:* Greater than 300 mL.

Child: *Bladder capacity and urinary flow vary with age.*

Description

Cystometry or cystometrogram (CMG) evaluates the neuromuscular function of the bladder. After the instillation of a measured quantity of fluid, this test measures the efficiency of the detrusor muscle, the intravesical pressure and capacity, and the effect of thermal stimulation. CMG is used for evaluating bladder dysfunction caused by neurologic disorder or disease, such as spinal cord injury, stroke, multiple sclerosis, or diabetes mellitus, and it also includes stress incontinence, urinary/stress incontinence, and the effects of drugs the client is taking.

Urethral pressure profile (UPP) is frequently performed during the cystometry. A special catheter that had been inserted is slowly withdrawn as the urethral pressures are measured. These tests may be conducted in a urologist's office or clinic.

Cystometry is contraindicated for a client with a urinary tract infection (UTI).

Purposes

- To evaluate the detrusor muscle function and tonicity of the bladder.
- To measure the urethral pressures.
- To determine the cause of bladder dysfunction.

Clinical Problems

Abnormal Findings/Causes: Stress incontinence; neurogenic bladder from spinal cord injury, stroke, multiple sclerosis, diabetes mellitus; postoperative urinary dysfunction, and bladder and prostate obstruction.

Procedure

- Obtain a signed consent form from the client.
- No food or fluid restriction.
- Have the client urinate into a container attached to a machine that records the force of the urinary flow, amount, and the completion time.
- Insert a retention catheter to measure residual urine volume.
- Test for thermal sensation: Instill 30–50 mL of room-temperature normal saline solution (NSS) into the bladder. Client should report the sensation that is felt. The NSS is then withdrawn. Instill 30 mL of 30–40°C of NSS. Again, the client reports his or her sensations as a feeling of warmth, flushing, need to void, and/or discomfort. The bladder is then drained.
- Connect the catheter to a cystometer (a tube to monitor bladder pressures). Normal saline solution, sterile water, or gas (carbon dioxide) is *slowly* instilled into the bladder. The cystometer graphically records the data. The client tells when he or she can no longer hold the urine without voiding; the liquid instillation is stopped, and the catheter is removed. Client is to void, but not strain when voiding. Again, the voiding pressure is recorded. If gas is used, the gas is withdrawn and the pressure from the urethral wall is obtained.
- The cholinergic drug bethanechol (Urecholine), a urinary stimulant, may be administered during the cystometric procedure to enhance the bladder tone.
- This test takes approximately 45 minutes to 1 hour.

Factors Affecting Diagnostic Test

- Antihistamines cause relaxation of the bladder muscle and wall, thus bladder function can be inhibited.

NURSING IMPLICATIONS WITH RATIONALE

- Obtain a history of the client's urinary problem and what drugs the client is taking daily.
- Check vital signs, which may be the baseline for the posttest.
- Discuss the procedure with the client.

Client Teaching

- Inform the client that he or she may have a strong urge to urinate during the test and that this is not abnormal. Tell the client to let the urologist know what sensations he or she has at various times during the test.

Posttest
Client Teaching

- Inform the client that he or /she may have bladder spasms after the test. An analgesic is usually prescribed. After 24 hours, if the bladder spasms continue, the health care provider should be called.
- Notify the health care provider if blood in the urine occurs 4–6 hours posttest or after the third voiding.
- Explain to the client who received carbon dioxide gas that it may cause posttest discomfort.
- Instruct the client to report fever, dysuria, or urinary frequency to the health care provider. Urinary tract infection (UTI) may have resulted from this procedure and needs to be reported and treated.
- Encourage the client to increase fluid intake. Measurement of intake and output may be requested.

Cystoscopy, cystography (cystogram)

Normal Finding

Normal structure of the urethra, bladder, prostatic urethra, and ureter orifices.

Description

Cystoscopy is the direct visualization of the bladder wall and urethra with the use of a cystoscope (a tubular lighted telescopic lens). Usually this diagnostic test is performed by a urologist. Small renal calculi can be removed from the ureter, bladder, or urethra with this procedure, and a tissue biopsy can be obtained. In addition, *retrograde pyelography* (injection of contrast dye through the catheter into the ureters and renal pelvis) may be performed during the cystoscopy.

Cystoscopy is performed in a cystoscopy room of a hospital or in a urologist's office under general or local anesthesia. Premedications are administered an hour prior to the test.

Cystography is the instillation of a contrast dye into the bladder via a catheter. This procedure can detect a rupture in the bladder, a neurogenic bladder, fistulas, and tumors. The test is useful when x-rays are needed and a cystoscopy or retrograde pyelography is contraindicated.

Purposes

- To detect renal calculi and renal tumor.
- To remove renal stones.
- To determine the cause of hematuria or urinary tract infection (UTI).

Clinical Problems

Abnormal Findings: Hematuria or urinary tract infection; renal calculi (stones), tumors, or prostatic hyperplasia.

Procedure

- A consent form should be signed by the client.
- The client can have a full liquid breakfast the morning of the test if local anesthetic is used. Several glasses of water may be ordered. If general anesthesia is to be administered, the client should be NPO for 8 hours before cystoscopy.
- Record baseline vital signs.
- A narcotic analgesic (meperidine, morphine) may be ordered an hour before the cystoscopy. The procedure is done under local or general anesthesia.
- The client is placed in a lithotomy position (feet or legs in stirrups). A local anesthetic is injected into the urethra. Water may be instilled to enhance visualization. A urine specimen may be obtained.
- The cystoscopy takes approximately 30 minutes to 1 hour.

Factors Affecting Diagnostic Results

- None reported.

NURSING IMPLICATIONS WITH RATIONALE

Pretest

- Obtain history concerning the presence of cystitis or prostatitis, which could result in sepsis.
- Explain the procedure to the client. Answer questions or refer questions you cannot answer to the urologist.
- Check with the urologist about the form of anesthesia the client will receive—local or general. Inform the client that a local anesthetic will be injected into the urethra several minutes before the cystoscope is inserted.
- Check that the consent form has been signed before administering the premedications. Normally the drugs are given 1 hour before the test.
- Check with the client concerning hypersensitivity to anesthetics.
- Assess urinary patterns, such as amount, color, odor, and specific gravity of the urine.
- Take baseline vital signs.

Client Teaching

- Inform the client that there may be some pressure or burning discomfort during and/or following the test.

Posttest

- Recognize the complications that can occur as a result of the cystoscopy, such as hemorrhaging, perforation of the bladder, urinary retention, and infection.
- Monitor vital signs. Compare with baseline VS. VS may be ordered every half hour until stable.

- Monitor the urinary output for 48 hours following a cystoscopy. If urine output is less than 200 mL in 8 hours, encourage fluid intake. Anuria could indicate urinary retention due to blood clots or urethral stricture. Report findings to the urologist. An indwelling catheter may be ordered.
- Report and record gross hematuria. Inform the client that blood-tinged urine is not uncommon after a cystoscopic examination.
- Observe for signs and symptoms of an infection (e.g., fever, chills, an increased pulse rate, and pain). Antibiotics may be given before and after the test as a prophylactic measure.
- Apply heat to the lower abdomen to relieve pain and muscle spasm as ordered.

Client Teaching

- Advise the client to avoid alcoholic beverages for 2 days after the test.
- Instruct the client to increase water intake for several days after the test.
- Inform the client that a slight burning sensation when voiding for a day or two is considered normal. Usually the urologist leaves an order for an analgesic.

Dilation and Curettage (D & C) (uterus)

Normal Findings

No cancer cells, absence of abnormal bleeding.

Description

Dilation and curettage (D & C) is frequently performed to obtain cells from the endometrium of the uterus and to diagnose abnormal bleeding. The D & C procedure differs from an endometrium biopsy (see *Biopsy—endometrium*). The biopsy does not require general anesthesia whereas the D & C does. During the D & C, the cervical canal is dilated and the entire endometrium is scraped.

D & C is done to obtain cells to test for possible cancer, abnormal uterine bleeding, dysmenorrhea, incomplete abortion (miscarriage), and uterine polyps. This procedure is also done to insert a radium device for treatment of cancer.

Purpose

- To scrape (curettage) the endometrium of the uterus to obtain cells, correct abnormal uterine bleeding, and to remove the products of miscarriage and uterine polyps.

Clinical Problems

Positive: Uterine bleeding, cancer cells, uterine polyps, miscarriage, dysmenorrhea.

Procedure

- No food or fluid for 12 hours prior to the procedure.
- Client should void before the procedure.
- Vital signs are recorded before and throughout the surgery.

NURSING IMPLICATIONS WITH RATIONALE

- Obtain a history of the medical problem the client is having, such as abnormal uterine bleeding, an incomplete abortion, etc.
- Obtain baseline vital signs. During the D & C, vital signs will be taken frequently.
- Explain the procedure for the D & C. The client will be under general anesthesia.

Client Teaching

- Tell the client that she may have some cramping following the D & C.
- Advise the client to immediately call the physician if she has an elevated temperature above 102°F or excessive bleeding, purulent vaginal drainage, or vaginal pain.
- Inform the client that the physician will give her the result of the uterine specimen. If she has not heard after a week, she should give the physician a call.

E

Echocardiography (echocardiogram)*

M-mode; Two-Dimensional; Spectral Doppler; Color Flow Doppler; Transesophageal, Contrast, and Stress Echocardiography

Normal Findings

Normal heart size and structure; normal movements of heart valves and heart chambers.

Description

Echocardiography (echocardiogram) is a noninvasive ultrasound test used to identify abnormal heart size, structure, and function, and valvular disease. A handheld transducer (probe) is moved over the chest in the area of the heart and other specified surrounding areas. The transducer sends and receives high-frequency sound waves. The sound waves that are reflected (echo) from the heart back to the transducer produce pictures. These pictures are viewed live on the video monitor and are digitally recorded and can be transmitted electronically offsite.

There are several types of echocardiographic studies, which include M-mode; two-dimensional; spectral Doppler; color Doppler; and transesophageal, contrast, and stress echocardiography. Transesophageal echocardiography (TEE) is gaining popularity for diagnosing and managing a wide range of cardiovascular diseases, such as valvular heart dysfunction, aortic pathology, and source of embolic stroke and is useful in the evaluation of endocarditis. Stress echocardiography is a valuable tool for assessing myocardial ischemia without the need of an IV; it is less expensive, and involves less nuclear exposure, than nuclear stress tests.

DEFINITY is a perflutren lipid microsphere, which is a contrast used to enhance echocardiographic images. Once activated and injected intravenously, the acoustic properties provide contrast enhancement of the endocardial borders of the left ventricle. New contrast agents may allow visualization of the coronary arteries and perfusion to the myocardium. Use is contraindicated

---

*Updated by Dr. Anthony W. Clay, DO FACC Cardiologist, Newark/Wilmington, Delaware.

in clients with known or suspected right-to-left cardiac shunts. Serious cardiopulmonary reactions have occurred with the risk of these events happening in clients with pulmonary hypertension or worsened or unstable heart failure (HF).

M-Mode Echocardiography: M-mode echocardiography, the earliest type of echocardiography, is used to record the motion of various heart structures (M is for *motion*). This test assesses the dimension of the left ventricle and its degree of dilatation and contractility related to myocardial disease or volume overload. It is useful for measuring the thickness of the right and left ventricles (hypertrophy). M-mode echocardiography is also used to assess the cardiac valves and valvular movements for stenosis or prolapse.

Two-Dimensional Echocardiography: This test records motion and provides two-dimensional (cross-sectional) views of the heart structure. It is used to evaluate the size, shape, and movement of the chambers and values of the heart and is useful in detecting valvular disease and in assessing congenital heart disease.

Spectral Doppler Echocardiography: Spectral Doppler measures the amount, speed, and direction of blood flow passing through the heart valves and heart chambers. A swishing sound is heard as the blood flows throughout the heart. This test can detect turbulent blood flow through the heart valves, which may indicate valvular disease. Septal wall defects may also be detected.

Color Doppler Echocardiography: Color Doppler (red and blue) echocardiography shows the direction of blood flowing through the heart. It can identify leaking heart valves (regurgitation) or hardened valves (stenosis), malfunction of prosthetic valves, and the presence of shunts (holes) in the heart. The use of the color Doppler complements 2D echocardiography and the spectral Doppler study.

Transesophageal Echocardiography: With transesophageal echocardiography (TEE), a transducer (probe) is attached to an endoscope and is inserted into the esophagus to visualize adjacent cardiac and extracardiac structures with greater acuity than most echocardiography studies, including transthoracic (TTE). TEE is ordered when the traditional echocardiogram fails to report a probable diagnosis. It records ultrasound images of the heart. TEE can be used in the intensive care unit, emergency department, and operating room, as well as in cardiac testing facilities. This type of echocardiography is useful for diagnosing mitral and aortic valvular pathology; determining the presence of a possible intracardiac thrombus in the left atrium; detecting suspected acute dissection of the aorta and endocarditis; monitoring left ventricular function before, during, or after surgery; and evaluating intracardiac repairs during surgery.

This test is contraindicated if esophageal pathology (e.g., strictures, varices, trauma) exists. Also, TEE should not be performed if undiagnosed active gastrointestinal bleeding is occurring or if the client is uncooperative. A light sedative is frequently given prior to testing. TEE can be performed on an unconscious client. TEE is tolerated well, with approximately 1% of clients being intolerant of the esophageal probe. The rate of complications is less than 0.2%.

Contrast Echocardiography: This test assists in determining intracardiac communications, myocardial ischemia, and perfusion defects. Microbubbles are injected into the venous circulation for the purpose of recording showers of echoes by M-mode or 2D tests. The microbubbles pass through the right atrium and ventricle, where they are absorbed in the lung; they do not pass to the left side of the heart. If the microbubbles are detected on the left side of the heart, an intracardiac communication or shunt is present.

Stress Echocardiography: It may be necessary to evaluate the function of the left ventricle under stress. Before starting an exercise, a baseline two-dimensional and Doppler echocardiogram is performed for the evaluation of regional and global left and right ventricular systolic function, left ventricular diastolic functions, and valvular assessment. The client then exercises using a standardized protocol until the predicted maximum heart rate is achieved, symptoms appear, or electrocardiographic or echocardiographic signs of myocardial ischemia occur. Immediately after exercise, the client returns to a left lateral decubitus position for reimaging (ideally obtained in less than 1 minute). Then these are compared to those at baseline for any wall motion changes.

The stress modalities used in conjunction with echocardiography include exercise on a treadmill or bicycle; for clients who are unable to exercise, a pharmacologic agent such as Dobutamine is used.

Purposes

- To detect viable myocardium.
- To obtain a risk stratification following an acute myocardial infarction (AMI).
- To measure ejection fraction.
- To identify abnormal heart size, structure, and function.
- To detect cardiac valvular disease and detect shunts.
- To determine the function of prosthetic heart valves.
- To assess the effects of congenital heart disease.
- To monitor left ventricular function before, during, and after surgery.
- To evaluate the client's ejection fraction while he or she is undergoing chemotherapy.
- To evaluate and rule out coronary artery disease based primarily on wall motion abnormalities.
- To evaluate the pericardium and diagnosis and treatment of pericardial fusion.
- To evaluate the ascending aorta for pathology.
- To evaluate right-sided heart chambers for pulmonary pathology and possible pulmonary hypertension.

Clinical Problems

Indications: To detect heart size, structure, and function; heart valvular disease (regurgitation or stenosis of the aortic or mitral valves); congenital heart disease; heart wall damage after a myocardial infarction; cardiomyopathy; mural thrombi; pericardial effusion; aortic pathology; and endocarditis.

DIAGNOSTIC TESTS	INDICATIONS TO DETERMINE/DETECT
M-mode echocardiography	Dimension of the left ventricle
	Degree of ventricular dilatation and contractility
	Ventricular hypertrophy
	Function of cardiac valves
Two-dimensional (2D) echocardiography	Cardiac valvular disease
	Dimension of the left ventricle
	Degree of ventricular dilatation and contractility and ejection fraction
	Ventricular hypertrophy
Spectral Doppler echocardiography	Blood flow through heart chambers and valves
	Septal wall defects
	Atrial and ventricular septal wall defects
Color Doppler echocardiography	Direction of blood flow through the heart
	Function of cardiac valves—stenosis or regurgitation
	Function of prosthetic valves
	Presence of shunting in the heart

(Continued)

DIAGNOSTIC TESTS	INDICATIONS TO DETERMINE/DETECT
Transesophageal echocardiography	Function of left ventricle before, during, or after surgery Cardiac valvular disease Presence of intracardiac thrombus in left atrium Aortic disease (e.g., dissection of aorta) Presence of endocarditis Visualize the atrium septum
Contrast echocardiography	Perfusion defects Better visualization of the endocardium for wall motion analysis
Stress echocardiography	Function of left ventricle under stress Perfusion defects

Procedure

Transthoracic Echocardiography (THE)

- A consent form should be signed by the client.
- There is no food or fluid restriction.
- No medications should be omitted before the test unless indicated by the institution or health care provider.
- The client undresses from the waist up and wears a hospital gown. For the test, the client will be positioned on his or her left side or in the supine position.
- Vital signs are recorded. Three electrode patches are applied to the chest area to monitor heart rate and changes in cardiac rhythm.
- Water-soluble gel is applied to the skin areas that are to be scanned. The transducer (probe), with slight pressure, is moved over different areas of the chest. Some clients may require that pictures be taken under the neck.
- The 2D echo takes about 20–30 minutes, and the 2D echo with Doppler studies takes approximately 30–45 minutes.
- The cardiologist interprets the test result and submits a report to the client's health care provider, who gives the test results to the client.

Transesophageal Echocardiography (TEE)

- The client should be NPO for at least 4 hours prior to the test.
- A light sedative is given prior to the test.
- An IV sedative (e.g., Versed) is given.
- The endoscopic transducer is inserted into the esophagus.
- The test takes 15–30 minutes.
- The client is monitored (Dinamap) during recovery for 1–2 hours.

Contrast Echocardiography

- An IV line is inserted for injection of contrast media.

Stress Echocardiography

- The client should be NPO for 4 hours before the test.
- The client may be placed on a treadmill or receive a pharmacologic agent.
- Images are acquired during rest (pretest) and then during stress or immediately following stress (posttest).

Factors Affecting Diagnostic Results

- Large body habitus may cause poor image quality.
- Severe respiratory disease may affect test results.

NURSING IMPLICATIONS WITH RATIONALE

Pretest

- Obtain a history of the client's physical complaint(s). Complete the pretest form provided by the institution, if available.
- Check that the consent form has been signed.
- Check the client's vital signs and obtain an electrocardiogram if indicated by the institution or health care provider. These baseline values are used for comparison purposes.

Client Teaching

- Explain the procedure to the client (see *Procedure*). Inform the client that the test does not cause pain or discomfort. The test takes approximately 30 minutes, more time if additional testing is done.
- Inform the client that he or she will be positioned on his or her back and/or left side during the test procedure. The client may be asked to change body position during testing. If the client is in an uncomfortable position, he or she should tell the technician.
- Inform the client that a gel will be applied to the skin over the area that is to be studied. The gel may feel cool. The transducer (probe) is placed on the gel area and moved to different positions. The sound waves are transmitted and viewed on the video monitor and digitally recorded.

Posttest

- Explain to the client that the test results will be submitted to his or her health care provider. If the client does not hear from the health care provider in 1 week, the client should call him or her.
- Answer the client's questions. Refer questions to appropriate health professionals as necessary.

E

Echoencephalography

See Ultrasonography

Electrocardiography (electrocardiogram—ECG or EKG), vectorcardiography (vectorcardiogram—VCG)*

Normal Finding

Normal electrocardiogram deflections (P, PR, QRS, ST, and T).

---

*Updated by Dr. William F. Bilski, Delaware

Description

An electrocardiogram records the electrical impulses of the heart by the means of electrodes and a galvanometer (ECG machine). These electrodes are placed on the legs, arms, and chest. Combinations of two electrodes are called bipolar leads (i.e., lead I is the combination of both arm electrodes, lead II is the combination of the right-arm and left-leg electrodes, and lead III is the combination of the left-arm and left-leg electrodes). The unipolar leads are AVF, AVL, and AVR; the A means augmented, V is the voltage, and F is left foot, L is left arm, and R is right arm. There are at least six unipolar chest or precordial leads. A standard ECG consists of 12 leads: 6 limb leads (I, II, III, AVF, AVL, AVR) and 6 chest (precordial) leads (V_1, V_2, V_3, V_4, V_5, V_6).

With each cardiac cycle or heartbeat, the sinoatrial node (SA or sinus node) sends an electrical impulse through the atrium, causing atrial contraction or atrial depolarization. The SA node is called the pacemaker, because it controls the heartbeat. The impulse is then transmitted to the atrioventricular (AV) node and the bundle of His (a collection of heart muscle cells specialized for electrical conduction) and travels down the ventricles, causing ventricular contraction or ventricular depolarization. When the atria and the ventricles relax, repolarization and recovery occurs.

The electrical activity that the ECG records is in the form of waves and complexes: P wave (atrial depolarization); QRS complex (ventricular depolarization); and ST segment, T wave, and Unit wave (ventricular repolarization). An abnormal ECG indicates a disturbance in the electrical activity of the myocardium. A person could have heart disease and have a normal ECG as long as the cardiac problem did not affect the transmission of electrical impulses (Figure 2-1).

P Wave (Atrial Contraction): The normal time is 0.12 seconds or three small blocks. An enlarged P wave deflection could indicate atrial enlargement, which could be the result of mitral stenosis. An absent or altered P wave could suggest that the electrical impulse did not come from the SA node.

PR Interval (from the P Wave to the Onset of the Q Wave): The normal time interval is 0.2 seconds or five small blocks. An increased interval could imply a conduction delay in the AV node. It could be the result of rheumatic fever or arteriosclerotic heart disease. A short interval could indicate Wolff-Parkinson-White syndrome.

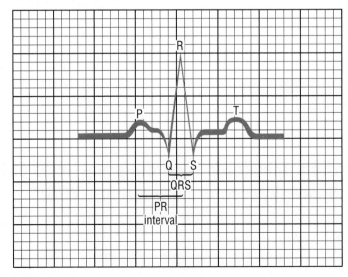

Figure 2-1   ECG graph.

QRS Complex (Ventricular Contraction): The normal time is less than 0.12 seconds or three small blocks. An enlarged Q wave may imply an old myocardial infarction. An enlarged R-wave deflection could indicate ventricular hypertrophy (enlargement). An increased time duration may indicate a bundle-branch block.

ST Segment (Beginning Ventricular Repolarization): A depressed ST segment indicates myocardial ischemia (decreased supply of oxygen to the myocardium). An elevated ST segment can indicate acute myocardial infarction or pericarditis. A prolonged ST segment may imply hypocalcemia or hypokalemia. A short ST segment may be due to hypercalcemia.

T Wave (Ventricular Repolarization): A flat or inverted T wave can indicate myocardial ischemia, myocardial infarction, or hypokalemia. A tall, peaked T wave, greater than 10 mm or 10 small blocks in precordial leads, or greater than 5 mm or five small blocks in limb leads, can indicate hyperkalemia.

Vectorcardiogram (VCG): The VCG records electrical impulses from the cardiac cycle, making it similar to the ECG. However, it shows a three-dimensional view (frontal, horizontal, and sagittal planes) of the heart, whereas the ECG shows a two-dimensional view (frontal and horizontal planes). The VCG is considered more sensitive than the ECG for diagnosing a myocardial infarction. It is useful for assessing ventricular hypertrophy in adults and children.

Purposes

- To detect cardiac dysrhythmias.
- To identify electrolyte imbalance (e.g., hyperkalemia [peaked T wave]).
- To monitor ECG changes during the stress/exercise tests and the recovery phase after a myocardial infarction.

Clinical Problems

Abnormal Findings: Cardiac dysrhythmias, cardiac hypertrophies, myocardial ischemia, electrolyte imbalances (potassium, calcium, and magnesium), myocardial infarction, and pericarditis.

Procedure

- Food, fluids, and medications are not restricted, unless otherwise indicated.
- Clothing should be removed to the waist, and the female client should wear a gown.
- Nylon stockings should be removed, and trouser bottoms should be raised.
- The client should lie in a supine position.
- The skin surface should be prepared. Excess hair should be shaved from the chest if necessary.
- Electrodes with Electro Paste or pads are strapped to the four extremities. The color-coded lead wires are inserted into the correct electrodes. Chest electrodes are applied. The lead selector is turned to record the 12 standard leads unless the ECG machine automatically records the lead strips.
- The ECG takes approximately 15 minutes.

Factors Affecting Diagnostic Results

- Body movement and electromagnetic interference during the ECG recording could distort the tracing.
- Poor electrode-to-skin contact will distort tracing.

NURSING IMPLICATIONS WITH RATIONALE

- Record the list of medications the client is taking. The health care provider may want to compare ECG readings to check for improvement and changes; therefore, knowing the drugs the client is taking at the time of the ECG would be helpful.

Client Teaching

- Instruct the client to relax and to breathe normally during the ECG procedure. Tell the client to avoid tightening the muscles, grasping bed rails or other objects, and talking during the ECG tracing.
- Tell the client that the ECG should not cause pain or any great discomfort.
- Inform the client to tell you if he or she is having chest pain during the ECG tracing. Mark the ECG paper at the time the client is having chest pain.
- Allow the client time to ask questions. Refer questions you cannot answer to another health care provider, for example, a physician or cardiologist.
- Inform the client that the ECG takes about 15 minutes.

Posttest

- Remove the adhesive gel electrode pads that were applied to the chest wall when the ECG is completed Assist the client with dressing, if necessary.

Electroencephalography (electroencephalogram—EEG)

Normal Finding

Adult and Child: Normal tracing, regular short waves.

Description

The electroencephalogram measures the electrical impulses produced by brain cells. Electrodes, applied to the scalp surface at predetermined measured positions, record brain-wave activity on moving paper. EEG tracings can detect patterns characteristic of some diseases (e.g., seizure disorders, neoplasms, cerebral vascular accidents, head trauma, and infections of the nervous system). At times, recorded brain waves may be normal when there is pathology.

Another use for the EEG is to determine cerebral death. If the EEG recording gives a flat or straight line for many hours, this usually indicates severe hypoxia and brain death. The cardiovascular functions are usually being maintained through the use of life-support systems (e.g., a respirator, oxygen, and IVs). The neurologist interprets the EEG readings and gives suggestions.

Purposes

- To detect a seizure disorder.
- To identify a brain tumor, abscess, or intracranial hemorrhage.
- To assist in the determination of cerebral death.

Clinical Problems

Abnormal Tracing: Epilepsy, seizures (grand mal, petit mal, psychomotor), brain neoplasms (tumors), brain abscesses, head injury, intracranial hemorrhage, encephalitis, unconsciousness, coma, and "brain death."

Procedure

The procedure may be performed while the client is (1) awake, (2) drowsy, (3) asleep, (4) undergoing stimuli (hyperventilation or rhythmic flashes of bright light), or (5) a combination of any of these.

Pretest

- The hair should be shampooed the night before the test. Instruct the client not to use oil or hairspray on the hair.
- The decision concerning withdrawal of medications before the EEG is made by the health care provider. Sleeping pills and other sedatives may not be given the night before the test because they can affect the EEG recording.
- Food and fluids are not restricted except *no* coffee, tea, cola, and alcohol before the test.
- The EEG tracing is usually obtained with the client lying down; however, the client could be seated in a reclining chair.
- For a sleep recording, keep the client awake 2–3 hours later the night before the test and wake the client up at 6 AM. A sedative such as chloral hydrate may be ordered.
- The EEG test takes approximately 1½–2 hours. Flat electrodes will be applied to the scalp.

Posttest

- Remove the collodion or paste from the client's head. Acetone may be used to remove the paste.
- The client should resume normal activity unless he or she has been sedated.

Factors Affecting Diagnostic Results

- Drugs (e.g., sedatives, barbiturates, anticonvulsants, and tranquilizers) can affect test results.
- Alcohol could decrease cerebral impulses.
- Oily hair or the use of hairspray can affect test results.

NURSING IMPLICATIONS WITH RATIONALE

Pretest

- A consent form should be signed by the client.
- Explain the procedure to the client, step by step. List the important steps on paper for the client if needed.
- Report if the client is taking medications that could change the EEG result.
- Check with the health care provider and/or EEG department in regard to the type or types of recordings ordered (i.e., awake, sleep, stimuli).
- Be supportive of the client. Answer questions and permit the client to express concerns.
- Report to the health care provider and inform the EEG laboratory if the client is extremely anxious, restless, or upset.
- Observe for seizures and describe the seizure activity—the movements and how long they last. Have a tongue blade by the bedside at all times. Chart all seizure activity and the time of its occurrence, because it is very important for the technologist and electroencephalographer to know this.

E

Client Teaching

- Inform the client that he or she will *not* get an electric shock from the machine (electro-encephalograph) and that the machine does not determine the client's intelligence and cannot read the client's mind. Many clients are apprehensive and fearful of this test.
- Encourage the client to eat a meal before the test. Hypoglycemia should be prevented because it can affect normal brain activity. Coffee, tea, cola, and any other stimulants should be avoided. Alcohol is a depressant and can affect the test result.
- Inform the client that the test does not produce pain.
- Advise the client to be calm and to relax during the test. If rest and stimuli (flashing lights) recordings are ordered, inform him or her that there will be a brief time when there are flashing lights. Prepare the client, but do not increase his or her apprehension, if possible.
- Inform the client that the test takes 1½–2 hours. The room is quiet where the EEG recording is made and is conducive to rest and sleep.
- Instruct the client, after the test, that normal activity can be resumed.

E

Electromyography (electromyogram—EMG)

Normal Finding

At Rest: Minimal electrical activity.

Voluntary Muscle Contraction: Markedly increased electrical activity.

Description

Electromyography (EMG) measures electrical activity of skeletal muscles at rest and during voluntary muscle contraction. A needle electrode is inserted into the skeletal muscle to pick up electrical activity, which can be heard over a loudspeaker, viewed on an oscilloscope, and recorded on graphic paper all at the same time. Normally there is no electrical activity when the muscle is at rest; however, in motor disorders abnormal patterns can occur. With voluntary muscle contraction there is a loud popping sound and increased electrical activity (wave) is recorded.

The test is useful in diagnosing neuromuscular disorders. The EMG can be used to differentiate between myopathy and neuropathy.

Purpose

- To diagnose neuromuscular disorders, such as muscular dystrophy.

Clinical Problems

Abnormal Findings: Muscle disorders (muscular dystrophy), neuromuscular disorders (peripheral neuropathy [i.e., diabetes mellitus, alcoholism], myasthenia gravis, myotonia), and central neuronal degeneration (amyotrophic lateral sclerosis [ALS], anterior poliomyelitis).

Procedure

- A consent form should be signed by the client.

- Food and fluids are not restricted, with the exceptions of *no* coffee, tea, colas, or other caffeine drinks, and *no* smoking for at least 3 hours before the EMG.
- Medications such as muscle relaxants, anticholinergics, and cholinergics should be withheld before the test with the approval of the health care provider. If the client needs the specific medication, the time for the test should be rearranged.
- The client lies on a table or stretcher or sits in a chair in a room free of noise. The EMG takes 1 hour but could take longer if a group of muscles is to be tested.
- Needle electrodes are inserted in selected or affected muscles. If the client experiences pain, the needle should be removed and reinserted.
- If serum enzyme tests are ordered (i.e., AST [SGOT], CPK, LDH), the samples should be drawn before the EMG or 5–10 days after the test.

Posttest
- If residual pain occurs, analgesic may be given.

Factors Affecting Diagnostic Results

- Pain could cause false reports.
- Age of the client: electrical activity may be decreased in some elderly persons.
- Drugs: muscle relaxants, anticholinergics, and cholinergics could affect the results.
- Fluids that contain caffeine can affect results.

E

NURSING IMPLICATIONS WITH RATIONALE

- Ask the health care provider about withholding client medications that could affect EMG results. If the client takes drugs that could interfere with test results prior to the test, the drugs should be listed on the request slip and recorded in the chart.
- Check the health care provider's order for a serum enzyme request. Blood needed for serum enzyme determinants (i.e., AST [SGOT], CPK, LDH) should be drawn before the EMG test.

Client Teaching

- Explain the procedure to the client. Inform the client that the test will not cause electrocution; however, there may be a slight temporary discomfort when the needle electrodes are inserted. If pain persists for several minutes, the client should tell the technician.
- Instruct the client to follow the technician's instructions (i.e., to relax the specified muscle[s] and to contract the muscle[s] when requested). An analgesic may be ordered before and after the test.
- Inform the client that the EMG test usually takes 1 hour, but it could take longer.

Electroneurography (ENoG)
Nerve Conduction Studies

Normal Finding

No evidence of peripheral nerve injury or disease.

Description

Electroneurography (ENoG) evaluates and identifies peripheral nerve injury or disease. A common cause is diabetic neuropathy. A stimulus is applied to the affected area. The result of the stimulus is shown on a monitor.

Neuropathies, trauma, and contusion will cause a slowing of conduction velocity. However, a velocity greater than normal does not indicate a pathologic problem. This test is usually performed along with electromyography.

Purpose

- To identify peripheral nerve injury or disease, such as diabetic neuropathy.

Clinical Problems

Diabetic neuropathy, carpal tunnel syndrome, peripheral injury or trauma, Guillain-Barré syndrome, myasthenia gravis.

Procedure

- The test may be performed at the bedside or a specific laboratory.
- Have the client in a supine position or a sitting position if indicated.
- Inform the client that electrode gel and electrode(s) will be placed at the affected sites. The nerve(s) will be shocked, and the time between nerve impulse and electrical contraction will be measured.

Factors Affecting Diagnostic Results

- The client is unable to remain still during the procedure.

NURSING IMPLICATIONS WITH RATIONALE

- Obtain a history from the client of the location of the pain or severe discomfort.
- Have the client describe the pain or severe discomfort.

Client Teaching

- Explain the procedure of the test; that electrode gel and electrodes are applied to the affected area. The nerves will be stimulated by a shock emitter device, which may cause some discomfort. The conduction velocity is measured.
- Answer the client's questions about the test and if unknown, refer them to a health care provider.

Electronystagmography (ENG)

Electronystagmogram

Normal Finding

Normal nystagmus with stimulation; normal vestibular-ocular reflex.

Description

Electronystagmography (ENG) is used to detect physiologic and pathologic nystagmus. This test helps to determine if the problem/abnormality that occurs is in the brain stem, the temporal lobe of the cerebral cortex, auditory nerve, or vestibular-cochlear area. If nystagmus (involuntary rapid eye movement) does not occur with stimulation, the health problem may be due to infection, tumor, ischemia to the surrounding tissues, or degeneration. The pattern of nystagmus helps in differentiating between peripheral and central vertigo.

ENG helps in determining if unilateral hearing loss is caused by the middle ear defect or nerve injury. If nystagmus does not occur with stimulation, the hearing loss is due to auditory nerve damage and not a middle ear problem.

Purposes

- To aid in the diagnosis of lesions in the brain stem or cerebellum.
- To identify oculovestibular lesions or abnormalities.

Clinical Problems

Abnormal Findings: Brain stem lesion, cerebellum lesion, 8th cranial nerve injury, vestibular lesion, head trauma, middle ear infection, congenital disorder, and peripheral lesions.

Procedure

- A signed consent form is required.
- The client should avoid applying facial makeup before the test.
- Nothing by mouth after midnight. Vomiting frequently occurs with this procedure; thus, NPO for 8 or more hours reduces the chance of vomiting.
- Eardrum should be free of wax.
- Avoid consuming caffeine drinks or alcohol 24 hours prior to the test.
- Avoid sedatives and antivertigo drugs prior to the test.
- The client is seated or is lying in a darkened room.
- Small electrodes are applied around the eyes.
- Test takes about 1 hour.
- Various techniques may be used to stimulate nystagmus, for example, positional, pendulum tracking, gaze position, calibration, and water caloric test.

Positional Technique

- Obtain a baseline recording of eye movement.
- With head erect and eyes looking forward, turn the head quickly to the right and then to the left; repeat the procedure with the eyes closed.
- Various positions are requested, such as lying down quickly from a sitting position and sitting up quickly from a lying position.

Pendulum Tracking Technique

- Client looks ahead and follows a pendulum.
- With the eyes closed, the client stares straight ahead for 30 seconds.

Gaze Technique

- The client is given a math problem.
- The client closes eyes and solves the math problem in 30 seconds while eye motion is recorded.
- The client looks straight ahead with eyes fixed and head straight; again, eye motion is recorded.

Caloric (Water) Test Technique: The test is to evaluate the vestibular part of the 8th cranial nerve. *Note:* The client's eardrum should not be perforated.
- The client's head is elevated to 30 degrees and the eyes are to be closed.
- The external auditory canal is irrigated with hot and cold water.
- The client's eyes are opened and the procedure is repeated for 60 seconds. Then the eyes are closed and the procedure is again repeated. The total time is 3 minutes.
- The client may encounter nausea and vomiting during the procedure. Following the test, the client should rest until these symptoms have subsided.

Factors Affecting Diagnostic Results
- Sedatives and other central nervous system (CNS) depressants.
- Blinking of the eyes.
- Loose electrodes.

Caution: Test is contraindicated for clients with pacemakers. Check with the facility.

NURSING IMPLICATIONS WITH RATIONALE

Pretest
- Obtain a history of the client's health problems and drugs that are taken daily.
- Explain the procedure(s) to the client. Refer questions with unknown answers to other health professionals.
- Check that the client is not wearing facial makeup and has not had food in the last 8 hours.
- Record baseline vital signs.
- Ask the client if he or she has a pacemaker or a perforated eardrum. The test is contraindicated if either is present.

Client Teaching
- Inform the client that the room will be dark and electrodes will be placed around the eyes.
- Tell the client that nausea and vomiting may occur during the test. If this feeling occurs, the operator should be informed.
- Explain to the client that several positions and procedures may occur during the test. The client is asked to cooperate.
- Tell the client that bed rest may be ordered following the test if nausea or vertigo is present.
- Inform the client that the test takes 1 hour or less.
- Be supportive of the client and answer questions or refer the unknown questions to health professionals.

Endoscopic retrograde cholangiopancreatography (ERCP)*

Normal Finding
Normal biliary and pancreatic ducts.

*Updated by Dr. Warren G. Butt, Gastroenterology-Stomach-Colon-Liver, Newark, Delaware.

Description

Endoscopic retrograde cholangiopancreatography (ERCP) is an imaging technique in which the biliary pancreatic ducts are examined endoscopically after contrast medium is injected into the duodenal papilla. The purpose for this procedure is to identify the cause of a biliary obstruction, which could be stricture, cyst, stones, or tumor. Jaundice is usually present.

ERCP is performed following abdominal ultrasound, computed tomography, liver scanning, and/or biliary tract x-ray studies to confirm or diagnose a hepatobiliary or pancreatic disorder. However, endoscopic ultrasound and MRI are usually preferred to ERCP.

Purposes

- To detect biliary stones, stricture, cyst, or tumor.
- To identify biliary obstruction, such as stones or stricture.
- To confirm a biliary or pancreatic disorder.

Clinical Problems

Indications: Biliary stones, stricture, cyst, or tumor; primary cholangitis; cirrhosis; pancreatic stones, stricture, cysts or pseudocysts, or tumor; chronic pancreatitis; pancreatic fibrosis; or duodenal papilla tumors.

Procedure

- Food and fluids are restricted for at least 8 hours before the test.
- The consent form should be signed by the client prior to premedication.
- Obtain baseline vital signs. Have the client void.
- Premedicate with mild narcotic or sedative. Atropine may be given prior to or after insertion of the endoscope. Atropine relaxes gastrointestinal motility and will cause dryness of mouth.
- Local anesthetic is sprayed in back of throat (pharynx) to decrease the gag reflex prior to the insertion of the fiberoptic endoscope.
- Secretin may be given intravenously to paralyze the duodenum. Contrast medium is injected after the endoscope is at the duodenal papilla and the catheter is in the pancreatic duct.

Factors Affecting Diagnostic Results

- Inability to cannulate biliary and/or pancreatic duct.

NURSING IMPLICATIONS WITH RATIONALE

Pretest

- Obtain a client history of allergies to seafood, iodine, and contrast dye. Report allergic findings.
- Determine whether the anxiety level may interfere with the client's ability to absorb information concerning the procedure.
- Check that the consent form has been signed prior to premedications.
- Explain to the client that when the contrast medium is injected, there usually is a transient flushing sensation.

E

- Be supportive of the client prior to and during the test procedure.
- Monitor the vital signs during the test and compare them to baseline vital signs. An increase in the pulse rate could be due to atropine. Rupture within the gastrointestinal tract caused by endoscope perforation could cause shock.

Client Teaching

- Inform the client that the endoscope will not obstruct breathing.
- Inform the client that atropine will make the mouth dry and the tongue feel large or swollen.
- Inform the client that the test takes approximately 1 hour and that lying still on the x-ray table is important.

Posttest

- Monitor vital signs. A rise in temperature might indicate infection (bacteremia or septicemia). Check respirations for respiratory distress resulting from anesthetic spray and/or the endoscope.
- Check skin color. Increased or decreased jaundice is an indicator of a disease process or the result of therapy.
- Check the gag reflex before offering food or drink.
- Check signs and symptoms of urinary retention caused by atropine.

Client Teaching

- Suggest warm saline gargle and/or lozenges to decrease throat discomfort.
- Explain to the client that he or she may have a sore throat for a few days after the test. This is due to the endoscope.

Endoscopic ultrasound (EUS)*

Normal Findings

Normal ultrasonographic views; no irregular borders.

Description

Endoscopic ultrasound (EUS) is an imaging technique that allows fine visualization of structures outside the gastrointestinal tract. An endoscope is attached to an ultrasound transducer providing both a view of the lumen and ultrasound imaging of deeper structures. EUS is one of the newest diagnostic tests of ultrasonography that improves accuracy by reducing artifacts from anatomic structures and gas.

This technique is mostly utilized for early detection of cancer, staging of cancer, and visualization of the biliary tree. Fine needle aspiration under EUS guidance allows for pathologic evaluations.

*Written by Dr. Warren G. Butt, Gastroenterology-Stomach-Colon-Liver, Newark, Delaware.

Purposes

- Detect and staging of tumors.
- Obtain pathology.
- Visualize bile duct stones.

Clinical Problems

Positive Findings: Tumors, staging tumors, lymph node metastasis, bile duct stones.

Procedure

- Food and fluids are restricted for 6–8 hours before the test.
- Obtain a signed consent form before the procedure.
- Obtain vital signs.
- Anesthesia is given. The scope is then introduced into the mouth or anus.
- Obtain a biopsy when indicated.

Factors Affecting Diagnostic Test

- Food in the stomach.
- Prior surgery.

E

NURSING IMPLICATIONS WITH RATIONALE

- Obtain a history of prior surgery, especially cholecystectomy.
- Obtain a signed consent form. Discuss the risks of the procedure before client signs.
- Record client's vital signs before, during, and following the procedure.
- Determine the client's anxiety level to see if it may interfere with the client's ability to absorb information.
- Remove dentures, glasses, jewelry.

Client Teaching

- Explain the procedure to the client.
- Inform the client that the test will take approximately 1 hour.
- Inform the client that his or her mouth may feel dry and the tongue large or swollen. This will subside.
- Explain to the client that he or she may have a sore throat for a few days after the test. This is due to the endoscope. Suggest warm saline gargle and/or lozenges to decrease throat discomfort.

Esophageal acidity
See Esophageal Studies

Esophageal manometry

See Esophageal Studies

Esophageal studies*

Esophageal Acidity, Esophageal Manometry, Acid Perfusion (Bernstein test)

Normal Finding

Esophagus secretions of pH 5–6.

Description

Esophageal studies may be performed to determine cause of pyrosis (heartburn) and dysphagia (difficulty in swallowing). Most esophageal problems result from the reflux of gastric juices into the lower part of the esophagus caused by inadequate closure of the cardioesophageal (low esophageal) sphincter.

Gastric secretions are highly acidic, with a pH of 1–2.5, whereas the pH in the esophagus is 5–6. Backflow of gastric juices causes esophageal irritation or esophagitis.

Esophageal acidity, esophageal manometry, and acid perfusion (Bernstein test) are three common studies performed.

Esophageal Acidity: *One-Time Measurement:* A pH electrode attached to a catheter is passed into the lower esophagus to measure esophageal acidity. Measurement of pH in the esophagus is taken. If there is no acid reflux, hydrochloric acid (HCl) 0.1N is instilled into the stomach. Analysis of esophageal acidity is repeated. A pH less than 2 indicates acid reflux, which is most likely caused by an incompetent lower esophageal sphincter. The one-time measurement of esophageal acidity has largely been replaced by the 24-hour pH monitoring. *24-Hour pH Monitoring:* A pH electrode probe is passed through the nostril into the lower esophagus to measure esophageal acidity. The probe is connected to a recording device, which is worn by the client. The client keeps a diary of all symptoms and activities as they occur and marks them by an indicator on the recorder. After 24 hours, the data are analyzed and interpreted.

Esophageal Manometry: This procedure measures esophageal sphincter pressure and records peristaltic contractions (duration and sequence). It detects esophageal motility disorder (e.g., achalasia). The baseline cardioesophageal sphincter pressure is approximately 20 mm Hg. In achalasia, the baseline sphincter pressure could be as high as 50 mm Hg (baseline cardio-esophageal sphincter pressure is approximately 20 mm Hg), and the relaxation pressure could be around 24 mm Hg. This indicates that peristalsis is weak and that food and fluid cannot pass into the stomach until the weight of the contents is increased. For spasms of the esophagus, the sphincter is normal and peristalsis has irregular motility and force.

---

*Updated by Dr. Warren Butt, Gastroenterology-Stomach-Colon-Liver, Newark, Delaware.

Acid Perfusion (Bernstein Test): This test is useful to distinguish between gastric acid reflux causing "heartburn" or esophagitis, and cardiac involvement (i.e., angina, myocardial infarction). Saline and HCl 0.1N are dripped through tubing, one at a time, into the esophagus. If the client complains of symptoms of esophagitis (i.e., epigastric discomfort, heartburn after ½ hour of IV HCl drip), then the cause is acid reflux. Additional gastrointestinal studies, such as barium swallow and esophagogastroduodenoscopy, are needed to confirm the suspected diagnosis.

Esophageal Impedance: This test is usually performed in conjunction with 24-hour pH studies. With this study, nonacid reflux can be assessed.

Purposes

- To distinguish between gastric acid reflux and cardiac involvement.
- To diagnose gastric acid reflux.
- To determine the cause of heartburn or difficulty in swallowing.

Clinical Problems

Esophageal Acidity: Incompetent lower esophageal sphincter, chronic reflux esophagitis.

Esophageal Manometry: Spasm of esophagus, achalasia, esophageal scleroderma.

Acid Perfusion (Bernstein Test): Esophagitis, epigastric pain or discomfort.

Procedure

- A consent form should be signed.
- Food and fluids are restricted 8–12 hours prior to the test. Avoid alcohol intake 24 hours before the test.
- Place client in high Fowler position.
- Monitor pulse during test procedure to detect arrhythmias from catheter insertion.
- Withhold antacids and autonomic nervous system agents (i.e., anticholinergics, cholinergics, adrenergic blockers, glucocorticoids, and H_2 blockers [cimetidine, ranitidine]) for 24 hours before the test as indicated, or note on the laboratory slip the last time administered and dosage.
- Withhold proton pump inhibitors 1 week prior to the test.

Esophageal Acidity: One-Time Measurement
- Catheter with pH electrode is inserted into the esophagus through the client's nostril.
- The client is asked to stimulate acid reflux by performing a Valsalva maneuver or lifting the legs.
- If there is no acid reflux, then 300 mL of HCl 0.1N is administered over 3 minutes, and the Valsalva maneuver or lifting of the legs is repeated.

Esophageal Acidity: 24-Hour pH Monitoring and Impedance Monitoring
- The client should be NPO of solid foods for 8 hours.
- The catheter with the pH probe is inserted into the esophagus through the client's nostril.
- The probe is taped securely at the nose.
- Secure the recorder to the client's belt or provide a shoulder strap.
- The client records symptoms and activities in a diary and on the recorder over a 24-hour period.

Esophageal Manometry

- A manometric catheter with a pressure transducer is inserted through the nostril into the esophagus.
- Esophageal sphincter pressure is measured before and after swallowing.
- Peristaltic contractions are recorded.

Acid Perfusion (Bernstein Test)

- A catheter is passed through the nose into the esophagus.
- Saline solution is dripped (6–10 mL/min) through the catheter.
- The client is told to indicate when pain occurs.
- HCl 0.1N is dripped through the catheter for ½ hour.
- The client is told to indicate when pain occurs.
- As soon as pain or discomfort is reported, the HCl line is turned off, and saline solution is started until symptoms have subsided.

Factors Affecting Diagnostic Results

- Antacids, anticholinergics, H_2 antagonists, and proton pump inhibitors may increase pH, thus reducing acidity and causing false test results.
- Cholinergics, adrenergic blockers, alcohol, or corticosteroids may decrease pH, thus increasing acidity and relaxing the lower esophageal sphincter.

NURSING IMPLICATIONS WITH RATIONALE

- Explain the test procedure(s) to the client (see *Procedure*). Answer the client's questions, or refer the questions to appropriate health professionals.
- Assess communications for verbal–nonverbal expressions of anxiety and fear about tests and/or the potential or actual problem.
- Monitor pulse and blood pressure during procedure. Baseline vital signs should be recorded. Report irregularity of pulse rate immediately to the health care provider. Check for signs of respiratory distress during catheter insertion.

Client Teaching

- Inform the client that food and fluids are restricted for 8–12 hours before the test. Alcoholic beverages should be avoided for 24 hours prior to the test.
- Explain to the client that certain drugs taken (e.g., antacids, anticholinergics, adrenergic blockers, cholinergics, cimetidine) may be withheld for 24 hours. If these drugs are not withheld, the drug name and dose and the last time the drug was taken should be recorded on the laboratory slip.
- Instruct the client to sit in the high Fowler position for insertion of the catheter.

Esophageal Activity—Client Teaching

- Inform the client that a catheter (with electrode) will be swallowed, and the pH of the esophagus secretions are recorded.

- Tell the client to perform the Valsalva maneuver (bear down and hold breath) or to lift legs to stimulate gastric acid reflux as directed by the health care provider.
- Instruct the client to inform the health care provider of any pain or discomfort.

Esophageal Acidity: 24-Hour pH Monitoring—Client Teaching

- Instruct the client that he or she can have a regular diet during the 24 hours of recording unless otherwise indicated.
- Inform the client that a catheter (with electrode) will be inserted through the nostril and the pH of the esophageal secretions will be recorded.
- Inform the client that the catheter will be attached to a recording device. He or she will wear the recorder for 24 hours.
- Instruct the client that a diary will be provided. Symptoms and activities should be noted in the diary at the time they occur.
- Instruct the client not to operate the microwave oven during the 24 hours.
- Inform the client that the recorder should not get wet. A sponge bath rather than a shower is suggested.
- Instruct the client to return to the department in 24 hours to have the probe removed.

Esophageal Manometry—Client Teaching

- Inform the client that a manometric catheter is to be swallowed. The esophageal pressure and peristaltic contractions are recorded.
- Tell the client that drinking water will be requested.

Acid Perfusion (Bernstein Test)—Client Teaching

- Inform the client that a catheter is to be inserted through the nose into the esophagus.
- Tell the client there will be two IV solutions, and that only one will be dripping into the catheter at a time.
- Instruct the client to inform the health care provider immediately when pain or discomfort occurs during the procedure.

Esophagogastroduodenoscopy, esophagogastroscopy*

Gastroscopy, Esophagoscopy, Duodenoscopy, Endoscopy

Normal Finding

Normal mucous membranes of the esophagus, stomach, and duodenum; absence of pathology.

Description

Esophagogastroscopy includes gastroscopy and esophagoscopy. If duodenoscopy is included with the endoscopic examination, the term is *esophagogastroduodenoscopy*. A flexible fiberoptic endoscope is used for direct visualization of the internal structures of the esophagus, stomach,

---

*Updated by Dr. Warren G. Butt, Gastroenterology-Stomach-Colon-Liver, Newark, Delaware.

and duodenum. Biopsy forceps or a cytology brush can also be inserted through a channel of the endoscope. Suction can be applied for the removal of secretions and foreign bodies.

This test is performed under local anesthesia or IV sedation (benzodiazepine or narcotics), in a gastroscopy room of a hospital or clinic, usually by a gastroenterologist. This procedure can be done on an emergency basis for removal of foreign objects (a bone, a pin, etc.) and for diagnostic purposes. The major complications that can occur from esophagogastroduodenoscopy are perforation and hemorrhage.

Purposes

- To visualize the internal esophagus, stomach, and duodenum.
- To obtain a cytologic specimen.
- To confirm the presence of gastrointestinal pathology.

Clinical Problems

Esophageal: Esophagitis, hiatal hernia, esophageal stenoses, achalasia, esophageal neoplasms (benign or malignant tumors), esophageal varices, Mallory-Weiss tear.

Gastric: Gastritis, gastric neoplasm (benign or malignant), gastric ulcer (acute or chronic), gastric varices.

Duodenal (Small Intestine): Duodenitis, diverticula, duodenal ulcer, neoplasm (benign or malignant).

Procedure

- A consent form should be signed by the client.
- The client should be NPO for 8–12 hours before the test. When this procedure is used during an emergency and NPO cannot be enforced, the client's stomach is lavaged (suctioned) to prevent aspiration.
- The client may take prescribed medications at 6 AM on the day of the test. Check with laboratory or health care provider for any changes.
- A sedative/tranquilizer, a narcotic analgesic, and atropine may be given an hour before the test, or they can be titrated intravenously immediately prior to the procedure and during the procedure as needed.
- A local anesthetic may be used.
- Dentures, jewelry, and clothing should be removed from the neck to the waist.
- Record baseline vital signs. The client should void before the procedure.
- Specimen containers should be labeled with the client's name, the date, and the type of tissue.
- Emergency drugs and equipment should be available for hypersensitivity to medications (premedications and anesthetic) and for severe laryngospasms.
- The test takes approximately 1 hour or less.
- The client should not drive self home following the test because of possible after effects of sedation.

Factors Affecting Diagnostic Results

- Barium from a recent gastrointestinal imaging series can decrease visualization of the mucosa. This test should not be performed within 2 days after such tests. An x-ray film of the abdomen can be taken to see if barium is in the stomach or duodenum.

NURSING IMPLICATIONS WITH RATIONALE

Pretest

- Recognize that a gastroscopy test for visualizing the esophageal, gastric, and duodenal mucosa is actually an esophagogastroduodenoscopy. These names are frequently used interchangeably.
- Check that the client's dentures, eyeglasses, and jewelry are removed. Give the client a hospital gown.
- Have the client void. Take vital signs.
- Check that a consent form has been signed before giving the client premedications. Once the sedative and the narcotic analgesic are given, the client should remain in bed with the bed sides up. Tell him or her that these medications will cause drowsiness.
- Be a good listener. Allow the client time to ask questions and to express concerns or fears. Refer questions you cannot answer to the gastroenterologist or health care provider.
- Check that the client has not had food or fluids 8–12 hours before the tests.

Client Teaching

- Explain the procedure to the client. Inform the client that the instrument is flexible; the procedure will be done under local anesthesia (the throat will be sprayed); premedications will be given before the test, and usually IV sedation is given with the test; dentures and jewelry should be removed; and food and fluids will be restricted for 8–12 hours before the test.

Posttest

- Explain to the client that he or she may feel some pressure with the insertion of the endoscope and may feel some fullness in the stomach when air is injected for better visualization of the stomach and intestine areas.
- Check the gag reflex before offering food and fluids by asking the client to swallow or by touching the posterior pharynx with a cotton swab or tongue blade if the throat was sprayed with an anesthetic.
- Keep the client NPO for 2–4 hours after the test or as ordered.
- Monitor vital signs (blood pressure, pulse, respirations) as ordered.
- Give the client throat lozenges or analgesics for throat discomfort. Inform the client that he or she may have flatus or "burp-up gas," which is normal. This is caused by the instillation of air during the procedure for visualization purposes.
- Observe the client for possible complications (e.g., perforation in the gastrointestinal tract from the endoscope). Symptoms could include pain (epigastric, abdominal, back pain), dyspnea, fever, tachycardia, and subcutaneous emphysema in the neck.

Client Teaching

- Be supportive of the client and family.

Fetal biophysical profile
Fetal Activity: Ultrasound

Normal Finding
Score of 8–10 points, the total for five parameters.

Description
Fetal biophysical profile evaluates fetal status by five parameters with ultrasound: (1) fetal heart rate, (2) fetal breathing movement, (3) gross fetal movements, (4) fetal muscle tone, and (5) amniotic fluid volume, according to Pagana and Pagana (2011). The fetal nonstress test measures primarily the fetal heart rate, whereas the ultrasound measures these parameters of fetal status. Each of the five parameters are rated as 0–2. A perfect score for the five parameters is 10.

The *fetal heart rate reactivity* is measured, and a score of 2 is given if the rate is at least 15 beats per minute above baseline for 20 minutes. If the fetal heart rate would be nonreactive, the score would be 0. The *fetal breathing movements* are given a rating of 2 for 1 fetal breathing in 1 minute. Fetal breathing usually does not become regular until after 36 weeks of gestation. Also fetal breathing movements increase after meals and at bedtime. Lack of breathing movement can indicate hypoxemia and the score would be 0. If the pregnant female smokes or drinks alcohol, the fetal breathing rate decreases. The *fetal body movement* is determined by the frequency of fetal movement. A score of 2 is given if the fetus moves at least 3 times in 30 minutes. If fewer fetal movements occur in 30 minutes, the score is 0. Fetal movement is increased during the mother's meals. The *fetal muscle tone* is assessed according to the fetal positions in flexion and extension of the arms, legs, and head. When there is one extension and returned flexion, the score is 2. If there is only a partial extension and no flexion, the score would be 0. The *amniotic fluid volume* is measured by a pocket or quadrant of amniotic fluid. A rating of 2 is given if the pocket or quadrant of amniotic fluid measures 1 cm. Too little amniotic fluid could indicate uterine growth retardation, fetal anomalies, or postterm pregnancy. The score of 0 would be given if the pocket of amniotic fluid is less than 1 cm.

If the total score is less than 2, immediate delivery would be indicated.

Purpose
- To assess the fetal status according to five parameters (see *Description*).

Clinical Problems
Abnormal findings: Fetal distress because of fetal hypoxemia, congenital anomalies, oligohydramnios (lack of amniotic fluid), postterm pregnancy, fetal stress, and fetal death.

Procedure
- A consent form may or may not be required.
- There is no food or fluid restriction.
- Prepare the pregnant mother for an ultrasound.

Factors Affecting Diagnostic Tests

- If no movement is noted visually, the fetus could be asleep.
- If the mother has recently eaten or is taking CNS stimulants, the fetal activities could be increased.

NURSING IMPLICATIONS AND RATIONALE

- Obtain a history from the pregnant mother of any fetal or physical problems that are occurring.
- Explain the procedure and the five parameters to be noted by ultrasound to the mother.
- Record and monitor vital signs.

Client Teaching

- If the fetal findings are abnormal, which the health care provider has indicated, be supportive to the mother. Permit her to ventilate her feelings and concerns.

Fetal fibronectin (fFN)
Cervicovaginal Fluid Analysis

F

Normal Finding

Negative to less than 0.05 mcg/mL.

Description

The fetal fibronectin is detected in cervicovaginal secretions during the first 22 weeks of pregnancy. fFN is secreted in early pregnancy to help attach the fertilized egg to the endometrium (uterus). It diminishes during the 24th–34th weeks of gestation. The highest concentration of fFN is in the amniotic fluid. There is a high risk of preterm (premature) birth if fFN is present in the vaginal secretions after 24 weeks.

The test for fFN on vaginal secretions is usually done after 24 weeks, when there are questionable symptoms of early labor. The membranes should be intact and cervical dilation should be less than 3 cm. An early drug intervention such as corticosteroids or tocolytic agent may be prescribed to prevent preterm labor. There is a 35% chance that pregnant women who test positive for fFN will still deliver a full-term infant.

Purposes

- To detect the presence of fetal fibronectin in the cervicovaginal fluid during 24–34 weeks of gestation.
- To prevent preterm labor following a positive fFN test after 24 weeks of gestation with medical and drug intervention.

Clinical Problems

Abnormal Findings: Increase in fFN, greater than 0.05 mcg/mL after 24 weeks of gestation; prelabor symptoms with an increase in fFN.

Procedure

- There is no food or fluid restriction.
- Obtain cervicovaginal secretions by rotating a Dacron swab in the cervix and vagina areas, rotating the swab for approximately 10 seconds to absorb the secretions.
- Place the swab into a buffered collection tube. Send the specimen to the laboratory.

Factors Affecting Diagnostic Results

- Sexual intercourse within 24 hours of the test.
- Ruptured membranes and cervical dilation >3 cm.
- Vaginal bleeding.
- Contamination of vaginal area with use of lubricants, disinfectants during the collection of secretions.

NURSING IMPLICATIONS WITH RATIONALE

- Ask the female if she has had any symptoms of prelabor, the number of weeks of gestation, and previous pregnancy history.
- Obtain vital signs (VS). Keep a chart of her VS.
- Explain the procedure to the client.

Client Teaching

- Inform the client of symptoms of prelabor, such as uterine cramps or contractions, pelvic pressure, back pain, vaginal discharge, and any recent changes in the pregnancy.
- Inform the client that there should not be any discomfort except when the speculum is introduced into the vagina.
- Tell the client the test results may not be available for 2 days.
- Be available to the client for her to express concerns. Be supportive of the client and family.

Fetal nonstress test (NST) and contraction stress test (CST)*

Normal Finding

Normal (negative) result.

NST: Expressed as a *reactive* (reassuring) NST; evidenced by acceleration in fetal heart rate (FHR) occurring either spontaneously or in response to fetal movement in utero. The American College of Obstetricians and Gynecologists (ACOG) criteria for a *reactive* NST is the presence of two or more accelerations of fetal heart rate of at least 15 beats per minute (bpm) or more above the baseline FHR of 120–160 bpm (each acceleration having a duration of at least 15 seconds) within a 20-minute period of monitoring.

---

*Prepared by Jane Purnell Taylor, Associate Professor, Neumann College, Aston, Pennsylvania.

Reactive (reassuring) NST implies presence of adequate fetal oxygenation and an intact central and autonomic nervous system.

CST: Expressed as a *negative* (reassuring) test; evidenced by detecting *no* late decelerations during a 10-minute period when three "good" quality contractions of 40 seconds or more occur. Additionally, the CST result is expressed as negative if contractions are 3 minutes apart, of palpable intensity, and of 40- to 60-second duration, and the fetus shows no late decelerations.

Negative (reassuring) CST implies presence of uteroplacental sufficiency such that the fetus is considered likely to be able to withstand the stressors associated with labor contractions with decreased risk for intrauterine asphyxia.

Description

The fetal nonstress test and the contraction stress test are two diagnostic tests used to help evaluate fetal functioning and well-being in response to either fetal movement (NST) or to spontaneous or induced uterine contraction (CST). The **NST** is inexpensive, rapidly accomplished, lacks side effects, and is helpful in identifying at-risk fetuses of mothers who exhibit high-risk pregnancy conditions, including diabetes, intrauterine growth retardation, pregnancy-induced hypertension, and report by mother of decreased fetal movements, among others. Only minimal equipment is required (external transducer for fetal heart rate monitoring); testing occurs 1–2 times per week depending on the reason for doing the testing. The **CST** is also employed at 32–34 weeks in evaluating high-risk pregnancies, particularly pregnancy conditions that may place the fetus at risk if there is poor placental perfusion, including diabetes, intrauterine growth retardation, and postterm gestation over 42 weeks. In addition, certain fetuses who exhibit a nonreactive NST in the presence of additional data may also have a CST performed. Contraindications to CST testing include presence of a classical uterine incision, presence of placenta previa, multiple gestation, and vaginal bleeding, among others. Equipment required for CSTs includes an external transducer (for FHR monitoring), together with a tocodynamometer (toco) for monitoring uterine contractions. The NST and CST are able to be performed in hospital, office, and clinic settings; the NST may also be conducted in the home care setting with supervision.

Fetal Nonstress Test (NST): NST is a noninvasive test that monitors FHR with fetal movement. According to the ACOG, the FHR should increase by 15 bpm within a 20-minute interval. If there is no fetal movement or increased FHR in 20 minutes, the mother's abdomen may be rubbed or a loud noise made close to the abdomen to stimulate fetal movement. If after 40 minutes there is no acceleration of FHR, the NST is nonreactive and a CST may be ordered. With a nonreactive NST after 40 minutes, fetal distress may be considered; however, the fetus may be in a sleep cycle or the mother may have taken a CNS depressant drug. The NST is usually performed at 30 weeks of gestation to allow for sufficient CNS maturation, after which heart rate accelerations in response to movement become more fully established.

Contraction Stress Test: There are two types of CST; the nipple stimulation test and the oxytocin challenge test (OCT). The nipple stimulation test is a noninvasive test that stimulates the hypothalamus, which promotes the release of oxytocin. This can cause uterine contractions, and a normal result would be that the FHR does not show late deceleration. The OCT is somewhat noninvasive but could induce labor in some clients. Oxytocin, a uterine stimulant, is well diluted in IV fluids and thus does not cause continuous contractions. There should be three moderate contractions occurring within 10 minutes, and the FHR should not show any late deceleration. If there is a late deceleration of FHR with contractions, the test indicates that hypoxia may result during labor due to insufficient placental function. The CST with oxytocin is performed at 32 weeks, preferably 34 weeks of gestation. In case this test would induce labor, the fetus would have a better chance to survive.

Purposes

- To evaluate fetal functioning and well-being.
- To evaluate sufficiency of uteroplacental function to support the fetus in labor.
- To screen high-risk pregnancies.

Clinical Problems

Abnormal Findings: Fetal distress, fetal death, and placental dysfunction.

Procedure

- A signed consent form is required.
- Baseline vital signs are taken for future comparison.
- Position mother in semi-Fowler or lateral position with roll/wedge under right hip to displace uterus to the left slightly.
- Apply transducer (NST) or transducer and toco (CST).
- Monitor maternal blood pressure during the procedure for occurrence of hypotension.

Nonstress Test

- The client presses the pressure transducer when she feels the body move.
- Monitor for FHR acceleration. There should be 15 bpm that last for 15 seconds. If the FHR does not increase, rub the mother's abdomen or thump/hit a pan that is close to her abdomen to stimulate fetal movement. If there is no fetal movement in 40 minutes and no acceleration in FHR, the test indicates a nonreactive fetus.

Contraction Stress Test

Nipple Stimulation:

- The client stimulates one nipple with water-soluble ointment until a contraction occurs. Contraction should occur within 2 minutes, and if it does not, nipple stimulation could continue for 15 minutes.
- If there is no late deceleration occurring during three contractions in FHR, the test result is considered normal. If there are late decelerations during any contractions, the appropriate health care provider should be notified, for it can indicate that the fetus is receiving insufficient blood supply from the placenta.

Oxytocin Challenge Test

- Vital signs and FHR are taken at frequent intervals.
- NPO may be suggested in case labor begins.
- Administer oxytocin by IV infusion pump, dosage will be ordered. The oxytocin rate may be slowly increased until the client has a moderate contraction. If contraction occurs before the oxytocin infusion, withhold the drug.
- A normal test result is no late deceleration of FHR. If late deceleration occurs, it could indicate placental dysfunction that could cause the fetus to receive insufficient oxygen during labor.
- Test should be conducted in a health facility.
- Monitor FHR for 30–60 minutes after oxytocin infusion has been stopped.
- Test takes approximately 1–2 hours.

Factors Affecting Diagnostic Results

- NST is often nonreactive before 30–32 weeks due to central nervous system immaturity.
- NST may be classified as falsely nonreactive because of the occurrence of fetal sleep cycles.
- NST may be more commonly classified as falsely reactive in diabetic clients, postterm pregnancies, and pregnancy-induced hypertension associated with intrauterine growth retardation.
- NST may be falsely nonreactive when smoking has occurred prior to the NST; also in the event of CNS depressant drugs or beta blockers taken by the client.
- NST and CST's equipment difficulties and/or inexperienced operators may mean difficulty obtaining or accurately interpreting tracings.

NURSING IMPLICATIONS WITH RATIONALE

- Obtain a gestation history from the client.
- Determine mother's knowledge level related to high-risk pregnancy condition and purposes of NST/CST testing and what these measure.
- Incorporate the family into the discussion and testing process as much as possible and desired.
- Remain with the client during testing as often as possible if other supports are lacking.
- Attempt to schedule testing times at client's convenience; follow up on missed appointments.
- Position client correctly to prevent hypotension.
- Monitor blood pressure and other vital signs at stated intervals consistent with agency protocols.
- Report abnormal changes.

Client Teaching

- Use testing opportunity (NST) to teach importance of observing fetal movement.
- Encourage the client to rest following the test procedure.
- Inform the client to report bleeding, continuous contractions, and lack of fetal movement.

Fetoscopy*

Percutaneous Umbilical Blood Sampling (PUBS), Cordocentesis

Normal Finding

Absence of abnormalities as presented in *Clinical Problems, Abnormal Findings*.

Description

Fetoscopy: Fetoscopy is the direct visualization of the fetus by means of an endoscope inserted through the maternal abdominal wall into the uterine cavity for the purpose of obtaining a blood or skin sample or for visualization of external developmental abnormalities. It is rarely used now

---

*Prepared by Jane Purnell Taylor, MS, RN, Associate Professor, Neumann College, Aston, Pennsylvania.

for blood sampling due to 2–5% risk of serious complications. As a result of possible complications, this technique has evolved (particularly in high-risk perinatal centers) into the increased use of *percutaneous umbilical blood sampling or PUBS*, which is known as *cordocentesis.*

Cordocentesis or PUBS: It is a technique in which an ultrasound-guided 22–26 gauge needle is used to puncture the umbilical cord to obtain fetal blood samples. Reports indicate that many operators find a site about 1 cm from the placenta to be an optimal site for obtaining fetal blood from the umbilical vein. Cordocentesis has been done as early as 12 weeks, but more commonly after 18 weeks until 36 weeks. Early procedures carry a higher risk to the fetus. The amount of blood removed is between 1 and 4 mL; after 20 weeks of gestation, 5 mL may be safely removed. Ultrasound is used to ascertain gestational age of the fetus, position of the fetus, the thickness and location of the placenta, position of tissues to be visualized or sampled, and placement of the needle tip used to obtain the sample. While fetoscopy is less used today for purposes of fetal blood sampling, the endoscopic technique does allow for direct visualization of aspects of the fetus determined at risk for external abnormalities involving the spine, extremities, face, and genital areas; also for visual access to preferred skin biopsy sites, including the back, thighs, or scalp to aid in diagnosis of selected skin disorders of genetic origin unable to be otherwise detected. In the event that fetal blood sampling is desired but the umbilical cord is unable to be punctured to obtain fetal blood, a safe alternative for consideration is ultrasound needle-guided *fetal heart puncture.* These procedures, their benefits and risks for fetoscopy, cordocentesis (PUBS), or fetal heart puncture should be discussed with the client and family.

Purposes

(Overall purpose is to aid in diagnosis, treatment, and monitoring of fetal disease.)
- To detect inherited blood disorders, including hemophilia A or B, hemoglobinopathies (measurement of hemoglobin concentration to assess fetal anemia), and fetal thrombocytopenia (measurement of fetal platelet count to assess and treat potential risks for perinatal cerebral bleeding).
- To perform rapid fetal karyotyping.
- To detect fetal chromosome abnormalities.
- To detect fetal infection (including CMV, toxoplasmosis, rubella).
- To validate suspected fetal hypoxia or acidosis.
- To treat fetal anemia by transfusion.
- To assess and treat isoimmunization.

Clinical Problems

Abnormal Findings: Hemophilia A and B, fetal anemia, fetal thrombocytopenia, chromosome abnormalities, fetal hypoxia, fetal acidosis, fetal infection, isoimmune hemolytic disorders.

Procedure (Cordocentesis)

- A consent form should be signed and witnessed.
- Health care providers should schedule this diagnostic test within ready access to a room suitable for delivery if necessity should arise. Steroid therapy may need to be administered to the mother prior to the procedure.
- Should the need arise, respiratory support (anesthesiologist/anesthetist) should be quickly available in the setting.
- Monitor maternal vital signs prior to and throughout the test.

- Position mother to reduce opportunity for occurrence of supine hypotension; she must remain still during the procedure.
- Ultrasound scanning of abdomen is performed to visualize chosen area and identify an approach that will protect fetal parts and avoid maternal vessels.
- Skin insertion site is cleansed with agency protocol-specified antiseptic.
- Local anesthetic is injected into the skin and onto the abdominal and uterine peritoneum.
- Use of prophylactic antibiotics varies by setting; rationale for use generally is to avoid amnionitis (infection to amniotic fluid). It has been suggested that this invasive procedure to the fetus might be avoided in the case of a known infected mother depending on benefit-to-risk ratio.
- A paralytic drug, intravascular pancuronium bromide, may be used to prevent the fetus from moving during the sampling procedure.
- The mother may be given medication to assist her to relax during the procedure; however, it is important that the mother not become sedated to the point she exhibits deep breathing. Deep breathing could, as a result of the movement created by her diaphragm, interfere with the puncture of the umbilical vein during the procedure.
- Real-time ultrasound is used for confirmation that the needle tip is correctly placed in the umbilical vein (approximately 1 cm from the placenta cord insertion site). This allows for removal of the stylet from the needle and subsequent aspiration of designated quantity of blood into a syringe containing anticoagulant.

Posttest

- Observe the puncture site (using ultrasound) for bleeding after removal of the needle.
- Employ fetal heart rate monitoring for 30 minutes (minimal) postprocedure, followed by an additional ultrasound 1 hour postprocedure to verify no evidence of bleeding/hematoma.

Factors Affecting Diagnostic Results

- Degree of experience of operator with ultrasound-guided needle procedures.
- Incorrect placement of needle tip resulting in need for additional manipulation; aspiration of sample at wrong time; amniotic fluid contamination of sample (the amniotic fluid has a coagulation effect), or failure to actually obtain a sample.
- Amount of sedation received by mother; degree of hyperventilation; adequacy of placental perfusion (as related to incorrect maternal positioning with resultant supine hypotension). These factors may affect fetal oxygenation levels and outcome of diagnostic studies.
- Placement of sample into incorrect container or container having insufficient or incorrect anticoagulant; loss of portion of the sample; sample contamination; improper labeling of sample.

NURSING IMPLICATIONS WITH RATIONALE

- Obtain a history of the client's health problems, familial health disorders, medications, and any past or present pregnancy problems.
- Monitor vital signs. Monitor fetal heart rate.
- Monitor maternal anxiety level.
- Check medical record to determine if the mother is Rh negative and not sensitized and if the father is Rh positive or negative or unknown. Plan to administer an IM injection of Rh IgG globulin (RhoGAM) following cordocentesis, unless the mother is found to be previously sensitized.

- Have the health care provider or an appropriate health professional discuss the benefits and risks of this procedure. A genetic counselor should also be included.
- Be available to answer questions and concerns, and if unable, refer the questions to other health professionals.
- Assist the mother with proper positioning for the test; assist the mother to relax using relaxation exercises and guided imagery.
- Prevent oversedation of the mother for the procedure to reduce chance of occurrence of deep breathing with diaphragm movement that may interfere during the puncture procedure.

Posttest

- Monitor the mother's vital signs and the fetal heart rate.

Client Teaching

- Instruct the client that she will be ultrasonically monitored for bleeding once the needle is removed.
- Instruct the mother to expect to have fetal monitoring for 30 minutes or more postprocedure.
- Instruct the mother that if intravascular pancuronium bromide (Pavulon) is used during the procedure, she may not detect the amount of fetal movement she has become accustomed to for a few hours.
- Instruct the Rh negative mother to expect, if not sensitized previously, that she will receive an injection of RhoGAM postprocedure.
- Instruct the client to report any pain or bleeding that might occur.
- Instruct her to rest for at least a day following the procedure and to do no heavy lifting.
- Encourage her to increase fluid intake.
- Inform her to notify the health care provider with any questions or concerns.

Fluoroscopy

Fluoroscopic Examination

Normal Finding

Normal size, structure, and physiologic function of the organ(s) being examined (chest, heart, intestines).

Description

The fluoroscopic examination allows the radiologist and health care provider to view in motion the physiologic function of organs on a fluorescent screen. Usually the client is between the x-ray tube and the fluorescent screen. The x-ray beam penetrates the client and then strikes the screen. Unfortunately, the client can receive substantially more radiation than he or she would receive from standard radiography. Today, fluoroscopy is used with many diagnostic tests for visualization and for guidance.

During cardiac catheterization, the fluoroscopic procedure is essential for visualizing the coronary arteries. The moving images can be recorded on videotape and can be a valuable aid to diagnosis.

During fluoroscopic examination, the room is darkened for contrast and visualization purposes. If the radiologist and assistant remain in the room, aprons should be worn.

Purpose

- To view the functions of organs in motion.

Clinical Problems

TEST AREA	INDICATIONS/PURPOSES
Thorax	To visualize lung expansion, diaphragm movement or paralysis, bronchiolar obstruction
Abdomen	To detect bowel obstruction (stricture or tumor), filling defects, active bleeding and ulceration (peptic ulcer), Meckel diverticulum, intra-abdominal hernias
Heart	To detect coronary occlusion (partial or total)

Procedure

Thorax

- Food and fluids are usually not restricted.
- Jewelry should be removed. A gown should be worn.
- The client should breathe deeply and cough as instructed.

Abdomen

- The client should be NPO after midnight.
- A gown should be worn.
- The client swallows a chalky substance, barium sulfate.
- Food and fluids are permitted after the examination.
- A laxative is usually ordered after the test or that evening.

Heart

- The client should be NPO after midnight.
- Follow the procedure for cardiac catheterization (see *Cardiac Catheterization*).

Factors Affecting Diagnostic Results

- Jewelry and metal objects.
- Nausea and vomiting.
- Medications: narcotics, barbiturates.

NURSING IMPLICATIONS WITH RATIONALE

Client Teaching

- Explain the procedure to the client.
- Inform the client that the fluoroscopic examination should *not* cause discomfort.
- Discuss the client's anxiety and fears. Refer questions you cannot answer to other appropriate health professionals.
- Explain to the client that the chest fluoroscopy should take approximately 10 minutes, and the abdominal fluoroscopy 30 minutes to 1 hour.

- Determine if the client is pregnant or if pregnancy is suspected. Report findings immediately. Fluoroscopy should not be done during pregnancy.
- Inform the client that the radiologist or x-ray personnel will give step-by-step instructions during the procedure. Tell the client to ask questions if he or she has any.
- Determine if the client has had extensive exposure to x-rays in the last few years or during his or her lifetime. Excessive radiation can be cumulative. Notify the health care provider of previous prolonged exposure to radiation.

Gastric analysis (basal and stimulation with tube), tubeless gastric analysis

Normal Finding

Fasting: 1–5 mEq/L/h.

Stimulation: 10–25 mEq/L/h.

Tubeless: Detectable dyes in the urine.

Description

The gastric analysis test examines the acidity of the gastric secretions in the basal state (without stimulation) and the maximal secretory ability (with stimulation; i.e., with histamine phosphate, betazole hydrochloride [Histalog], pentagastrin). An increased amount of free hydrochloric acid (HCl) could indicate a peptic ulcer (stomach or duodenal), and an absence of free HCl (achlorhydria) could indicate gastric atrophy (possibly caused by gastric malignancy) or pernicious anemia. In addition, gastric contents can be collected for cytologic examination.

Gastric analysis by tube (basal and stimulation) and tubeless gastric analysis (urine examination after a resin dye and stimulant are administered) are the methods used for evaluating gastric secretions.

Basal Gastric Analysis (Tube): Gastric secretions are aspirated through a nasogastric tube after a period of fasting. Specimens are obtained to evaluate the basal acidity of the gastric content first, and the gastric stimulation test follows.

Stimulation Gastric Analysis (Tube): The stimulation test is usually a continuation of the basal gastric analysis. After samples of gastric secretions are obtained, a gastric stimulant (i.e., Histalog or pentagastrin) is administered, and gastric contents are aspirated every 15–20 minutes until several samples are obtained.

Tubeless Gastric Analysis: This test is for screening purposes to detect the presence or absence of HCl; however, it will *not* indicate the amount of free acid in the stomach. A gastric stimulant (caffeine, Histalog) is given, and an hour later a resin dye (Azuresin, Diagnex Blue) is taken orally by the client. The free HCl releases the dye from the resin base; the dye is absorbed by the gastrointestinal tract and is excreted in the urine. Absence of the dye in the urine 2 hours later is indicative of gastric achlorhydria. This test method saves the client the discomfort of being intubated with a nasogastric tube; however, it does lack accuracy. There is controversy over the usefulness of gastric acid secretory tests; however, they are still used to document gastric acid hypersecretions (e.g., Zollinger-Ellison syndrome and hypergastrinemia).

Purposes

- To evaluate gastric secretions.
- To detect an increase or decrease of free HCl.

Clinical Problems

Decreased Level: Pernicious anemia, gastric malignancy (atrophy), atrophic gastritis.

Increased Level: Peptic ulcer (duodenal), Zollinger-Ellison syndrome.

Procedure

Basal Gastric Analysis (Tube)
- The client should be NPO for 8–12 hours prior to the test. Smoking should be restricted for 8 hours.
- Certain groups of drugs (i.e., anticholinergics, cholinergics, adrenergic blockers, antacids, steroids) and alcohol and coffee should be restricted for at least 24 hours before the test. It should be noted on the request slip if the drugs cannot be withheld.
- Baseline vital signs should be recorded.
- Loose dentures should be removed.
- A lubricated nasogastric tube is inserted through the nose or mouth.
- A residual gastric specimen and four additional specimens taken 15 minutes apart should be aspirated and labeled with the client's name, the time, and a specimen number. The nasogastric tube may be attached to low intermittent suction.

Stimulation Test: A continuation of the basal gastric analysis.
- A gastric stimulant is administered (i.e., betazole hydrochloride [Histalog] or histamine phosphate intramuscularly; pentagastrin subcutaneously).
- Several gastric specimens are obtained over a period of 1–2 hours (histamine four 15-minute specimens in 1 hour and Histalog eight 15-minute specimens in 2 hours). Specimens should be labeled with the client's name, the date, the time, and specimen numbers.
- Vital signs should be monitored. Emergency drugs such as epinephrine (Adrenalin) should be available.
- The test usually takes 2½ hours for both parts (basal and stimulation).

Tubeless Gastric Analysis
- The client should be NPO for 8–12 hours before the test.
- The morning urine specimen is discarded.
- Certain drugs are withheld for 48 hours before the test (i.e., antacids, electrolyte preparations [potassium, calcium, sodium, magnesium], quinidine, quinine, iron, vitamin B complex), with the health care provider's permission.
- Give the client caffeine sodium benzoate 500 mg in a glass of water.
- Collect a urine specimen 1 hour later. This is the control urine specimen.
- Give the client the resin dye agent (Azuresin or Diagnex Blue) in a glass of water.
- Collect a urine specimen 2 hours later. The urine may be colored blue or blue-green for several days. Absence of color in the urine usually indicates absence of HCl in the stomach.

G

Factors Affecting Diagnostic Results

- Incorrect labeling of specimens could affect test results.
- Drugs—antacids, anticholinergics, and histamine blockers (cimetidine, ranitidine) could decrease HCl levels; adrenergic blockers, cholinergics, steroids, and alcohol could elevate HCl levels; antacids, electrolyte and iron preparations, vitamin B complex, and quinidine could falsely elevate the Diagnex Blue level.
- Stress, smoking, and sensory stimulation could increase HCl secretion.

NURSING IMPLICATIONS WITH RATIONALE

- Notify the health care provider if the client is receiving the following categories of drugs: antacids, antispasmodics, anticholinergics, adrenergic blockers, cholinergics, and steroids. Drugs from the above groups and a few others should be withheld for 24–48 hours before the gastric analysis. Drugs that cannot be withheld should be listed on the request slip.
- Monitor vital signs. Observe for possible side effects from use of stimulants (e.g., dizziness, flushing, tachycardia, headache, and a lower systolic blood pressure).
- Label the specimens (gastric or urine) with the client's name, the date, the time, and the specimen number.
- Be supportive of the client. Encourage the client to express his or her concerns or fears. Answer questions or refer them to appropriate health professionals.

Client Teaching

- Explain the purpose and procedure of the tube or tubeless gastric analysis test to the client. Check with the health care provider before you give your explanation to find out whether he or she will perform both basal and stimulation gastric analysis (see *Procedure*). List the steps of the test on paper for the client, if needed.
- Tell the client how the nasogastric tube is inserted (i.e., the tube is lubricated and passes through the nose or mouth) and that he or she will be asked to swallow or will be given sips of water as the tube is passed into the stomach. The end of the tube may be attached to low intermittent suction.

Gastrointestinal (GI) series, upper GI series, barium swallow, small bowel series, hypotonic duodenography

Normal Finding

Normal structure of the esophagus, stomach, and small intestine, and normal peristalsis.

Description

Upper gastrointestinal (GI) and small-bowel series are fluoroscopic and x-ray examinations of the esophagus, stomach, and small intestine. Oral barium meal (barium sulfate) or a water-soluble contrast agent, Gastrografin (meglumine diatrizoate), is swallowed. By means of fluoroscopy, the barium is observed as it passes through the digestive tract, and spot films are taken. Inflammation, ulcerations, and tumors of the stomach and duodenum can be detected through this procedure.

Upper GI series are performed in hospitals or in private laboratories. A preparation sheet is given or sent to the client prior to the test.

If increased peristalsis, a spastic duodenal bulb, or a space-occupying lesion is observed or suspected in the duodenal area during the GI series, a *hypotonic duodenography* procedure can be performed by giving glucagon, atropine, or propantheline (Pro-Banthine) to slow down the action of the small intestine. Preparations for the hypotonic duodenography are similar to those for the upper GI series. Because of the anticholinergic effect of the drug, the client should be observed closely for urinary retention.

Purposes

- To detect an esophageal, gastric, or duodenal ulcer.
- To identify polyps, tumor, or hiatal hernia in the GI tract.
- To detect foreign bodies, esophageal varices, or esophageal or small bowel strictures.

Clinical Problems

Abnormal Findings: Hiatal hernia; esophageal varices; esophageal or small-bowel structures; gastric or duodenal ulcer; gastritis or gastroenteritis; gastric polyps; benign or malignant tumor of the esophagus, stomach, or duodenum; diverticula of the stomach and duodenum; pyloric stenosis; malabsorption syndrome; volvulus of the stomach; foreign bodies.

Procedure

- The client should be NPO (food and fluids) and should refrain from smoking for 8–12 hours before the test. A low-residue diet may be ordered for 2 or 3 days before the test.
- Withhold medications 8 hours before the test unless otherwise indicated. Narcotics and anticholinergic drugs are withheld for 24 hours to avoid intestinal immobility.
- Laxatives may be ordered the evening before the test.
- The client swallows a chalky flavored (chocolate, strawberry) barium meal or meglumine diatrizoate (Gastrografin) in the calculated amount (16–20 oz).
- Spot films are taken during the fluoroscopic examination. The procedure takes approximately 1–2 hours but could take 4–6 hours if the test is to include the bowel series. A 24-hour x-ray film (post-GI series) may be requested.
- A laxative is usually ordered after the completion of the test to get the barium out of the GI tract.

Factors Affecting Diagnostic Results

- Barium in the GI tract from a recent barium study.
- Retention of foods and liquids, which would decrease visualization.
- Excessive air in the stomach and small intestine.

NURSING IMPLICATIONS WITH RATIONALE

- Record vital signs. Note in the chart any epigastric pain or discomfort.

Client Teaching

- Explain the procedure to the client concerning diet and medication restrictions; no smoking; the length of time required to complete the procedure; and the posttest laxative, if ordered (see *Procedure*).
- Inform the client that all of the chalky flavored liquid must be swallowed. Tell the client the tests should not cause pain or any significant discomfort.
- Encourage the client to ask questions or to express any concerns. Refer questions you cannot answer to other appropriate health professionals.

Posttest

- Check with the radiology department that the upper GI series and/or small bowel studies are completed before giving the late breakfast or late lunch. Usually the x-ray department will send a slip with the client stating that the test is finished or that a 24-hour x-ray film will be needed.
- Administer the ordered laxative (e.g., milk of magnesia) after the test.

Client Teaching

- Inform the client that the stools should be light in color for the next several days. Instruct the client to notify the health care provider if he or she does not have a bowel movement in 2–3 days. Barium can cause fecal impaction.

Gastroscopy

See Esophagogastroduodenoscopy

Holter monitoring

Ambulatory Electrocardiography, Dynamic Electrocardiography

Normal Finding

No abnormal electrocardiographic findings.

Description

Holter monitoring (ambulatory electrocardiography) evaluates the client's heart rate and rhythm during normal daily activities, rest, and sleep over 24 hours (occasionally 48 hours). The Holter monitor consists of a continuous electrocardiogram (ECG) recording on a cassette tape that is boxed inside an approximately 1 lb monitor. After 24 hours, the monitor with the tape is returned to the cardiac center and is scanned or reviewed for abnormal findings such as cardiac dysrhythmias.

Holter monitoring began in 1962, and it is still widely used today. The Holter recorder contains a clock that is coordinated with the tape recorder and an event marker for the client to use when having symptom(s). The client is given a diary to record the symptoms such as palpitations, chest pain, shortness of breath, syncope, or vertigo, and the time of the symptoms.

The primary purpose for Holter monitoring is to identify suspected and unsuspected cardiac dysrhythmias, which can be correlated between the recorder, event marking of symptoms, and transient symptoms marked in the diary. It is infrequently ordered for clients having Prinzmetal variant angina, a form of myocardial ischemia that results from spasms of the coronary arteries. Holter monitoring is more sensitive for identifying the cause of the symptoms than a routine ECG.

Purpose

- To identify cardiac dysrhythmias related to cardiac symptoms as marked on the monitor and recorded in the diary.

Clinical Problems

Indications: Suspected and unsuspected cardiac dysrhythmias (supraventricular and ventricular), correlation of symptoms with the ECG tape, mitral valve prolapse causing dysrhythmia, hypertrophic obstructive cardiomyopathy causing atrial and ventricular dysrhythmias, pacemaker malfunction.

Procedure

- A signed consent form may be required.
- There is no food or fluid restriction.
- The skin is cleansed and shaved as needed, and electrodes are placed over bony areas to eliminate artifacts that could be caused by skeletal muscle movements.
- Five to seven electrode patches are placed on the chest. For a five-lead electrode placement, two negative electrodes are secured at the upper right and left manubrial border of the sternum, and two positive electrodes are placed below the sternum, one placed at 2 cm right of the xiphoid process on the rib margin and the second at the left anterior axillary line—sixth rib. A ground electrode is secured at the lower right rib margin over the bone.
- The client is given a diary to record what he or she was doing when symptom(s) such as palpitations, chest pain, and shortness of breath occurred.
- The client should not shower, take a bath, or swim until the electrodes are removed. The client should also avoid vigorous exercise and sweating.

Posttest

- The client returns the Holter monitor the next day (24 hours later) with the diary.
- The nurse/technician reviews the diary with the client for any needed clarification.
- The tape is scanned (reviewed) and the cardiologist submits a written report to the personal health care provider. The client's health care provider explains the ECG monitoring results to the client.

Factors Affecting Diagnostic Results

- The client does not record activities correlated with symptoms in the diary.
- The electrodes fall off the chest.

NURSING IMPLICATIONS WITH RATIONALE

Pretest

- Review client's history of cardiac disorders and/or symptoms.
- Check that a baseline ECG has been received. A comparison of the baseline ECG with the 24-hour ECG monitoring could be requested.

H

Client Teaching

- Explain to the client that this test does not cause pain or any major discomfort. Tell the client that the monitor device weighs approximately one pound.
- Instruct the client that the monitor device will be attached either by a shoulder strap or as a belt.
- Review the procedure for Holter monitoring with the client (see *Procedure*). Answer questions the client may have or refer the questions to appropriate health professional.
- Emphasize the importance of pushing the event marker button on the monitor when symptoms occur and recording in the diary the time, symptoms, and activity that is taking place at the time of symptoms.
- Inform the client that the monitor should *not* get wet. Bathing, showering, and swimming should be avoided. The client should not use an electric razor or electric toothbrush during the 24 hours of monitoring to avoid possible ECG artifacts.
- Instruct the client to return the Holter monitor at approximately the same time that the test was started. The electrodes will be removed. The diary should be given to the nurse or technician, and the client should not leave until the diary has been briefly reviewed for any needed clarifications.
- Explain to the client that the cardiologist will submit a written report to his or her health care provider. The health care provider or other health care providers will notify the client of the findings.

Hysterosalpingography (hysterosalpingogram)
Uterosalpingography

Normal Finding

Normal structure of the uterus and patent fallopian tubes.

Description

Hysterosalpingography is a fluoroscopic and x-ray examination of the uterus and fallopian tubes. A contrast substance, either oil-base Ethiodol or Lipiodol or water-soluble such as diatrizoate or iodinated contrast dye, is inserted into the cervical canal. It flows through the uterus and into the fallopian tubes and spills into the peritoneal cavity where it is absorbed if there is no obstruction. The flow of the contrast medium is radiographically visualized. This test is frequently ordered as part of an infertility study. Usually the procedure is performed by the radiologist and the health care provider (gynecologist).

The hysterosalpingogram should be done on the 7th to the 9th day after the menstrual cycle. The client should not be pregnant or have active bleeding, or an acute infection; if any of these conditions exists, the test should be canceled.

There may be some abdominal cramping, and sometimes there are chills and transient dizziness as the contrast substance spills into the abdominal area. Normally the spillage is not harmful and is expected.

The amount of radiation exposure is high because of the fluoroscopic examination. Today ultrasonography is replacing hysterosalpingography, except that the latter test is more effective in determining tubal patency.

This test should not be performed if there is an infection in the uterus or fallopian tubes, or during a normal pregnancy.

Uterotubal insufflation tests (Rubin's test) is a test used primarily to determine the patency of the fallopian tubes. This test is described in detail later in this part of the text.

Purposes

- To identify uterine fibroids, tumor, or fistula.
- To identify fallopian occlusion, such as internal scarring, obstructed adhesions, kinked tubing, mucous plugs, tubal pregnancy.
- To evaluate repeated fetal losses.
- To determine if tubal ligation is effective.

Clinical Problems

Abnormal Findings: Uterine masses (i.e., fibroids, tumor), uterine fistulas, fallopian tubal occlusion (i.e., adhesions, stricture), extrauterine pregnancy, evaluation of repeated fetal losses.

Procedure

- A consent form for hysterosalpingography should be signed by the client.
- Food and fluids are not restricted.
- A cleansing enema and douche may be ordered prior to the test.
- A mild sedative (e.g., diazepam [Valium]) may be ordered prior to the test.
- The client lies on an examining table in the lithotomy position. The gynecologist, health care provider, or radiologist inserts the speculum into the vaginal canal, and the contrast substance is injected into the cervix under fluoroscopic control. X-rays are taken throughout the 15- to 30-minute procedure.
- Baseline vital signs (VS) should be taken, and VS should be frequently monitored. Baseline ECG may be taken.

Factors Affecting Diagnostic Results

- The client is uncooperative or does not remain still during the procedure.
- The client has allergies to the contrast medium (dye). This should be known before the tests.
- The client has an undiagnosed bleeding problem or renal insufficiency.
- Tubal spasm may cause tubal stricture, which could give the appearance of a partial or complete tubal obstruction in a normal fallopian tube.

NURSING IMPLICATIONS WITH RATIONALE

- Check that the consent form is signed.
- Obtain a history of clinical problems related to the uterus or fallopian tubes.
- Ask the client if she has had any recent barium or contrast dye procedures.
- Record when the client had her last menstrual period. The procedure should *not* be performed on pregnant clients.
- Tell the client that vital signs (VS) will be taken frequently during the procedure.
- Have the client void before the procedure.
- Inform the client that the procedure lasts approximately 30 to 45 minutes.

Client Teaching

- Explain to the client that the purpose of the test is to visualize the uterus and tubes for any abnormalities or to determine the patency of the fallopian tubes.

- Explain the procedure to the client. The procedure may differ slightly in your institution, so check before explaining to the client.
- Encourage the client to ask questions and to express concerns. Be a good listener. Refer questions and concerns you cannot handle adequately to other appropriate health professionals.

Posttest

- Check for signs and symptoms of infection following the test, such as fever, increased pulse rate, and pain. Notify the health care provider.

Client Teaching

- Inform the client that she may experience some abdominal cramping and some dizziness. Explain that this is normal but that if there is continuous and severe cramping, she should call the physician.
- Advise the client that any abnormal symptoms, such as difficulty in breathing, fast heart rate, chest pain, or abdominal pain, should be reported to the health care provider.
- Inform the client that sexual intercourse is not advised until 2 weeks after the test. The time frame may differ with some physicians.
- Inform the client that there may be some bloody discharge for several days following the test. If it continues beyond 3–4 days, she should notify her health care provider.
- Instruct the client to call the health care provider if a high fever is present.

Hysteroscopy

Normal Finding

Normal uterine cavity; normal endometrial uterine tissue.

Description

Hysteroscopy allows visualization of the entire endometrial cavity of the uterus. This test is considered to be more effective for viewing and obtaining endometrial pathology than the D & C (dilatation and curettage) or hysterosalpingography. With D & C, scraping of the endometrial tissue is done without visualization, which may result in failure to harvest the pathologic tissue. With the use of the hysteroscope, a biopsy could be taken and polyp(s) removed.

Hysteroscopy is contraindicated if there is cervical or vaginal infection, pelvic inflammatory disease, or purulent vaginal discharge, or if cervical surgery has been performed previously. Risks of hysteroscopy include perforation of the uterus or infection.

Purposes

- To visualize the uterine cavity.
- To obtain a biopsy of the endometrial lining of the uterus.
- To remove a uterine polyp.

Clinical Problems

Abnormal Findings: Hyperplasia of the endometrial tissue in the uterus; endometrial cancer; polyps.

Procedure

- A consent form should be signed by the client.
- Restrict food and fluid for 8 hours prior to the test.
- Have the client void before the procedure.
- The client is placed in the lithotomy position.
- A hysteroscope is placed through the cervical os into the endometrial cavity of the uterus. Carbon dioxide is usually instilled to distend the uterine cavity.
- Biopsy of tissue can be obtained.
- The test takes approximately 30 minutes.

Factors Affecting Diagnostic Results

- None reported.

NURSING IMPLICATIONS WITH RATIONALE

Pretest

- Obtain a signed consent form from the client.
- Obtain a menstrual history. The test should be performed after menstruation and prior to ovulation.

Client Teaching

- Explain the procedure to the client.
- Explain that discomfort following the carbon dioxide instillation is possible. Lower abdominal distention (uterus) and bloating can result.

Posttest

- Monitor vital signs.
- Check for excessive bleeding or discharge.

Client Teaching

- Inform the client that cramping may occur following the test. Use of a mild analgesic decreases discomfort.
- Sexual intercourse or douching should be avoided for 2 weeks or as instructed by the health care provider.
- Instruct the client to report severe discomfort or shortness of breath immediately to the health care provider.

Intravenous pyelography (IVP)

Intravenous Pyelogram, Excretory Urography

Normal Finding

Normal size, structure, and function of the kidneys, ureters, and bladder.

Description

Intravenous pyelography is more properly called *excretory urography*, because it visualizes the entire urinary tract and not just the kidneys and pelvis. A radiopaque substance (sodium diatrizoate or meglumine diatrizoate [Renografin-60]) is injected intravenously, and a series of x-rays are taken at specific times. The test usually takes 30–45 minutes.

Excretory urography is useful for locating stones and tumors and for diagnosing kidney diseases (i.e., polycystic kidney, renovascular hypertension). A few clients may be hypersensitive to the radiopaque iodine dye, especially if they have a history of allergy to many substances. Emergency drugs (epinephrine, vasopressors, etc.), a tracheostomy set, a suction machine, and oxygen should be available for treating anaphylactoid reaction if it should occur.

Purposes

- To identify abnormal size, shape, and functioning of the kidneys.
- To detect renal calculi, tumor, cyst.

Clinical Problems

Abnormal Findings: Renal calculi, neoplasm (tumor) of the kidney or bladder, and kidney diseases (polycystic kidney, hydronephrosis, renovascular hypertension).

Procedure

- A consent form for IVP should be signed by the client or an appropriate member of the family.
- The client should be NPO for 8–12 hours before the test. In the morning, the client may be slightly dehydrated; however, this will help the kidney to concentrate the dye.
- A laxative is ordered the night before, and a cleansing enema(s) is ordered the morning of the test. These preparations may vary, so check with the radiology department for exact preparations.
- An antihistamine or a steroid may be given prior to the test to clients who are hypersensitive to iodine, seafood, and contrast dye used in other diagnostic tests as well as to those who have histories of asthma and severe allergies.
- Baseline vital signs should be recorded.
- The client lies in the supine position on an x-ray table. X-rays are taken 3, 5, 10, 15, and 20 minutes after the dye is injected.
- Emergency drugs and equipment should be available at all times.
- The test takes approximately 30–45 minutes. A delay in visualizing the kidneys could indicate kidney dysfunction.
- The client voids at the end of the test, and another x-ray is taken to visualize the residual dye in the bladder.

Factors Affecting Diagnostic Results

- Feces, gas, and barium in the intestinal tract can decrease visualization of the kidneys, ureters, and bladder.

NURSING IMPLICATIONS WITH RATIONALE

Pretest

- Obtain a client history of known allergies. Notify the health care provider if the client is allergic to seafood, iodine preparations, or contrast dye. As a precaution, an antihistamine or

a steroid drug may be ordered if the client has an allergic reaction to drugs. A skin test may be performed to determine how hypersensitive the client is to the radiopaque contrast dye.
- Check the blood urea nitrogen (BUN). If BUN levels are greater than 40 mg/dl, notify the health care provider. Normally the test would not be done.

Client Teaching

- Explain to the client that the purpose of the test is to detect any kidney disorder or to observe the size, shape, and structure of the kidney, ureters, and bladder.
- Explain the procedure to the client. As a reminder, the procedural steps could be listed for the client.
- Instruct the client that he or she is not to eat or drink after dinner. Mild dehydration usually occurs. This could be harmful to clients with poor renal output, especially the aged and the debilitated. Sips of water or a glass of water may be indicated to avoid complications.
- Inform the client that he or she may feel a transient flushing or burning sensation and a salty or metallic taste during or following the IV injection of the contrast dye.
- Encourage the client to ask questions and to express any concerns before and during the procedure to the nurse, radiologist, and technician.

Posttest

- Monitor vital signs and urinary output.
- Observe, report, and record possible delayed reactions to the contrast dye (e.g., dyspnea, rashes, flushing, urticaria [hives], tachycardia, and others).
- Check the site where the dye was injected (usually it is in the antecubital fossa vein). If pain, warmth, or redness at the injection site is present, apply warm compresses, with permission.
- Administer oral antihistamines or steroids as ordered to treat dye reactions.

Laparoscopy

Pelviscopy, Peritoneoscopy

L

Normal Findings

Normal abdominal and pelvic organs; no pathology noted.

Description

Laparoscopy is the insertion of a laparoscope through the abdominal wall into the peritoneum to visualize the abdominal and pelvic organs. A light camera is usually attached to the scope for visualization. The peritoneal cavity is filled with carbon dioxide gas to increase the view and separate the abdominal wall from the organs.

The **laparoscopy** and **pelviscopy** are useful for diagnosing endometriosis, ovarian cyst, tubal pregnancy, uterine fibroids, benign and malignant tumors, pelvic inflammatory disease (PID), salpingitis, cause of infertility, and adhesions. Surgical procedures can be performed with laparoscopy, such as biopsy specimens, tubal ligation, release of adhesions, and laser treatment for endometriosis.

Peritoneoscopy is primarily prescribed to view the liver and to stage cancers, including lymphomas. It can be used for surgical procedures, such as cholecystectomy, appendectomy, hernia repairs including hiatal hernia, bowel resection, and biopsies. Laparoscopy and peritoneoscopy overlap somewhat with their surgical procedures. These tests are usually performed with general anesthesia.

Contraindications for a laparoscopy include advanced abdominal wall cancer, severe bleeding disorder, and severe respiratory and/or cardiac disorders.

Purposes

- To visualize the abdominal and pelvic organs.
- To perform surgical procedures within the abdominal and pelvic region.

Clinical Problems

Abnormal Findings: Endometriosis, ovarian cysts, tumors, abscesses, ectopic pregnancy, uterine fibroids, liver nodules, cirrhosis, adhesions in the abdominal area, PID.

Procedures

Pretest

- A signed consent form is required.
- NPO after midnight or 8–12 hours prior to the test procedure.
- Anticoagulant therapy should be discontinued 5–7 days prior to the test.
- Laboratory tests are ordered by the physician prior to the test.
- Administer cleansing enemas as ordered the night before the procedure and/or in the morning.
- Client should void before the procedure.
- IV infusion started. IV medications may be given through the IV line.

Test Procedure

- Small surgical incision is made below the umbilicus.
- The peritoneal cavity is filled with carbon dioxide gas so that the organs can easily be visualized.
- Laparoscope is inserted through a trocar.
- After the procedure, carbon dioxide escapes; however, not all of the gas is removed but will be slowly eliminated from the body over a period of 24 hours.

Posttest

- Vital signs are monitored and bleeding from the small incisional area is checked periodically.
- Analgesics for pain and for shoulder or subcostal discomfort caused by carbon dioxide gas may be given every 4–6 hours.
- Physical activity should be minimized for 4–7 days posttest or as instructed by the health care provider.

Factors Affecting Diagnostic Results

- Excessive adhesions.
- Severe obesity.

NURSING IMPLICATIONS WITH RATIONALE

Pretest

- Obtain a history of the client's health problem. Relate findings to other health professionals.
- Check baseline vital signs. These vital signs are compared with those during the test procedure and during the posttest time.
- Report gas pains that remain beyond 24–36 hours and any frank bleeding from incision site.
- Follow the posttest procedure.

Client Teaching

- Explain to the client to take analgesics as ordered to relieve pain and discomfort due to the gas that was inserted in the abdomen. Inform the client that all the gas in the abdomen is not always released from the procedure; it may take 24 hours.
- Instruct the client to report pain that lasts for 48 hours or more and any bright bleeding that occurs at the incisional site.
- Answer the client's questions and if unable to, refer the questions to the primary health care provider or other professionals.

Lymphangiography (lymphangiogram)

Lymphography

Normal Finding

Normal lymphatic vessels and lymph nodes.

Description

Lymphangiography is an x-ray examination of the lymphatic vessels and lymph nodes. A radiopaque iodine contrast oil substance (e.g., Ethiodol) is injected into the lymphatic vessels of each foot; the dye can also be injected into the hands to visualize axillary and supraclavicular nodes. Fluoroscopy is used with x-ray filming to check on lymphatic filling of the contrast dye and to determine when the infusion of the contrast dye should be stopped. The infusion rate is controlled by a lymphangiographic pump, and approximately 1½ hours are required for dye to reach the level of the 3rd and 4th lumbar vertebrae.

This test is useful to identify malignant lymphoma (Hodgkin disease) and metastasis to the lymph nodes. Lymphangiograms are also used for staging malignant lymphoma, from stage I (a single lymph node area of involvement) to stage IV (diffuse extranodal involvement). Other tests, such as ultrasonography, computed tomography, and/or biopsy, may be used to confirm the diagnosis and to stage lymphoma involvement.

Lymphangiography is usually contraindicated if the client is hypersensitive to iodine or has severe chronic lung disease, cardiac disease, or advanced liver or kidney disease. Persons with possible allergies to iodine and/or contrast dye used in other diagnostic tests (e.g., IVP) should receive

L

antihistamines or steroids before the test, and emergency drugs should be available during the test. Lipid pneumonia may occur if the contrast dye flows into the thoracic duct and sets up microemboli in the lungs. The small emboli that can occur will gradually disappear after several weeks or months.

Purposes

- To detect metastasis of the lymph nodes.
- To identify malignant lymphoma.
- To determine the cause of lymphedema.
- To assist with the staging of malignant lymphoma.

Clinical Problems

Indications: Malignant lymphoma (Hodgkin disease), metastasis to the lymph nodes, lymphedema (primary [decreased number of lymphatic vessels] or secondary [tumor or surgical removal]), and staging of malignant lymphoma.

Procedure

- A consent form should be signed by the client.
- Food and fluids are not restricted.
- Antihistamines and a sedative may be ordered prior to the test.
- Contrast dye (blue) is injected intradermally between several toes of each foot, staining the lymphatic vessels of the feet in 15–20 minutes. This is for visualization of the lymphatic vessels.
- A local skin anesthetic is injected, and small incisions are made on the dorsum of each foot.
- A 30-gauge lymphangiographic needle with polyethylene tubing is inserted carefully into the identified lymphatic vessel. The contrast dye is slowly infused with the aid of the infusion pump over a period of 1½ hours until it reaches the 3rd and 4th lumbar vertebrae. The client should remain still during the procedure. X-rays are taken of the lymphatics in the leg, pelvis, abdomen, and chest. The entire test takes 2½–3 hours.
- Twenty-four hours later, a second set of films is taken to visualize the lymph nodes. X-ray filming usually takes 30 minutes. The contrast dye remains in the lymph nodes for 6 months to a year; thus, repeated x-rays can be taken to determine the disease process and the response to treatment.

Factors Affecting Diagnostic Results

- None known.

NURSING IMPLICATIONS WITH RATIONALE

Pretest

- Explain the purpose and procedure to the client. Be available to answer questions, and be supportive of the client and family.
- Check that the consent form was signed by the client before giving the sedative for the test.
- Obtain a client history of allergies to seafood, iodine preparations, or contrast dye used in another x-ray test.
- Record baseline vital signs, and have the client void before the test.

Client Teaching

- Instruct the client to remain still during the test. Inform the client that there may be some discomfort with the injection of the local skin anesthetic into each foot. The sedative is given to promote relaxation and to decrease movement during the test.
- Inform the client that the blue contrast dye will discolor the urine and stool for several days and could cause the skin to have a bluish tinge for 24–48 hours.
- Inform the client that the test takes 2½–3 hours and that he or she will be told to return the next day for additional x-rays. Tell the client that the procedure will *not* be repeated the next day; only x-rays will be taken.

Posttest

- Keep the client on bed rest for 24 hours or as ordered.
- Monitor vital signs until stable and as indicated.
- Observe for dyspnea, pain, and hypotension, which could be due to microemboli from the spillage of the contrast dye.
- Assess the incisional site for signs of an infection (i.e., redness, oozing, and swelling). Report and record findings. The dressing is usually not changed for the first 48 hours.
- Check for leg edema. Elevate lower extremities as indicated.

Magnetic resonance imaging (MRI)*

Nuclear Magnetic Resonance (NMR) Imaging

Normal Findings

Normal tissue, structure, and blood flow.

Description

Magnetic resonance imaging (MRI) produces cross-sectional images similar to those produced by computed tomography (CT); however, unlike CT, it does not use ionizing radiation and thus is free of the hazards presented by exposure to x-rays. The cost of MRI is approximately one third more than the cost of CT.

The MRI scanner consists of a magnet encased in a large, doughnut-shaped cylinder Magnetic field is everywhere in the MRI suite. The client lies on a narrow table and is guided into the cylinder until the body part to be imaged is within the magnetic field. The hydrogen nuclei of the cells of the body respond like magnets to the magnetic field and align. When a radio frequency wave is applied, the protons in the nuclei resonate, and when the radio frequency wave is removed, the energy released by the protons as they relax is detected as a radio signal. This signal is interpreted by a computer and translated into cross-sectional images.

M

*Reviewed by Dr. Garth Koniver, Delaware; Updated by Dr. Stephen Grahovac, Christiana Care, Newark, Delaware.

Since the introduction of MRI in 1983, the quality of images produced by this technique has greatly improved, and MRI is now the most sensitive technique for defining the structure of internal organs and for detecting edema, infarction, hemorrhage, blood flow, tumors, infections, and plaques on the myelin sheath that cause multiple sclerosis. Many of these conditions would be difficult to distinguish using CT or conventional x-rays. It can differentiate between edema and tumor. MRI excels in diagnosing pathologic problems associated with the central nervous system (CNS), such as tumors, hemorrhage, edema, cerebral infarction, and subdural hematoma. Early after an ischemic stroke, diffusion weighted imaging can detect the stroke's location and extent and can determine the severity of the damage to the brain tissue. MRI can visualize bone, joint, and soft tissue injuries. Bone artifacts do not occur, and MRI can identify a tumor adjacent to or within bony structures (e.g., pituitary gland tumor).

Pacemakers, wires left in the chest from a previous pacemaker, some aneurysm or some surgical intracranial clips, and certain hearing aids are contraindications to undergoing an MRI procedure. Jewelry, watches, keys, credit cards, and hair clips must be removed prior to the procedure. Insulin pump should be taken off. Piercing from any part of the body should be removed. When an emergency situation occurs during imaging, the client must be moved from the MRI room so that resuscitation equipment can be used. MRI is difficult to use to study critically ill clients on life-support systems because of the effect of the magnet on the equipment.

MRI and CT can be used for similar tissue studies. MRI involves the use of contrast media in certain circumstances, but the IV contrast for MRI is chemically unrelated to the iodinated contrast used in CT and conventional radiography. Presently the only commercially available contrast for MRI is gadolinium-DTPA. Gadolinium is frequently used to evaluate problems of the brain, base of the skull, and spine. This contrast agent can cross the "leaky" blood-brain barrier. Imaging can occur 5–60 minutes after the start of the gadolinium infusion.

Magnetic Resonance of the Brain and Spine (Intracranial [IC] MRI): Intracranial MRI gives cross-sectional images of the brain and spine. It can detect neuropathology, such as visualizing fluid (edema) within soft tissues. The IC-MRI can identify cerebral thrombosis caused by cerebral vascular accident (stroke), cerebral tumors, abscesses or aneurysms, cerebral hemorrhage, and demyelinated nerve fibers (myelin sheaths) causing multiple sclerosis (MS). It can also detail the abnormalities of the spinal cord and degenerated discs.

Magnetic Resonance of the Heart and Coronary Arteries: Cine MRI, or ultrafast MRI, is a fast-moving MRI procedure that can image the heart in a continuous motion. It is useful for perfusion imaging, and it can determine the patency of coronary arteries following coronary grafts. Also, it is used to detect the viability of the myocardium and to assess chambers' volumes. The echo-planar MRI (EPI), like cine MRI, is used for rapid imaging of the heart and coronary arteries.

Magnetic Resonance Angiography: Magnetic resonance angiography (MRA) is a noninvasive means of displaying vessels by imaging. It maximizes the signals in structures containing blood flow and reconstructs only the structures with flow. It is useful for evaluating vascular lesions. Other structures of lesser interest are subtracted from the image by the computer.

Magnetic Resonance Spectroscopy: This MRI technique uses a scanner that can evaluate and detect ischemic heart disease and the effects of cancer treatment on tumors. It is especially useful in detecting residual tumors and radiation necrosis. It allows biochemical sampling of the tissue that is being imaged so that one can distinguish between a demyelinating condition and a neoplasm versus an infection without need for a biopsy. It can also confirm the presence of Alzheimer dementia, determine the extent of head injury due to trauma and stroke, and identify the cause of coma.

Purpose

- To detect a central nervous system lesion, vascular problem (blood flow, hemorrhage), cardiac perfusion problem, injury, tumor, or edema.

Clinical Problems

Abnormal Findings: Tumors, blood clots, cysts, edema, hemorrhage, abscesses, infarctions, aneurysms, demyelinating disease (multiple sclerosis), dementia including Alzheimer disease, muscular disease, skeletal abnormalities, congenital heart disease, intervertebral disc abnormalities, spinal cord compression, acute renal tubular necrosis (ARTN), blood flow abnormalities.

Procedure

- A consent form should be signed.
- Inform the client that there will be no exposure to radiation.
- Instruct the client to empty bladder prior to the test.
- Remove all jewelry, including watches, glasses, hearing aids, hairpins, cosmetics that may contain metallic fragments, and any metal objects. The magnetic field can damage watches. Those with pacemakers are not candidates for MRI; some with metal prosthetics, and those with nerve stimulating devices may not be candidates for MRI. Remove dentures as advised.
- Occupational history is important. Metal in the body, such as shrapnel or flecks of ferrous metal in the eye, may cause critical injury, such as retinal hemorrhage or globe rupture.
- Contraindications include clients in the first trimester of pregnancy. MRI could cause excess heat in the amniotic fluid.
- With the closed MRI, the client must lie absolutely still on a narrow table with a cylinder-type scanner around the body area being scanned.
- Sedation may be needed if the client, receiving closed MRI, is extremely claustrophobic. A client receiving a sedative should not drive home; therefore, a family member or friend should be available to drive.
- Open MRI may be ordered for clients who are claustrophobic, obese, or confused or for children; a family member or friend may be present. A mirror is available to see outside during the procedure. Clients need to remain still during the open MRI. Open MRI uses a lower-field magnet, whereas the closed MRI uses a higher-field magnet; hence lesser-quality images are usually produced by open MRI.
- Certain MRI studies require a noniodinated contrast media (gadolinium DTPA), which usually is injected intravenously. Use of MR contrast media may be contraindicated for those with kidney dysfunction; the contrast media is excreted by the kidneys.
- There is no food or fluid restriction for adults. NPO for 4 hours for children.
- The procedure takes approximately 45 minutes to 1½ hours.

Blood Flow: Extremities
- The limb to be examined is rested in a cradlelike support. Reference sites to be imaged are marked on the leg or arm, and the extremity is moved into a flow cylinder.
- The procedure takes approximately 15 minutes for arms and 15 minutes for legs.

Factors Affecting Diagnostic Results

- Movement during the procedure will distort the imaging.

M

- Ferrous metal in the body could cause critical injury to the client and distorts the images.
- Nonferrous metal may produce artifacts that degrade the images if in close proximity to the area being scanned.

NURSING IMPLICATIONS WITH RATIONALE

Pretest

- Elicit any problems with claustrophobia. Relaxation techniques or a sedative might be used.
- Ascertain from the client the presence of a pacemaker, wire left in the body from a previous pacemaker, any metal prosthetics, or shrapnel left in the body, which could cause serious tissue injury as the result of the magnetic pull.
- Alert the physician or health care provider if client is on an IV pump. MRI can disrupt IV flow.
- Provide emotional support.
- Assess for body tattoos, especially red in color, because they may get warm during MRI.

Client Teaching

- Explain the procedure. Inform the client that various loud noises (clicking, thumping) from the scanner will be heard. Earplugs are available. Inform the client that the MRI personnel will be in another room but can communicate via an intercom system. With the open MRI, a family member or friend may be in the room with the client while the MRI scanning is taking place. This is also possible with closed MRI.
- Inform the client to remain still during the procedure as indicated.
- Explain to the client that there is no exposure to radiation. The contrast media that might be used is not iodinated contrast.
- Instruct the client to remove watches, credit cards, hairpins, jewelry, and makeup. The magnetic field can damage a watch.
- Inform the client that the MRI procedure is painless. Encourage the client to relax during the testing.
- Caution clients with cardiac pacemakers not to approach the MRI unit.
- Inform the client who has metal fillings in teeth that a "tingling sensation" may be felt during imaging.

Posttest

- Monitor any effects resulting from the MRI. Answer any questions that the client has following the MRI or refer the questions to appropriate health professionals.

M

Mammary ductoscopy

Ductoscopy, Breast Ductal Lavage

Normal Finding

No abnormal or atypical cells. No malignant cells.

Description

Most breast cancer begins in the cells of milk ducts of the breast. A ductoscopy is performed for women who have complaints of nipple discharge. Ductoscopy is an endoscopy procedure in which the ductoscope is passed into the breast nipple. The scope can visualize the breast duct for a camera light is attached to the ductoscope. During the procedure, water is injected to dilate the ducts. It can identify abnormal cells and those that are at the beginning stages of cancer.

This test is usually not performed if the breast exam and mammogram are normal. Also it is not performed if the client is not at high risk for breast cancer (no family history of breast cancer or no positive mutations in BRCA-1 ad BRCA-2).

Breast ductal lavage collects possible abnormal and atypical cells from the nipple of the milk ducts. This procedure is usually performed on women at high risk for breast cancer. A cytologic examination is done of the lavage cells to identify abnormal cells. If abnormal or atypical cells are identified, the risk of breast cancer could occur 5–10 years later. To prevent this risk, the woman and her health care provider may need to discuss several methods for prevention.

Purpose

- To determine the presence of abnormal or atypical breast cells.

Clinical Problems

Increased Level: Abnormal or atypical breast cells, hyperplasia of breast cells, noninvasive ductal cancer, invasive breast cancer cells.

Procedure

- A consent form should be signed by the client.
- Nothing by mouth 8–12 hours before the procedure, especially if it is performed under general anesthesia.
- If the procedure is performed with local anesthesia, topical anesthetic should be applied to the nipple area 30 minutes before the test.
- Aspirate some of the fluid from the breast duct for cytologic examination.

Factors Affecting Diagnostic Results

- Breast tissue infection before the procedure.
- Inability to access the breast duct because of duct occlusion.

NURSING IMPLICATIONS WITH RATIONALE

- Explain the procedure for the mammary ductoscopy or the breast ductal lavage.
- If the test is performed with general anesthesia, the client should be NPO before the test.
- Check that the consent form is signed.
- Obtain vital signs before the test.

Client Teaching

- Answer the client's questions about the test. If answers are unknown, refer to appropriate health professional.

M

- Explain that the procedure will take about 1 hour.
- Inform the client that there may be some breast discomfort following the procedure. For any redness, breast pain, and fever, contact the health care provider.
- Inform the client that the test results may not be available for several days or a week. If she has not heard from the physician or health care provider after a week, she should call the office.
- Be supportive to the client. Allow the client time to express her fears and concerns.
- Encourage the client to continue with self-examination of the breast once a month and a mammogram once a year. Demonstrate breast examination if necessary.

Mammography (mammogram)

Normal Finding

Normal ducts and glandular tissue; no abnormal masses.

Description

Mammography is an x-ray examination of the breasts to detect cysts or tumors. Benign cysts are seen on the mammogram as well-outlined, clear lesions and tend to be bilateral, whereas malignant tumors are irregular and poorly defined and tend to be unilateral. A breast mass (neoplasm) is not clinically palpable until it is 1 cm in size, so it may take 5 years or longer to grow and be detectable. A mammogram can detect a breast lesion approximately 2 years before it is palpable.

The second most common cause of cancer deaths in women in the United States is breast cancer (cancer of the lung being the most common cause). Eighty to 85% of breast cancer occurs in women over 50 years of age. The majority of those women do not have any other identifiable risk factors.

There is much controversy over how often a woman should receive a mammogram and whether this x-ray test should be only for symptomatic women having a palpable mass, nipple discharge, skin thickening of the breast, or a markedly asymmetric breast, rather than for those who are asymptomatic.

The American Cancer Society and the American College of Radiologists have suggested that women between 35 and 40 years of age have a mammogram every 2 years, and women over 40 years have an annual mammogram. Radiation received is very low dose.

The mammogram can detect approximately 90% of breast malignancies; however, the test carries a 10% false-positive rate. A positive test should be confirmed by biopsy.

There have been technical improvements in the equipment, mammographic units, and the recording system used for mammography. The use of radiographic grids has improved the imaging quality of mammograms by decreasing image density. With the use of grids, the visibility of small cancers is increased. Also, the use of magnification mammography has improved the capability to identify cancers; however, the magnification increases the client's radiation dose by prolonging exposure time.

Purposes

- To screen for breast mass(es).
- To detect breast cyst or tumor.

Clinical Problems

Indications: A breast mass (cyst or tumor); periodic examination of the breast, as indicated by the health care provider.

Procedure

- Food and fluids are not restricted.
- The client removes clothes and jewelry from the neck to the waist and wears a paper or cloth gown that opens in the front. Powder and ointment on the breast should be removed to avoid false-positive results. No deodorants should be used.
- The client is standing, and each breast (one at a time) rests on an x-ray cassette table. As the breast is compressed, the client will be asked to hold her breath while the x-ray is taken. Two x-rays are taken of each breast.
- The procedure usually takes 15–30 minutes.

Factors Affecting Diagnostic Results

- Previous breast surgery can affect the reading of the x-ray film.
- Jewelry, metals, ointment, and powder could cause false-positive results.

NURSING IMPLICATIONS WITH RATIONALE

- Ascertain whether the client is pregnant or is suspected of being pregnant. A mammogram is contraindicated during pregnancy.
- Ask the client to identify the lump in the breast if one is present.
- Be supportive of the client. Allow the client time to express her fears and concerns. Notify the health care provider of her concerns, especially if they cause her great anxiety.
- Answer the client's questions when possible or refer the question(s) to other health care professionals.

Client Teaching

- Explain the procedure to the client. Explain that the test will not hurt but may cause a little discomfort when the breast is compressed during the x-ray.
- Inform the client that the test takes 15–30 minutes; however, the client will be asked to wait until the x-rays are developed and readable. Inform the client not to be alarmed if an additional x-ray is needed.
- Instruct the client not to use ointment, powder, or deodorant on the breast or under the arms on the day of the mammogram.
- Instruct the client to perform a self-examination of the breast after each menstrual period. Demonstrate breast examination, if necessary.

M

Mediastinoscopy

Normal Finding

Normal mediastinal structure and lymph nodes; absence of disease process.

Description

This is a surgical procedure in which a mediastinoscope is inserted through a small incision at the suprasternal notch. The test is to visualize mediastinal structure and lymph nodes. These mediastinal lymph nodes receive lymphatic drainage from the lungs. They are examined to detect lymphoma (e.g., Hodgkin disease, sarcoidosis, lung metastasis, and for staging of lung cancer).

Mediastinoscopy is an invasive procedure and is usually performed when x-rays, sputum cytology, and lung scans (computed tomography and nuclear) have not confirmed a diagnosis. Complications from this test may include perforation of the trachea, esophagus, aorta, or other blood vessels; pneumothorax; laryngeal nerve damage; and infection.

Purposes

- To view mediastinal structure and lymph nodes.
- To obtain lymph node biopsy.

Clinical Problems

Abnormal Findings: Lymphoma (e.g., Hodgkin disease), sarcoidosis, lung metastasis to mediastinal lymph nodes, granulomatous infection, and mediastinal tuberculosis.

Procedure

- Food and fluids are restricted 8–12 hours prior to the test.
- Consent should be signed by the client before premedication or by the designated family member.
- Obtain baseline vital signs and have client void prior to the surgical procedure.
- Complete a preoperative checklist.

Factors Affecting Diagnostic Results

- None known.

NURSING IMPLICATIONS WITH RATIONALE

Pretest

- Check that the consent form is signed before the client is premedicated for surgery.
- Record baseline vital signs. Check to be sure that the preoperative checklist is completed.

Client Teaching

- Encourage the client to express concern about the mediastinoscopy. Answer questions, and refer questions you cannot answer to appropriate health professionals.
- Explain the procedure to the client. It is a surgical procedure, and the client will receive general anesthesia. Ask the client if he or she is allergic to any anesthetic. Explain that this test procedure will take approximately 1 hour.
- Be available to family members and provide time for them to express concerns and ask questions.

Posttest

- Monitor vital signs until stable and as indicated. Report changes (i.e., increase in pulse rate [tachycardia], increase in respirations and dyspnea, decrease in blood pressure).
- Check breath sounds. Report absence of breath sounds if noted.
- Check dressing for bright blood or increased blood on dressing.
- Report if crepitus is detected at chest or neck area. This could be due to air leaking into the subcutaneous tissue as the result of perforated lung.
- Be supportive to client and family members. Provide comfort measures as needed (i.e., position change, medication).

Myelography (myelogram)

Normal Finding

Normal spinal subarachnoid space; no obstructions.

Description

Myelography is a fluoroscopic and radiologic examination of the spinal subarachnoid space (spinal canal) using air or a radiopaque contrast agent (oil and water soluble). With clients who are hypersensitive to iodine and seafood, air is the contrast agent used. This procedure is performed in an x-ray department by a radiologist, a neurologist, and/or a neurosurgeon. After the contrast dye is injected into the lumbar area, the fluoroscopic table is tilted until the suspected problem area can be visualized, and spot films are taken.

If the contrast agent is an oil (i.e., Pantopaque or iophendylate), then the contrast agent must be removed at the end of the test. Because oil is heavier than spinal fluid, it does not mix and tends to sink to the lower part of the spinal canal. Water-soluble contrast agents (e.g., metrizoate sodium [Amipaque]) do not have to be removed; however, after the procedure the client should remain in a high Fowler position (60-degree elevation of the head) for 8 hours.

The myelogram is usually performed to detect spinal lesions (i.e., intervertebral disks, tumors, or cysts). This procedure is contraindicated if increased intracranial pressure is suspected.

Purposes

- To identify herniated intervertebral disks.
- To detect cysts or tumor at or within the spinal column.
- To detect spinal nerve root injury.

Clinical Problems

Abnormal Findings: Herniated intervertebral disks, metastatic tumors, cysts, astrocytomas and ependymomas (within the spinal cord), neurofibromas and meningiomas (within the subarachnoid space), spinal nerve root injury, and arachnoiditis.

M

Procedure

- A consent form should be signed by the client.
- The client should be NPO for 4–8 hours before the test. If the myelogram is scheduled for the afternoon, then the client may have a light breakfast or clear liquids in the morning, as ordered.
- A cleansing enema may be ordered the night before or early in the morning of the test to remove feces and gas for improved visualization.
- Premedications include a sedative and/or narcotic analgesic and usually atropine. The drugs are prescribed by the health care provider.
- The client is placed in the prone position on a fluoroscopic table and is secured to the table with the use of several straps. A spinal puncture is performed, and contrast dye is injected. As the dye enters the spinal canal, the table is tilted.
- The myelogram takes approximately 1 hour.

Posttest
- After the test the radiopaque oil is removed, and the client should remain flat for 6–8 hours. If a water-soluble radiopaque agent was used, then the client's head should be elevated at 60 degrees for 8 hours.

Factors Affecting Diagnostic Results

- Gas or fecal material in the gastrointestinal tract.

NURSING IMPLICATIONS WITH RATIONALE

Pretest

- Obtain a client history of allergies to iodine, seafood, and radiopaque dye used in other x-ray tests. Inform the health care provider, because air or oxygen can be used as the contrast agent instead of the dye. A skin test may be performed.
- Follow the prescribed pretest regimen (i.e., NPO, a cleansing enema, and premedications [sedative or narcotic analgesic]). Check that the consent form has been signed before giving a sedative or narcotic.
- Allow the client the time to ask questions and to express concerns or fears. Refer questions you cannot answer to other health professionals.
- Recognize conditions in which myelography would be contraindicated (i.e., multiple sclerosis [could cause an exacerbation] and increased intracranial pressure [↑ ICP]). The radiologist and/or neurosurgeon should be notified if they are unaware of the client's condition.
- Record baseline vital signs.

M

Client Teaching

- Explain the procedure to the client. Inform the client that he or she will most likely lie on the abdomen and will be strapped to a table. The health care provider will tilt the table as the dye circulates in the spinal canal.
- Inform the client that he or she may have a transient burning sensation and/or a flushed, warm feeling as the dye is injected; the sensation may last for a short time afterward.

- Instruct the client to let the health care provider know of any discomfort (e.g., pain down the legs). The test takes about 1 hour.

Posttest

- Monitor vital signs until stable and as indicated.
- Monitor urinary output. The client should void in 8 hours.
- Observe for signs and symptoms of chemical or bacterial meningitis (e.g., severe headache, fever, stiff neck, irritability, photophobia, and convulsions).

Client Teaching

- Instruct the client to lie in the prone and/or supine position for 6–8 hours, as ordered. If the client received a water-soluble contrast agent or if all the contrast oil was not removed, the head of the bed should be elevated at a 60-degree angle for 8 hours or longer.
- Encourage the client to increase fluid intake. The fluids will help restore the cerebrospinal fluid loss. Increased fluid intake may decrease a post-lumbar-puncture headache, which could be due to a loss of spinal fluid.
- Instruct the client about prevention measures for avoiding back injury (i.e., principles of good body mechanics, such as flexing the knees and keeping the back straight when lifting).

Nephrotomography

Normal Finding

Normal size and shape of kidney; no abnormality noted in kidney tissue.

Description

Nephrotomography visualizes the kidney in detail by combining the use of tomography and intravenous pyelography. Tomography is a radiographic examination in which each sequence of x-ray film represents a slice of a single layer of tissue. Flat-plate x-ray cannot give detailed visualization of tissue from various angles and depth as can tomography. Contrast medium is injected prior to the tomographic examination. The purpose of this test is to differentiate between a solid renal tumor and a renal cyst. The thickness of the mass and its interior are recorded on film.

Purpose

- To differentiate between a renal tumor and a renal cyst.

N

Clinical Problems

Abnormal Findings: Solid renal tumors, renal cysts, renal sinus-related lesions, adrenal tumors, renal trauma, renal areas of nonperfusion.

Procedure

- Food and fluids are restricted for 8 hours before the test.
- A consent form should be signed by the client.
- Check that the client is not allergic to contrast medium used in other x-ray tests, iodine, or seafood. Notify the health care provider if the client has allergies to these substances.
- During the test, changes in positions to prone, supine, and lateral might be requested. The x-ray tube moves rapidly during the test procedure.
- Contrast medium is injected intravenously (by infusion or bolus), and tomographic filming takes place while the dye is perfusing the kidney and while the kidney is excreting dye.

Factors Affecting Diagnostic Results

- Recent use of barium sulfate for a gastrointestinal series or barium enema might decrease detailed visualization of the kidney.

NURSING IMPLICATIONS WITH RATIONALE

Pretest

- Obtain baseline vital signs prior to the test.
- Check client's history for allergy to contrast dye, iodine, or seafood. The health care provider should be notified of any past allergic reaction or sensitivity to the above substances.

Client Teaching

- Explain the procedure to the client (see *Procedure*). Inform the client that the test takes approximately 1 hour and that there should be no discomfort except for lying on the x-ray table.
- Inform the client that several x-rays are taken first, then dye is injected, and more x-rays are taken.
- Tell the client that a flush may be felt as the dye is injected. The contrast medium can be given as an infusion or as a bolus injection.
- Inform the client that changing body positions, such as back to side, may be requested by the radiologist.
- Allow time for the client to express concern about the test and unknown findings. Answer the client's questions or refer the questions to appropriate health professionals.

Posttest

- Monitor vital signs and urine output. Changes in pulse rate (tachycardia) should be reported immediately to the health care provider.
- Observe for allergic reaction to contrast medium (i.e., rash, itching, dysphagia, or urticaria [hives]).

N

Nuclear scans (bone, brain, brain perfusion, heart, kidney, liver and spleen, colon and ovary, gastroesophageal reflux, gastrointestinal bleeding, gastric emptying, gallbladder, lung, and thyroid studies)*

Radionuclide Imaging, Radioisotope Scans

Normal Finding

Adult: Normal; no observed pathology.

Description

Nuclear medicine is the clinical field concerned with the diagnostic and therapeutic uses of radioactive nuclides (one or more isotopes of the same chemical element but with different atomic weights). A radioactive isotope is an unstable isotope of an element that decays or disintegrates, emitting radiation or energy. Radioisotopes are referred to as *radionuclides*. Radioactive materials are concentrated by certain organs of the body, and their distribution in normal tissue differs from the distribution in diseased tissue. Equal or uniform gray distribution is normal, but lighter or brighter areas, referred to as *hot spots*, indicate hyperfunction, and darker areas, *cold spots*, indicate hypofunction. *Note:* The hot spots can be lighter or darker areas depending on the equipment, display of the images, and the film. Hyperfunction (or hot spots) means that more of the tracer is concentrated in the area and can be displayed as light spots on a black screen or dark spots on a white screen.

Nuclear medicine imaging began in the early 1950s with the use of a rectilinear scanner. This type of scanner was replaced in the late 1960s by the gamma scintillation camera, also called the Anger camera, after its inventor, Hal Anger. The gamma scintillation camera converts photons emitted by the radionuclide to a signal that forms an image of the distribution of radionuclide. The more photons detected in a particular area, the brighter the "hot spot."

The two types of imaging systems are (1) planar imaging, which projects images acquired from two or three different angles, and (2) single photon emission computed tomography (SPECT), in which the scintillation camera rotates and projects images in an arc of 180 degrees (for cardiac imaging) to 360 degrees, acquiring 32 or more images. This produces a 3D image. SPECT became available in the 1980s. The advantage of SPECT over planar imaging is that with SPECT the images are not obscured by overlying organs, tissue, or bone. SPECT uses a conventional Anger camera detector head with a collimator (the part of the camera that absorbs photons), which fits in a rotating gantry. This camera orbits around a client lying on a special table. Also with SPECT, the images are enhanced with computer processing. The use of a two- or three-headed imaging gamma camera increases the sensitivity and specificity of the SPECT system. With the use of filtering and three-dimensional computer reconstruction of the images, the data analysis can be of great diagnostic value. Nuclear medicine imaging is moving toward a new era with the use of high-speed computers and new radiopharmaceuticals.

N

---

*Reviewed by Dr. Garth Koniver, Delaware; updated by Theresa Riggle, BS, CNMT, ARRT(N), NCT, Nuclear Medicine, Christiana Care Health Services, Newark, Delaware.

The use of radionuclides as radiopharmaceuticals is considered safe. Reactions are uncommon and adverse. Reactions are rare (occurring 1–10 per 100,000 administrations). The radionuclide used in most studies is technetium 99m (Tc-99m), which accounts for 70% of the nuclear imaging procedures. Other radionuclides used for studying the function, anatomy, and morphology of organs include iodine 123 (I-123), thallium (T-201), xenon (Xe-133), indium 111 (In-111)-labeled white blood cells, and gallium (Ga-67) citrate.

The purposes and methods of various imaging organs are discussed in detail below. Positron emission tomography (PET) is discussed separately later in the text.

Clinical Problems

ORGAN/STUDY	INDICATIONS/PURPOSES
Bone	To detect early bone disease (i.e., osteomyelitis, ankylosing spondylosis); carcinoma metastasis to the bone; bone response to therapeutic regimens (i.e., radiation therapy, chemotherapy [antineoplastic agent])
	To determine unexplained bone pain
	To detect fractures and abnormal healing of fractures; degenerative bone disorders such as arthritis
Brain	To detect an intracranial mass (i.e., tumors [malignant or benign], abscess, cancer metastasis to the brain, head trauma [subdural hematoma], cerebral vascular accident [stroke] after the 3rd or 4th week, aneurysms)
Brain perfusion study	To diagnose Alzheimer disease, brain death, AIDS dementia
	To diagnose Parkinson disease vs. essential tremors
	To detect frontotemporal dementia (Pick disease)
	To locate seizure foci
	To determine the location and size of cerebral ischemia
Heart (cardiac) (MUGA*)	To identify cardiac hypertrophy (cardiomegaly)
	To quantify cardiac output (ejection fraction), wall motion especially following chemotherapy
	To detect coronary artery disease (CAD)
	To detect heart failure (HF), and aneurysm
Kidney (renal)	To detect parenchymal renal disease (i.e., tumor, cysts, glomerulonephritis), obstruction of the urinary tract
	To evaluate differential function for renovascular hypertension
	To assess the function of renal transplantation
	To determine the extent of pyelonephritis and scarring due to urinary reflux
Liver and spleen	To detect tumors, cysts, or abscesses of the liver or spleen; hepatic metastasis; splenic infarct
	To assess for chronic liver or spleen disease, including metastasis, jaundice, cirrhosis, hepatocellular disease, hepatitis, or elevated laboratory results
	To assess liver response to therapeutic regimens (i.e., radiation therapy, chemotherapy)
	To identify hepatomegaly and splenomegaly
	To identify liver position and shape
Colon and ovary (monoclonal antibodies for cancer)	To detect colon and ovarian cancer cells in the body

ORGAN/STUDY	INDICATIONS/PURPOSES
Gastrointestinal reflux	To detect esophageal reflux syndrome
	To detect failure to thrive in infants
Gastrointestinal bleeding	To detect the localization of gastrointestinal (active and occult) and nongastrointestinal bleeding sites
Gastric emptying	To diagnose gastric obstruction and the cause of dysmotility
Gallbladder (cholecytokinin hepatobiliary)	To diagnose acute or chronic cholecystitis, cystic or common bile duct obstruction
	To evaluate for biliary dyskinesia
	To detect biliary atresia in infants
	To evaluate after gallbladder surgery for suspected biliary leakage
	To detect hypercholestosis conditions
Lung	To detect pulmonary emboli; tumors; pulmonary diseases with perfusion changes (i.e., emphysema, bronchitis, pneumonia, COPD, pulmonary hypertension)
	To assess arterial perfusion changes secondary to cardiac disease
	To detect right and left cardiac shunt
Thyroid	To detect thyroid mass (i.e., tumors); diseases of the thyroid gland (i.e., Graves, Hashimoto thyroiditis)
	To determine the size, structure, and position of the thyroid gland
	To evaluate thyroid function resulting from hyperthyroidism and hypothyroidism
	To evaluate and manage thyroid cancer

*For nuclear stress tests see the Procedure for Heart (Cardiac) Scanning section, below.

Procedure

The radionuclide (radioisotope) is administered orally, inhaled, or given intravenously. The interval from the time the radioactive substance is given to the time of the imaging can differ according to the radionuclide and organ in question. The scintillation camera detects the radiation that comes from the organ. Normally masses such as tumors absorb more of the radioactive substance than does normal tissue. This is because of tumors being more metabolically active than normal tissue.

For diagnostic purposes, the dose of radionuclide is low (less than 30 mCi) and should have little effect on visitors, other clients, and nursing and medical personnel. There are some food, fluid, and medication restrictions with some procedures. Check with the nuclear medicine staff first.

The procedures for the organ scans are listed according to the radionuclides used, the method of administration, the waiting period after injection, the food and fluids allowed, and other instructions.

1. **Bone:** Bone scanning can detect abnormalities weeks to months before conventional skeletal radiography. The use of SPECT improves the sensitivity and specificity of the bone scan.
   a. Radionuclides: Tc-99m-labeled phosphate compound (Tc-99m diphosphonate).
   b. *Administration:* Intravenously.
   c. *Waiting period after injection:* Waiting period is 2–4 hours after injection before imaging.
   d. *Food and fluids:* No restrictions; for Tc-99m, water is encouraged during the waiting period (at least three glasses).

N

e. *Other instructions:* The client should void before the imaging begins and be well hydrated. Any metal objects, such as jewelry or keys, should be removed. Scanning usually occurs 2–4 hours after IV injection of the radionuclide and takes ½–1 hour to complete. A sedative or pain medication may be ordered if the client has difficulty lying quietly during imaging. Both anterior and posterior views are obtained.

2. **Brain:** Scanning is done for cerebral blood flow—dynamic and static imaging. Many abnormalities of the central nervous system alter the blood-brain barrier and permit localization of the radioactive tracer dose. Radionuclide brain scanning is effective for identifying metastatic disease, strokes, subdural abscesses, and hematomas.

a. *Radionuclides:* Tc-99m glucoheptonate, Tc-99m-O$_4$, Tc-99m diethylenetriamine pentaacetic acid (Tc-99m-DTPA), Tl-201 NaCl, Tc-99m-HMPAO (Ceretec), Tc-99m-ECD (Neurolite).

b. *Administration:* Intravenously.

c. *Waiting period after injection:* Tc-99m-O$_4$, 1–3 hours; Tc-99m-DTPA, 45 minutes to 1 hour. With Ceretec or Neurolite, imaging is started immediately. Frequently a few images are taken during the injection to image initial blood flow to the brain.

d. *Food and fluids:* No restrictions.

e. *Other instructions:* When Tc-99m-O$_4$ is used, the client may be given 10 drops of Lugol's solution the night before or at least 1 hour before the injection of potassium perchlorate, 200 mg to 1 g, 1–3 hours before the scheduled scan. These drugs block the uptake of Tc-99m-O$_4$ in the salivary glands, thyroid, and choroid plexus. Blocking agents are not needed with the other radionuclide. The client should remain still during the imaging (½–1 hour).

3. **Brain Perfusion Study:** The perfusion study is done to diagnose Alzheimer disease and extrapyramidal disorders (e.g., Parkinson disease) and locate seizure foci and cerebral ischemia.

a. *Radionuclides:* Tc-99m-hexamethylpropyleneamineoxime (Tc-99m-HM-PAO), Tc-99m-ECD (ethyl cysteinate dimer) Neurolite. New drug, I-123, Ioflupane (DaTscan).

b. *Administration:* Intravenously.

c. *Waiting period after injection:* Scanning begins 45–60 minutes after injection.

d. *Food and fluids:* No restriction.

e. *Other instructions:* The imaging room should be quiet and lights dimmed. The IV line should be inserted before the test. The client lies still 15 minutes before the Tc-99m-HM-PAO injection. During imaging the client is in the supine position with the head in a head holder. The entire brain including the cerebellum is imaged.

4. **Heart (Cardiac) MUGA:** (For myocardial perfusion imaging studies with stress imaging, see *Stress/Exercise Testing.*)

Multigated acquisition (MUGA) scanning is a rapid, safe method to evaluate the heart size, ventricle wall motion, and ejection fraction. The blood is tagged with a radioactive tracer, such as technetium-99m, which permits the heart and its function to be visualized. There are multiple projections of the heart taken during MUGA scanning. MUGA identifies changes occurring with contraction and expansion of the ventricles of the heart. With cardiac disease, the heart's ability to pump blood sufficiently may be reduced. The amount of radiation exposure is comparable to that of a CT scan.

a. Radionuclides: Tc-99m-O_4-tagged red blood cells (RBCs).

b. *Administration:* Intravenously.

c. *Waiting period after injection:* None.

d. *Food and fluids:* None.

e. *Other instructions:* The electrocardiogram is monitored. The client is in a supine position with a gamma camera over the chest. The radioactive tracer (containing no dye) allows visualization of the heart and its function.

5. **Kidney (Renal):** The renal scan is performed to evaluate renal function and perfusion and to detect renovascular diseases associated with glomerular filtration problems. This test can identify renal obstruction, trauma, acute and chronic renal failure, renal artery stenosis, and renal transplant rejection. Two drugs may be used with renal imaging: furosemide (Lasix), for determining renal excretory function, and Captopril, for identifying renovascular hypertension.

a. Radionuclides: Tc-99m-pertechnetate, Tc-99m-glucoheptonate, and Tc-99m-dimercapto-succinic acid (DMSA) for renal cortical and tubular disorders; Tc-99m-diethylene-triamine penta-acetic acid (Tc-99m-DTPA) for evaluating renal function and perfusion disorders; Tc-99m glucoheptonate and I-131 hippuran for renal perfusion studies; Tc-99m mercaptylacetyltriglycine (Tc-99m-MAG3) for evaluating renal clearance related to renal insufficiency.

b. *Administration:* Intravenously.

c. *Waiting period after injection:* Renal perfusion study: Imaging is done immediately after the radiopharmaceutical is given intravenously. Renogram curves are plotted. Renal cortical studies have an initial delay of 1 hour before imaging and may require additional imaging up to 24 hours post injection.

d. *Food and fluids:* No restrictions. The client should be well hydrated before an injection of radionuclide. He or she should drink at least two or three glasses of water 30 minutes before the scheduled scan. Dehydration could lead to false test results.

e. *Other instructions:* The client should void before the scan. If the client has had an IVP or renogram, the scan should be delayed 24 hours. The client should lie quietly 30 minutes to 1 hour during imaging. Usually there are a combination of diagnostic renal tests performed along with radionuclide renal scanning to determine the cause of the renal disorder. Radionuclide renal scanning is useful for clients allergic to contrast.

6. **Liver and Spleen:** Liver imaging can detect 90% of hepatic metastases and 85% of hepatocellular diseases. It is useful for screening the liver and spleen for lacerations and hematomas following trauma. SPECT improves lesion/mass detection. Also it is useful in diagnosing liver hemangiomas.

a. Radionuclides: Tc-99m-labeled RBCs, Tc-99m sulfur colloid.

b. *Administration:* Intravenously.

c. *Waiting period after injections:* Tc-99m sulfur colloid, 15 minutes. A spleen scan can be done at the same time. Tc-99m-labeled RBCs must wait 1 hour.

d. *Food and fluids:* No restrictions.

e. *Other instructions:* The client should lie quietly for 30 minutes to 1 hour during the imaging. The client may be asked to turn from side to side and onto his or her abdomen during the imaging.

N

7. **Colon and Ovary:** Colorectal cancer is the third most common malignancy. Ovarian cancer is the fourth most frequent cause of cancer death in women. Radiolabeled monoclonal antibodies are used to identify colon and ovarian cancer cells in areas of the body. The radiolabeled monoclonal antibodies attach to cancer cells, and the cancer cells can then be detected with use of a gamma camera.
   a. Radionuclides: Monoclonal antibodies labeled with indium 111 (In-111).
   b. *Administration:* Intravenously. Infusion takes 5–30 minutes.
   c. *Waiting period after injection:* 1–3 days after radiolabeled monoclonal antibodies. Usually two sets of images are taken at different times using the nuclear gamma camera, up to 5 days apart.
   d. *Food and fluids:* Light breakfast or lunch.
   e. *Other instructions:* Regular medications can be taken. Client voids prior to the test. Allergic reaction to the monoclonal antibodies, though uncommon (less than 4%), may occur. Monoclonal antibodies are obtained from mice (human cancer cells are injected into the mice to produce antibodies).

8. **Gastroesophageal Reflux:** Esophageal clearance is determined following a swallowed radioactive tracer. Numerous esophageal tests, such as endoscopy, barium esophagoscopy, and acid reflux testing may be performed to detect esophageal reflux syndrome. The radionuclide gastroesophageal reflux scan is highly sensitive (99%) for esophageal reflux.
   a. Radionuclides: Solution containing 150 mL of orange juice, 150 mL of 0.1 N hydrochloric acid, and 300 μCi Tc-99m sulfur colloid (Tc-99m-SC). Child: 250 μCi Tc-99m-SC in 10 mL of sterile water via a feeding tube.
   b. *Administration:* Orally.
   c. *Waiting period:* 30 seconds.
   d. *Food and fluids:* Fasting for at least 4 hours prior to the study.
   e. *Other instructions:* The client is in an upright or semi-recumbent position. The procedure may require that the client perform a Valsalva maneuver.

9. **Gastrointestinal (GI) Bleeding:** Upper GI bleeding sites are more difficult to detect than lower GI bleeding sites. Tc-99m-labeled (tagged) RBCs are most effective for detecting active bleeding sites. The radionuclide GI bleeding study is more sensitive than angiography. For a positive test result, the client must be actively bleeding at the time of imaging for accurate identification of the bleeding site.
   a. Radionuclides: Tc-99m-labeled RBCs.
   b. *Administration:* Intravenously by bolus injection. For Tc-99m-labeled (tagged) RBCs, withdraw 1–3 mL of whole blood into a shielded syringe containing Tc-99m sodium pertechnetate. After processing the blood, Tc-99m-labeled RBCs are injected as a bolus.
   c. *Waiting period after injection:* Imaging begins immediately after injection and continues until the site of bleeding is located. If negative after 2 hours, imaging may be repeated when client begins active bleeding or imaging at different time periods during the 24 hours after injection.
   d. *Food and fluids:* NPO unless otherwise indicated.

N

e. *Other instructions:* The client is in the supine position. Imaging is usually over the abdominal and pelvic areas. This test may be done as an emergency study, before surgery to locate the site of intestinal bleeding, or before angiography. Sequential images are acquired for 90 minutes. If the test is negative for bleeding sites, imaging can be taken within 2–4 hours or when active bleeding is suspected.

10. **Gastric Emptying:** Delayed gastric emptying could be due to acute disorders, such as trauma, postoperative ileus, gastroenteritis, or chronic disorders, such as diabetic gastroparesis, peptic ulcers, pyloric stenosis, and Zollinger-Ellison syndrome.
    a. Radionuclides: In-111 DTPA or Tc-99m-labeled juice and Tc-99m sulfur colloid-labeled eggs.
    b. *Administration:* The client ingests a scrambled egg sandwich and juice (all radiolabeled). Tc-99m-sulfur colloid-labeled instant oatmeal may be ordered instead of eggs.
    c. *Waiting period after oral meal:* Immediately after ingesting the oral meal and continuously for 1 hour. A 2- and 4-hour image is required following the oral meal.
    d. *Foods and fluids:* NPO for at least 4 hours and no smoking before or during the test.
    e. *Other instructions:* The client is in a mid-Fowler position for the meal and during imaging. The test should be performed in the morning because during the day the gastric emptying time can vary.

11. **Gallbladder (Hepatobiliary Scan):** Hepatobiliary radioactive scanning is more sensitive for diagnosing acute cholecystitis than other standard gallbladder diagnostic tests. With hepatobiliary scanning, accurate imaging of the biliary tract can be performed even when there is marked hepatic dysfunction and jaundice.
    a. Radionuclides: Tc-99m disofenin, Tc-99m mebrofenin, or other Tc-IDA derivatives.
    b. *Administration:* Intravenously, cholecytokinin (CCK), a hormone that stimulates the gallbladder (GB) to contract and empty, may be used with normal saline solution as an infusion to promote GB emptying for imaging purposes. CCK may be given prior to imaging if the client has been NPO for more than 24 hours.
    c. *Waiting period after injection:* Immediately after CCK and radionuclide infusions.
    d. *Foods and fluids:* NPO for at least 4 hours before the test with use of CCK.
    e. *Other instructions:* Usually CCK is given before the radiopharmaceutical injection to stimulate the gallbladder for clients who have not eaten. CCK is short acting (20–30 minutes). The normal value for gallbladder ejection fraction (GBEF) is greater than 35%. Lower values indicate chronic cholecystitis. Higher values usually indicate hypercholestosis conditions. Nausea and abdominal discomfort may occur for a few minutes after the CCK infusion.

12. **V/Q Lung (Pulmonary):** Lung perfusion and ventilation scannings are sensitive for detecting pulmonary emboli (PE) and obstructive pulmonary disease. Both types of lung scans may be performed to identify the pulmonary disorder.
    a. Radionuclides: *Perfusion study:* Tc-99m compounds: macroaggregated albumin (Tc-99m-MAA), Tc-99m human albumin microspheres (Tc-99m-HAM). Ventilation study: Xe-133 (more commonly used), Xe-127 (not commonly used), krypton (Kr) 81m, and Tc-99m-DTPA aerosol.
    b. *Administration:* Intravenously (perfusion) or inhaled (ventilation).

N

c. *Waiting period after injection:* Tc-99m compounds, 5 minutes after the injection of the radionuclide.

d. *Food and fluids:* No restrictions.

e. *Other instructions:* A chest radiograph is usually ordered for comparison with the nuclear medicine study. The ventilation and perfusion lung scan procedure takes 30 minutes. The camera will be moving around the client to take multiple images.

13. **Thyroid:** Thyroid scintigraphy is effective for determining the functional status of the thyroid nodules and for detecting post-thyroidectomy residual thyroid tissue and metastases. Radioactive iodine is the most frequently used radionuclide because iodine is easily taken up in the thyroid gland. Iodine is a precursor in thyroid hormone synthesis.

a. *Radionuclides:* I-131 sodium iodide, I-123, Tc-99m-pertechnetate.

b. *Administration:* I-123, I-131 (oral: liquid or capsule), Tc-99m-pertechnetate (intravenously).

c. *Waiting period after injection:* I-123, I-131—2 to 24 hours. I-123 is the radionuclide most commonly used because it has a shorter half-life. Tc-99m-pertechnetate, 30 minutes.

d. *Food and fluids:* No breakfast and NPO for 2 hours following oral iodine.

e. *Other instructions:* Three days before the scan (imaging), iodine preparations, thyroid hormones, phenothiazines, corticosteroids, aspirin, sodium nitroprusside, cough syrups containing iodides, and multivitamins are usually discontinued with the health care provider's permission. Seafood and iodized salt should be avoided. If the drugs cannot be withheld for 3 days, the drugs should be listed on the nuclear medicine request slip. The client should lie quietly for 30 minutes during the imaging procedure.

Factors Affecting Diagnostic Results

- Antihypertensives may affect results.
- Two radionuclides administered in 1 day may interfere with each other.
- Movement by the client may distort the image.
- A distended bladder could decrease visibility of the pelvic (bone) area.
- Diet and drugs containing iodine could interfere with the results of the thyroid scan (see *Procedure for the Thyroid*).
- Too short or too long a waiting period after injection of the radionuclide could affect the results.
- Dehydration prior to imaging.

NURSING IMPLICATIONS WITH RATIONALE

Pretest

- Explain to the client the procedure for the ordered study. Procedures will differ according to the type of study (see *Procedure*). In most cases, food and fluids are not restricted. Check with the nuclear medicine staff about preparations. For the bone scan (Tc-99m), water is encouraged during the waiting period. For the renal scan, the client should be well hydrated before the scheduled scan. Blocking agents (i.e., Lugol's solution and potassium perchlorate) are usually ordered before studies that use radioiodine, except for the thyroid scan.

N

- Obtain a signed consent form, if required.
- Obtain a brief health history in regard to recent exposure to radioisotopes (radionuclides), allergies that could cause an adverse reaction, being pregnant, breastfeeding, and drugs.
- Adhere to the instructions from the nuclear medicine laboratory concerning the client and the radionuclide procedure. The client should arrive on time. This is especially true if he or she has received the injection. The waiting periods for each study have specified times.
- Be supportive of the client and family. Answer questions, or refer questions you cannot answer to appropriate health care personnel.
- Advise the client to ask questions and to communicate any concerns. Be available when the client wishes to discuss concerns and fears.
- Report to the health care provider if the client is extremely apprehensive. The health care provider may wish to see the client and/or order a sedative.
- Notify the dietitian and/or dietary department not to send foods high in iodine content for 3 days to the client who is to receive a thyroid scan, unless otherwise indicated. This also includes iodized salt. Instruct the client not to eat foods rich in iodine (e.g., seafood, table salt).
- List restricted drugs containing iodine that the client is taking on the nuclear medicine slip (see *Procedure for the Thyroid*). This is important if the radionuclide is iodine.

Client Teaching

- Explain to the client that the dose of radiation he or she will receive from radionuclide imaging is usually less than the amount of radiation received from diagnostic x-rays.
- Inform the client that the injected radionuclide should not affect the family, visitors, other clients, or staff members. The radioactive substance usually leaves the body in 6–24 hours. The dose of radionuclide is very low.
- Inform the client that there could be a waiting period after the injection of the radioactive substance. Some of the tissues take longer than others to concentrate the substance.
- Instruct the client to void before the study. Voiding will diminish bladder activity and increase visibility.
- Explain to the client that the detection equipment will be moved over a section or sections of the body; however, there should not be any discomfort from the imaging equipment.
- Inform the client that he or she may be asked to change body positions during the test. Other than that, he or she should lie still during the procedure. Cardiac imaging requires the left arm be raised for approximately 25 minutes, which can be uncomfortable.
- Inform the client that the imaging may take 30 minutes to 1 hour, depending on which organ is being studied. The client should be informed that he or she may need to return for additional imaging at specified intervals.
- Instruct the client to remove jewelry or any metal object in the area of the study.
- Inform the client that the personnel in nuclear medicine will give step-by-step directions concerning the procedure. Tell the client to ask questions if he or she does not understand.
- Inform the client that heart (cardiac) imaging may be done during the stress test as part of the testing for ischemic heart disease.

N

Oculovestibular reflex study (OVR study)
Caloric Study

Normal Findings
Nystagmus with irrigation.

Description
This test is used to evaluate the vestibular area of the 8th cranial nerve. The auditory (ear) canal is stimulated by irrigating the canal with cold water, thus causing nystagmus (involuntary rapid eye movement) away from the ear being irrigated. If hot water is used, nystagmus occurs toward the side of the ear being irrigated. If there is no nystagmus, there is likely disease of the 8th cranial nerve or the labyrinth, such as Ménière syndrome.

This test should not be conducted if the eardrum is perforated. Cold air may be used instead of cold water. The test is contraindicated if there is Ménière syndrome. It should not be performed during an acute attack.

Purpose
- To determine the presence of disease to the 8th cranial nerve or the labyrinth.

Clinical Problems

Positive Findings: 8th cranial nerve neuritis, Ménière syndrome, vestibular or cochlear inflammation or tumor, and brain stem or cerebellar inflammation or tumor.

Procedure
- NPO of solid foods 6–8 hours before the test to prevent the urge to vomit.
- Eardrum should be free of wax to ensure that water can flow freely.
- The external auditory canal is irrigated until nystagmus occurs or the client complains of nausea and/or dizziness, which is about 15–30 seconds. If there is no sign of nystagmus after 3 minutes, irrigation is stopped.
- If the test is negative after 5 minutes, the procedure can be repeated on the other ear.

Factors Affecting Diagnostic Results
- Wax or blockage in the auditory canal.
- Presence of nystagmus before the test.

NURSING IMPLICATIONS WITH RATIONALE
- Check that there is no blockage in the auditory canal.
- Obtain a history of the client's health problems.

P

Client Teaching

- Inform the client that he or she may experience nausea and/or dizziness.
- Inform the client that the test takes approximately 15 minutes.
- Encourage the client to rest for 1 hour following the test. This can prevent any reaction, such as nausea or dizziness.

Pacemaker (remote) monitoring*

Normal Finding

A regular heart rate and rhythm. Pacemaker capture verified with magnet placement during **transtelephonic** testing. Normal pacemaker diagnostic values with **home remote monitor interrogations.**

Description

Pacemaker technology has developed rapidly in the last two decades. In general, there are two types of pacemakers: dual and single chamber. Aside from the basic function of cardiac electrical stimulation, each pacemaker may have multiple programmable settings. The flexibility determines which chambers (atrium and ventricle) are sensed and a variety of pacemaker responses. Once it has been established that the client has a conduction disorder and warrants permanent pacing, the decision of a single or dual chamber device and its programming is based on the following: client's underlying pathology or conduction disturbance, associated medical problems, exercise capacity, and chronotropic response to exercise.

Single chamber ventricular pacing is usually reserved for clients with chronic atrial fibrillation or flutter. Dual chamber pacing is indicated for clients with sick sinus syndrome or AV conduction disease (i.e., heart block). The ICHD codes (i.e., VVl, DDD, etc.) were designed to indicate pacemaker function and whether single or dual chambers are being paced and/or sensed. This code has been widely adopted and is used universally.

Transtelephonic Transmission of the client's heart rate and rhythm over the telephone is still used for routine pacemaker follow-up. The ECG is the universally recognized test for detecting abnormal pacemaker function and/or cardiac arrhythmias. The magnet rate provided is for the determination of battery and electronic status and confirms normal pacer function as evidenced by capture (the heart's contraction in response to the pacemaker's electrical stimulation). Proper sensing (the pacemaker's ability to recognize the client's intrinsic heart rhythm) can also be assessed on the ECG. Transtelephonic monitoring is easy to use and provides safety for the client in determining normal pacer function in between office follow-up. The guidelines for follow-up have been largely established by Medicare regulations.

The transtelephonic monitoring consists of wristband electrodes (some of the older boxes have axillary electrodes), a cradle for the client to place his or her telephone handset into, and a magnet. This monitor box is powered by a 9-volt battery.

---

* Written by Leigh Sibert, MSN, APN, Clinical Specialist, Christiana Care Cardiology Consultants, Newark, Delaware.

P

Remote Home Monitors Transtelephonic monitoring used to be the standard of care for remote follow-up of pacemakers, but this has been largely replaced by a new internet-based technology called remote transmissions.

Remote monitoring, both wireless and those used with analog phone lines, are now recognized by the Heart Rhythm Society as the standard of care in monitoring both pacemakers and other cardiac implanted electronic devices (CIEDs, ICDs). This internet-based technology offers clinicians 24/7 access to a comprehensive report of a client's device comparable to an in-office pacer interrogation. There is no ability to reprogram a pacemaker remotely, which ensures safety for the client. These devices transmit full programming and diagnostic stored in the pacemaker to a secure network that can only be accessed by the client's physician and/or device support staff. The home remote monitors for each company may look different, but all include a power source, a power display light, a transmission button, and some have a wand to be held externally over the pacemaker. They can be used from any location in the United States, and some have capability when clients travel abroad.

Purposes

- To assess normal pacer function.
- To evaluate the client's heart rate and rhythm.
- To evaluate the pacemaker battery status.
- To assess the client's arrhythmia burden.

Clinical Problems

- Failure to pace. The client could experience symptoms of syncope, presyncope, or lightheadedness.
- Failure to sense. The client may experience palpitations or "pacemaker syndrome," which is associated with fatigue, shortness of breath, dizziness, or hypotension. These symptoms are associated with loss of AV synchrony.
- Atrial and ventricular arrhythmias. The client may experience palpitations, dizziness, shortness of breath, or even syncope.

Procedure

- No consent necessary with either type of pacemaker testing and monitoring.
- Client may eat and drink without restriction prior to transmission.

Transtelephonic

1. Client should open monitoring box.
2. The client should dampen the inside of his or her wrists with water prior to putting on the wristband electrodes.
3. The client should verify that the wristband electrodes are on the proper wrists (they are labeled left and right) and that the hand electrode on the band is against the inside of the client's wrists.
4. The client establishes telephone contact with the monitoring nurse or technician. Usually the client is called at a prearranged time by the monitoring clinician.
5. Instruct the client to turn on the monitoring box via the on/off button.
6. Instruct the client to place his or her telephone handset into the cradle located on the monitoring box. The cradle is labeled so that the receiver must be placed correctly at one end.

P

The client is instructed that once the telephone is placed in the cradle, he or she should wait 40 to 45 seconds before picking the telephone back up. The client can time him- or herself by using the second hand on a clock or watch or by simply counting slowly.

7. The client should then pick up the telephone handset and verify that the ECG tracing transmitted is acceptable.
8. Instruct the client to place his or her telephone handset back into the monitor cradle and then place the magnet (included with the monitor box) directly over the pacemaker. It is helpful for the client to locate the pacemaker on the chest wall with one hand before applying the magnet with the other hand. Again, the client should wait 40 to 45 seconds with the magnet in place before picking the telephone back up.
9. Verify that the magnet ECG tracing is acceptable.
10. Repeat step 8. The client should then pick up his or her telephone handset and verify that the ECG tracing was acceptable. This will then conclude the transmission procedure.
11. The client should place the magnet back in the monitoring box and turn off the box.

Remote Home Monitors

1. The client should keep the monitoring box plugged in and turned on at all times. This allows wireless devices to get routine software updates via the secure wireless network.
2. The client should keep the box within 10–15 feet of where he or she sleeps, if possible. The device will automatically transmit at programmed intervals to those pacemakers that have a wireless chip in them.
3. Clients who do not have a pacemaker with wireless chip technology will be instructed to send a transmission on a given day at any time convenient for the client. The client will then stand in front of the monitor and press the Transmit button while holding a small wand (located on top of the device) over the pacemaker. There is a series of lights on the programming box to indicate whether the transmission was successful.
4. Clients with pacemakers that have wireless chip technology do not have to do anything except to keep their monitoring boxes plugged in, and transmissions are programmed by the caregivers at designated time intervals largely regulated by Medicare guidelines. Alert transmission for lead problem detections or certain arrhythmias will download to the caregivers' secure network site automatically. This technology continues to change yearly, and if the client has any uncertainty of how to use the remote monitoring box, he or she should call the client services phone number (made available by all manufactures).

Factors Affecting Diagnostic Results

- If the telephone is not in good working order.
- If the client forgets to wet his or her wrists prior to putting on the wristband electrodes.
- If the battery in transtelephonic monitoring box is depleted.
- If the client's telephone handset is placed on the transtelephonic box cradle backward.
- Fluorescent lights, TV, radios, and computers that are turned on in close proximity to the transtelephonic monitoring box could cause interference with ECG transmission.
- If the client has a condition such as uncontrolled shaking or involuntary muscle movements (e.g., Parkinson disease), this could produce a poor baseline on the ECG, making it difficult to assess.
- Home remote monitor box is not plugged in.

P

- There is no wireless/cellular signal in the area where the home monitoring box is placed. May need to move it to a window or area in home with an improved Wi-Fi signal.
- In nonwireless home remote monitors: If the telephone is not in good working order or there is no analog signal.

NURSING IMPLICATION WITH RATIONALE

- Explain the telephone monitoring box and its components to the client. This equipment is usually given to the client in the hospital prior to discharge or at his or her first follow-up office visit. Some clients' physicians use a monitoring company, which may mail the telephone box or remote monitoring box to the client.
- Assess the client's level of understanding on the use of home remote monitoring box and provide reassurance that transmission is easy and can be re-explained each time the client transmits from home.
- Involve family members or support persons in the teaching of the telephone transtelephonic or home remote monitoring procedure, especially if the client suffers from dementia or short-term memory loss.
- Obtain history concerning the presence of symptoms that may be related to pacemaker malfunction and/or may correlate with abnormal findings on the ECG or via diagnostic recordings on the home remote monitoring printout.

Client Teaching

Pretest

- Answer any questions that the client may have regarding proper transmission, and verify that the client has the monitor box in front of him or her and that the wristbands have been applied.
- Help the client troubleshoot placement of home monitoring box if a signal cannot be obtained for transmission.
- Remind the client of sources of transmission interference.

Posttest

- Instruct the client to turn off the transtelephonic monitoring box and remove the wrist leads. The magnet should stay in the monitoring box so that it is not displaced or lost.
- Instruct the client to keep the home remote monitoring box plugged in and turned on at all times.
- Inform the client that the transmission will be reviewed by the advanced practice clinician or monitoring physician and that the client will be contacted via telephone or letter with his or her results.
- Inform the client of his or her next scheduled transmission date if he or she does not have a wireless remote device.
- Remind the client that he or she should never attempt telephone transmission without establishing contact with the monitoring clinicians or company.

Papanicolaou smear (Pap smear)*

Cytology Test for Cervical Cancer

Normal Finding

No abnormal or atypical cells.

Description

The Pap (Papanicolaou) smear became nationally known and used in the early 1950s for detecting cervical cancer and precancerous tissues. Dr. George Papanicolaou developed the cytology tests in 1928 after spending 18 years in research. Today he is referred to as the father of modern cytology. The use of the Pap test in the United States as a screening tool for cervical cancer has dramatically increased cure rates.

Because malignant tissue changes usually take many years, yearly examination of exfoliative cervical cells (cells that have sloughed off) allows detection of early, precancerous conditions. It is suggested that women have their first Pap test within 3 years of the onset of sexual intercourse or at age 21. Women younger than 30 should have yearly standard Pap tests, but every 2 years is recommended if a liquid-based thin prep system is used. HPV testing with the Pap test begins at age 30. Women older than 30 should have a different screening frequency depending on their risk factors:

1. Women with a history of two normal yearly Pap tests in a row can be screened every 2–3 years with cessation of screening in low-risk women at age 65 years.
2. Women with a normal Pap test and a human papillomavirus (HPV) test that is negative for high-risk HPV type can be screened every 3 years. More often than every 3 years is not necessary because these women are at low risk for abnormal cervical cell changes.
3. Women with the following risk factors require yearly or more frequent screening:
   - Using birth control pills.
   - Having sex with someone who has multiple sexual partners.
   - Having three or more sexual partners in a lifetime.
   - Starting sexual intercourse before age 18.
   - Sexual intercourse with partners who have HPV.
   - Cigarette smoking.
   - Being infected with chlamydia.
   - Being infected with high-risk type HPV.
   - Having an impaired immune system.
   - A history of treatment for abnormal cervical cell changes or cervical cancer.
   - Infection with HIV (two Pap tests in first year after diagnosis and yearly after that).
   - Exposure to diethylstilbestrol (DES) in utero (rare).

The Pap smear (cytology) results are reported by The Bethesda System (TBS). General categories of The Bethesda System are as follows:

I. Within normal limits. TBS will also identify if the sample is adequate.
II. Abnormal changes

---

*Updated by Ellen K. Boyda, RN, MSN, CRNP-BC, Family Nurse Practitioner, PA and Instructor, Widener University, Pennsylvania.

P

A. Benign cellular changes
  1. Differentiate reactive (such as normal cell repair process, radiation, and IUD) or inflammatory (such as chlamydia, bacterial vaginosis, trichomoniasis) changes from true dysplastic changes.
  2. Most important features of the TBS.
  Management: Repeat smears yearly or as determined by the client's health care provider.

B. Epithelial abnormalities
  1. Atypical squamous cells of undetermined significance (ASCUS): favoring a neoplastic process or a reactive process.

  Management: Repeat smears at closer intervals, recall for colposcopy and/or combine repeat cytology with cervicography or HPV-DNA type.
  2. Low-grade squamous intraepithelial lesion (LSIL): Shows the earliest abnormal nuclear changes; combines diagnosis of HPV, mild dysplasia, and cervical intraepithelial neoplasia (CIN 1).

  Management: Repeat cytology at close intervals, recall for colposcopy.
  3. High-grade squamous intraepithelial lesion (HSIL): Includes moderate and severe dysplastic changes, carcinoma in situ (CIS 1), CIN 2, and CIN 3.

  Management: Recall for colposcopy.
  4. Squamous cell carcinoma: Changes consistent with invasive cancer.

  Management: Recall for colposcopy.
  5. Glandular cell abnormalities
    a. Atypical cells of undetermined significance, atypical endocervical cells, or endometrial cells.

    Management: In young women, check for endocervicitis, repeat smear, refer for colposcopy. In older women, refer for colposcopy with endocervical sample.
    b. Adenocarcinoma

    Management: Refer for colposcopy.

For suggestive or positive Pap smears, colposcopy and/or a cervical biopsy are frequently ordered to confirm the test results. Atypical cells can occur following cervicitis and after excessive or prolonged use of hormones.

Purposes

- To detect precancerous and cancerous cells of the cervix.
- To assess the effects of sex hormonal replacement.
- To identify viral, fungal, and parasitic conditions.
- To evaluate the response to chemotherapy or radiation therapy to the cervix.

Clinical Problems

Positive Findings: Precancerous and cancerous cells of the cervix; cervicitis; viral, fungal, and parasitic conditions.

Procedure

- Food and fluids are not restricted.
- The client should not douche, insert vaginal medications, or have sexual intercourse for at least 24 hours (preferably 48 hours) before the test. The test should be done between menstrual periods.
- The client is generally asked to remove all clothes, because the breasts are examined before the Pap smear is taken. A paper or cloth gown is worn.
- Instruct the client to lie on the examining table in the lithotomy position (heels in the stirrups).
- A speculum is inserted into the vagina. The speculum may be lubricated with warm running water.
- A curved spatula (Pap stick) or spatula/brush combination is used to scrape the cervix. Specimens are obtained from the exocervix and endocervix. The obtained specimen is transferred onto a slide and sprayed with a commercial fixation spray, or the whole stick is immersed in a container of liquid-based fixative. Label the slide or container with the client's name and date.
- The Pap smear procedure takes approximately 10 minutes.

Factors Affecting Diagnostic Results

- Allowing cells to dry on the slide before using the fixative solution or spray.
- Douching, use of vaginal suppositories, or sexual intercourse within the 24 hours before the test.
- Menstruation can interfere with the test results.
- Drugs (e.g., digitalis preparations, tetracycline, female hormones) could change the cellular structure.
- Lubricating jelly on the speculum can interfere with the test results.
- Inadequate specimen. It should be noted that liquid-based collection reduces the rate of inadequate results by 90%.

NURSING IMPLICATIONS WITH RATIONALE

Pretest

- Explain the procedure to the client. Emphasize to the client that she should not douche, insert vaginal suppositories, or have sexual intercourse for at least 24 hours before the Pap smear. Douching could wash away the cervical cells.
- Obtain a client history regarding menstruation and any menstrual problems (i.e., the date of the first day of the last menstrual period, bleeding flow, vaginal discharge, itching, whether she is taking hormones or oral contraceptives, or previous abnormal Pap test).
- Answer the client's questions, and refer questions you cannot answer to other health professionals. Try to alleviate the client's anxiety, if at all possible. Be a good listener.
- Label the slide or container with the client's name and date. The laboratory slip should include the client's age and the specimen site(s).

Client Teaching

- Inform the client that a manual examination of the vagina, lower abdomen, and breast will precede the Pap smear. Emphasize that a pelvic exam is different than a Pap smear and that both are important.
- Explain to the client that the frequency of the test depends on her risk factors and as determined by her health care provider. (See section on Risk Factors under Description.) Usually women over 30 years old should have a Pap smear once a year.
- Inform the client that test results should be back in 7–10 days. Physicians and health care providers differ in the way they report test results; some send cards to the client stating that the Pap smear is normal, while others send cards only if the test is abnormal.

Pericardial fluid analysis

Pericardiocentesis

Normal Finding

Appearance: Clear, pale yellow, straw color.

Abnormal Findings

Bacteria present, red and white blood cells, blood streaks, milky appearance.

Description

The pericardial membrane surrounds the heart and contains a small amount of serous fluid that is produced and absorbed at the same rate. When there is an excess of fluid in the pericardium, a pericardiocentesis is usually ordered. The procedure involves the insertion of a needle through the intercostal space into the lower part of the pericardium. Echocardiography helps to locate the site for the needle insertion. Excess fluid is aspirated; the fluid is evaluated to determine the cause of the problem.

This procedure is contraindicated if the client is taking an anticoagulant, has a bleeding disorder, or has thrombocytopenia. Potential complications might occur, such as air embolism, coronary artery or mycoardial laceration, dysrhythmias, excess bleeding, pleural infection, pneumothorax, and ventricular fibrillation.

Purposes

- To identify the cause of pericardial fluid excess.
- To determine the presence of a bacterial infection.

Clinical Problems

Abnormal Findings: Pericarditis, bacterial infection, metastatic cancer, heart failure, cardiac trauma, cardiac surgery, heart transplant rejection, acute rheumatic fever, and tuberculosis.

Procedure

- Obtain a signed consent form.
- Restrict fluids and food for 6–8 hours.

P

- Start an IV line for possible IV medications.
- Start an ECG; echocardiography may be used to guide the insertion of the needle.
- Insert pericardial fluid in a red- or lavender-top tube (according to the policy).

Factors Affecting Diagnostic Results

- Blood from the insertion of the needle into the heart chamber.

NURSING IMPLICATIONS WITH RATIONALE

Pretest

- Obtain a history of cardiac problems.
- Record the medications the client is taking.
- Take baseline vital signs. Record on chart.
- Check that consent form has been signed.
- Note any signs or symptoms of chest pain, dizziness, shortness of breath (SOB) during the procedure.
- Have the client void before the test.
- Monitor ECG during and after the procedure.

Client Teaching

- Monitor vital signs. Record VS on chart.
- Inform the client that the procedure should take 30–45 minutes.
- Explain the importance of remaining still during the procedure.
- Explain to the client that a local anesthetic will be administered prior to the insertion of the needle.
- Answer client's and/or family's question(s) before and after the test or refer questions to appropriate health professionals.

Posttest

- Monitor vital signs following the procedure. Note any changes.
- Assess the puncture site for bleeding and any discharge.
- Note any chest pain, SOB, or nausea following the test.

Peritoneal fluid analysis

Paracentesis, Peritoneal Tap

Normal Findings

Appearance: Clear, pale yellow, light yellow.

Red Blood Cells: None to less than 100,000 mm^3.

Protein: Less than 4 g/dL.

Glucose: Same as serum glucose.

Amylase: Same as serum amylase.

Alkaline phosphatase: Same as serum alkaline phosphatase.

Bacteria: None.

Description

The peritoneal cavity contains two layers of serous membranes (the peritoneum) that lines the walls of the abdominal and pelvic cavities. The fluid between these two layers of membrane is called the serous fluid; excess fluid is known as the ascites fluid. Normally there is a small amount of fluid present; the fluid production and absorption are about the same. The procedure to remove excessive amounts of fluid is called paracentesis. A needle or catheter is inserted into the peritoneal cavity to remove ascites fluid for therapeutic purpose (relief of client's symptoms) and/or for diagnostic purpose (cause of the effusion of fluid).

The client with cirrhosis of the liver may develop ascitic fluid, which causes shortness of breath (SOB) and abdominal distention. Removal of the fluid can help alleviate these symptoms. Excessive amount of fluid removal may cause fluid recurrence in the peritoneal cavity. For diagnostic purposes, the fluid that has been removed is analyzed to determine the cause of the peritoneal effusion. It could also be caused by infectious or neoplastic conditions. Bloody fluid could be the result of the needle penetrating a blood vessel, which may be referred to as a traumatic tap.

Purposes

- To remove peritoneal fluid for therapeutic purposes.
- To remove peritoneal fluid for diagnostic purposes.

Clinical Problems

Abnormal Findings: Cirrhosis of the liver, heart failure (HF), portal hypertension, nephrotic syndrome, hypoproteinemia, metastatic cancer, peritonitis, pancreatitis, trauma, and gastrointestinal diseases.

Procedure

- Obtain a signed consent form.
- There is no food or fluid restriction.
- Have client void prior to the procedure to prevent an accidental bladder tap.
- Have client in a high Fowler position.
- Use strict sterile technique to clean skin and during needle insertion and collection of fluid. A scalpel may be needed to allow needle or catheter insertion.
- Send the specimen(s) immediately to the laboratory.
- Usually 2 liters (2,000 mL) of fluid is removed at one time. Excessive amounts of fluid removal could cause hypovolemia.
- Antibiotic therapy may be ordered following the procedure.

Factors Affecting Diagnostic Results

- Bloody fluid as the result of a traumatic tap.

P

NURSING IMPLICATIONS WITH RATIONALE

Pretest

- Obtain baseline vital signs; continue monitoring vital signs.
- Measure abdominal girth.
- Record client's weight before and after the procedure.
- Have client urinate before the procedure.
- Obtain the necessary equipment. Keep a sterile field.
- Observe the client for signs and symptoms of hypovolemia (excess fluid loss). Watch for signs of hypotension and rapid pulse during the procedure.

Client Teaching

- Inform the client that a local anesthetic will be used to eliminate the pain during the needle insertion. The client may feel some pressure during the insertion of the needle.
- Instruct the client to report any excessive abdominal pain.
- Inform the client that the procedure usually takes 30–45 minutes.
- Be supportive of the client. Answer questions or refer to appropriate health professionals.

Posttest

- Continue to observe the client for signs and symptoms of hypovolemia.
- Monitor vital signs. Report any signs of hypotension and rapid pulse rate.
- Check dressing for blood or leaking of ascetic fluid after the procedure.

Positron emission tomography (PET)*

Normal Findings

Normal brain, heart, lung, and gastrointestinal activities and blood flow.

Description

Positron emission tomography, a relatively noninvasive test, measures the body's abnormal molecular cell activity. Myocardial perfusion abnormalities can be determined at rest and after administration of dipyridamole (Persantine). Devices for imaging positron-emitting radioactivity were in existence as early as the 1950s; however, it was not until the mid-1970s that tomographic imaging of positron-emitting radiotracers began. PET scanning has greatly improved since the 1970s.

Early use of PET was primarily to study the brain and heart. Today PET is also used to study the lungs and abdominal organs, and for oncologic purposes. In oncology, PET has recently been approved for lung nodules and colorectal cancer imaging. PET's greatest advances have been in oncology. For brain studies, PET assesses normal brain function; regional cerebral blood flow

---

*Reviewed by Dr. Garth Koniver, Delaware; updated by Susan L. Chudzik, CRNP, Delaware Heart Group PA, Newark, Delaware.

P

and volume; glucose, protein, and oxygen metabolism; blood-brain barrier function, neuroreceptor–neurotransmitter systems; and the pathophysiology of neurologic and psychiatric disorders. For heart studies, PET assesses cardiac perfusion or blood flow; glucose and oxygen metabolism; and receptor functions. PET perfusion imaging provides information concerning the severity of coronary artery disease.

Most PET imagers have several radiation detector rings. Each detector group represents a profile or one-dimensional projection of the radioactivity distribution in a tomographic slice. These profiles are combined to produce a cross-sectional (tomographic) image. The two-dimensional (2D) PET images are reconstructed from projection data derived from the detector rings. Three-dimensional (3D) PET imaging is a new approach in which 3D images are generated from the 2D images.

The client receives a substance tagged with a radionuclide (i.e., radioactive glucose, rubidium 82, oxygen 15, nitrogen 13). Fluorodeoxyglucose (FDG) is the most common radioisotope used in PET. Tomographic slices from cross-sections of tissue are detected and visually displayed by computer. PET is most effective in determining blood flow to the brain and heart. Radiation from PET is a quarter of that received from computed tomography.

Purposes

- To detect a decreased blood flow or perfusion with coronary artery disease.
- To determine the size of infarct and myocardial viability.
- To detect transient ischemia.
- To detect viable myocardium.
- To detect decreased oxygen utilization and decreased blood flow with brain disorders such as cerebral vascular accident (CVA).
- To differentiate between types of dementia, for example between Alzheimer disease and parkinsonism.
- To identify stages of cranial tumors.
- To identify lung nodules and colorectal metastasis.
- To differentiate between benign and malignant lesions.
- To stage malignant lesions and disease.
- To monitor a response to therapy.

Clinical Problems

Abnormal Findings: Hypoperfusion to brain and heart, stroke, epilepsy, migraine, Parkinson disease, dementia, Alzheimer disease, acute myocardial infarction (AMI) for first 72 hours, malignant lesions.

Procedure

- A consent form should be signed by the client.
- Nothing by mouth 4–6 hours prior to the study.
- No coffee, alcohol, or tobacco is allowed for 24 hours before the test.
- CT or MRI scans less than 6 weeks old should be available for the purpose of comparison.
- Any laboratory or biopsy reports should be available. Glucose levels are required if a study with fasting glucose is being performed.
- Start two IVs—one for radioactive substance and the second to draw blood gas samples.

- For certain brain studies, a blindfold may be used to keep the client from being distracted.
- For brain studies, the client's head is placed in a holder to restrict movement. For heart or abdominal studies, Velcro straps are used to restrict body motion.
- No sedatives are given, since client needs to follow instructions.
- Empty the bladder 1–2 hours before the test if imaging the pelvis.
- Test takes 1–2 hours.

Factors Affecting Diagnostic Results

- Anxiety could interfere with test results.
- Sedatives given might prevent client from following directions.

NURSING IMPLICATIONS WITH RATIONALE

Pretest

- Check that a consent form has been signed.
- Assess the IV site; monitor vital signs.
- Listen to the client's concerns.

Client Teaching

- Instruct the client to follow instructions given during the test.
- Inform the client that a head holder or Velcro straps could be used for the restriction of body movement during imaging.

Posttest

- Continue to monitor vital signs.
- Avoid postural hypotension by slowly moving the client to an upright position.
- Increase fluid intake to remove radioisotope from the bladder.

Client Teaching

- Explain to the client that the radiation from the test is short-lived and that the test is considered to be relatively noninvasive.
- Encourage the client to remain relaxed and to avoid stress. The client should not sleep but should remain quiet and still.
- Instruct the client to take fluids posttest to help eliminate the radioactive substance.

Postcoital test

Sims-Huhner Test, Cervical Mucus Sperm Penetration Test

Normal Findings

Number of motile sperm: 6–20 active sperm per high-power field (HPF).

P

Description

Postcoital test is frequently referred to as the Sims-Huhner test, which exams the number and the motility of the sperm cells in the endocervical mucus of a woman after intercourse. This test assists in the determination of infertility. Also, it measures the quality of the cervical mucus. The test is performed 1–2 days before ovulation because of the increase in estrogen in the cervical mucus, which enhances sperm survival and penetration. It may be performed during ovulation. It could detect the presence of antisperm antibodies in the cervical mucus, which could explain why the sperm cells lack penetration. Also, this test could determine if there is a hormonal problem that is causing infertility. If the sperm cells are inactive under a microscopic HPF, the cause could be an unsuitable cervical mucus for the sperm survival.

The postcoital test is usually requested when prior infertility tests, such as semen analysis, are normal. This test may be repeated during the next ovulatory cycle if the test results have been inconclusive.

Purposes

- To determine the quality of the cervical mucus for sperm penetration.
- To analyze the motility of the sperm cells under a microscopic high-power field.
- To aid in determining the cause of infertility.

Clinical Problems

Abnormal Findings: Infertility because of inadequate or abnormal cervical mucus, antisperm antibodies, insufficient sperm cells.

Procedure

- There is no food or fluid restriction.
- A consent form is usually not necessary. Check the policy on consent forms associated with your institution.
- The man should not ejaculate for 3 days before the test.
- The test should be performed 1–2 days before ovulation or during ovulation according to the health care provider. An elevated body temperature usually indicates ovulation.
- The woman should remain in recumbent position 10–15 minutes after coitus and be examined by the health care provider within 1–2 hours following coitus.
- The woman will be in lithotomy position, and an unlubricated speculum is used with a rubber tube attached to a syringe for the aspiration of the endocervical mucus substance.
- Take the specimen in the syringe to the laboratory, where the cervical mucus is assessed and a drop of mucus is placed on a microscope slide to count the number of active sperm cells.

Factors Affecting Diagnostic Tests

- The cervical mucus specimen is not obtained within 5 hours.

NURSING IMPLICATIONS WITH RATIONALE

- Obtain a history related to the probable infertility problem.
- Explain the procedure (see *Procedure*). Tell the client that it is important that she has the test done within 1–2 hours after coitus for best findings.

P

- Take vital signs.
- Explain to the client that she should not use any vaginal lubrication or douche before the test.
- Tell her that discomfort may occur with the insertion of the speculum.

Client Teaching

- Answer the client's questions or refer them to the appropriate health professional.
- Permit the client time to express her concerns and fears. Show understanding and be supportive.

Pulmonary function tests*
Pulmonary Diagnostic Tests

Normal Findings

Normal values according to patient's age, sex, and height; greater than 80% of the predicted value. Also 95% confidence levels are being used; these confidence ranges give a normal and a low or minimal normal value. This is done to account for physiologic differences in body types.

Description

Pulmonary function tests (PFTs) are useful in differentiating between obstructive and restrictive lung diseases and in quantifying the degree (mild, moderate, or severe) of obstructive or restrictive lung disorders. Other purposes for PFTs include establishing baseline test results for comparison with future tests; evaluating pulmonary status before surgery; determining pulmonary disability for insurance; tracking the progress of lung disease; assessing the response to therapy; pulmonary evaluation; determining pulmonary status before rehabilitation; and postrehabilitation to document outcomes.

In pulmonary physiology testing, the lungs are monitored by many complex devices and tests. The most basic device is the spirometer; it is used to measure flows, volumes, and capacities.

A number of pulmonary tests are conducted, because no single measurement can evaluate pulmonary performance. The most frequently performed PFTs are the slow vital capacity tests; lung-volume tests; forced vital capacity, flow-volume loop, and diffusion-study tests; bronchodilator response studies; exercise studies; and nutritional studies.

Results of testing are based on predicted values. These predicted values can have a large range of ±10% from the mean. Another method is to compare serial study results over time or trending the date. This could play an important role in demonstrating responses to therapy or progression of the disease over a period of time. Predicted values are influenced by height, weight, and age. Extremes in these values may cause predicted values to fall apart and become useless. Highly conditioned persons may have very high values compared to the normal population. In these persons, significant changes that are considered abnormal in the general population would

---

* Written by David C. Sestili, CRTT, RPFT, LRCP, Albert Einstein Medical Center, Pulmonary Diagnostic Laboratories and Pulmonary Rehabilitation Program, Philadelphia, Pennsylvania.

P

actually be normal. Normal baseline may be 120–130% of predicted values in these individuals, yet a drop to 100–110% of predicted would indicate an abnormal response or hyperreactive airways.

Pulmonary Rehabilitation: Many pulmonary laboratories incorporate pulmonary rehabilitation into their outpatient programs because it is important for clients with pulmonary diseases to keep active. Activities and exercises prescribed in the pulmonary rehabilitation program have been demonstrated to reduce the amount of oxygen required for muscle use. Other benefits gained from exercise for clients with pulmonary disease include a decrease in the sedentary lifestyle that can lead to depression, decrease in dyspnea, increase in activities of daily living, lesser dependence on significant others to assist in basic care; a decrease in complications and increase in the recovery time for clients having transplant and lung reduction surgery (pre- and postoperatively); and improvement in respiratory status for clients with interstitial fibrosis, cystic fibrosis, asthma, emphysema, primary pulmonary hypertension, or alpha-1-antitrypsin deficiency. Pulmonary rehabilitation incorporates a multidisciplinary approach. Specialists in the program include the dietitian; exercise physiologist; nurse; occupational, physical, and respiratory therapists; and social worker.

Purposes

- To assess pulmonary/respiratory function.
- To detect the occurrence of pulmonary dysfunction.
- To differentiate between obstructive and restrictive lung diseases.
- To evaluate the response to drug therapy (i.e., some cardiac drugs and chemotherapy may induce hyperactivity or fibrosis where response to bronchodilator therapy and steroids may increase function).
- To be informed of program(s) for improving respiratory status for clients with pulmonary dysfunction or for clients prior to or following lung surgery.

Pulmonary Function Tests

1. Slow Vital Capacity (SVC) Tests
   - *Tidal volume (TV, V_t):* The amount of air inhaled and exhaled during rest or quiet respiration or normal breathing.
   - *Inspiratory capacity (IC):* The maximal inspired amount of air from end-expiratory tidal volume in normal breathing.
   - *Expiratory reserve volume (ERV):* The maximal amount of air that can be exhaled from end-expiratory tidal volume in normal breathing.
   - *Inspiratory reserve volume (IRV):* The maximal amount of air that can be inspired from end-inspiratory tidal volume in normal breathing.
   - *Vital capacity (VC):* The maximal amount of air exhaled after a maximal inhalation:

$$VC = ERV + IC$$

Note: These pulmonary measurements are done slowly, without force. Individuals with obstructive lung disease will be able to expire more volume with this test than during the forced vital capacity maneuver that may lead to early airway closure and air trapping known as hyperinflation.

2. Lung Volume Studies

- *Lung volume tests using indicator gas:* Helium dilution and nitrogen washout are special studies that use the data generated in the slow vital capacity test to obtain the lung volumes. Tracer gases such as 10% helium and 100% oxygen are required. Using one of the gases, the person breathes in and out as the tracer gas is equilibrated in the lung; the functional residual capacity (FRC) is calculated from the changes. This method will tend to underestimate persons with advanced obstructive lung disease. This underestimation is a result of the trapped air in the lung, which does communicate with the airways.
- *Lung volumes by plethysmography method:* Lung volumes can be obtained by total body plethysmography. Body plethysmography uses a device that resembles an airtight telephone booth in which the subject sits. This method is a more accurate means to measure total volume of the lungs than the tracer gas method. Volumes measured in the box will be larger than by the indicator gas method. The body plethysmography is able to measure trapped air that does not communicate with the airways.
- *Lung volume measurements:* See Figure 2-2.
- *Residual volume (RV):* The amount of air that remains in the lungs after maximal expiration.

$$RV = FRC - ERV$$

- *Functional residual capacity (FRC):* The amount of air left in the lungs after tidal or normal expiration.

$$FRC = ERV + RV$$

In obstructive disorders, FRC is increased because of hyperinflation and/or air trapping in the lungs. This value may normalize in clients with asthma postexacerbation but will not for clients with COPD. In classical restrictive disorders, FRC, TLC, and RV are all reduced.

- *Total lung capacity (TLC):* The total amount of air that is in the lungs at maximal inspiration.

$$TLC = VC + RV \text{ or } TLC = FRC + IC$$

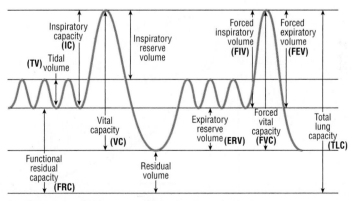

Figure 2-2 Graphic of lung volume and capacity.

P

3. Lung Volumes and Capacity (see Figure 2-2).

- *Forced vital capacity (FVC):* The maximal amount of air that can be forced out of the lungs as hard, as fast, and as long as possible before a forceful inspiration. In obstructive lung disease, the FVC is decreased; in restrictive lung disease, the FVC is normal or decreased.

$$FVC = IC + ERV$$

- *Forced inspiratory volume (FIV):* The greatest amount of air inhaled after a maximal expiration.
- *Forced expiratory volume timed (FEVT):* This value reflects the air flow through the bronchial tubes from the greatest to the smallest. It is reported as a time-based value as in 0.5 second $FEV_{0.5}$, 1 second FEV_1, 2 seconds FEV_2, and 3 seconds FEV_3. See Figure 2-3. The American Thoracic Society (ATS) has suggested reporting the FEV_6, which is the amount of air expired in 6 seconds. This reflects the minimum exhalation time suggested for a force vital capacity maneuver. The parameter of choice for evaluation of asthmatics and other obstructive lung disease and to evaluate the response to bronchodilator therapy is still FEV_1. An improvement of greater than 15% after bronchodilator therapy is considered significant and indicates the presence of reversible airway obstruction, such as bronchospasm.

4. Flow-Volume Loop (FVL)

Another method to visualize FVC measurement is by graphing flow versus volume, as seen in Figure 2-4. Abnormal FVLs in Figure 2-5 indicate types of pulmonary problems. This test yields the same basic information as the FVC test, but in addition provides useful visual information, such as concerning small-airway disease and upper-airway obstruction. Its usefulness in screening people with some types of sleep disorder problems has been recently documented. It is used as a noninvasive tool to evaluate clients who may have some type of upper-airway obstruction from thermal injury, polyps on the vocal cords, vocal cord paralysis, edema of the epiglottis, scar tissue from old tracheotomy site, and floppy trachea.

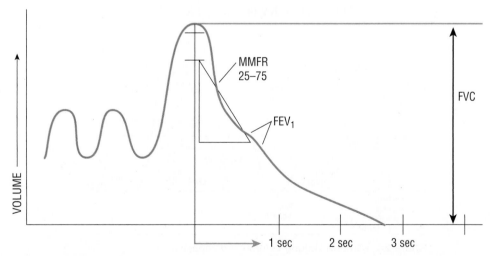

Figure 2-3 Graphic of forced expiratory volume timed. *[Courtesy of David C. Sestili. CRTT. RPTT.]*

P

Figure 2-4   Flow-volume loop [FVL] and forced expiratory flow
[FEF].   *[Courtesy of David C. Sestili, CRTT, RPF.T.]*

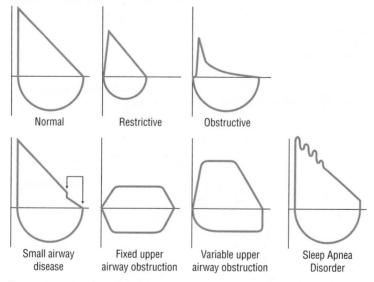

Figure 2-5   Abnormal flow-volume loops [FVL].   *[Courtesy of David
C. Sestili, CRTT, RPFT.]*

- *Peak expiratory flow (PEF):* The highest flow rate achieved at the beginning of the FVC;
  reported in liters per second. *Note:* Peak flow meters measure in liters per minute.
- *Peak inspiratory flow (PIF):* The highest flow rate achieved at the beginning of the forced
  inspiratory capacity.

P

- *Forced expiratory flow (FEF):* Figure 2-4 demonstrates the rate of flow at selected points on the flow-volume loop. The FEF looks at flow at the 25%, 50%, and 75% of the FVC and evaluates flow in various-size airways. It can evaluate the effectiveness of bronchodilator therapy. FEF 25% reflects flow through large airways; FEF 50% reflects flow through medium airways; and FEF 75% reflects flow through small airways. Decreased FEF 75% indicates small-airway disease.

5. Impulse oscillometry spirometry (IOS)/Forced oscillatory technique (FOT)

IOS, also known as FOT, is a noninvasive test that employs sound waves to measure the resistance, impedance, and reactance of the airways. This testing modality has been gaining popularity with the commercial availability of equipment (1997). The device generates a sound signal that is superimposed on the normal tidal breathing of the subject. Du Boise et al. first described this technique in 1956 as a noninvasive method to measure resistance to breathing. As a historical note, the total body plethysmograph was also developed at the same time.

The computer creating small impulses of air at random frequencies between 3 and 40 hertz oscillates a base speaker. The reflected returning signals from the airways are analyzed using the Fast Fourier Transformation equation. The FOT device is compared to the plethysmography method of airway resistance measurement; see Figure 2-6. Total body plethysmography makes a single measurement of the total respiratory system resistance. In contrast, FOT is a spectral analysis, which reflects the resistances of the central and peripheral airways. The measurements for these airways are in two well-published values: R20, which reflects the resistance in the large airways, and R5, which reflects the resistance in the peripheral airways.

Figure 2-6   Forced oscillometry device.
[Courtesy of David C. Sestili, CRTT, RPFT.]

P

The test requires the patient to perform normal tidal breathing only for a minimum of 30 seconds. The subject is required to hold his or her cheeks, or an operator will hold them, while breathing through a filter mouthpiece, and a nose clip is required. What is unique about this testing method is that, unlike spirometry, complicated breathing maneuvers are not required. An added advantage for clients with obstructed disease is FOT, which will not alter the tone of their airway, which can lead to air trapping and increased hyperinflation of the lungs.

The IOS/FOT method has demonstrated great potential in its ability to test very young children and adults who may have difficulty in performing spirometry or more complicated testing. IOS/FOT has shown great promise of being more sensitive than spirometry testing. Asthmatics may have normal spirometry yet have higher airway resistances than normal subjects. FOT can also be used to determine bronchodilator reversibility or evaluate airway hyperreactivity as part of a bronchial challenge study with exercise, cold air, hypertonic saline, methacholine, or other drugs.

The downside of this method is the small percentage of the population used to develop the predicted normal rates. The more practical approach would be to use the client as his or her own control by serial testing change. Unfortunately, most laboratories use a predicted group that is decided on more by preference or by the numbers in the device manual than on a universal standard that everyone agrees on. The power in monitoring a trend of the pulmonary data is that one is able to see a change in the client's data after establishing a mean to follow over a period of time.

Preparation for the Test The client preparation for testing requires the subject not to use inhaled bronchodilator medication unless so directed by the ordering practitioner and not to perform any exercise prior to the testing. Also, the client should refrain from caffeine, smoking, and large changes in temperature. Instructions to the client should include that the test does not hurt; it will require him or her to perform relaxed normal tidal breathing only for a minimum of 30 seconds. The IOS unit makes light popping sounds like popcorn. During testing, the subject will be required to hold his or her cheeks, or an operator can hold them. He or she will be breathing through a filter mouthpiece, and a nose clip is required. Total test time is between 30 and 45 minutes.

6. Exhaled Nitric Oxide (eNO)

In the lungs, inflammatory processes can lead to increased production of the nitric oxide gas in the bronchial tree. Nitric oxide (NO) is released by the leukocytes in the bronchial wall as a response to inflammation. Normal lung nitric oxide levels are less than 12 parts per billion (ppb). Abnormal levels of exhaled nitric oxide (eNO) has been published as greater than 30 ppb in clients with diseases such as asthma and interstitial disease. In moderate to severe chronic obstructive pulmonary disease (COPD) clients, eNO may be downregulated from normal levels and may be much lower than 12 ppm. This is thought to be the result of the destruction of airways and the alveolar capillary bed.

In the sinus cavity, normal nasal NO levels are greater than 200 ppb. Nitric oxide is also elevated in the stomach. In geographic locations where there is high air pollution, such as cities, atmospheric NO levels have been recorded at greater than 300 ppb. Studies have been published demonstrating the inspired atmospheric nitric oxide levels do not affect the expired NO. Nevertheless, it is recommended that atmospheric or inspired NO levels be

P

monitored and recorded in the client data report. Some laboratories use NO scrubbers on the inspired side of the valve.

The most popular method of measuring eNO is via the chemiluminescent technique. There are two methods of collecting the NO sample. In one method, the sample is collected in a special Mylar bag and is measured offline at a later time. The second method is the online method. NO is measured in real time as the subject exhales through the valve. The same type of valve configuration is used to collect the samples in both methods.

The client is instructed to take a deep breath in through a one-way valve. On the exhalation side is a restrictor to help maintain a predetermined exhalation rate at a constant pressure. The client is instructed to exhale at a target pressure and/or until flows are displayed on a monitor for greater than 6 seconds. No nose clip is used, as the back pressure generated by the subject as he or she exhales is used to close the velum of the nose. This prevents contamination of the exhaled nitric oxide (eNO) in the sinus cavity to mix with the exhaled lung gas. The client must be able to follow commands and be able to exhale for more than 6 seconds.

For more detailed information on the methods and uses, the American Thoracic Society has published recommendations for the collection of exhaled nitric oxide in adults and children, which is available at www.ats.org.

Exhaled nitric oxide is useful in monitoring subjects with asthma, allergic reactions, interstitial fibrosis, and cystic fibrosis, just to name a few. By monitoring exhaled nitric oxide in asthmatic subjects, compliance to prescribed therapy can be monitored and adjusted.

Preparation of the Client for Exhaled Nitric Oxide (eNO) Preparation for the exhaled nitric oxide is extensive and should be documented via a client questionnaire or checklist.

The client must be able to follow commands and be able to exhale for more than 6 seconds.

The client must abstain from some foods and drinks that may alter the exhaled nitric oxide values, including alcohol (including mouthwash), water, salads, and foods with nitrates (e.g., lunchmeats, pickled products, bacon, ham, and hot dogs). The client should refrain from smoking and taking medications that block nitric oxide production and other medications. The client is also required to not exercise and to limit his or her exposure to cold air or sudden changes in temperature, as this may also affect the eNO levels.

7. Diffusion Capacity Test
   Diffusion tests can be done using a number of techniques. The most commonly used is the single-breath test. This requires the client to inspire from RV to TLC. The gas inhaled is a mixture of helium 10%, carbon monoxide 0.3%, oxygen 21%, and the balance is nitrogen. The client holds his or her breath for 10 seconds prior to expiration. After the first 750 mL is discarded to wash out dead-space gas, an alveolar sample is collected in a bag and analyzed for helium and carbon monoxide concentration. Results of this reflect the state of the alveolar capillary barrier.

   Decreased diffusing capacity occurs in such disease states as interstitial fibrosis, pulmonary edema, and emphysema. It will also decrease in persons with abnormal hemoglobin, such as occurs in anemias including methemoglobin and increased carboxyhemoglobin in smokers. Cardiac output can affect this result. Increased DLCO values can be caused by pulmonary hemorrhage.

8. Bronchial Provocation Studies

   Inhalation of pharmacological and antigenic substances is used to test the sensitivity or hyperreactivity of the airways. Types of challenge would include methacholine, histamine, ASA, cold air, hypertonic saline, antigens, and others. Serial spirometry tests are performed to document the amount or degree of reactivity (a drop in FEV_1 greater than 20% of baseline spirometry). A baseline test followed by a challenge substance is given first, followed by a bronchodilator to assure reversal. Indications for these tests are (1) normal spirometry test, (2) a history of symptoms such as wheezing or coughing without a cause, and (3) symptoms related to exposure to industrial substances.

   Methacholine chloride is usually the testing drug of choice because it causes rapid bronchoconstriction. The client inhales progressively larger doses of the drug until all levels are administered without change in FEV_1 or a drop of 20% of baseline FEV_1 is reached. The drug is then reversed by administration of a bronchodilator.

9. Exercise Studies

   Pulmonary function studies are done at a resting or static state. Exercise studies evaluate the patient during an active or dynamic state. These tests are performed by having the subject walk on a treadmill or pedal an ergometer to a set protocol to stimulate activity at progressive workloads. During this test, the heart rate and rhythm are monitored by a 12-lead electrocardiogram (ECG). The client will also be breathing through a mouthpiece during the test to measure ventilation, expired carbon dioxide (VCO_2), and oxygen consumption (VO_2). Blood gases may be drawn at rest and at peak exercise. Pulse oximetry may also be monitored, as well as blood pressure. These tests are used to determine the amount of disability and to evaluate persons with exertion dyspnea. This information can be used to develop an exercise prescription for activities for fitness programs and pulmonary and cardiac rehabilitation.

   Another important role of exercise testing is evaluating subjects with obstructive lung disease for dynamic hyperinflation. This process of air being trapped in the lungs can limit activity. This trapped air is described as a feeling of "no air movement" in and out of the chest or no room to breathe. This can be treated with medications, breathing retraining, and exercise in a pulmonary rehabilitation program to help prevent and reduce the air trapped in the lungs. Other treatments for hyperinflation are lung volume reduction surgery, lung transplantation, and nonsurgical lung volume reduction using endobronchial valves or by other methods.

   Types of exercise testing can be designed to simulate activity-related problems, of which *exercise-induced bronchospasm (EIB)* is an example. A common complaint of clients active in sport activities is bronchospasm. Several theories suggestive of the cause include allergy-triggered airway, production of nitric oxide by the airway, hyperreactivity in association with physical activity, and mouth breathing required when the participant increases activity. When the individual breathes rapidly in and out through the mouth, the nose, which warms and filters air, is bypassed. This dry air causes chilling of the airway, leading to instability of the airways and can lead to bronchoconstriction in some persons.

10. Pulse Oximetry (POX)

    This is a noninvasive procedure to measure the oxygen saturation (SaO_2) of the blood. The device measures the SaO_2 by passing two wavelengths of infrared light through an extremity, such as a finger. The device (sensor probe) measures the saturation of oxyhemoglobin in

P

the pulsatile fraction of blood. This method is an excellent noninvasive trending device; when values vary, a blood gas analysis of the partial pressure of oxygen (PO_2) and/or CO-oximetry to measure oxyhemoglobin (%HbO_2) and SaO_2 should be done to validate the results. A note of caution: Blood gas analyses normally do not measure SaO_2; they are calculated. Check with your blood gas laboratory for this information.

Pulse oximetry is a very useful test, but it has some drawbacks. It should be trusted after direct comparison to CO-oximetry is done. Abnormal hemoglobin levels (i.e., carboxyhemoglobinemia, methemoglobinemia, and sulfhemoglobinemia) could fool the device. These abnormal levels are detected at the same infrared wavelengths as O_2 and may be falsely interpreted by the oximeter to be oxygen. Impeded blood flow to an area will also affect the pulse oximetry. Correlation with the client's true pulse will assist in correcting this problem. Light sources may also affect the results; thus, the area should be guarded against external light sources.

11. Nutritional Studies

Indirect calorimetry is the measurement of oxygen consumption (VO_2) to derive energy expenditure (EE) and carbon dioxide production (VCO_2), allowing us to derive respiratory quotient (RQ). Respiratory quotient obtained from the calorimetry yields the type and amount of substrate used in metabolism (carbohydrate, protein, fats). It is calculated as follows:

$$RQ = VO_2 / VCO_2$$

This noninvasive test gives useful information as to the resting energy expenditure (REE), the amount of calories needed for minimal existence expressed in kilocalories per 24 hours. What it measures is the output side of the nutrition question since we know and measure the input side. The RQ will indicate the type of fuel substrates being metabolized. For example, an RQ of 1 indicates carbohydrates; RQ of 0.80 indicates mixed carbohydrates, fats, and protein; where an RQ of 0.75 indicates lipids metabolism; and an RQ of 0.65 could be seen in an individual in ketosis. If 24-hour urine urea nitrogen is known, nonprotein R can be calculated along with the actual amount of carbohydrates, fats, and protein metabolized in grams and percent of EE.

12. Body Plethysmography (body box)

Body plethysmography is a method to measure the exact amount of air in the thorax. This is accomplished by having the subject sit inside an airtight box and breathe through a flow-measuring device. A panting maneuver is employed, and a shutter is closed to measure pressure at the mouth, and a second pressure measures the changes of the box. By measuring the mouth and box pressure, the measurements can be applied to Boyle's Law. The thoracic gas volume (TGV), which correlates to functional residual capacity, can be measured. The compliance of the lungs can be measured, but it requires the subject to swallow an esophageal balloon. This device can also measure airway resistances of the lung. Advantages are that the body box measures all air in the thorax that causes volumes to be larger in box studies than by other methods. Disadvantages to the body box test are that some clients have claustrophobia, and persons with perforated eardrums will tend to have readings much higher than normal, which could be misleading. Obese clients may not be able to be tested due to weight limitations of the equipment. This test requires total client cooperation and ability to follow commands.

P

Clinical Problems

Obstructive Diseases: Emphysema, chronic bronchitis, bronchiectasis, bronchospasm, bronchial secretions, airway inflammation caused by bacterial or viral infections, and asthma.

Restrictive Diseases: Pulmonary fibrosis, pneumonia, lung tumors, kyphoscoliosis, neuromuscular diseases, chest trauma, obesity, scleroderma, pulmonary edema, surgical removal of lung tissue, and high abdominal incisions.

Procedure

For most pulmonary testing, the following are good guidelines. It is always wise to contact the laboratory for specific restrictions, as they vary.

- Eating a heavy meal before the test should be discouraged.
- Smoking should be avoided 4–6 hours before the test.
- The client should wear nonrestrictive clothing.
- Record the client's age, height, and weight, which may be used to predict the normal range.
- Bronchodilator therapy is normally restricted prior to the test, because it is usually administered in the pulmonary function laboratory to evaluate response to the drug.
- Usually sedatives and narcotics are not given. Other medications are given prior to the test unless otherwise indicated by the health care provider.
- Postpone procedure if the client has an active cold, is running a fever, or is under the influence of alcohol.
- Dentures may be left in during testing if they are tight fitting.
- A nose clip is applied and the client is instructed to breathe in and out through his or her mouth while attached to a mouthpiece.
- Practice sessions on fast-and-deep breathing. Normally the test is repeated until two efforts are reproducible and the best tracing is used. Check with your laboratory to find out the length of time the client may be in the laboratory as it may take anywhere from 1 to 4 hours for testing according to the tests ordered.
- The test or tests may be repeated after using a bronchodilator.

Bronchial Provocation Studies: The routine test is methacholine. Make sure to contact the pulmonary laboratory to check for restrictions and the type of test used at your facility.

- Informed consent is needed for this test.
- It is recommended that the client has a pre- and post-bronchodilator test done before being referred for this test. History of severe reactions, hives, anaphylaxis, and so on may be contradictive for this test.
- There are many restrictions associated with this test, and the laboratory should be contacted. Some restrictions include exercise, smoking, or caffeine (coffee, cola, or chocolate) consumption for a minimum of 6 hours before testing. Any bronchodilator or antihistamine therapy (PO or inhaled) should be discontinued; some may need to be withheld up to 72 hours prior to testing.
- Avoid methacholine challenge testing for women who are pregnant and breastfeeding or who are trying to become pregnant. Its safety has not been documented. Other testing, such as cold air challenge, may be employed.

Nutritional Studies

- The client should be NPO for 12 hours prior to and until completion of the test.
- Physical activity must be restricted before the test.

P

- Nutritional studies are usually performed ½ hour after awakening, if possible.
- The client's exhalation is analyzed for oxygen consumption (VO_2) and carbon dioxide production (VCO_2). Clients on ventilators, receiving continuous hyperalimentation, and/or tube feeding can be tested as long as there are no changes in the diet or ventilator settings until the test is completed.
- Clients with a leaking endotracheal tube, tracheotomy tube, or chest tubes cannot be tested as the gas leaking will alter the results. Clients weaning on various ventilator modalities may also have variations in their metabolic rate. Clients on dialysis of any type cannot be tested because of CO_2 removal and variation in metabolic status. Check with your laboratory for restrictions.

Exercise Studies: Exercise-induced bronchospasm (EIB) stress testing is a form of broncho-provocation testing that can be performed by one of the two methods:

In the first method:
- The client refrains from pulmonary medications, caffeine, exposure to cold air, and physical exercise, as in the methacholine procedure, prior to testing.
- A 12-lead ECG is applied.
- A baseline spirometer test is done, which acts as the control.
- The client exercises on a treadmill or a bicycle ergometer until the target heart rate of 85% of maximum is met or the client has symptoms limiting the exercise.
- Exercise is terminated and serial spirometry is performed immediately postexercise and at 1, 3, and 5 minutes, and then every 5 minutes for a period of up to 45 minutes postexercise. A drop of greater than 10–15% of the FEV_1 indicates a positive response.

In the second method, the procedures of the first method are followed with the following additions:
- The client inhales cold (–20°C), dry air, which is generated by a chilling device driven by compressed air prior to and during the exercise test.
- Spirometry is performed the same as above; see the first method.

Factors Affecting Diagnostic Results

- Use of bronchodilator 4 hours before the pulmonary function test may produce falsely improved pulmonary results. Other medications used may also cause other changes. Check with the health care provider to see what is being diagnosed and the pulmonary laboratory regarding the medication list.
- Activity/exercise may cause bronchodilation.
- Sedatives and narcotics given before the test could decrease test results.
- Lack of cooperation by the client due to not understanding the specific test procedure or malingering may affect results.

NURSING IMPLICATIONS WITH RATIONALE

- List on the request slip oral/inhaled bronchodilators and steroids the client is taking. Record client's age, height, and weight.
- Record vital signs.
- Assess for signs and symptoms of respiratory distress, that is, breathlessness, dyspnea, tachycardia, severe apprehension, and gray or cyanotic color. Notify the health care provider and the laboratory. If the client is too ill or a recent exacerbation has occurred,

pulmonary testing may yield little useful information. These tests require total client effort, cooperation, and ability to follow instructions. The majority of this type of testing is performed on an outpatient basis.

- Be supportive of the client, and answer the client's questions if you can or contact the laboratory for more information. Many laboratories will come and access clients prior to testing. Clients with recent mental status changes, uncontrolled blood pressure, acute myocardial infarction (MI), or stroke may not do well with these procedures.

Client Teaching

- Instruct the client to eat a light breakfast, except in nutritional studies; to take medications, except for bronchodilators, sedatives, narcotics, and others as stated by the health care provider; and to avoid smoking for 4–6 hours before test. For any questions, contact the pulmonary laboratory.
- Explain to the client that the test should not be performed if he or she has an active cold, is running a fever, or has a communicable disease such as active TB, unless approved by the health care provider and the pulmonary laboratory chief.
- Practice breathing patterns for pulmonary function tests with the client (i.e., normal breathing, rapid breathing, and forced deep inspiration and forced deep expiration).

Radioactive iodine (RAI) uptake test

I-131 Uptake Test, Radioiodine Thyroid Uptake Test

Normal Finding

Adult: *2 Hours:* 1–13% (thyroid gland). *6 Hours:* 2–25% (thyroid gland). *24 Hours:* 15–45% (thyroid gland).

Description

The radioactive iodine (RAI) uptake test is used to determine the metabolic activity of the thyroid gland by measuring the absorption of I-131 or I-123 in the thyroid. The uptake test is one of the tests used in diagnosing hypothyroidism and hyperthyroidism. It is also useful for differentiating between hyperthyroidism (Graves disease) and an overactive adenoma. This test tends to be more accurate for diagnosing hyperthyroidism than for diagnosing hypothyroidism.

A calculated dose of I-131 or I-123 (in capsule or liquid form) is given orally. The client's thyroid is scanned at three different times. The tracer dose has a small amount of radioactivity and is considered harmless. The client's urine output may be checked for radioactive iodine excretion.

Purposes

- To determine the metabolic activity of the thyroid gland.
- To diagnose hypothyroidism and hyperthyroidism.
- To differentiate between hyperthyroidism and an overactive adenoma.

R

Clinical Problems

Decreased Level: Hypothyroidism (myxedema). *Drug Influence:* Lugol's solution, vitamins, expectorants (i.e., SSKI), antithyroid agents, cortisone preparation, ACTH, aspirin, antihistamines, phenylbutazone (Butazolidin), anticoagulants (i.e., warfarin [Coumadin]), thiopental sodium (Pentothal). *Foods:* Seafood, cabbage, ionized salt.

Elevated Level: Hyperthyroidism (Graves disease), thyroiditis, cirrhosis of the liver. *Drug Influence:* Barbiturates, estrogens, lithium carbonate, phenothiazines.

Procedure

- The client should be NPO for 8 hours prior to the test. The client can eat 1 hour after the radioiodine capsule or liquid has been taken.
- The amount of radioactivity in the thyroid gland is measured three times (after 2, 6, and 24 hours).
- The client should return to the nuclear medicine laboratory at specified times to allow measurement of the I-131 uptake level with the scintillation counter.

Factors Affecting Diagnostic Results

- Certain drugs can affect test results (see *Drug Influence*). Foods containing iodine (seafood, ionized salt) could cause a false-negative result.
- Drugs and foods (see *Clinical Problems*).
- Severe diarrhea, intestinal malabsorption, and x-ray contrast media studies may cause a decreased I-131 uptake level, even in normal thyroid glands.
- Rapid diuresis during the test could cause iodine excretion and a low iodine uptake in the thyroid gland.
- Renal failure could cause an increased iodine uptake.

NURSING IMPLICATIONS WITH RATIONALE

Pretest

- Explain to the client the purpose and procedure for the test.
- Ask the client if he or she is allergic to iodine products.
- Inform the client that a technician from the nuclear medicine laboratory will give the radioactive substance and that he or she must go to the laboratory 2, 6, and 24 hours after taking the iodine preparation. Explain to the client that the procedure is to determine the percentage of I-131 or I-123 uptake, that the test should not be painful, and that the amount of radiation received should be harmless. Emphasize the importance of being on time for each determination.
- List on the request slip for the I-131 uptake test the x-ray studies and drugs the client has received in the last week that could affect test results. These drugs should, if possible, be discontinued for 3 or more days before the test (see *Drug Influence*).
- Draw blood for thyroid hormone (T_3 and/or T_4) tests, if ordered, before the client takes the radioiodine capsule or liquid.
- Answer the client's questions. Encourage the client to communicate concerns.

- Observe for signs and symptoms of hyperthyroidism (e.g., nervousness, tachycardia, excessive hyperactivity, exophthalmos, mood swings [euphoria to depression], and weight loss). Report these to the health care provider, and record them in the client's chart.

Client Teaching

- Inform the client that he or she may eat an hour after the radioiodine capsule or liquid has been taken, according to the nuclear medicine laboratory's procedure.
- Instruct the client to return to the nuclear medicine laboratory at specified times. The testing should be done on time.
- Inform the client that the radioactive substance should not harm family members, visitors, or other clients, since the dosage is low and gives off very little radiation. Women who are pregnant definitely should not be given this test or any other radioactive tests.

Retrograde pyelography (retrograde pyelogram)
Retrograde Ureteropyelography

Normal Finding

Normal size and structure of the bladder, ureters, and kidneys.

Description

A retrograde pyelography test may be performed after or in place of intravenous pyelography. The contrast dye is injected through a catheter into the ureters and the renal pelvis. The visualization of the urinary tract is exceptionally good because the dye is injected directly. Usually this test is done in conjunction with cystoscopy.

Although retrograde pyelograms are not done too frequently today, this test is still performed when there is a suspected nonfunctioning kidney, an unlocated calculus, or an allergy to IV contrast dye. Only a small amount of the dye that is injected directly into the ureters will be absorbed through the membranes.

Purposes

- To view the urinary tract.
- To check for a nonfunctioning kidney.

Clinical Problems

Abnormal Findings: Renal calculi, neoplasm (tumor), renal stricture, and nonfunctioning kidney.

Procedure

- A consent form should be signed by the client.
- The client should be NPO for 8 hours before the retrograde pyelography. The client should not be dehydrated before the test.

R

- Laxatives and cleansing enemas may be ordered prior to the test.
- Baseline vital signs should be recorded.
- Sedatives/tranquilizers and narcotic analgesics are given approximately 1 hour before the test.
- The client is usually placed in the lithotomy position (feet and legs in stirrups).
- Radiopaque contrast dye is injected through a ureteral catheter into the renal pelvis and x-rays are taken. As the catheter is removed, additional x-rays may be taken.
- This procedure is usually done under local or general anesthesia, and the test takes approximately 1 hour.

Factors Affecting Diagnostic Results

- Barium in the gastrointestinal tract could interfere with good visualization. Barium studies should be done after a retrograde pyelogram.

NURSING IMPLICATIONS WITH RATIONALE

Pretest

- Record baseline vital signs.
- Obtain a client history of allergies to seafood, iodine, and/or radiopaque dye used in other diagnostic tests.
- Administer laxatives, cleansing enemas, and premedications as prescribed. If the client is not hospitalized, check that the prescribed orders were completed at home or in another institution. Check that the consent form has been signed before giving premedications.

Client Teaching

- Explain to the client that the purpose of the test is to identify kidney stones or to determine the cause of his or her kidney problems, or give a similar response related to the symptoms.
- Explain the procedure to the client. Explain to the client that he or she will be placed in stirrups. If the client is having the test done under local anesthesia, tell the client that he or she will most likely feel pressure and the urge to urinate with insertion of the cystoscope.
- Inform him or her that there should be little to no pain or discomfort. Tell the client that the test takes about 1 hour.
- Inform the client that food and fluids are restricted for 8 hours before the test. Some health care providers may not restrict water unless the client is to have general anesthesia. Check for symptoms of dehydration (e.g., dry mouth and mucous membranes, poor skin turgor, decreased urine output, and fast pulse and respirations). Report symptoms to the health care provider and record them on the client's chart.

Posttest

- Monitor vital signs until stable or as ordered.
- Observe for allergic reactions to the contrast dye (e.g., skin rash, urticaria [hives], flushing, dyspnea, and tachycardia).

- Monitor urinary output. Report and record gross hematuria. Blood-tinged urine is usually normal. Report to the health care provider if the client has not voided in 8 hours or the urinary output is less than 200 mL in 8 hours.
- Give an analgesic for discomfort or pain. Report severe pain.
- Observe for signs and symptoms of infection (sepsis; i.e., fever, chills, abdominal pain, tachycardia, and, later, hypotension).
- Be supportive of the client and family. Answer the client's questions, or refer them to urologist or appropriate health professional.

Saliva ferning test

Ovulation Test (Home Test)

Normal Finding

Ovulation occurring.

Description

There are various methods used to determine when ovulation is occurring. The oldest method is to track increases in body temperature. The saliva ferning test kit was approved by FDA in 2002. It is a home test that gives the approximate time of ovulation. The kit contains a mini-microscope for the woman to exam her dry saliva. Women's estrogen levels increase just before ovulation and remain increased during ovulation. Ferning occurs with the presence of estrogen to indicate ovulation. The saliva is dried, and under the mini-microscope it gives a frosted appearance, which is ferning. Estrogen occurs 3–4 days before ovulation and lasts 2–3 days after ovulation.

The sperm lives for approximately 3–5 days in an estrogen cervical mucus. The egg lives 24 hours or less after ovulation. This method may be used for pregnancy or it could be used to prevent pregnancy. There are other ovulation tests that can be used.

Purpose

- To assess when ovulation occurs.

Clinical Problems

Positive test: Ovulation is appending or occurring.

Procedure

- There is no food or fluid restriction.
- The client purchases a saliva ferning test kit. The client should follow directions given by the kit.

NURSING IMPLICATIONS WITH RATIONALE

- Discuss various methods used to determine ovulation.
- Obtain a history of the client's problem related to pregnancy.
- Encourage the client and her partner or spouse to make an appointment with the health care provider to discuss methods for achieving pregnancy. Various pregnancy tests may be suggested.

Client Teaching

- Be supportive to the client concerning her reproductive problems. Allow her time to ventilate her feelings.

Scans

See Nuclear Scans

Schilling test (urine)

Co-57-Tagged Vitamin B_{12} (cobalt-57-tagged cyanocobalamin)

Reference Values

Adult: Greater than 7% excretion of radioactive vitamin B_{12} within 24 hours. Usual range is 10–40% of vitamin B_{12} excretion. *Pernicious Anemia:* Excretion of vitamin B_{12} is less than 3%. *Intestinal Malabsorption:* Excretion is 3–5%.

Description

The Schilling test is primarily ordered to diagnose pernicious anemia, a macrocytic anemia. The test determines if the client lacks the intrinsic factor in the gastric mucosa that is necessary for the absorption of vitamin B_{12} from food. With impaired absorption due to the lack of the intrinsic factor or from intestinal malabsorption, little to no vitamin B_{12} is absorbed and therefore less is excreted in the urine.

A vitamin B_{12} deficiency affects the bone marrow, the gastrointestinal tract, and the neurologic system. The bone marrow becomes hyperplastic, having many bizarre red blood cell forms. The leukocytes (white blood cells) are large but reduced in number; likewise, the platelets are bizarre in form and reduced in number. The gastrointestinal mucosa atrophies, and there is a decrease in hydrochloric acid. Classic symptoms of pernicious anemia include a beefy red tongue, indigestion, abdominal pain, diarrhea, and tingling and numbness of the hands and feet.

The test consists of collecting a 24-hour urine specimen after the client has taken a radioactive capsule of vitamin B_{12} administered by a technician from the nuclear medicine laboratory and an injection of intramuscular vitamin B_{12} given by the nurse. The intramuscular vitamin B_{12} will saturate the liver and the protein-binding sites, thus permitting the absorption of the capsule cobalt-tagged vitamin B_{12} by the small intestines and its excretion in the urine. There are various types of radioactive cobalt (Co-57, Co-56, Co-60), but Co-57 is preferred because of its shorter half-life and its low-energy gamma radiation. Usually a Schilling test is performed after a plasma vitamin B_{12}, RIA assay test; however, the Schilling test aids in diagnosing pernicious anemia.

Purposes

- To determine if there is a vitamin B_{12} deficiency.
- To detect pernicious anemia and intestinal malabsorption syndrome.

Clinical Problems

Decreased Level: Pernicious anemia, intestinal malabsorption syndrome, liver diseases, hypothyroidism (myxedema), pancreatic insufficiency, and sprue.

Procedure

- Obtain a signed consent form.
- The client should be NPO for 8–12 hours before the test. Food and fluids are permitted after the IM vitamin B_{12} dose.
- Avoid ingestion of B vitamins for 3 days prior to the test and laxatives for 1 day prior to the test.
- A sample of urine (25–50 mL) should be collected before cobalt-tagged vitamin B_{12} is given to determine if there are radionuclide contaminants.
- The radioactive Co-57-tagged vitamin B_{12} capsule(s) of liquid is/are administered orally by a technician from nuclear medicine.
- Vitamin B_{12} (usually 1 mg) is given IM by the nurse 1–2 hours after the radioactive dose.
- Collect urine in a large container for 24 hours, according to the institution's procedure. No preservative is needed in the urine container. The container may or may not be iced or refrigerated; check with the laboratory's policy.
- Label the urine container with the client's name, the room number, the date, and the time.
- Rubber gloves should be worn to handle the urine for the 24-hour specimen.

Factors Affecting Laboratory Results

- A recent radionuclide scan within 7 days prior to the test.
- Food and fluid taken within 1–8 hours before the test.
- Inadequate urine output due to renal insufficiency or old age.
- Partial gastrectomy can decrease the amount of intrinsic factor, so less vitamin B_{12} could be absorbed.
- If IM vitamin B_{12} is not given on time, the Co-57-vitamin B_{12} can be absorbed in the liver.

NURSING IMPLICATIONS WITH RATIONALE

- Obtain a history of chronic diseases or conditions that could decrease renal function or gastrointestinal absorption of the radioactive capsule, such as diabetes mellitus, hypothyroidism, liver disease, or pancreatic insufficiency.

- Assess for signs and symptoms of pernicious anemia, such as beefy red tongue, indigestion, abdominal pain, diarrhea, and tingling numbness of the hands and feet.
- Assess urine output; low urine output affects test results. If the urine output is less than 25 mL/h or 600 mL/day, the health care provider should be notified.
- Do not administer laxatives the night before the test. Laxatives could decrease the absorption rate.
- Determine the time of administration of the radioactive vitamin B_{12} capsule. The nurse administers the IM vitamin B_{12} 1–2 hours after the technician administers the capsule.
- Observe the client for at least 1 hour for possible anaphylactic reaction to radionuclide.
- Administer the nonradioactive vitamin B_{12} injection at the *specified* time.
- Notify the dietary department to release the breakfast tray after the nonradioactive vitamin B_{12} is given.
- Label the urine container and laboratory slip with the exact dates and times of collection (e.g., 2/3/20 at 8:00 AM to 2/4/20 at 8:00 AM).

Client Teaching

- Explain the procedure to the client. Tell the client that he or she is to have nothing by mouth for 8–12 hours before the test. Breakfast will be given after the IM injection is given. Urine will be collected for 24 hours.
- Instruct the client to avoid putting feces or toilet paper in the urine. Inform the client that the hands should be washed thoroughly with soap and water after handling the urine.
- Tell the client's family or visitors not to throw away the urine. Inform the family that hands should be washed thoroughly with soap and water after handling the urine.
- Explain to the client that the radioactive substance should not be harmful to family members, visitors, or self unless the person is pregnant. Notify the nursing staff when urine needs to be emptied.
- Instruct the client that foods high in vitamin B_{12} are mostly animal products, such as milk, eggs, meat, and liver. Vegetables are low in vitamin B_{12}. Discuss dietary needs with the client and refer the dietitian to the client as needed.

Sex chromatin mass, buccal smear, Barr body analysis

Normal Finding

Barr body in 25–50% of the female buccal mucosal cells.

Description

The sex chromatin test is a screening method to detect the presence or absence of Barr chromatin body (an inactivated X chromosome in a mass lying at the periphery of the cell nucleus) in the buccal mucosal cells. Buccal smears are used to check for Barr body when chromosomal abnormalities are suspected (e.g., Turner syndrome [absent or less than 20% Barr body in females] and Klinefelter syndrome [presence of Barr body in males]). This test is also indicated if amenorrhea or abnormal sexual development is present.

Abnormal findings should be followed up by chromosome analysis (karyotype). The sex chromatin test should not be used for sex determinations.

Purposes

- To detect Barr chromatin body.
- To check for the presence of Turner syndrome or Klinefelter syndrome.

Clinical Problems

Abnormal Findings: Turner syndrome (female): absence of Barr body, amenorrhea, sterility, and underdeveloped breasts. Klinefelter syndrome (male): presence of Barr body, small penis and testes, sparse facial hair, gynecomastia, and sterility.

Procedure

- There is no food or fluid restriction.
- The client should rinse his or her mouth well.
- A wooden or metal spatula is used to scrape the buccal mucosa twice; the first scraping is discarded, and the second is spread over a glass slide. The slide should be sprayed with a fixative solution and sent to the laboratory for identifying a Barr body in the cells. The specimen should be labeled with the client's name, sex, and age, as well as the date and the specimen site.
- Check that the specimen is not saliva. The smear is stained and examined under a microscope.
- The procedure usually takes 10–20 minutes.

Factors Affecting Diagnostic Results

- If the specimen is saliva and not cells, the test result could be inaccurate.
- Failure to use a preservative spray on the buccal smear specimen will cause cell deterioration.

NURSING IMPLICATIONS WITH RATIONALE

- Record in the chart any abnormal sexual characteristics or problems and note them on the request slip (e.g., amenorrhea, gynecomastia).
- Be supportive of the client and his or her family. Be a good listener. Answer questions or refer them to the appropriate health professionals.

Client Teaching

- Explain to the client and/or parents that the purpose of the test is to determine the cause of abnormal sexual development. Inform them that this is a screening test and that other tests, such as chromosome analysis, may be indicated.
- Explain the procedure to the client and parents. Inform the client that the cells from inside the mouth (buccal smear) are used because they are easy to obtain. Tell them that the test has a high percentage of accuracy. The procedure usually takes 10–20 minutes; however, the results from the test may take several weeks.
- Inform the client that there should be a minimal amount of discomfort. Light pressure will be applied when scraping the mucosa.

Sigmoidoscopy*

Normal Finding

Normal mucosa and structure of the rectum and sigmoid colon.

Description

Sigmoidoscopy is an examination of the anus, rectum, and sigmoid colon using a flexible sigmoidoscope to visualize the descending colon. This test is usually performed for screening for colon polyps and can be performed in a physician's office, clinic, or hospital. It may be part of an annual physical examination. Sigmoidoscopy may be requested when the client does not want a colonoscopy. With this procedure, the rectum and distal sigmoid colon can be visualized, and specimens can be obtained with biopsy forceps or a snare.

Purposes

- To examine the anus, rectum, and sigmoid colon.
- To detect blood, polyps, or tumor in the sigmoid colon.
- To obtain a culture of tissue or secretion for cytologic study.

Clinical Problems

Abnormal Findings: Hemorrhoids; rectal and sigmoid colon polyps; fistulas, fissures; rectal abscesses, benign or malignant neoplasms; ulcerative or granulomatous colitis; and infection and/or inflammation of the rectosigmoid area.

Procedure

- A consent form should be signed by the client.
- The client should follow the pretest preparation given by the physician or health care provider. The client is usually allowed a light dinner the night before the test and then NPO afterward. Usually heavy meals, vegetables, and fruits are prohibited within 24 hours of the test.
- No barium studies should be performed within 3 days of the test.
- Fleet enema(s) (hypertonic salt enema[s]) are given the morning of the test. If enemas are contraindicated, then a rectal suppository such as bisacodyl (Dulcolax) may be prescribed. Fecal material must be evacuated before the examination. Preparation with GoLYTELY could be used. Oral cathartics are seldom used, because they may increase fecal flow from the small intestine during the test.
- The client should assume a Sims (side-lying) position.
- A lubricated flexible endoscope is inserted into the rectum. The client should be instructed to breathe deeply and slowly. Air may be injected into the bowel to improve visualization.
- Specimens can be obtained during the procedure.
- The procedure takes approximately 15–30 minutes.

*Updated by Dr. Warren G. Butt, Gastroenterology-Stomach-Colon-Liver, Newark, Delaware.

Factors Affecting Diagnostic Results

- Barium can decrease the visualization, and so barium studies should be performed a week before the test or afterward.
- Fecal material in the lower colon can decrease visualization.

NURSING IMPLICATIONS WITH RATIONALE

Pretest

- Explain the purpose of the sigmoidoscopy to the client. The test could be a part of the routine physical examination for preventive health care, or to determine the cause of symptoms such as bright blood or mucus in stools, constipation, and bowel changes.
- Explain the procedure to the client.
- Check the chart to determine if the client has had a barium study. If so, notify the physician.
- Obtain a client's history in regard to health problems and pregnancy. Caution should be taken with some health problems, such as ulcerative colitis.
- Record baseline vital signs before the test and following the test.
- Allow the client time to ask questions and express concerns. Refer questions you cannot answer to a physician or to the appropriate health professional.

Client Teaching

- Inform the client that the procedure may cause some discomfort but should not cause severe pain. Encourage the client to breathe deeply and slowly and to relax during the test. Explain that there may be some gas pains if a small amount of air is injected during the procedure for better visualization.

Posttest

- Monitor vital signs as indicated.
- Observe for signs and symptoms of bowel perforation, for example, pain, abdominal distention, and rectal bleeding. These problems rarely occur. Report all symptoms immediately to the physician or health care professional.
- Be supportive of the client and his or her family.

Client Teaching

- Encourage the client to rest for several hours or as indicated after the test. This procedure may be done in a physician's office, clinic, or hospital. If the test is done on an outpatient basis, the client should rest for 1 hour before leaving.

Sinus endoscopy

Normal Finding

Normal sinuses; no infection or structural abnormalities noted.

Description

Sinus endoscopy examines the anterior ethmoids and the middle meatus of the sinuses. The primary purposes are to correct structural abnormalities and alleviate an infectious process. Sinus endoscopy is frequently prescribed for clients with chronic sinusitis who are nonresponsive to antibiotic therapy.

The sinus endoscopy may be performed in the health care provider's office or in an outpatient department.

Purpose

- To diagnose the presence of a chronic sinus infection or structural abnormality.

Clinical Problems

Acute or chronic sinusitis, cysts, sinus erosion, and structural abnormality.

Procedure

- A consent form should be signed by the client.
- Food and fluids are restricted after midnight or for 12 hours prior to the procedure.
- Dentures, jewelry, and hairpins, if present, should be removed.
- Intravenous fluids are usually started prior to the procedure.
- Eye pads may be used to protect the eyes from injury during the procedure.
- The nostrils are sprayed with a topical anesthetic.
- A fiberoptic endoscope is frequently used.
- Computed tomography may be needed during the procedure to visualize the sinus area.
- Nasal packing may be inserted into the nostril(s) following the procedure.

Factors Affecting Diagnostic Results

- Severe nasal septal defect.

NURSING IMPLICATIONS WITH RATIONALE

- Obtain a history of the sinus problem(s) from the client.
- Check that the consent form is signed.
- Monitor vital signs.

Client Teaching

- Explain the procedure for sinus endoscopy (see *Procedure*). Answer questions that the client may have or refer questions to appropriate health professionals.

Posttest

- Continue monitoring the client's vital signs until stabilized.
- Check for excessive bleeding or discharge.

Client Teaching

- Instruct the client to call the health care provider if excessive bleeding or discharge occurs and if body temperature becomes elevated.
- Instruct the client to take prescribed drugs (antibiotic and pain medication). Discuss posttest care as indicated by the health care provider.

Skin tests (tuberculin, blastomycosis, coccidioidomycosis, histoplasmosis, trichinosis, and toxoplasmosis)

S

Normal Finding

Negative results.

Description

Skin testing is useful for determining present or past exposure to an infectious organism: bacterial (tuberculosis), mycotic (blastomycosis, coccidioidomycosis, histoplasmosis), or parasitic (trichinosis and toxoplasmosis). The types of skin tests include scratch, patch, multipuncture, and intradermal. The antigen of the organism is injected intradermally (under the skin), and if the test is positive in 24–72 hours, the injection site can become red, hard, and/or edematous.

Bacterial Organism and Disease: *Tuberculosis:* The tuberculin (antigen) skin test indicates whether a person has been infected by the tubercle bacilli. A negative test usually rules out the disease. The methods for skin testing include the following:

1. *Mantoux test:* Purified protein derivative (PPD) tuberculin is injected intradermally. PPD has several strengths, but the intermediate strength is usually used unless the client is known to be hypersensitive to skin tests. The client should not receive PPD if there has been a previous positive test. The test is read in 48–72 hours.
2. *The tine test or Mono-Vacc test:* These are multipuncture tests that use tines impregnated with PPD. This method is used for mass screening. The tine test is read in 48–72 hours, and the Mono-Vacc test is read in 48–96 hours. When the result is uncertain, the Mantoux test should be done.
3. *Vollmer patch test:* This patch resembles a Band-Aid; however, the center piece is impregnated with concentrated old tuberculin (OT). The patch is removed in 48 hours, and the test is read 48 hours later.

Mycotic Organisms and Diseases: *Blastomycosis:* The organism *Blastomyces dermatitidis* causes blastomycosis. The antigen blastomycin is injected intradermally, and if an erythematic area greater than 5 mm in diameter develops, the test is positive. The skin test should be read in 48 hours. Positive sputum and tissue specimens will confirm the blastomycin skin test. *Coccidioidomycosis:* The coccidioidin skin test is useful for diagnosing coccidioidomycosis, a fungus disease caused by *Coccidioides immitis.* The antigen coccidioidin is injected intradermally, and the skin test should be read in 24–72 hours. A client treated for coccidioidomycosis may remain positive during his or her life span. *Histoplasmosis:* Histoplasmosis is caused by the organism *Histoplasma capsulatum,* which on a lung x-ray resembles tuberculosis. The histoplasmin skin test for histoplasmosis is not always reliable. The antigen is injected intradermally and should be read in 24–48 hours. A positive test result occurs when an erythematic area is over 5 mm in diameter. To confirm the skin test results, sputum and tissue specimens should be obtained.

Parasites: *Trichinosis:* The parasitic organism *Trichinella spiralis* causes trichinosis. This organism is present in uncooked meat, especially pork. Symptoms occur approximately 2 weeks after ingesting the organism; the client complains of nausea, diarrhea, pain, colic, fever, and swelling of the muscles. The antigen is injected intradermally, and the test should be read in 15–20 minutes. A positive test is a blanched wheal with an erythematic area surrounding it. *Toxoplasmosis: Toxoplasma gondii* is the organism causing toxoplasmosis. This organism is found in the eye ground and brain tissue of humans. It can cause blindness and brain damage. The antigen toxoplasmin is injected intradermally, and the test result should be read in 24–48 hours. A positive test is an erythematic area greater than 10 mm in diameter.

Purposes

- To determine the present or past exposure to an infectious organism.
- To determine if the client has been infected by the tubercle bacilli using the tuberculosis skin test.

Clinical Problems

ANTIGEN SKIN TEST	ORGANISM	DISEASE
Tuberculin	Tubercle bacilli	Tuberculosis
Blastomycin	*Blastomyces dermatitidis*	Blastomycosis
Coccidioidin	*Coccidioides immitis*	Coccidioidomycosis
Histoplasmin	*Histoplasma capsulatum*	Histoplasmosis
Trichinellin	*Trichinella spiralis*	Trichinosis
Toxoplasmin	*Toxoplasma gondii*	Toxoplasmosis

Procedure

- Food and fluids are not restricted.
- Cleanse the inner aspect of the forearm with alcohol and let it dry.
- Inject intradermally 0.1 mL of the antigen into the inner aspect of the forearm.
- Record the client's name, the name of the test, the site on the arm of the skin test, the date, and the time it should be read (see *Description* for readings of individual tests).

Factors Affecting Diagnostic Results

- Steroids and immunosuppressants given within 4–6 weeks can cause false-negative skin test results.
- A skin test performed before the body's incubation period (infectious process) can cause a false-negative result.
- Test results read several days after the designated time can give an inaccurate reading.

NURSING IMPLICATIONS WITH RATIONALE

- Obtain a client history about hypersensitivity to skin tests. Ask the client if the skin test was performed before and, if so, whether the skin test result was positive or negative. The skin test should be repeated only if it was negative.
- Report if the client has taken steroids (e.g., cortisone) or immunosuppressant drugs in the last 4–6 weeks, because false test results could occur.

- Record the client's abnormal signs and symptoms. Ask the client about his or her contact with bacterial, fungal, or parasitic organisms, if known.
- Be supportive of the client and family, and allow them time to express their concerns.

Client Teaching

- Explain to the client that the purpose of the skin test is to determine the presence of an organism. The organism and the type of skin test should be discussed.
- Explain the procedure to the client. Tell the client that a pin prick will be felt as a small needle with a small amount of solution is injected under the skin.
- Inform the client that the result of the skin test must be read during the stated time.
- Inform the client that a positive skin test does not always indicate active infectious disease. However, the positive test does indicate that the organism is present in the body in either an active or a dormant state. If the results are positive, other studies are performed (i.e., x-rays, sputum and tissue cultures, and serum tests).

Sleep studies
Polysomnography (PSG)

Normal Findings

Normal sleep pattern with normal ECG, EEG, EMG, O_2 saturation.

Description

Normal sleep is composed of two phases: four stages of nonrapid eye movement (NREM) sleep and rapid eye movement (REM) sleep. Both NREM and REM occur cyclically during sleep at approximately 90-minute intervals.

A sleep disorder such as insomnia occurs more frequently in women and increases with age. Older adults have a decrease in stages 3 and 4 of NREM sleep and have frequent waking periods. Children have few REM sleep periods and longer periods of stages 3 and 4 NREM sleep. REM sleep periods become longer during the sleep process and if the person is aroused from REM sleep, he or she may recall a vivid, bizarre dream. Sleepwalking or nightmares occur in children most frequently during NREM sleep. Sleep disorders occur in 75% of psychiatric clients, which also includes those clients with anxiety and mood and panic problems.

Sleep studies, primarily called polysomnography (PSG), determine the cause of sleep disorders, including daytime sleepiness, obstructive sleep apnea (OSA; also called sleep disordered breathing), insomnia, nocturnal awakening, and snoring problems. OSA occurs when there is no ventilation for 10 seconds. It may be attributed to oxygen desaturation, cardiac dysrhythmia, or sleep interruption. Also, PSG is indicated for persons having difficulty staying awake during the day who fall asleep at inappropriate times, pregnancy-associated sleep disorders, "short" sleepers (hyposomniac-sleep duration less than 5 hours), and "long" sleepers (hypersomniac-sleep duration greater than 10 hours).

Testing for sleep disorders is performed in a sleep laboratory at night over an 8-hour period of time. The client is monitored during the night by electrocardiogram, pulse oximetry to determine heart rate and oxygen saturation, electroencephalogram (EEG), electrooculogram (EOG), electromyogram (EMG), airflow monitoring, and snoring sensor. All these testing devices may not be indicated.

Purpose

- To determine the cause of the sleep disorder.

Clinical Problems

Abnormal Findings: Obstructive sleep apnea, insomnia, nocturnal awakening, and snoring.

Procedure

- A consent form should be signed by the client.
- The client should keep a sleep log for 1–2 weeks prior to the PSG test.
- The client should avoid caffeine products, alcohol, sedatives, and naps 1–2 days before testing.
- Omit prescribed medications until the sleep studies are completed, if indicated.
- Sleep studies are scheduled in the sleep laboratory at night usually 10 or 11 PM until 6 or 7 AM (8-hour period of time).
- Attach electrodes for ECG, EEG, EMG.
- Attach the pulse oximetry.
- Place a commode by the bedside. Electrode leads may inhibit bathroom use.
- Lights are turned off.
- In the AM, have the client evaluate his or her sleep experience.

Factors Affecting Diagnostic Results

- Defective electrodes or those that become loose or fall off.
- Inability to sleep.
- Drugs such as sedatives, caffeine taken prior to the test.

NURSING IMPLICATIONS WITH RATIONALE

- Obtain a history from the client in regard to medications, past stroke, head injury, headaches, seizures.
- Review the sleep log that the client has given.
- Check vital signs. Note if there is respiratory distress.

Client Teaching

- Explain to the client that electrodes will be attached to the head, chest, and legs.
    ECG: selected leads attached.
    EEG: two sets of electrodes to the scalp.
    EOG: one electrode to canthus eye.
    EMG: electrodes attached to the leg muscles.
    Pulse oximeter: attached to the finger to determine heart rate and oxygen saturation.
- Answer the client's questions or refer the questions to other health professionals.

Stress/exercise tests: treadmill exercise electrocardiology, exercise myocardial perfusion imaging test (thallium/technetium stress test), nuclear Persantine (dipyridamole) stress test, nuclear dobutamine stress test*

S

Normal Finding

Normal electrocardiogram (ECG) with little or no ST-segment depression with exercise. Normal myocardial perfusion.

Description

Treadmill stress testing is based on the theory that clients with coronary artery disease (CAD) will have marked ST-segment depression on the ECG when exercising. Depression of the ST segment and depression or inversion of the T wave indicate myocardial ischemia. In 1928, Fiel and Siegel reported on the relationship of exercising and ST-segment depression in clients complaining of angina. Master used an exercise test (two-step) in 1929 to demonstrate ischemia but used only pulse and blood pressure (BP) to note changes. In 1931, Wood and Wolferth felt exercise was a useful tool for diagnosing coronary disease but that it could be dangerous. Later it was discovered that ST-segment depression usually occurred before the onset of pain and was still present for some time after the pain had subsided. Mild ST-segment depression after exercise can occur without CAD.

Treadmill and Bicycle Electrocardiology: In 1956, Bruce established guidelines for performing stress testing on a treadmill. Master's step test (1955) was also accepted as a method for stress testing. Another method used today is the bicycle ergometer test; however, the treadmill seems to be the choice for testing cardiac status. The body muscles do not seem to tire with the treadmill method as much as leg muscles do with the bicycle ergometer. For clients who cannot walk (e.g., paraplegics, amputees), an arm ergometer or pharmacologic stress testing (to be discussed later) can be used. With the treadmill stress test, the work rate (load) is changed every 3 minutes by increasing the speed slightly and the degree of incline (grade) by 3% each time (3%, 6%, 9%). The clients will exercise until they are fatigued, develop symptoms, or reach their maximum predicted heart rate (MPHR).

Exercise Thallium Perfusion Test: The radioisotope thallium 201, which accumulates in the myocardial cells, is used during the stress test to determine myocardial perfusion during exercise. With severe narrowing of the coronary arteries, there is less thallium accumulation in the heart muscle. If a coronary vessel is completely occluded, no uptake of thallium will occur at the myocardial area that the vessel supplies. The presence of thallium is most effective for assessing myocardium viability.

Clients with coronary artery disease may have normal thallium perfusion scans at rest; however, during exercise, when the heart demands more oxygen, myocardial perfusion decrease. The client returns in 2 or more hours to take a second scan of the heart at rest. Frequently second scans are done to differentiate between an ischemic area and an infarcted or scarred area of the

---

*Updated by Susan L. Chudzik, CRNP, Delaware Heart Group PA, Newark, Delaware.

myocardium. In the resting state, blood flow in a coronary artery with stenosis remains normal until the stenosis exceeds 85%.

Uses for the stress/exercise test or the exercise myocardial perfusion test include screening for CAD, evaluating myocardial perfusion, evaluating the work capacity of cardiac clients, developing a cardiac rehabilitation program, and preoperative assessment for noncardiac surgery.

Exercise Technetium Perfusion Test: For detection of myocardial ischemia, technetium Tc-99m-laced compounds, such as Tc-99m-sestamibi (Cardiolite), are commonly used for perfusion scanning because they are trapped in the myocardium and do not redistribute. Technetium compounds provide more clinical information by allowing the assessment of perfusion, wall motion, and ejection fraction in one test procedure. Other technetium agents approved by the U.S. Food and Drug Administration (FDA) are Tc-99m-teboroxime and Tc-99m-tetrofosmin.

Cardiolite imaging is perhaps the most useful noninvasive test for diagnosing and following CAD at the present time. Positive stress Cardiolite scanning should be considered strong presumptive evidence of CAD. The more markedly abnormal the scan, the more likely the client has serious CAD. It is important to correlate the scan findings with the ECG, the exercise stress test, and the client's symptoms. The use of gated single positron emission (SPECT) (gated refers to the synchronizing of images with the computer and the client's heart rhythm) greatly improves the sensitivity and specificity of the Cardiolite scan.

Nuclear Persantine (Dipyridamole) Stress Test: This is an alternative stress test usually ordered when the client is not physically able to exercise or to walk on a treadmill. Persantine is administered intravenously to dilate the coronary arteries and increase blood flow to the myocardium. Arteries that have become narrowed because of CAD cannot expand like normal arteries. Thallium, Cardiolite, or other Tc-based compounds, administered intravenously, detect decreased blood flow to the heart muscle (myocardium). The isotope is administered 3 minutes after the 4-minute IV Persantine infusion.

The client must avoid foods, beverages, and medications containing xanthines (caffeine and theophyllines), such as colas, chocolate, and tea, 24 hours prior to the test, and theophylline preparations 36 hours prior to the test.

Nuclear Persantine stress testing is contraindicated for clients who have severe bronchospastic lung disease, such as asthma, or advanced atrioventricular heart block. Additional unfavorable conditions in which this test is not indicated include acute myocardial infarction within 48 hours of the test, severe aortic or mitral stenosis, resting systolic blood pressure less than 90 mm Hg, and allergy to dipyridamole.

Nuclear Dobutamine Stress Test: Dobutamine is an adrenergic (sympathomimetic) drug that increases myocardial contractility, heart rate, and systolic blood pressure, which increases the myocardial oxygen consumption and thus increases coronary blood flow. If the client has heart block or asthma and takes a theophylline preparation daily, this test may be ordered instead of the nuclear Persantine (dipyridamole) stress test. Dobutamine is an alternative stressor test.

Nuclear dobutamine stress testing can identify clients with CAD and identify those who are at high risk for severe ischemic changes prior to vascular surgery.

Contraindications for nuclear dobutamine stress testing include clients having acute myocardial infarction within 10 days, acute myocarditis or pericarditis, unstable angina pectoris (prolonged episodes, episodes at rest), ventricular or atrial dysrhythmias, severe hypertension or hypotension, severe aortic or mitral stenosis, hyperthyroidism, and acutely severe infections. Propranolol (Inderal) should be available for any possible adverse reaction to the dobutamine infusion.

Purposes

- To screen for CAD.
- To evaluate myocardial perfusion.
- To differentiate between an ischemic area and an infarcted or scar area of the myocardium.
- To develop a cardiac rehabilitation program.
- To evaluate cardiac status for work capability.
- To evaluate drug efficacy.

Clinical Problems

Abnormal Findings: Positive: Greater than 2 mm ST depression, coronary artery disease, and myocardial hypoperfusion.

Procedure

- A consent form should be signed by the client.
- The client should be NPO 2 or 3 hours before the test. The client should not consume alcoholic and caffeine-containing drinks and should avoid smoking for 2–3 hours before the test. Milk could cause nausea.
- Medications should be taken, unless otherwise indicated by the health care provider.
- Comfortable clothes should be worn (i.e., shorts or slacks with a belt and sneakers or tennis shoes with socks). Most bedroom slippers are not suitable.
- The chest is shaved as needed, and the skin is cleansed with alcohol.
- Electrodes are applied to the chest according to the lead selections.
- Baseline ECG, pulse rate, and BP are taken and then are monitored throughout the test.
- The test is stopped if the client becomes dyspneic, suffers severe fatigue, complains of chest pain, has a rapid increase in pulse rates and/or BP, or develops life-threatening arrhythmias (i.e., ventricular tachycardia, premature ventricular contractions [PVCs] greater than 10 PVC in 1 minute).
- Usually the test is not stopped abruptly unless this is necessary. Vital signs and ECG tracings are recorded at the end of the testing or the recovery stage.
- The test takes approximately 30 minutes, which includes up to 10–15 minutes of exercising.

Treadmill Stress Test: Usually there are 5 stages. In the first stage, the speed is 2 mph at a 3% grade or incline for 3 minutes. In the second stage, the speed is 3.3 mph at a 6% grade for another 3 minutes. Normally the speed does not go beyond 3.3 mph. With each stage the grade is increased 3% and the time is increased by 3 minutes, unless fatigue or adverse reactions occur. The power-driven treadmill has support rails to help the client maintain balance.

Bicycle Ergometer Test: The client is instructed to pedal the bike against an increased amount of resistance. The bike handlebars are for maintaining balance and should not be gripped tightly for support. The client should not shower or take a hot bath for 2 hours after testing.

Exercise Thallium Perfusion Test: An IV line is inserted. Exercise time for the stress test is determined. The client obtains the maximal exercise level, and thallium is injected intravenously 1 minute before the test ends. The client continues to exercise for 1–2 more minutes. A scan is then taken by gamma camera, which visualizes thallium perfusion of the myocardium.

Client returns in 2 or more hours for a second scan.

Exercise Technetium Perfusion Test: With the Cardiolite stress test, the client receives two injections intravenously, one at rest and one at stress. The client should be NPO for 2–3 hours prior to the test. Any medications that may affect the blood pressure or heart rate should be discontinued 24–48 hours prior to the test (unless the test is being performed to evaluate the efficacy of cardiac medications). The client should be physically able to exercise on a treadmill. The total time for the test is 3 hours, which is shorter than thallium imaging.

Persantine (Dipyridamole) Stress Test: The client remains NPO after midnight except for water. A diabetic client may have a light breakfast of juice and toast and half of the insulin dose but should first check with the health care provider. Caffeine-containing drugs, food, and beverages such as colas must be avoided 24 hours prior to the test. Decaffeinated beverages should also be avoided. Theophylline preparations (Theo-Dur, Theolair-SR, Bronkodyl, Elixophyllin SR, and others) should be stopped 36 hours before the test.

The client is in a supine position during the test. The client receives a total of 0.56 mg/kg/ dose of IV Persantine (dipyridamole) over a period of 4 minutes. Three minutes after the Persantine infusion, the isotope (thallium, Cardiolite, or other Tc-based compound) is injected intravenously. Aminophylline should be available to reverse any adverse reaction to Persantine. Imaging procedure begins 15–30 minutes after the isotope infusion. Heart rate, blood pressure, and ECG will be monitored before and during the test.

The test is terminated if any of the following occur: ventricular tachycardia, second degree (heart block, severe ST-segment depression, severe hypotension [less than 90 mm Hg], or severe wheezing). The asthmatic client may use the beta-agonist inhaler if necessary during the procedure.

Nuclear Dobutamine Stress Test: The client remains NPO after midnight except for water. Beta blockers, calcium channel blockers, and angiotensin-converting enzyme (ACE) inhibitors should be discontinued 24 hours prior to the test. Nitrates should not be taken 4–6 hours before the test. Dobutamine is administered intravenously using an infusion pump. The dobutamine is mixed in a liter of normal saline solution and the dose and infusion rate is increased until the client's heart rate reaches approximately 85% of his or her maximum predicted heart rate. If the heart rate is less than 110 beats/min, IV atropine sulfate may be given. The isotope is injected when the maximum heart rate is achieved.

The test is terminated if any of the following occur: atrial or ventricular tachycardia, atrial flutter or fibrillation, severe ST-segment depression, progressive anginal pain, severe hypotension (less than 90 mm Hg systolic), and severe hypertension (greater than 220 mm Hg systolic or greater than 120 mm Hg diastolic). Nitroglycerin may be given for angina pain. Propranolol (Inderal) should be available for adverse reaction to dobutamine. Imaging procedure occurs 15 minutes after the completion of the dobutamine infusion.

Factors Affecting Diagnostic Results

- Certain drugs (e.g., digitalis preparations) can cause a false-positive test result.
- Leaning on support rails of the treadmill or the handlebars of the bicycle.

Nuclear Persantine (Dipyridamole) Stress Test
- Taking theophylline preparations within 24 hours of the test.
- Ingesting caffeine products (beverages, chocolates) 6 hours before the test.
- Ingesting decaffeinated beverages 4 hours before the test.

Nuclear Dobutamine Stress Test
- Taking beta blockers, calcium channel blockers, ACE inhibitors 24 hours before the test.
- Taking nitrates 4 hours before the test.
- Ingesting a full meal 4 hours before the test.

NURSING IMPLICATIONS WITH RATIONALE

Pretest

- Recognize when the stress/exercise test is contraindicated (i.e., with recent myocardial infarction; severe, unstable angina; uncontrolled cardiac dysrhythmias; heart failure; or recent pulmonary embolism).
- Check that the consent form has been signed.
- Recognize whether a treadmill stress test or pharmacological stress test is appropriate.
- Review medications that may interfere with the test, for example, beta blockers to decrease heart rate.

Client Teaching Treadmill Stress Test

- Explain the procedure to the client in regard to NPO 2–3 hours prior to test; not smoking, continuing with medications; the clothing and shoes that should be worn; shaving and cleansing the chest area; electrode application; continuous monitoring of the ECG, pulse rate, and BP; and not leaning on the rails of the treadmill or the handlebars of the bike.
- Instruct the client to inform the cardiologist or technician if he or she experiences chest pain, difficulty in breathing, or severe fatigue. The risk of having a myocardial infarction during the stress test is less than 0.2%.
- Inform the client that after 10–15 minutes of testing or when the heart rate is at a desired or an elevated rate, the test is stopped. It will be terminated immediately if there are any severe ECG changes (i.e., multiple PVCs, ventricular tachycardia).
- Allow the client to ask questions. Refer questions you cannot answer to other appropriate health professionals (i.e., a cardiologist, a specialized technician, or a nurse in the stress test laboratory).
- Instruct the client to continue the walking exercise at the completion of the test for 2–3 minutes to prevent dizziness. The treadmill speed will be decreased. Tell the client that he or she may be perspiring and may be "out of breath." Profuse diaphoresis, cold and clammy skin, severe dyspnea, and severe tachycardia are not normal and the test will be terminated if these occur.
- Inform the client that an ECG and vital signs are taken 5–10 minutes after the stress test (recovery stage) until returning to baseline.
- Encourage the client to participate in a cardiac/exercise rehabilitation program as advised by the health care provider/cardiologist. Tell the client of the health advantages—constant heart monitoring, improved collateral circulation, increased oxygen supply to the heart, and dilating coronary resistance vessels.
- Discourage the client over 35 years of age from doing strenuous exercises without having a stress/exercise test or a cardiac evaluation.
- Inform the client that he or she can resume activity as indicated.
- Explain to the client that a written report is submitted to the client's personal physician from the cardiologist. The client should check with the health care provider for the test results.

S

Exercise Thallium Perfusion Test

- Explain the procedure for the test (see *Procedure*). Explain that the difference between the routine stress test and the exercise thallium perfusion test is an injection of thallium 201 during the routine stress test followed by scans and/or x-rays. Nursing implications are the same for both tests.
- Instruct the client to return for additional pictures in 2–4 hours as indicated by the technician or cardiologist.

Exercise Technetium Perfusion Test

- Explain the procedure (see *Procedure*).
- The client should lie quietly for approximately 30 minutes during the imaging.
- Inform the client that the test should last no more than 3 hours.
- Instruct the client taking medications that affect the blood pressure or heart rate to check with the health care provider about discontinuing the medications for 24–48 hours prior to testing.

Nuclear Persantine (Dipyridamole) Stress Test

- Explain the procedure for the test to the client (see *Procedure*). The client should be NPO after midnight except for water.
- Instruct the client to avoid food, beverages, and drugs that contain caffeine. Beverages and foods rich in caffeine include colas (Coke and Pepsi), Dr. Pepper, Mountain Dew, Tab, chocolate (syrup and candy), tea, and coffee. Decaffeinated coffee and tea should also be avoided. Drugs containing caffeine include Anacin, Excedrin, NoDoz, Wigraine, Darvon compound, Cafergot, Fiorinal. Theophylline preparations should be avoided 36 hours before the test; the client should check with the health care provider in case it is not possible to discontinue the theophylline drug for that period of time.
- Explain to the client that first Persantine will be given intravenously and then an isotope. The client is positioned under a camera with his or her left arm over the head. The camera will be moving very close to the chest for taking pictures (imaging). The imaging takes approximately 20–30 minutes.
- Instruct the client to return for additional pictures in 2–4 hours as indicated by the technician or cardiologist.
- Explain to the client that a written report is submitted to the client's personal health care provider from the cardiologist.

Nuclear Dobutamine Stress Test

- Explain the procedure for the test to the client (see *Procedure*). The client should be NPO after midnight except for water.
- Instruct the client to discontinue drugs that are beta blockers, calcium channel blockers, or ACE inhibitors for 36 hours prior to the test with the health care provider's approval. Give the client the date and time for stopping the drug. Nitrates should not be taken 6 hours before the test unless necessary (check with the health care provider).
- Inform clients of side effects that may occur, such as chest pain, palpitations, headache, paresthesia, nausea, tremor, ventricular arrhythmias, ST-segment depression, and hypotension, which resolve with the discontinuation of the infusion.

Thermography (breast)
Mammothermography

Normal Finding

No hot "white" spots; symmetric appearance of the breasts (photograph).

Description

Mammothermography (breast thermography), an infrared photographic test, measures and records heat energy from the skin surface of the breast. Lesions of the breast, especially cancerous ones, cause increased breast metabolism, resulting in an increased breast surface temperature and vascularity. If hot spots are recorded, then additional tests (such as low-dose mammography, ultrasonography, and/or biopsy) should be performed to confirm breast cancer.

Approximately 80% of positive thermograms are accurate for diagnosing lesions of the breast (35% of positive thermograms show benign breast lesions). The remaining 20% of the tests give false-positive results. Because one fifth of the results are false positive, mammothermography is not commonly used, except for screening purposes. Usually it cannot detect small or deep breast cancer lesions. Mammothermography should be used in conjunction with a physical examination of the breast.

Purpose

- To aid in the diagnosis of a breast lesion.

Clinical Problems

Indications: Cancer of the breast, abscesses of the breast, and fibrocystic disease of the breast.

Procedure

- Food and fluids are not restricted. Immediately before the test, hot or very cold drinks should be avoided.
- The client should remove jewelry and clothes from the neck to the waist. The client is given a cloth or paper gown, and the gown should be worn with the opening in the front.
- Ointment or powder on the breast should be removed before the test.
- The client usually sits in a cool room (68°F) for 10–15 minutes before the test. This helps to equalize body temperature.
- The client is seated and will be asked to place her hands over her head or on her hips.
- Usually three photographs of different angles are taken of each breast. The procedure takes about 15 minutes.
- The films are checked for readability before the client dresses.

Factors Affecting Diagnostic Results

- Ointment, powder, and recent sunburn could change skin temperature and cause false-positive results.
- Fluctuations in room temperature could affect the test results.
- Menstruation (immediately before or during) could increase vascular engorgement of the breasts.

NURSING IMPLICATIONS WITH RATIONALE

- Obtain a menstrual history. Ask the client when she had her last menstrual period. She should not have the thermogram if she is pregnant or if she is menstruating or close to her period. The vascularity of the breasts increases at these times.

Client Teaching

- Explain the procedure to the client. Procedure in hospitals and in private laboratories may differ slightly, so check before discussing the procedure with the client. Tell the client the test is not painful.
- Instruct the client not to use ointment or powder on the breast the day of the test. These could cause false-positive results. Check the skin for recent exposure to sunlight.
- Inform the client that the test takes about 15 minutes; however, she will be asked to wait for several minutes after the pictures are taken to be sure they are readable. Tell the client not to be alarmed if one of the pictures needs to be repeated.
- Encourage the client to express her concerns. Answer questions, if possible, or refer questions to other appropriate health professionals.
- Inform the client that the mammothermography is generally a screening test and that if the test is positive, other tests will be conducted to confirm the test results. Inform the client that approximately one third of the positive results are benign lesions and one fifth of the positive results could be false-positives.
- Encourage the client to perform breast examination after each menstrual period and to keep routine medical appointments. If necessary, demonstrate the breast examination technique.

Thoracoscopy

Normal Finding

Free of pleural and lung disease.

Description

With thoracoscopy, an endoscope (thoracoscope) tube is inserted into the thoracic cavity to visualize the pleural space, thoracic wall, pericardium, and the mediastinum. This test is replacing the thoracotomy procedure. Biopsies and fluid can be obtained with this procedure; also, fluid can be drained. Wedge resection to remove blebs or diseased tissue and laser procedure may be performed during this test.

Purposes

- To obtain biopsy specimens.
- To assess tumor growth, pleural effusion, pleural and pulmonary infections, emphysema.
- To perform laser procedure to the thoracic area.

Clinical Problems

Abnormal Findings: Pleural or lung tumors, metastatic cancer in the lungs and/or pleura, emphysema, empyema, and inflammatory process in the thoracic cavity.

Procedure

- A signed consent form is required.
- Nothing by mouth for 8–12 hours prior to the test.
- Pretest requirements: Pulmonary function tests, chest x-ray, ECG (EKG), selected laboratory tests. These tests should be completed before the thoracoscopy.
- IV line is inserted for IV medications.
- Client is anesthetized, and an endobronchial tube is inserted.
- The lung on the operative side is collapsed.
- The thoracoscope is inserted through a trocar to view the thoracic cavity.
- Following the thoracoscopic procedure, the lung is reexpanded, and a chest tube is placed in the thoracic cavity with a water-sealed drainage tube attached (closed drainage system).
- The thoracoscopy takes approximately 1 hour.

Factors Affecting Diagnostic Results

- Previous thoracic surgery can inhibit the test procedure.

NURSING IMPLICATIONS WITH RATIONALE

- Obtain a history of the client's health problems and drugs that are taken daily.
- Obtain vital signs.
- Check that the client has completed the pretest orders. Report any abnormal findings.

Client Teaching

- Explain the procedure to the client and refer questions to which answers are unknown to other health professionals.
- Inform the client that pain medication will be available if the client has discomfort following the procedure.
- Inform the client that he or she will have a chest tube with a drainage system after the test. The chest tube is to assure that any fluid left in the chest will be removed.

Posttest

- Monitor vital signs every 15 minutes for 1 hour, then every 30 minutes for 2 hours, and then hourly for 2 more hours.
- Check frequently or as ordered for patency of the drainage tube.
- Assess respiratory status.
- Report frank bleeding that appears in the drainage tube.
- Administer analgesics for pain as ordered and as needed.
- A chest x-ray will be ordered to determine if the lung has expanded. Chest tube remains in the thoracic cavity until the lungs have expanded.

Ultrasonography (abdominal aorta, brain, breast, carotid, Doppler—arteries and veins, eye and eye orbit, gallbladder, heart, kidney, liver, pancreas, pelvis [uterus, ovaries, pregnant uterus], prostate, scrotum, spleen, thoracic, and thyroid)*

Ultrasound, Echography (echogram), Sonogram

Normal Finding

A normal pattern image of the organ or normal Doppler analysis.

Description

Ultrasonography (ultrasound or sonogram) is a diagnostic procedure used to visualize body tissue structure or wave-form analysis of Doppler studies. An ultrasound probe called a transducer is held over the skin surface or in a body cavity to produce an ultrasound beam in the tissues. The reflected sound waves or echoes from the tissues can be transformed by a computer into scans, graphs, or audible sounds (Doppler).

Ultrasonography diagnostic, a dynamic, nonionizing test, is relatively inexpensive and fast and does not cause any known harm to the client. It is also referred to as a *sonogram*. There are limitations because it cannot be used to determine bone abnormalities or for air-filled organs. The ultrasound beam cannot penetrate air. In obese persons, it is difficult for sound waves to pass through fat layers. Ultrasound is particularly useful in children because of their small size, and it does not require ionizing radiation.

Ultrasound can detect tissue abnormalities (i.e., masses, cysts, edema, stones). Most ultrasound studies (e.g., gallstones) do not need other modalities for confirmation; however, computed tomography, magnetic resonance imaging, or radionuclide scanning may be used to confirm certain ultrasound results.

Some of the body structures that this procedure examines are the abdominal aorta, the brain, the arteries and veins (Doppler), the gallbladder, the heart, the kidney, the liver, pregnant uterus (pelvic), the pancreas, the spleen, and the thyroid.

Abdominal Aorta: The area for abdominal scanning includes the xyphoid process to the umbilicus. Ultrasonography can detect aortic aneurysms with 98% accuracy and determine whether they are fusiform, saccular, or dissecting types.

Arteries and Veins with Doppler: An arterial study is indicated for clients with symptoms of claudication, rest pain, or a persisting open wound in the lower extremity. Doppler ultrasonography can determine the presence or absence of flow, flow direction, and flow character. The Doppler effect can detect decreased blood flow caused by partial arterial occlusion or by deep-vein thrombosis. It can be used in fetal monitoring during labor and delivery. The Doppler instrument

---

*Updated by Dr. Beth Bilski, Newark Delaware; previously updated by Dr. Sharon W. Gould, Department of Medical Imaging, DuPont Hospital for Children, Wilmington, Delaware.

is available to nurses for monitoring blood flow for those who have altered circulation. Low-frequency waves usually indicate low-velocity blood flow. This procedure may also be used to evaluate the patency of a graft.

Brain: Echoencephalography is an ultrasound of the brain. Neonatal neurosonography is also ultrasound of the brain. If the ventricles are dilated and/or shifted to one side, then pathologic findings, such as intracranial lesions or intracranial hemorrhage, may be suspected. This test is most useful for evaluating hydrocephalus and intracranial hemorrhage in newborns. (See *echoencephalography* for detailed data.)

Breast: Ultrasonography of the breast is helpful for (1) diagnosing breast lesions in women who have dense breasts, (2) differentiating between cystic and solid lesions, (3) follow-up of fibrocystic breast disease, and (4) evaluating women with silicone breast implants for breast lesions. Breast ultrasonography may be suggested for pregnant women as well as any woman with a palpable breast mass. X-ray mammography remains the *screening* examination of choice as ultrasonography cannot detect microcalcification. Still, ultrasonography serves as a valuable adjunctive tool.

Carotid Artery with Doppler: Blood flow in the carotid artery can be measured by using Doppler technique to determine carotid stenosis. During a carotid sonogram, vertebral arteries can be visualized by this Doppler technique to determine antegrade or retrograde blood flow through these vessels.

Eye and Eye Orbit: Ultrasonography of the eye and eye orbital area may be used to (1) determine abnormal tissue of the eye (vitreous adhesions, retinal detachment) when opacities within the eye are present, and (2) detect orbital lesions. With this test, orbital lesions can be distinguished from orbital inflammation.

Gallbladder and Bile Ducts: Gallbladder ultrasonography is accurate in delineating the anatomy of the gallbladder and biliary system. It can evaluate the size, structure, and position of the gallbladder and can determine the presence of gallstones. It may be used in conjunction with nuclear medicine.

Heart (Cardiac): Echocardiography is ultrasound of the heart. It can determine the size, shape, and position of the heart and the movement of heart valves and chambers. The methods commonly used are the M-mode method, which records the motion of the intracardiac structures, such as valves, and the two-dimensional method, which records a cross-sectional view of cardiac structures. The echocardiogram is useful in detecting mitral stenosis, pericardial effusion, congenital heart disease, and enlargement of a heart chamber. (See *echocardiography* for detailed data.)

Intravascular Ultrasonography: An ultrasound transducer mounted on a catheter is used to assess pathologic changes to the arterial wall and to evaluate vascular procedures such as angioplasty placement. This test is usually performed in large medical centers.

Kidneys (Renal): Ultrasonography is a reliable method of identifying and differentiating renal cysts and tumors. Cysts are echo free, and tumors and renal calculi record multiple echoes. This test is highly recommended when the client is hypersensitive to iodinated contrast dye used in x-ray tests (e.g., CT, intravenous pyelography). This test is most useful for depicting anatomic changes in the kidneys.

Liver (Hepatic): The liver was one of the first organs examined by ultrasound, because it is large and difficult to x-ray. Ultrasonography is useful for distinguishing between cysts and tumors and for determining the size, structure, and position of the liver. With cysts, the sonogram reflects an echo-free response, whereas with a tumor, multiple echoes are recorded. Ultrasonography is very

U

helpful in differentiating obstructive from nonobstructive jaundice. The client may have abnormal liver laboratory values, and the liver may still appear within normal limits.

Pelvis: *Uterus:* Ultrasonography may be used to distinguish between cystic, solid, and complex masses as well as to localize free fluid and inflammatory processes. *Ovaries:* The dimensions of the ovaries, as well as ovarian cysts and solid lesions, can be identified by pelvic sonography. Pelvic ultrasonography is a valuable tool but should not replace a gynecologic examination.

Pregnancy: In pregnancy, the amniotic fluid enhances reflection of sound waves from the placenta and fetus, thus revealing their size, shape, and position. Echoes from the pregnancy may be seen after as few as 4 weeks of amenorrhea. For visualization of pelvic structures, a full bladder is indicated in the nongravid and first-trimester pregnancy. The uterus is sometimes evaluated with a transvaginal transducer with the bladder empty.

Placenta Previa: Ultrasound is performed at 18 to 20 weeks gestation to determine many factors, including the location of the placenta in relationship to the cervical os. If the diagnosis of placenta previa is made, another ultrasound will be scheduled in the third trimester and may be followed with serial ultrasounds to determine the placenta's location with regard to the cervical os. The degree of placenta overlap of the os at term will determine the mode of delivery of the baby—vaginal versus caesarian section (C section).

A transvaginal sonography (TVS) may be used to locate the placenta at any time during the pregnancy and is more accurate than transabdominal sonography.

Pancreas: The pancreas is a more difficult organ to examine and may require distending the stomach with water to create an acoustic window. Ultrasonography does not measure pancreatic function, but it can determine overall size of the gland and detect pancreatic abnormalities, such as pancreatic tumors, pseudocysts, and pancreatitis. This test is useful for clients who are too thin for adequate CT scanning.

Prostate (Transrectal): Ultrasonography of the prostate gland is used to (1) evaluate palpable prostate nodules and seminal vesicles, (2) determine if urinary problems may be related to benign prostatic hypertrophy (BPH), (3) detect early small prostatic tumors, and (4) identify tumor location for biopsy and/or radiation purposes. A rectal examination and the laboratory test, prostate-specific antigen (PSA), should be included for diagnosing prostatic lesions.

Scrotum/Testes: Ultrasonography of the scrotum sac contents is helpful in diagnosing abscesses, cysts, hydroceles, spermatoceles, varicoceles, testicular tumors, torsion, and chronic scrotal swelling. Pulsed Doppler or color Doppler techniques may be used to assess testicular blood flow.

Spleen: Ultrasonography can be used to determine the size, structure, and position of the spleen. This procedure can identify splenic masses. In some cases, it is a useful tool for evaluating the need for splenectomy and follow-up of pathologies such as hematoma or abscess.

Thoracic: Ultrasonography is useful in identifying lesions, but it is not diagnostic in the air-filled lungs unless there is a lesion, outside the lungs, adherent to the chest wall. It may be used to identify pleural fluid, malposition of the diaphragm, and the presence of an abscess. Ultrasound of the thoracic area may be used in combination with x-ray and thoracic scans.

Thyroid: Ultrasonography of the thyroid is 85% accurate in determining the size and structure of the thyroid gland. This procedure can help differentiate between a cyst and a tumor and can determine the depth and dimension of thyroid nodules. Nuclear imaging is the test choice of thyroid pathology.

Purposes

- To evaluate the size, structure, and position of body organs.
- To evaluate the blood flow in arteries and veins.
- To detect cysts, tumors, and calculi.

Clinical Problems

ORGAN	ABNORMAL FINDINGS
Abdominal aorta	Aortic aneurysms, aortic stenosis
Arteries and veins (Doppler)	Arterial occlusion (partial or complete), deep-vein thrombosis, chronic venous insufficiency, arterial trauma
Brain	Intracranial hemorrhage, lesions (tumors, abscess), hydrocephalus
Breast	Cysts, tumors (benign or malignant), metastasis to the lymph nodes and muscle tissue
Carotid artery	Carotid plaque, thrombus, degree of stenosis
Eye and eye orbit	Vitreous opacities, detached retina, foreign bodies, orbital lesion, orbital inflammation, meningioma, glioma, neurofibroma, cyst, keratoprosthesis
Gallbladder	Acute cholecystitis, cholelithiasis, biliary obstruction
Heart (Cardiac)	Cardiomegaly, mitral stenosis, aortic stenosis and insufficiency, pericardial effusion, congenital heart disease, left ventricular hypertrophy, ischemic heart disease, septal defects
Kidney (Renal)	Renal cysts and tumors, hydronephrosis, perirenal abscess, acute pyelonephritis, acute glomerulonephritis
Liver (Hepatic)	Hepatic cysts, abscesses, tumor; hepatic metastasis; hepatocellular disease, congenital abnormalities
Pancreas	Pancreatic tumors, pseudocysts, acute pancreatitis
Pelvis	
Uterus	Uterine tumor, fibroids, hydatiform mole, endometrial changes
Ovaries	Ovarian cysts or tumor
Pregnancy	Fetal age, fetal death, placenta previa, abruptio placenta, hydrocephalus, breech fetal presentation
Prostate	Cancer of the prostate gland, benign prostatic hypertrophy (BPH), prostatitis
Scrotum	Hydrocele, spermatocele, varicocele, testicular tumors, torsion, orchitis, acute/chronic epididymitis, cyst, abscess, chronic scrotal swelling
Spleen	Splenomegaly; splenic cysts, abscesses, tumor, congenital anomalies
Thoracic	Pleural fluid, abscess formation, malposition of the diaphragm
Thyroid	Thyroid tumors (benign or malignant), thyroid goiters or cysts

Procedure

- Obtain a signed consent form, if necessary.
- Restrict food and fluids for 4–8 hours before test for abdominal aorta, gallbladder, liver, spleen, and pancreas ultrasound studies.
- The client should eat a fat-free meal the night prior to the test for abdominal, gallbladder, liver, pancreas, and kidney sonograms.

- Premedications are seldom given unless the client is extremely apprehensive or has nausea and vomiting.
- Conductive gel is applied to the skin surface at the site to be examined. The transducer is handheld and is moved smoothly back and forth across the oiled or gelled skin surface.
- The client's position may vary from supine to oblique, prone, semirecumbent, and erect.
- The average time for a procedure is 30 minutes.
- The client should not smoke or chew gum prior to the examination to prevent swallowing air.

Brain

- Remove jewelry and hairpins from neck and head.

Breast

- Handheld, real-time contact scanning over the palpable mass is the most widely used method for breast imaging.
- The automated system using full-breast water immersion and a reproducible, systematic survey is less widely used because of its higher cost, space requirements, and lack of real-time capability.
- No lotion or powder should be applied under the arm or on the breasts the day of the test.

Doppler

- The blood pressure will be taken at certain limb sites.

Eye and Eye Orbit

- Anesthetize the eye and eye area.
- With the contact method, the probe touches the corneal surface.

Heart and Liver

- Ask the client to breathe slowly and to hold breath after deep inspiration.

Gynecologic

- A transvaginal exam may be required. A slender probe is covered with a protective sleeve, and gel is placed on the sleeve. The client is asked to place the probe in the vagina.

Obstetrics (First Trimester), Pelvic and Renal

- The client should drink 24 ounces of water 1 hour prior to the examination, or three to four 8-ounce glasses of clear liquid 90 minutes prior to the test. The client should not void until the test is completed. Second and third trimester clients need not drink a large amount of water *unless* bleeding has occurred, in which case the above procedure is followed.

Prostate

- Administer an enema 1 hour before the test.
- The client should drink two 8-ounce glasses of clear fluid 1 hour before the test.
- The client should *not* void 1 hour before the test.
- The client lies on his left side.
- Rectal examination is usually performed before the transducer is inserted into the rectum. Lubricate the rectal probe and insert it into the rectum. The test takes approximately ½ hour.

Scrotum

- The penis is strapped back to the abdominal area or covered with a towel.
- Gel is applied and the transducer is passed over the scrotum.

Factors Affecting Diagnostic Results

- Residual barium sulfate in the GI tract from previous x-ray studies will interfere with ultrasound results. Ultrasonography should be performed before barium studies.
- Air and gas (bowel) will not transmit the ultrasound beam.
- Excess fecal material in the colon and rectum (prostate).

NURSING IMPLICATIONS WITH RATIONALE

- Obtain a signed consent form if needed.
- NPO for 6 hours prior to all abdominal studies, such as gallbladder, aorta, and others.
- Confirm that the client has not had any other tests that may interfere with test results, such as having an upper GI series.

Client Teaching

- Explain the purpose and procedure to the client (see *Description* and *Procedure* above). Tell the client that an oil or lubricant is applied to the skin surface at the site of the organ and that a probe will move with light pressure back and forth over the area.
- Inform the client that this is a painless procedure unless there has been trauma (injury) to the area. Tell the client that there will be no exposure to radiation, and that the ultrasound test is considered to be safe and fast.
- Instruct the client to remain still during the procedure. Inform him or her that the test usually takes 30 minutes or less, except for a few ultrasound tests (e.g., arterial, venous, and carotid ultrasonography), which could take 1 hour.
- Encourage the client to ask questions and to express any concerns. Refer questions you cannot answer to the ultrasonographer or the health care provider.
- Be supportive of the client and the family.

Eye

- Avoid rubbing the eyes until the anesthetic effect has worn off in order to avoid corneal abrasion.
- Inform the client that blurred vision may be present for a short time until the anesthetic has worn off.

Abdominal Studies

- Inform the client that she or he should be NPO for 6 hours prior to all abdominal studies.
- Confirm that the client has not had other tests that may interfere with the ultrasonography, such as upper GI series.

Uterotubal insufflation test
Rubin's Test

Normal Findings
Patent fallopian tubes
> Patency pressure: 80–100 mmHg
> (pressure decreases as CO_2 passes through the fallopian tubes)
> Partial patency pressure: 120–140 mmHg
> Occlusion of the fallopian tubes: >200 mmHg

Description

The uterotubal insufflation test (Rubin's test) is performed to determine the patency or occlusion of the fallopian tubes. The test uses a flowmeter with a pressure gauge to inflate the fallopian tubes with carbon dioxide (CO_2). If there is an occlusion in the fallopian tubes, the pressure rises. The CO_2 under pressure could dislodge any debris that may be in the tubes.

Today the **hysterosalpingography test** is usually prescribed to determine fallopian tube patency. However, dye is introduced with this test, and if the client is allergic to the dye, then the uterotubal insufflation might be recommended.

Purpose
- To determine the patency of the fallopian tubes.

Clinical Problem

Abnormal Findings: Partial or complete occlusion of the fallopian tube(s).

Procedure
- Client is placed in a lithotomy position. A vaginal speculum is inserted into the vaginal canal to expose the cervix.
- A sterile cannula is inserted into the cervical canal. Carbon dioxide is forced, and the pressures are recorded by a kymograph.
- Shoulder pain usually occurs if the tubes are patent, because of the gas, CO_2.
- The client may complain of nausea, vomiting, dizziness, and pain following the test.

Factors Affecting Diagnostic Results
- Fallopian tubes spasms due to anxiety and discomfort.

NURSING IMPLICATIONS WITH RATIONALE

- Explain the procedure to the client. Tell the client that the test is to determine the patency of the fallopian tubes.
- Have the client void before the test.
- Record vital signs on the chart.

Client Teaching

- Inform the client that there may be pain as the gas is introduced into the fallopian tubes. Usually the pain from the gas indicates patency of the tubes.
- Instruct the client to rest following the test for several hours. Her pelvis may be elevated to reduce discomfort following the test.
- Provide emotional support for the client as needed. Permit her time to ventilate her concerns. Answer her questions or refer them to appropriate health professionals.

Venography (lower limb)

Phlebography

Normal Finding

Normal, patent deep leg veins.

Description

Lower-limb venography is a fluoroscopic and/or x-ray examination of the deep leg veins after injection of a contrast dye. This test is useful for identifying venous obstruction caused by a deep-vein thrombosis (DVT). A thrombus formation usually occurs in the deep calf veins and at the venous junction and its valves. If DVT is not treated, it can lead to femoral and iliac venous occlusion, or the thrombus can become an embolus and cause pulmonary embolism.

This procedure is frequently done after Doppler ultrasonography to confirm a positive or questionable DVT. Radionuclide venography using iodine 125 (I-125)-tagged fibrinogen with scintillation scanning may be done for clients who are too ill for venography or are hypersensitive to contrast dye. The tagged fibrinogen, given intravenously, collects at the site of the thrombus. It may take 6–72 hours for the isotope to collect at the thrombus site; thus, the scanner will be used to check the leg daily for 3 days. This test should not be performed for screening purposes.

Purposes

- To detect DVT.
- To identify congenital venous abnormalities.
- To select a vein for arterial bypass grafting.

Clinical Problems

Abnormal Findings: DVT, congenital venous abnormalities.

Procedure

- A consent form should be signed by the client.
- The client should be NPO for 4 hours before the test; some hospitals permit clear liquids before the test.
- Anticoagulants may be temporarily discontinued.

- A skin test, antihistamine, and/or steroids may be ordered for clients who have a history of allergies to iodine, seafood, or x-ray dye from other tests (e.g., intravenous pyelography).
- The client lies on a radiographic table tilted at a 40- to 60-degree angle. A tourniquet is applied above the ankle, a vein is located in the dorsum of the foot, a small amount of normal saline is administered intravenously into the vein, and then the contrast dye is injected slowly over a period of 2–4 minutes. A cutdown may be necessary if a vein in the foot cannot be located or is not suitable. Fluoroscopy may be used to monitor the flow of the contrast dye, and spot films are taken.
- Normal saline is used after the procedure to flush the contrast dye from the veins.
- A sedative may be indicated prior to the test for clients who are extremely apprehensive and for those who have a low threshold of pain.
- The test takes 30 minutes to 1 hour.

Factors Affecting Diagnostic Results

- Weight on the leg being tested can cause a decrease in the flow of the contrast dye.
- Movement of the leg being tested can interfere with the clarity of the film.

NURSING IMPLICATIONS WITH RATIONALE

Pretest

- Obtain a client history of allergies to iodine, iodine substances (x-ray dye), and seafood. Antihistamines or steroids (e.g., cortisone) may be given for 2–3 days before the test.
- Record baseline vital signs. Have the client void before the test.

Client Teaching

- Explain the purpose and procedure to the client.
- Inform the client that he or she may have a slight burning sensation when the dye is injected. Inform the client not to move the leg being tested during the injection of the dye or during x-ray filming.

Posttest

- Monitor vital signs until stable and as ordered.
- Check the pulse in the dorsalis pedis, popliteal, and femoral arteries for volume intensity and rate.
- Observe for signs and symptoms of latent allergic reaction to the contrast dye (e.g., dyspnea, skin rash, urticaria [hives], and tachycardia).
- Observe the injection site for bleeding, hematoma, and signs and symptoms of infection (e.g., redness, edema, and pain). Report abnormal changes and problems to the health care provider, and record the observations on the client's chart.
- Elevate the affected leg as ordered. If the venogram is positive for DVT, the health care provider most likely will order bed rest, blood laboratory tests, heparin infusion, leg elevation, and warm, moist compresses.
- Be supportive of the client. Answer the client's questions, or refer him or her to the health care provider.

Ventilation scan (V/Q) scan*

Pulmonary Ventilation Scan

Normal Finding

Normal lung tissue with normal gas distribution in both lungs.

Description

The ventilation scan is a nuclear scan of the lungs. The client inhales a mixture of air, oxygen, and radioactive gas (xenon [Xe-127 or Xe-133] or krypton 81 [Kr-81]). A single-breath scan is taken first. Then three phases of scanning follow: (1) the wash-in (single inspiration) phase, which is the build-up of gas distribution in the lungs; (2) the equilibrium phase, in which radioactive gas reaches a steady state; and (3) the washout phase, in which room air is breathed to remove radioactive gas from the lungs.

The pulmonary ventilation scan is usually performed with the pulmonary perfusion scan to differentiate between a ventilatory problem and vascular abnormalities in the lung. The pulmonary perfusion scan indirectly evaluates problems related to blood flow to the lungs (e.g., pulmonary embolism). The radioactive substance used is technetium, and images are taken by a gamma camera. A ventilation scan can reveal decreased ventilation (uptake of radioactive gas) caused by chronic obstructive lung disease, atelectasis, and pneumonia, although the pulmonary perfusion scan is normal. However, pulmonary embolus can cause an abnormal perfusion scan and a normal ventilation scan.

Purposes

- To differentiate between a ventilatory problem and vascular abnormalities in the lung.
- To evaluate low blood oxygen saturation.
- To evaluate and stage persons with COPD, lung cancer, and bronchial obstruction.

Clinical Problems

Abnormal Findings: Chronic obstructive pulmonary disease, pulmonary emboli, tuberculosis, sarcoidosis, lung cancer, pulmonary hypertension, and right to left shunt.

Procedure

- There is no food or fluid restriction.
- Remove all metal objects (jewelry) from around the neck and chest.
- The client inhales the radioactive gas. The client will be asked to take a deep breath and to hold it for a short time (single breath) while the scanner takes an image of the lung. Other images will be recorded during three phases of the test: wash-in, equilibrium, and washout and lung perfusion. The client should breathe normally during all phases except the initial breath-hold phase.

---

*Updated by Theresa Riggle, BS, CNMT, ARRT(N), NCT, Nuclear Medicine Department, Christiana Care Health Services, Newark, Delaware.

Factors Affecting Diagnostic Results

- Metal objects could cause inaccurate recorded images.

NURSING IMPLICATIONS WITH RATIONALE

- Assess respiratory status. Note and report changes in rate and difficulty in breathing. Check breath sounds.
- Assess communications for verbal and nonverbal expressions of anxiety and fear about tests and/or potential or actual problems.
- Report if the client is having chest pain, especially if pulmonary embolism is suspected.
- Be supportive of the client and family members prior to the test. Answer questions, or refer the questions to appropriate health professionals.

Client Teaching

- Explain the procedure to the client (see *Procedure*). Tell the client that the amount of radioactive gas is minimal.
- Instruct the client to remove all jewelry from the chest and neck area.

Video capsule endoscopy (VCE)*

Normal Finding

Normal mucosa of the small bowel.

Description

Video capsule endoscopy (VCE) is a noninvasive diagnostic procedure allowing visualization of the small bowel. A metal pill is swallowed. This pill contains a camera and a transmitter. Images are transferred to a receiver and hard drive. The client wears the hard drive within a belt pack during the study. The pill-isomers is powered for approximately 8 hours by a battery contained within the pill.

The VCE is primarily used to evaluate gastrointestinal bleeding following a nondiagnostic upper and lower endoscopy and to diagnose Crohn disease of the small bowel.

Purposes

- To determine origin of gastrointestinal bleeding when prior studies do not indicate upper GI tract or colon bleeding.
- To determine whether chronic abdominal pain is due to small bowel disease.
- To detect Crohn disease.

---

*Written by Dr. Warren G. Butt, Gastroenterology-Stomach-Colon-Liver, Newark, Delaware.

Clinical Problems

Positive Findings: Crohn disease; origin of GI bleeding; small bowel disease.

Procedure

- Obtain a signed consent form.
- Withhold medications, for example, anti-inflammatory drugs that cause small bowel ulceration. Ideally, these medications should be stopped 90 days prior to the test.
- Electrical leads are attached to the client's chest similar to ECG (EKG) leads.
- Pill is activated then swallowed by the client.
- Client returns 8 hours later to return the belt pack containing the receiver and hard drive.
- Pill passes uneventfully into the stool. The pill is not reused.

Factors Affecting Test Results

- Delayed or slowed GI motility may limit passage of the pill camera.
- Retained food content and bile may interfere with viewing.

Complications

- Small bowel strictures may prevent the pill passage. This may cause a bowel obstruction.

NURSING IMPLICATIONS WITH RATIONALE

- Obtain a history of client's health problems.
- Record the medications that the client is taking. Note if a drug is an anti-inflammatory agent.
- Record baseline vital signs. Maintain a chart for vital signs.

Client Teaching

- Explain the procedure to the client. Stress that he or she will be awake throughout the test.
- Instruct the client not to eat for 2 hours after the pill camera is ingested.
- Explain to the client that normal activities of daily living may be performed during the test.
- Inform the client to return the belt pack after the test at a specified time.

Water loading test

Water Loading ADH Suppression Test

Normal Finding

1,000 mL of Water Intake: *Urine Output:* Greater than 500 mL in 4 hours. *Abnormal:* Less than 500 mL in 4 hours. *Urine Osmolality:* Less than 180 mOsm/kg. *Abnormal:* Greater than 230 mOsm/kg. *Serum Osmolality:* Greater than 280 mOsm/kg. *Abnormal:* Less than 280 mOsm/kg. *Plasma ADH:* (See *Antidiuretic Hormone.*)

Description

Water loading test is a diagnostic test for determining the presence of excess secretion of antidiuretic hormone (ADH), also called syndrome of inappropriate ADH secretion (SIADHs). This test is to suppress the secretion of ADH from the posterior pituitary gland or neurohypophysis through water loading. Normally, as fluid intake increases, urine output increases and urine osmolality decreases. With SIADHs, as water intake increases, the urine output does not increase, and the urine osmolality could be higher than serum osmolality (see *Abnormal Findings*). Caution in administering this test should be taken for clients with a history of heart failure.

SIADHs may be the result of ectopic hormone production caused by tumors, such as bronchogenic carcinoma, pancreatic carcinoma, brain tumors, and lymphoma. Other conditions that can cause SIADHs include tuberculosis, pneumonia, meningitis, thyroid and adrenal disorders, and certain drugs (thiazide diuretics, vincristine).

Purpose

- To detect the presence of SIADHs.

Clinical Problems

Abnormal Findings: SIADHs from ectopic hormone production due to malignant tumors (lung, pancreas, brain), respiratory conditions (pneumonia, tuberculosis), certain CNS disorders, and certain thyroid and adrenal disorders.

Procedure

- The client should be NPO after midnight. Check with the institution's policy.
- Hold diuretics for 12 hours prior to the test.
- Collect 7 mL of venous blood in a red-top tube. This blood specimen is for baseline serum osmolality. Collect a urine specimen for a baseline urine osmolality.
- Have the client drink 1 liter (1,000 mL) of water in 15–30 minutes.
- Collect 7 mL of venous blood and urine specimen every hour after water ingestion for 4–5 hours. (This may be a 4- or 5-hour test; check with the institution.) Refrigerate blood samples and urine specimens until test is completed.
- Blood specimens may also be ordered for serum sodium and plasma ADH. Check with the health care provider.

Factors Affecting Diagnostic Results

- Diuretics can dilute urine and cause a false test result. Diuretics should be held for at least 12 hours before the test and until the test is completed.
- Lithium carbonate can dilute the urine.
- Not collecting all blood and urine specimens.

NURSING IMPLICATIONS WITH RATIONALE

- Obtain a history of cardiac condition, including heart failure (HF).
- Assess for fluid retention, chest rales, peripheral edema.

- Administer 1 liter (1,000 mL) of water in 15–30 minutes.
- Collect blood samples and urine specimens hourly. Measure the urine output hourly and the total after 4–5 hours.

Client Teaching

- Explain the procedure to the client. It may be necessary that the procedure be written, step by step, for the client to follow. Emphasize the importance of collecting urine samples and blood specimens on time.
- Listen to the client's concerns.

X-ray (chest, heart, flat plate of abdomen, kidney, ureter, bladder, and skull)

Roentgenography, Radiography

Normal Finding

Chest: Normal bony structure and normal lung tissue.

Heart (Cardiac): Normal size and shape of the heart and vessels.

Flat Plate of Abdomen: Normal abdominal structures.

Kidney, Ureter, Bladder (KUB): Normal kidney size and structure.

Skeletal: Normal bone structures.

Skull: Normal structure.

Description

In 1895, Wilhelm Konrad Roentgen, a German physicist, discovered x-radiation for diagnosing diseases. Adequate control of the rays (roentgen rays) for the client and the operator did not occur until 1910, and it was then when the machines and techniques were greatly improved. Today x-ray studies cause only small amounts of radiation exposure because of the high quality of x-ray film and procedure.

There are four densities in the human body—air, water, fat, and bone—that will absorb varying degrees of radiation. Air has less density, causing dark images on the film, and bone has high density, causing light images. Bone contains a large amount of calcium and will absorb more radiation, thus allowing less radiation to strike the x-ray film; thus, a white structure is produced.

The chest x-ray is one of the diagnostic tests most often ordered by the health care provider. A skull x-ray is usually ordered following head trauma. The requests for cardiac, flat plate of abdomen, and kidney-ureter-bladder (KUB) x-rays have increased in the last two decades. X-ray studies are requested primarily for screening purposes and then are followed by other extensive diagnostic tests.

Purposes

- To identify bone structure and tissue in the body.
- To detect abnormal size, structure, and shape of bone and body tissues.

Clinical Problems

TEST	ABNORMAL FINDINGS
Chest	Atelectasis, pneumonias, tuberculosis, tumors, lung abscess, pneumothorax, sarcoma, sarcoidosis, scoliosis/kyphosis
Heart	Cardiomegaly, aneurysms, anomalies of the aorta
Abdominal (flat plate)	Abdominal masses, small bowel obstruction, abdominal tissue trauma, ascites
KUB (Kidney, ureter, bladder)	Abnormal size and structure of KUB, renal calculi, kidney and bladder masses
Skull	Head trauma (intracranial pressure, skull fractures), congenital anomalies, bone defects
Skeleton	Fractures, arthritic conditions, osteomyelitis

Procedure

Chest

- Food and fluids are not restricted.
- PA chest film is usually ordered with the client standing. An anteroposterior (AP) chest film may be ordered when PA film cannot be obtained. With an AP chest film, the client is sitting or lying down. A lateral chest film may also be ordered.
- Clothing and jewelry should be removed from the neck to the waist, and a paper or cloth gown should be worn.
- The client should take a deep breath and hold it as the x-ray is taken.

Heart

- Food and fluids are not restricted.
- Posteroanterior (PA) and left-lateral chest films are usually indicated for evaluating the size and shape of the heart. The left anterior oblique (LAO) 60-degree rotation with the PA position may be ordered for cardiac evaluation.
- Clothing and jewelry should be removed from the neck to the waist, and a paper or cloth gown should be worn.
- Client instructions will include body position (usually standing) and when to take a deep breath and hold it.

Abdomen and KUB

- Food and fluids are usually not restricted.
- X-rays should be taken before an intravenous pyelogram or gastrointestinal studies.
- Clothes are removed, and a paper or cloth gown is worn.
- The client lies in the supine position with his or her arms away from the body on a tilted x-ray table.
- The testes should be shielded as an added precaution.

Skull

- Food and fluids are not restricted.
- The client should remove hairpins, glasses, and dentures before the x-ray tests.
- The client will be asked to assume various positions so that different areas of the skull can be x-rayed. X-rays may include the facial bones and sinuses.

Skeletal

- The client should be NPO if a fracture is suspected.
- Immobilize suspected fracture site.

Factors Affecting Diagnostic Results

- Radiopaque materials for IVP and GI studies administered within 3 days of routine x-rays (i.e., chest, flat plate of abdomen, and KUB) could distort the pictures.
- Incorrect positioning of the client could produce distorted pictures.
- Obesity and ascites could affect the clarity of the x-ray film.

NURSING IMPLICATIONS WITH RATIONALE

- Describe the x-ray procedure to the client.

Client Teaching

- Inform the client that the x-ray test usually takes 10–15 minutes.
- Inform the client that there may be several x-rays taken, one or two chest films, or five skull films. The client may be asked to remain in the waiting room for 10–15 minutes after x-rays are taken to be sure the films are readable.
- Encourage the client to ask questions or to express his or her concerns to the nurse, physician, and the technician. Also, if the client does not understand the directions, he or she should ask to have them repeated.
- Ask the female client if she is pregnant or if pregnancy is suspected. X-rays should be avoided during the first trimester of pregnancy. If x-ray of the chest is necessary, the female client should wear a lead apron covering the abdomen and pelvic areas. Some dentists have women of childbearing age (12–48 years old) wear lead aprons.
- Explain to the client that the x-ray equipment and film today are of good quality and decrease the exposure to radiation.

Part II Situational Study Questions

Answers are not given, and if the answers are unknown, the student should check the diagnostic tests in the text (Part II).

SITUATION 1: Colorectal Cancer

E.H. noted blood in his stools. He had a sigmoidoscopy 4 years ago that was negative for polyps and cancer lesions. The physician ordered the following diagnostic tests: colonoscopy, computed tomography (CT) of the abdomen, and barium enema.

1. What does a sigmoidoscopy test include?
2. How does a colonoscopy test differ from a sigmoidoscopy? Explain.
3. What are the preparations for colonoscopy and sigmoidoscopy tests?
4. What is a virtual colonography? How does it differ from a colonoscopy?

E.H. had a CT of the abdomen.

5. What was the purpose for the CT of the abdomen?
6. What measures should be taken if contrast media is used for the CT scan?
7. Why would a barium enema be ordered?
8. Should a colonoscopy be performed before or after a barium enema? Explain.

A nuclear scan of the colon was not ordered for E.H.; however, it can be ordered to identify cancer cells.

9. Explain how nuclear scan is used to detect colon cancer.

SITUATION 2: Cardiac/Chest Pain (Angina Pectoris?)

S.W., age 65, complains of cardiac/chest pain that occurs "off and on." The physician/cardiologist ordered the following tests: 24-hour Holter monitoring, echocardiography, and stress/exercise test.

1. What is the purpose for S.W. to wear a Holter monitor for 24 hours?
2. What should S.W. be instructed to do when wearing the Holter monitor?

S.W. explains that she gets out of breath when exercising.

3. What type of stress test might be ordered if S.W. cannot have an exercise stress test?
4. Differentiate between an exercise thallium perfusion stress test and a nuclear Persantine (dipyridamole) stress test.

Also, S.W. had an echocardiogram performed.

5. What is the purpose for having an echocardiography (echocardiogram)?
6. Differentiate between a two-dimensional (2D) echocardiography, spectral Doppler echocardiography, transesophageal echocardiography, and stress echocardiography.
7. S.W. is having a 2D echocardiogram. What should S.W. be told concerning the procedure for this test?

Because S.W.'s chest/cardiac pain still persists, a cardiac catheterization was ordered.

8. S.W. asked you, "What is a cardiac catheterization?" What would your response be?
9. Differentiate between a right-sided and a left-sided cardiac catheterization.
10. S.W. is having a left-sided cardiac catheterization. What explanation would you give S.W. concerning the procedure?

SITUATION 3: Fetal Distress

T.J., age 32, gestation of 28 weeks, is experiencing a decrease in fetal movement. A fetal nonstress test (NST) is ordered.

1. How would you explain the fetal NST test to T.J.?
2. What is the difference between a fetal nonstress test (NST) and a contraction stress test (CST)?
3. Explain the two contraction stress tests and their procedures. Which CST is considered more invasive than the other? Explain.

A fetoscopy can be ordered to determine fetal well-being.

4. What is the purpose for a fetoscopy?
5. What is the difference between a fetoscopy and cordocentesis (percutaneous umbilical blood sampling [PUBS])?
6. What is external fetal monitoring? How does it differ from internal fetal monitoring? *Note:* See Part III: Reproductive function.

There are several laboratory tests ordered to determine fetal well-being.

7. When would a serum and/or urine estriol (E_3) be ordered? Why?
8. For what reason would an estetrol (E_4) be ordered? During what weeks of gestation would E_4 be prescribed?
9. What is the purpose for ordering an alpha-1-fetoprotein (AFP) test?

SITUATION 4: Peptic Ulcer

E.P., age 46, complains of pain in her upper abdomen. Her hemoglobin was 10.3 g/dL and hematocrit was 31%.

1. What are the reference values for hemoglobin and hematocrit (see Part I: Laboratory tests)?
2. What could E.P.'s hemoglobin and hematocrit values indicate?

The physician/health care provider ordered a gastric analysis, upper gastrointestinal (GI) series, and an esophagogastroscopy (gastroscopy).

3. Differentiate between the three types of gastric analysis. How do they differ?
4. How would you explain an upper GI test and procedure to E.P.?
5. E.P. asks what an abnormal upper GI series would mean. What would be your response?

An esophagogastroscopy was performed. Two ulcers were found in E.P.'s lower esophagus.

6. How would you explain the esophagogastroscopy procedure to E.P.?
7. How do you correlate E.P.'s hemoglobin and hematocrit values with the esophagogastroscopic findings?

SITUATION 5: Pulmonary Embolism (PE)

A.G., age 57, had a blood clot in her left leg. She was having shortness of breath (SOB), persistent coughing, and chest pain. Heparin IV was started. A nuclear lung scan was ordered.

1. What was the purpose for a nuclear lung scan?
2. How is the nuclear lung scan administered? Explain.
3. Does A.G. have any symptoms suggestive of pulmonary embolus? If so, explain.
4. As a nurse, give the client teaching points for nuclear lung scan that you will tell A.G.

A chest X-ray was ordered to compare the result with the nuclear lung scan.

5. Give the client teaching points that you would tell A.G. in preparing for an x-ray.

A CT and MRI might be prescribed for diagnosing a possible pulmonary embolus.

6. Give the advantage of each, CT and MRI, for diagnosing a pulmonary embolus.

Pulmonary angiography might be ordered to diagnose pulmonary embolus.

7. Would this be a first diagnostic test for PE? Explain.
8. Explain how this test is administered.
9. What are the pretest and posttest nursing implications that the nurse should follow?

SITUATION 6: Lung Cancer

B.T., age 63, has increased dyspnea and coughing in the last 6 months. He has been taking cough syrup and cough drops thinking it is a cold. He has smoked 1½ packs of cigarettes per day for the last 40 years.

The health care provider ordered a chest x-ray for B.T. The results showed a nodule in the lower right lobe of the lung. A bronchoscopy and lung biopsy were ordered.

1. Why do you think a bronchoscopy was ordered and for what purpose?
2. What pretest instructions would you give B.T.?
3. What are the two types of lung biopsies that can be performed? Which one uses a bronchoscope? Explain how a tissue specimen can be obtained.
4. What posttest assessment and nursing implications should follow the bronchoscopy?

B.T. has a chest CT scan and an MRI performed.

5. What was the purpose for prescribing a CT scan? For using IV iodinated contrast dye?
6. What pretest nursing implications for the chest CT scan would you include if you were B.T.'s nurse?
7. What are the advantages and contraindications with the use of an MRI?
8. How would the MRI help in diagnosing lung cancer?

PART THREE

Laboratory/Diagnostic Assessments of Body Function

Numerous laboratory and diagnostic tests are ordered to assist in the diagnosis of disease entities and to determine organ function. The purpose of Part III is to provide a listing of groups of tests, with explanations, used for diagnosing body dysfunction. Twelve categories related to organ, body structure, and clinical condition are presented. In each categoric section, the laboratory and diagnostic tests frequently performed are explained as they relate to the disorder. Nursing implications are at the end of each of the 12 categories.

For a more detailed description, procedure, and specific nursing implications of each test, the nurse should refer to Parts I and II of the text.

Cardiac function

LABORATORY TESTS	DIAGNOSTIC TESTS
Brain Natriuretic Peptide (BNP) (Plasma)	Cardiac Calcium Scoring ECG/EKG
Cardiac Enzymes:	Echocardiography
CK/CPK	Cardiac Calcium Scoring
AST/SGOT	Phonocardiography
LD	X-ray
High-Sensitivity C-Reactive Protein (hs CRP)	Exercise/Stress Tests
Homocysteine (Serum)	Thallium Perfusion
Myoglobin (Serum & Urine)	Persantine
Apolipoproteins	Dobutamine
Electrolytes (Serum)	Holter Monitoring
Lipoproteins (Serum Lipids)	Cardiac Catheterization (Cardiac Arteriography)
Troponins (Serum, Blood)	Nuclear Heart Scan
Clotting Times	Magnetic Resonance Imaging (MRI)
PT, INR	Positron Emission Tomography (PET)
PTT, APTT	Pacemaker Monitoring
Coagulation Time	Pericardial Fluid Analysis
ESR	
Antimyocardial Antibody (Serum)	
Anticardiolipin Antibody (ACA)	
Atrial Natriuretic Peptide (ANP)	
Cardiovascular Disease Genetic Test	
Hydroxybutyric Dehydrogenase (HBD)	
Glucose (Blood, Serum)	
Leukocytes (WBC)	
ABGs	
TDM	

Introduction

Numerous laboratory and diagnostic tests are performed to detect cardiac problems and the extent of myocardial injury. Serum enzyme levels are generally ordered immediately upon complaint of cardiac discomfort. Enzyme levels are frequently repeated later to determine if significant changes have occurred. Other tests ordered include serum electrolytes, blood glucose, blood lipids, sedimentation rate, INR, PT, PTT, ECG, cardiac x-ray, and cardiac catheterization, among others.

Laboratory Tests

Brain Natriuretic Peptide (BNP) (Plasma): Desired less than 100 pg/mL; positive greater than 100 pg/mL.

This test is useful in the diagnosis of heart failure.

Cardiac Enzymes: Because serum cardiac enzyme levels might be normal immediately following cardiac trauma, the first set of enzyme levels acts as the baseline measurement for comparison of changes. Following heart injury, creatine kinase (CK/CPK) and isoenzyme CK-MB band, lactate dehydrogenase (LD/LDH) and LD isoenzymes with an $LD_1:LD_2$ shift, and aspartate aminotransferase (AST/SGOT) increase in the blood in proportion to the extent of the injury. Each enzyme has its own time course of release after injury. Table 3.1 is a list of cardiac enzymes, including significant changes that can occur.

TABLE 3.1 Cardiac Enzyme Tests

ENZYME	REFERENCE VALUES	CHANGES	COMMENTS
Creatine kinase (CK) or creatine phosphokinase (CPK)	*Norms:* Male: 5–35 mcg/mL 30–180 IU/L 55–170 U/L at 37°C Female: 5–25 mcg/mL 25–150 IU/L 30–135 U/L at 37°C CPK-MB: 0–6%	Early detection after heart damage: 4–6 hours. Maximal levels for 24 hours. Maximum level rise is 5–8 times normal. CK-MB: 5–15 times normal. Return to normal 3–4 days.	Increased CK is an indicator of muscle damage (cardiac or skeletal). Differentiation between cardiac and skeletal involvement is determined by the CK isoenzymes: CK-MB (heart), CK-MM (skeletal muscle), CK-BB (brain)
Aspartate aminotransferase (AST) or (SGOT)	*Norms:* Average: 8–38 U/L Adult: 0–35 U/L 5–40 U/mL (Frankel) 4–36 IU/L 16–60 Karmen U/mL 30°C 8–33 U/L at 37°C, SI units	AST/SGOT increases within 6–10 hours after heart damage. Peaks within 24–48 hours. Returns to normal in 4–6 days. Rise is 3–5 times normal.	AST/SGOT is not the first enzyme to rise after severe heart damage
Lactic dehydrogenase (LD/LDH)	*Norms:* Adult, total: 100–190 IU/L 70–250 U/L 70–200 IU/L	LD elevation occurs 6–12 hours after heart damage. Peaks within 2–5 days. Returns to normal in 6–12 days.	Rise in LD is later than CK/CPK and AST/SGOT. The prolongation of serum level makes it valuable for diagnosing a late MI.
Isoenzymes: LD_1, LD_2	Isoenzymes: LD_1 14–26% LD_2 27–37%	Isoenzymes: 12–24 hours after heart damage. Flipped LD ratio LD_1: LD_2.	Normally LD_2 has a higher level than LD_1 with a ratio LD_2: LD_1. After acute myocardial infarction, LD_1 increase is greater than LD_2.

High-Sensitivity C-Reactive Protein (hs CRP): *Norms:* Adult: Less than 0.175 mg/L.

It is a highly sensitive test for detecting the risk of cardiovascular and peripheral vascular diseases. A positive hs CRP may indicate that the client is at high risk for coronary artery disease (CAD).

Homocysteine (Serum): *Norm:* 4–17 µmol/L (fasting).

It is useful to identify those persons at risk of CVD, such as MI or stroke. It may be helpful in diagnosing those with Alzheimer disease.

Myoglobin (Serum): *Norms:* 12–90 ng/mL; 12–90 mcg/L.

Myoglobin is a protein found in the skeletal and cardiac muscle cells. After an injury, this protein is released into circulation. After an acute myocardial infarction (AMI), it peaks in approximately 8–12 hours.

Apolipoproteins (Apo, Plasma): *Norm:* See text that includes Apo A-1, Apo B, Ratio, Apo E-4, and lipoprotein.

The apolipoproteins are protein components of lipoproteins. The major components of lipoproteins (HDL, LDL, etc.) are indicated according to the type of apolipoproteins.

Electrolytes (Serum): *Norms:* Potassium: 3.5–5.3 mEq/L. Sodium: 135–145 mEq/L.

Serum electrolyte levels could be normal immediately following myocardial damage. Cellular potassium is lost, and so the serum potassium level might be elevated if urinary output is decreased. It could be normal or decreased if urinary output is increased. Serum sodium level could be normal or decreased if sodium shifts into heart cells. Potassium-wasting diuretics (i.e., hydrochlorothiazide [HydroDIURIL], furosemide [Lasix]) used for treating heart failure could cause a loss of potassium and sodium.

Lipoproteins (Serum Lipids): *Norms:* Adult: Total: 400–800 mg/dL, 4–8 g/L (SI units). Cholesterol: 150–240 mg/dL. Triglycerides: 30–39 years: 20–150 mg/dL; 40–49 years: 30–160 mg/dL; greater than 50 years: 40–190 mg/dL. Phospholipids: 150–325 mg/dL. There could be laboratory differences with these ranges.

Elevated lipid levels (cholesterol, triglycerides, and phospholipids) could be the major factor in the cause of coronary artery disease. Because most lipids are bound to protein (lipoproteins), electrophoresis is used to separate the lipoproteins. Low-density lipoprotein (LDL) is composed of 45% cholesterol, and very-low-density lipoprotein (VLDL) is composed of 70% triglycerides. Both LDL and VLDL are strongly associated with CAD.

Troponins (cTn1) and (cTnT) (Serum, Blood): *Average range:* cTn1: less than 0.1–0.5 ng/mL; cTnT: less than 0.2 (check with institutions for their values). This test assists in diagnosing AMI and in differentiating between cardiac and noncardiac chest pain.

Clotting Times: The tests frequently used to monitor clotting time are prothrombin time (PT), international normalized ratio (INR), partial thromboplastin time (PTT), activated partial thromboplastin time (APTT), and coagulation time (CT) or Lee-White clotting time (LWCT). Table 3.2 explains these tests and gives the reference values and their purposes.

TABLE 3.2 Tests for Monitoring Clotting Times

TEST	REFERENCE VALUES	PURPOSE

Prothrombin time (PT)	*Norms:*
	11–15 seconds or 70%
	Anticoagulant therapy:
	  2–2.5 times control in
	  seconds or 20–30%
		PT is used to monitor clot formation and oral anticoagulant therapy. The PT is kept 2–2.5 times the control for anticoagulant therapy.

INR	2–3	
Partial thromboplast in time (PTT) or Activated partial thromboplastin time (APTT)	*Norms:* 60–70 seconds Anticoagulant therapy: 1.5–2.5 times the control *Norms:* 20–35 seconds	PTT and APTT are primarily used to detect clotting factor defects and to monitor heparin therapy. Following MI, many clients receive heparin therapy, and later some take oral anticoagulants.
Coagulation time (CT) or Lee-White clotting time (LWCT)	*Norms:* 3-tube method: 5–15 minutes	An infrequently used test to determine coagulation problems. It can be used to regulate heparin therapy. It is a time-consuming test.

Sedimentation (Sed) Rate, Erythrocyte Sedimentation Rate (ESR): *Norms:* Adult: Under 50 years (Westergren method): 0–10 mm/h; female: 0–20 mm/h. Over 50 years (Westergren method): male: 0–20 mm/h; female: 0–30 mm/h.

An elevated sedimentation rate might occur after MI or bacterial endocarditis.

Antimyocardial Antibody (Serum): *Normal:* None detected.

Antimyocardial antibodies occur because of a specific antigen in the heart muscle. This antigen can cause autoimmune damage to the heart.

Anticardiolipin Antibody (ACA) (Serum): *Normal:* Negative result.

ACA is an autoantibody found in some clients with systemic lupus erythematosus.

Atrial Natriuretic Peptide (ANP) (Plasma): *Norm:* 20–77 pg/mL.

ANH, secreted from the atrium of the heart, acts as an antagonist to renin and aldosterone. It has antihypertensive effects, lowering blood pressure.

Cardiovascular Disease Genetic Test: *Norm:* Negative to angiotensinogen (AGT) gene.

The angiotensinogen gene is a strong indicator of cardiovascular disease (CVD).

Hydroxybutyric Dehydrogenase (HBD) (Serum): *Norm:* 140–350 international unit/L. 114–290 unit/L.

HBD, an enzyme primarily in heart muscle, is similar to LD_1. Levels rise 8–10 hours following MI.

Blood Glucose: *Norm:* 60–100 mg/dL.

Serum or Plasma Glucose (Fasting): *Norm:* 70–110 mg/dL.

A slight-to-moderate increase in blood or serum glucose level (blood 150 mg/dL or serum 160–180 mg/dL) could be the result of stress caused by release of glucagon and catecholamines. A continuous elevation in blood or serum glucose level is a risk factor for CAD.

Leukocytes, White Blood Cells: *Norms:* 5,000–10,000 mm^3 (µL); 5–10 × 103/µL; 5–10 × 109/L (SI units).

An elevated WBC count could occur after MI because of an inflammatory response secondary to the infarction or could occur as the result of bacterial endocarditis.

Arterial Blood Gases (ABGs): *Norms:* Adult: pH: 7.35–7.45; $PaCO_2$: 35–45 mm Hg; PaO_2: 75–100 mm Hg; HCO_3: 24–28 mEq/L; BE: +2 to –2.

Abnormal ABGs could occur after an acute myocardial infarction; PaO_2 decreased; $PaCO_2$ decreased because of hyperventilation, normal or increased because of hypoventilation; and HCO_3 and base excess (BE) decreased.

Therapeutic Drug Monitoring (TDM): Drugs taken for cardiac conditions should be closely monitored through blood samples to determine therapeutic levels and peak time to avoid drug toxicity. Most drug levels should be checked after serum drug level is at a steady state, in approximately 12–72 hours. Lidocaine is usually checked in 12 hours after administration and then daily. Propranolol (Inderal), procainamide (Pronestyl), and quinidine are checked 24–72 hours after administration, and digoxin after 5 days. A schedule for TDM is suggested to maintain therapeutic levels and to prevent drug toxicity.

NAME OF DRUG	THERAPEUTIC RANGE	PEAK TIME	TOXIC LEVEL
Digitoxin	10–25 ng/mL	12–24 hours	Greater than 30 ng/mL
Digoxin	0.5–2 ng/mL	6–8 hours	2.5 ng/mL
Lidocaine	1.5–5 mcg/mL	10 minutes	Greater than 6 mcg/mL
Propranolol (Inderal)	50–100 ng/mL	1–2 hours	Greater than 150–1,000 ng/mL
Procainamide (Pronestyl)	4–10 mcg/mL	1 hour	Greater than 10 mcg/mL
Procainamide + NAPA	5–20 mcg/mL		Greater than 30 mcg/mL
Disopyramide (Norpace)	2–5 mcg/mL	2 hours	Greater than 7 mcg/mL
Quinidine	2–5 mcg/mL	1–3 hours	Greater than 5–6 mcg/mL
Diazepam (Valium)	400–600 ng/mL	1–2 hours	Greater than 1,000 ng/mL
Verapamil (Isoptin)	100–300 ng/mL	1–2 hours	Greater than 300 ng/mL
Nifedipine (Procardia)	50–100 ng/mL	30 minutes	100 ng/mL
Diltiazem (Cardizem)	50–200 ng/mL	2–3 hours	Greater than 200 ng/mL

Diagnostic Tests

Cardiac Calcium Scoring: *Norm:* 0.5% plaque in the coronary arteries. The amount of calcium in the coronary arteries can be scored using the multidetector CT (MDCT). (See *Cardiac Calcium Scoring*.)

Electrocardiography (ECG, EKG): Electrocardiography records the electrical impulses of the heart by means of electrodes attached at appropriate sites on the chest. Abnormal P waves, QRS complexes, ST segments, and/or T waves indicate a possible cardiac problem. A depressed ST segment and an inverted T wave could indicate myocardial ischemia.

Echocardiography, Ultrasound Cardiography: This test is useful in detecting enlargement of a heart chamber, changes in heart dimensions during cardiac cycle, and valvular disease (e.g., mitral stenosis, pericardial effusion, and congenital heart disease). It is considered a noninvasive test.

Phonocardiography, Phonocardiogram: Phonocardiography is the graphic recording of sounds from the heart. The phonocardiogram is considered superior to examination by stethoscope in that it can record low-frequency sounds (e.g., gallop sounds). It is useful to detect cardiac valvular damage and to record the shape of various murmurs heard.

X-ray of Heart and Chest: X-rays of the chest to determine heart size are taken in posteroanterior (PA) and left-lateral positions. The x-ray films from these positions are helpful for identifying cardiomegaly and anomalies of the aorta.

Exercise/Stress Testing: Stress testing is a diagnostic tool that provides information about the cardiac function during exercise (stress). From the results of the test, decisions can be made about the degree of work level considered safe and how soon the individual should return to work after the MI.

Thallium Perfusion Stress Test: The radioisotope thallium-201 is used during the stress test to determine myocardial perfusion during exercise. With severe narrowing of the coronary arteries, there is less thallium accumulation in the heart muscle.

Persantine (Dipyridamole) Stress Test: If the client is unable to exercise or to walk on a treadmill, Persantine (dipyridamole) is administered intravenously to dilate the coronary arteries. Narrowed coronary arteries respond poorly to the Persantine.

Dobutamine Stress Test: Dobutamine, an adrenergic or sympathomimetic, increases the myocardial contractility, myocardial oxygen consumption, heart rate, and systolic blood pressure. Dobutamine-thallium is an alternative stress test. This test can identify clients with CAD and those who are at high risk for severe ischemic changes prior to vascular surgery.

Holter Monitoring: Holter monitoring is a type of continuous ECG recorded on tape within a device known as the monitor. This test evaluates the heart rate and rhythm during normal daily activities, rest, and sleep for 24–48 hours.

Left Cardiac Catheterization, Cardiac Angiography/Arteriography: This is an invasive procedure to determine the patency of the coronary arteries and functions of aortic and mitral valves. Dye is injected to determine left ventricular functioning while video film is recording the activity of the coronary arteries and heart valves.

Nuclear Heart Scan: The radionuclides technetium 99m and thallium-201 are used to detect cardiomegaly, cardiac output, ischemic heart disease, and the presence of an aneurysm.

Magnetic Resonance Imaging (MRI): MRI, a noninvasive test, is useful for evaluating the cardiovascular system. It can detect atrial and ventricular septal defects, MI, aortic and ventricular aneurysms, plaque formation, and blood flow through coronary branches and through extremities.

Positron Emission Tomography (PET): This test is useful for studying myocardial perfusion imaging. It can evaluate myocardial perfusion 72 hours after MI; it can also be used to determine if the ischemic area in the myocardium is viable or is infarcted after an acute MI.

Pacemaker Monitoring (Transtelephonic): *Norm:* Regular heart rate and rhythm. The purposes for transtelephonic pacemaker monitoring are to assess normal pacemaker function and to evaluate the client's heart rate and rhythm and the status of the battery and magnet disc.

Pericardial Fluid Analysis: *Norm:* Pale yellow, clear fluid. A sample of fluid is obtained from the pericardium to determine the cause of the problem, such as bacterial infection.

NURSING IMPLICATIONS WITH RATIONALE

- Explain the purpose of the laboratory and diagnostic tests.
- Give a detailed explanation concerning the laboratory and diagnostic procedures and the need for the client's compliance with the procedure(s). Explanation might be brief or in depth depending upon the individual's unfamiliarity with the test.
- Explanation of the tests and procedures to the family members could be helpful with test compliance.
- Inform the client of any food, beverage, or drug restrictions (*see Parts I and II*).
- Listen to the client's expressed anxiety or fear concerning the tests and potential clinical problems. Clarification of test procedure might alleviate fear and anxiety and promote test compliance.
- Assess the client's chest discomfort by eliciting the intensity, duration, and location of the pain from the client. Check skin color and vital signs. Report findings immediately to the health care provider.
- Provide care to the client as prescribed by the health care provider (i.e., oxygen, drugs).
- Suggest to the client and family members the community resources available to them (e.g., American Heart Association).

Respiratory function

LABORATORY TESTS	DIAGNOSTIC TESTS
ABGs	Chest X-ray
Sputum Culture	Pulmonary Function Studies
α_1-Antitrypsin (Serum)	Tomography
Angiotensin-Converting Enzyme (ACE) (Serum)	Thoracic Computed Tomography (CT)
SARS	Cyanide
Skin Tests	Bronchoscopy
TDM Cyanide	Apnea Test
	Bronchography
	Mediastinoscopy
	Radionuclide Thoracic Scan
	Lung Scan
	Ventilation Scan
	Pulmonary Angiography/Arteriography
	Lung Biopsy
	Thoracentesis
	Thoracoscopy
	Magnetic Resonance Imaging (MRI)
	Pulmonary Function Tests (PFTs)
	Sinus Endoscopy

Introduction

Chest x-ray, arterial blood gases, and pulmonary function studies are usually ordered for respiratory problems. If abnormalities are reported, other diagnostic tests are performed (e.g., thoracic computed tomography [CT], radionuclide thoracic scan, bronchoscopy, and others).

Laboratory Tests

Arterial Blood Gases: *Norms:* pH: 7.35–7.45; $PaCO_2$: 35–45 mm Hg; PaO_2: 75–100 mm Hg; HCO_3: 24–28 mEq/L.

A decreased $PaCO_2$ less than 35 mm Hg and an elevated pH greater than 7.45 indicate respiratory alkalosis. An increased $PaCO_2$ greater than 45 mm Hg and a decreased pH less than 7.35 indicate respiratory acidosis. The latter acid–base imbalance is the result of many respiratory problems (e.g., chronic obstructive lung disease, pneumonia, drug-induced respiratory depression).

Cyanide: An increase in cyanide can occur from heavy cigarette smoking, end products of combustion from metal and plastic refineries, and cyanide poisoning. Respiratory distress can occur.

Culture (Sputum): Sputum specimens are useful for diagnosing microorganisms causing respiratory infection and for detecting malignant cells in lung tissue. Table 3.3 explains three studies conducted on sputum that are associated with respiratory problems.

α_1-Antitrypsin (Serum): *Norms:* Adult: 78–200 mg/dL; 0.78–2 g/L. Child: same as adult.

Antitrypsin inhibits proteolytic enzymes in destroying lung tissue. With a lack of this protein, the alveoli are damaged, resulting in chronic obstructive lung disease (i.e., emphysema). A nonsmoker with a decreased antitrypsin level could develop pulmonary emphysema.

TABLE 3.3 Uses of Sputum Culture

SPUTUM TEST	COMMENTS
Culture and sensitivity (C & S)	Sputum specimens are useful for diagnosing microorganisms causing respiratory infection and the appropriate antimicrobial sensitive to the pathogens.
Acid-fast bacilli (AFB)	When tuberculosis is suspected, sputum specimens are checked (over 3 days) to determine the presence of *Mycobacterium tuberculosis*.
Cytology	Cytologic examination of slough cells from the lung are checked. If malignant cells are *not* present, this means lung cancer is unlikely. However, the malignancy may be in its early stage and not shedding cancer cells.

Angiotensin-Converting Enzyme (ACE) (Serum): *Normal:* 11–67 unit/L.

ACE is found primarily in the lung epithelial cells and renal cells. ACE is elevated in pulmonary conditions such as pulmonary embolism, pulmonary fibrosis, tuberculosis, and sarcoidosis.

SARS: Negative. Severe acute respiratory syndrome (SARS) is a test that aids in identifying SARS clients. Positive findings are the presence of coronavirus antibodies and an elevated white blood cell (WBC) count.

Therapeutic Drug Monitoring; Theophylline: *Serum Theophylline: Therapeutic Range:* Adult: 5–20 mcg/mL; 28–112 μmol/L (SI units). *Toxic Level:* Adult: greater than 20 mcg/mL; greater than 112 μmol/L (SI units). Child: same as adult.

Clients with bronchoconstriction (i.e., asthma) are usually given one of the theophylline preparations (e.g., aminophylline, Theo-Dur, Slo-Phyllin). Serum theophylline levels should be closely monitored to maintain therapeutic levels and to avoid toxic levels.

Skin Tests: Skin tests are useful for determining the presence of suspected bacterial or mycotic organisms that can infect lung tissue. This test is one of the methods used to diagnose tuberculosis and histoplasmosis.

Diagnostic Tests

Apnea Test: The apnea test is ordered to determine the presence or absence of spontaneous breathing. This test is performed when the client is taken off the ventilator. If the adult client does *not* have spontaneous breathing after 10 minutes or a child after 15 minutes, the person is assumed brain dead.

Chest X-ray: Chest x-ray is a frequently ordered diagnostic test. It is useful in diagnosing pneumonia, neoplasms (malignant and benign tumors), lung abscess, tuberculosis, atelectasis, and pneumothorax.

Pulmonary Function Studies: These tests are routinely ordered for clients with respiratory disorders or for those suspected of having a respiratory problem. Pulmonary function studies are helpful for assessing the progression of lung disease and for evaluating the response to drug and rehabilitative therapies.

Tomography, Laminography, Planigraphy: Tomography is used to detect lung tumors and mediastinal lesions. The x-ray machine or tube and film moves around the client. Because it emits high radiation levels, this test is not used as a routine screening test to diagnose lung disorders.

Thoracic Computed Tomography: CT scanning is useful for detecting questionable chest masses—lesions and tumors. It identifies metastasis in the lung. Contrast media (dye) may or may not be used.

Bronchoscopy: Either a standard metal or flexible fiberoptic bronchoscope is inserted into the tracheobronchial tree to visualize the larynx, trachea, and bronchi for abnormalities (i.e., strictures, inflammation, tumors). Also, bronchial secretions may be aspirated for bacteriologic, cytologic, and histologic examination. To remove a foreign object or to excise a small lesion or growth, a large metal bronchoscope would be necessary. Complications as a result of the test procedure might be bleeding, infection, and pneumothorax.

Bronchography: A bronchography may be done in conjunction with bronchoscopy. Contrast media (radiopaque iodine dye) is injected through a catheter into the tracheobronchial tree, followed by x-rays. This test is not frequently performed because of newer, more effective diagnostic tests (e.g., CT scan). However, the purposes for the test are to detect bronchial obstruction, tumors, cysts, and bleeding sites.

Mediastinoscopy: The mediastinoscope is inserted through a small incision at the suprasternal notch for the purposes of examining mediastinal lymph nodes and of obtaining biopsy specimen(s). This test is frequently indicated when other diagnostic tests (e.g., chest x-ray, sputum cytology, bronchoscopy) fail to confirm a diagnosis. It is also useful to determine if the lung cancer is inoperable because of metastatic spread to the lymph nodes. Other uses of this test include detecting lymphoma (e.g., Hodgkin disease and sarcoidosis).

Radionuclide Thoracic Imaging (Scan): *Lung Scan:* Radionuclide imaging is useful for evaluating pulmonary blood perfusion and for diagnosing perfusion obstruction (i.e., pulmonary embolism). A radionuclide, such as technetium tagged with macroaggregated albumin or technetium tagged with human albumin microspheres, is injected into the client's peripheral vein. *Ventilation Scan:* When the perfusion problem is due to an airway obstruction causing decreased ventilation, a ventilation scan may be ordered. The client inhales radioactive gas, such as xenon. A nuclear scanner checks the distribution of the gas in the lungs at intervals.

Pulmonary Angiography/Arteriography: Contrast medium (radiopaque dye) is injected into the pulmonary arteries to detect vascular abnormalities (e.g., pulmonary embolus). Usually pulmonary angiography/arteriography is performed when other diagnostic tests fail to confirm a diagnosis.

Lung Biopsy: Biopsy specimens from the tracheobronchial tree and lymph nodes are usually obtained during bronchoscopy (if ordered) and mediastinoscopy. A transbronchial lung biopsy may be obtained through the use of a bronchoscope by wedging a small biopsy forceps into the lung tissue.

Thoracentesis; Pleural Fluid Aspiration: This test is used to remove fluid from the pleural cavity and to examine the fluid for the cause of pleural effusion.

Thoracoscopy: This endoscopic test uses a tube that is inserted into the thoracic cavity to visualize the pleural space, thoracic wall, pericardium, and the mediastinum, and to also obtain a biopsy or fluid sample as ordered. It can detect pleural and lung tumors, emphysema, and empyema.

Magnetic Resonance Imaging: MRI helps to supplement CT examination of the chest in cases of lung cancer. It can evaluate recurrent or residual lung masses.

Pulmonary Function Tests (PFTs): Various pulmonary studies evaluate pulmonary function. These include slow vital capacity groups, lung-volume groups, forced vital capacity, diffusion study, bronchodilator response studies, exercise studies, and nutritional studies.

Sinus Endoscopy: Sinus endoscopy examines the anterior ethmoids and the middle meatus sinus areas. The primary purposes are to correct structural abnormalities and alleviate an infectious process.

NURSING IMPLICATIONS WITH RATIONALE

- Explain the purpose of the laboratory and diagnostic tests.
- Give detailed explanation concerning the test procedures and the need for the client's compliance. The explanation may be brief or in depth, depending upon the client's familiarity with the test.
- Inform the client of any food, beverage, or drug restrictions (*see Parts I and II*).
- Elicit from the client or family member a history of any allergies, especially to contrast medium (dye), iodine, or seafood.
- Assess respiratory status in regard to breathlessness and dyspnea caused by acute and chronic lung diseases.
- Be supportive of the client with dyspnea during the procedure. Remain with the client and provide adequate time; this reduces anxiety and increases test compliance.
- Assist the client with breathing difficulty as needed.
- Check bleeding sites at incisional areas (e.g., mediastinoscopy test).
- Monitor vital signs before, during, and following invasive tests (e.g., bronchoscopy, pulmonary angiography).
- Listen to the client's expressed anxiety or fear concerning the tests and potential clinical problems. Clarification of the test procedure might alleviate fear and anxiety and promote compliance.

Renal function

LABORATORY TESTS	DIAGNOSTIC TESTS
Urinalysis	Kidney, Ureter, Bladder (KUB) X-ray
BUN	IVP
BUN/Creatinine Ratio (Serum)	Retrograde Pyelography
Creatinine (Serum)	Cystoscopy
Creatinine Clearance	Cystography
Inulin Clearance	Cystometry
Protein (24-Hour Urine)	Computed Tomography (CT) Scan
Electrolytes (Serum & Urine)	Nephrotomography
Osmolality (Serum & Urine)	Renal Ultrasound
Antidiuretic Hormone (Plasma)	Radionuclide Renal Scan

(Continued)

LABORATORY TESTS	DIAGNOSTIC TESTS
Complement C_3 (Serum)	Renal Angiography
Complement C_4 (Serum	Renal Biopsy
Beta$_2$ Microglobulin	
Aldosterone (Serum)	
Renin (Plasma)	
Urine Culture	
Antiglomerular Basement Membrane Antibody (Serum)	
Microalbumin (Urine)	
Uric Acid (Serum & Urine)	

Introduction

The first set of laboratory tests performed to determine renal function are urinalysis, blood urea nitrogen (BUN), and serum creatinine. These tests are ordered routinely when renal insufficiency is suspected. If any of these are abnormal, other laboratory and diagnostic tests would be necessary (e.g., creatinine clearance, inulin clearance, serum and urine osmolality, serum and urine electrolytes, intravenous pyelography [IVP], kidney, ureter, bladder [KUB] x-ray, renal ultrasound, renal computed tomography scan, and others).

Laboratory Tests

Urinalysis: A urinalysis is routinely performed in a variety of settings (hospitals, clinics, and health care providers' offices) for checking kidney and endocrine function. The components it measures are color, pH, specific gravity (SG), protein, glucose, and blood cells. Table 3.4 shows the components that are usually checked during urinalysis and their significant results. For more comprehensive data on urinalysis, see Part I.

TABLE 3.4   Urinalysis

COMPONENTS	RESULTS
Color	Color can indicate lack of body fluids (dark yellow), excess of body fluids (pale yellow), or the result of blood, drugs, and food (red, red-brown).
pH	Urine pH is usually 4.5–8. The urine would be acidic if pH is 4.5 and alkalotic if pH is >7.5. Bacteria multiply rapidly in alkalotic urine.
Specific gravity (SG)	A low SG is related to diluted urine, and a high SG is associated with concentrated urine.
Protein	Urine protein >8 mg/dL could indicate renal disorder. However, an athlete's urine protein (single sample) level might be 10–20 mg/dL. This could be normal after strenuous activity.
Glucose	Glycosuria could indicate diabetes mellitus. Normally glucose is not a measurable quantity in urine.
Blood cells (BCs)	Urine should not contain BCs (red or white blood cells). The presence of BCs in urine could indicate a renal disorder.

Blood Urea Nitrogen: *Norms:* 5–25 mg/dL. Child: 5–20 mg/dL.

Urea is a by-product of protein metabolism excreted by the kidneys. If the BUN is slightly elevated, 25–35 mg/dL, the cause could be dehydration caused by hemoconcentration. Elevated BUN that remains elevated after hydration is an indicator of renal disorder.

BUN/Creatinine Ratio (Serum): 10:1–20:1.

The BUN/creatinine ratio is useful for determining renal function. An increased ratio could be due to reduced renal perfusion, glomerular disease, or obstructive uropathy.

Creatinine (Serum): *Norms:*

ADULT	INFANT	2–6 YEARS	OLDER
0.5–1.5 mg/dL	0.7–1.7 mg/dL	0.3–0.6 mg/dL	0.4–1.2 mg/dL
45–132.5 µmol/L (SI units)			36–106 µmol/L (SI units)

Creatinine, a by-product of muscle creatinine phosphate, is excreted entirely by the kidneys. Serum creatinine is a more reliable test to determine renal function, because it is less affected, if at all, by dehydration or malnutrition than by BUN. After renal damage or insult, the serum creatinine would rise because the kidneys could not excrete this by-product. Monitoring serum creatinine is important for determining kidney function.

Creatinine Clearance: *Norms:*

PERSON	CREATININE CLEARANCE	URINE CREATININE
Adult:		
Male	85–135 mL/min	20–26 mg/kg/24 h 0.18–0.23 mmol/kg/24 h
Female	Somewhat lower values	14–22 mg/kg/24 h 0.12–0.19 mmol/kg/24 h
Child:		
Male	98–150 mL/min	
Female	95–123 mL/min	

The creatinine clearance test (12- or 24-hour) is performed to determine glomerular filtration rate (GFR) and renal insufficiency. Usually this test includes serum creatinine level on the morning of or at the beginning of the test. Serum and urine creatinine levels are assessed, and creatinine clearance rate is calculated (*see Part I*). If less than 40 mL/min, the test is suggestive of moderate to severe renal impairment.

Inulin Clearance: *Norms:* Male: 125 mL/min/1.73 m^2, 124 ± 15 mL/min. Female: 110 mL/min/1.73 m^2, 110 pm 15 mL/min.

Inulin, a small, inert sugar, which is not bound to protein, is freely filtered by the glomeruli and can be used to determine GFR. This is not a routine clinical test because it involves an initial IV injection of inulin and a continuous controlled infusion rate to achieve a constant plasma level. It is a reliable test for GFR and is often compared with other urine clearance procedures. Decreased levels are indicative of renal impairment.

TABLE 3.5 Serum and Urine Electrolytes

ELECTROLYTES	REFERENCE VALUES	CAUSE AND EFFECT
SERUM Potassium (K)	*Norms:* Adults: 3.5–5.3 mEq/L Child: 3.5–5.5 mEq/L Infant: 3.6–5.8 mEq/L	Primary cause of hyperkalemia: >5.5 mEq/L is renal insufficiency.
SERUM Sodium (Na)	*Norms:* Adult, child: 135–145 mEq/L Infant: 134–150 mEq/L	Hypernatremia, >145 mEq/L, might be caused by anuria due to acute renal failure. Hyponatremia, <135 mEq/L, might result from tubular disorders when there is an inability to reabsorb sodium.
URINE Potassium (K)	*Norms:* Adult: 25–120 mEq/24 h 25–120 mmol/24 h (SI units)	Decreased urine potassium level <25 mEq/24 h, with an increased serum potassium level, could be indicative of acute renal failure. Elevated urine potassium level could be due to chronic renal failure. *Note:* Urine potassium range depends on the amount of potassium consumed in the diet.
Sodium (Na)	*Norms:* Adult: 40–220 mEq/24 h 40–220 mmol/24 h (SI units)	A low urine sodium level occurring with oliguria could be due to acute renal failure from decreased perfusion of the kidneys. An increased urine sodium level could result from the inability of the kidney tubules to reabsorb sodium (i.e., polycystic disease, chronic pyelonephritis).

Protein (24-hour Urine): *Norms:* 25–150 mg/24 h. Random: 0–5 mg/dL.

If urinalysis report indicated proteinuria, a 24-hour protein-urine test might be ordered. The presence of protein in the urine, greater than 150 mg/24 h, could indicate glomeruli damage or disease.

Electrolytes (Serum and Urine): Both serum electrolytes and urine electrolytes are closely monitored in renal disorders. Table 3.5 explains the effects of serum and urine potassium and sodium as they relate to renal dysfunction.

Osmolality (Serum): *Norms:* Adult: 280–300 mOsm/kg. Child: 270–290 mOsm/kg.

Serum and urine osmolality are used in assessing distal tubular response to circulating antidiuretic hormone (ADH). An increased serum osmolality could be due to an inadequate ADH release or due to the distal renal tubules' inadequate response to circulating ADH.

Osmolality (Urine): *Norms:* Adult: 50–1,200 mOsm/kg (average 200–800 mOsm/kg). Child: same as adult. Newborn: 100–600 mOsm/kg.

Urine osmolality is a more accurate indicator of the kidneys' ability to concentrate and dilute urine than specific gravity. In advanced renal medullary disease, the urine osmolality could be decreased because of the inability of the kidneys to concentrate urine.

Antidiuretic Hormone (ADH) (Plasma): 1–5 pg/mL.

ADH, produced by the hypothalamus and stored and secreted by the posterior pituitary gland, promotes water reabsorption from the distal renal tubules in response to the serum osmolality.

With an increased serum osmolality (dehydration or hypovolemia) there is an increase in ADH secretion. More water is reabsorbed and conserved in the body.

Complement C₃ (Serum): *Norms:* Male: 80–180 mg/dL. Female: 76–120 mg/dL.

Complements contribute about 10% of the total plasma proteins and play an important role in the immunologic system. Serum C_3 (the most abundant complement) is decreased in certain renal conditions (e.g., glomerulonephritis and acute renal transplant rejection).

Complement C₄ (Serum): *Norm:* 15–45 mg/dL.

Serum C_4, the second most abundant component of the complement system, is significantly decreased in lupus nephritis and acute poststreptococcal glomerulonephritis.

Beta₂ Microglobulin (Blood, Serum, Urine): *Norm:* Less than 2 mcg/mL; 0.2 mg/dL.

This is a protein on the surface of many cells. The test is used to detect glomerular or tubular renal disease. Also, it can determine the progression of HIV to AIDS.

Aldosterone (Serum): *Norm:* Adult: 1–9 ng/dL (supine position).

An increased serum aldosterone level can be associated with renal disease and chronic renal failure.

Renin (Plasma): *Norm:* Adult: 1.3–4 ng/mL (upright position, normal salt intake).

Renin, an enzyme secreted by the kidneys, is a test used for diagnosing renal vascular hypertension. The result of this hypertension could lead to renal failure.

Urine Culture: Urine cultures are commonly performed to determine the type of microorganism present in the genitourinary tract. To avoid urine contamination, the urine should be obtained using the procedure for midstream specimen collection or by catheterization.

Antiglomerular Basement Membrane Antibody (AGBM): This test detects GBM antibodies that can damage the glomerular basement membrane in the glomeruli. Beta-hemolytic streptococcus is the major organism responsible for antibody response.

Microalbumin (MA) (Urine): *Norm:* 0.2–2 mg/dL.

Microalbumin is a test to determine the concentration of albumin in the urine. MA precedes nephropathy that is associated with diabetic nephropathy and renal disease.

Uric Acid (Serum and Urine): *Serum:* Male: 3.5–8 mg/dL. Female: 2.6–6.8 mg/dL. *Urine:* 250–500 mg/24 h (normal diet).

Serum and urine uric acid level is dependent upon renal function. Elevated serum uric acid can be attributed to renal disease, such as glomerulonephritis and renal failure. A decreased urine uric acid is associated with renal disease.

Diagnostic Tests

Kidney, Ureter, Bladder (KUB) X-ray: The KUB x-ray is a flat plate of the lower abdomen to identify the size, shape, and position of the kidneys, ureters, and bladder. If abnormalities (i.e., tumors, calculi, or malformations) are noted, more extensive diagnostic tests are performed. Usually the x-ray is taken while the client is in the supine position; however, an upright KUB film may be requested for better visualization of the area.

Intravenous Pyelography: During IVP, radiopaque contrast medium (dye) is injected intravenously. A series of x-rays is taken at specified times as the dye circulates and is collected by the renal glomeruli and passed throughout the urinary tract. The purpose is to visualize the kidneys, kidney pelvis, ureters, and bladder. This test is useful for determining kidney dysfunction and for locating renal tumors and calculi. A test dose of the dye is given first because some clients may be allergic to the dye.

Retrograde Pyelography: During the retrograde pyelography (pyelogram) test, contrast medium (dye) is injected through a ureteral catheter to visualize the ureters and kidneys. X-rays are taken. This test is usually done during cystoscopy to determine the cause of unilateral kidney disease (e.g., ureteral obstruction). The retrograde pyelogram gives better visualization of the ureter and problems than the IVP test.

Cystoscopy: A cystoscope, a lighted, telescopic tube, is transurethrally inserted into the bladder for numerous purposes, including the following: to visualize the bladder wall; to obtain tissue biopsy of the bladder, urethra, or prostate; to remove calculi from the bladder or urethra; to remove small lesions and/or growths; or to obtain a urine specimen directly from the kidney(s). If ureter examination is necessary, dye is injected through a ureteral catheter into the ureters and x-rays are taken (retrograde pyelogram).

Cystography: The bladder is instilled with contrast medium (dye) to detect a rupture in the bladder, a neurogenic bladder, fistulas, or tumors. X-rays are taken. The client voids, if able, or the dye is withdrawn through the catheter.

Cystometry: This test evaluates the neuromuscular function of the bladder. Bladder dysfunction can be caused by neurologic disorders such as spinal cord injury, stroke, multiple sclerosis, and diabetes mellitus.

Computed Tomography Scan: CT, also known as computerized axial tomography (CAT), provides an image of the kidneys for the purpose of identifying tumors, malformations, cysts, and calculi. Contrast medium (dye) might be used during the CT scan to enhance visualization of the kidneys. Usually renal CT scan is done after abnormal IVP results have been reported.

Nephrotomography: The nephrotomography test combines IVP and CT. It provides a clearer picture of the kidneys, identifying and differentiating between cysts and solid tumors.

Renal Ultrasound, Ultrasonography: Renal ultrasonography (considered a noninvasive test) passes high-frequency sound waves through a transducer to the kidneys and perirenal area. An image of the kidneys and surrounding structures is displayed on an oscilloscope screen. The purpose of this test is to detect abnormalities (i.e., masses [cyst, tumor]) or to clarify findings from other tests.

Radionuclide Renal Scan: A radionuclide, such as technetium compounds (Tc-99m), Tc-99m–pertechnetate, Tc-99m–diethylenetriamine-penta-acetic acid (Tc-99m–DTPA), and iodine-131 hippuran, is administered intravenously. The purpose of the test is to detect renal lesions or masses and to determine the presence of acute or chronic renal diseases. This test may be used instead of IVP for clients who are allergic to contrast medium (dye).

Renal Angiography: A contrast medium (dye) is injected into the renal artery to visualize renal arterial, capillary, and venous systems. Rapid-sequence x-ray filming detects renal vascular malformations (e.g., stenosis, nonfunctioning kidney, renal masses, and obstructive uropathy).

Renal Biopsy: Microscopic examination of kidney tissue provides data concerning renal disease (e.g., glomerulonephritis caused by streptococcal infection or lupus). The renal biopsy test is useful for diagnosing primary or metastatic cancer of the kidney. Complications that could result are hematuria, uncontrolled bleeding, and kidney damage.

NURSING IMPLICATIONS WITH RATIONALE

- Explain the purpose of the laboratory and diagnostic tests.
- Give a detailed explanation of the test procedures and the need for the client's compliance. The explanation might be brief or in depth, depending upon the client's familiarity with the test.
- Inform the client of any food, beverage, or drug restrictions (*see Parts I and II*).
- Collect specimen(s) at specific times according to the procedures.
- Elicit from the client a history of any allergies, especially to contrast medium (dye) or iodine.
- Assess renal function (i.e., changes in urinary output, abnormal laboratory results—elevated BUN and serum creatinine, hematuria).
- Monitor the client's intake and output and vital signs before and after laboratory and diagnostic tests.
- Listen to the client's expressed anxiety or fear about the tests and potential clinical problems. Clarification of test procedure might alleviate fear and anxiety and promote compliance.

Liver, gallbladder, and pancreatic function

LABORATORY TESTS	**DIAGNOSTIC TESTS**
Liver	
Bilirubin (Serum)	X-ray of Abdomen
Transcutaneous Bilirubin	Ultrasonography of Liver
Bilirubin (Urine)	
Urobilinogen (Urine)	Liver and Spleen Scan
Liver Enzyme Tests	CT, Liver
ALP and Isoenzyme (Serum)	Liver Biopsy
5′ N (Serum)	Hepatic Angiography
ALT SGPT (Serum)	Peritoneal Fluid Analysis
LAP	
LDH and Isoenzymes (Serum)	
GGT/GGTP (Serum)	
Protein (Serum)	
Protein Electrophoresis	
Ammonia (Plasma, Blood)	
Antimitochondrial Antibody (AMA) (Serum)	
Antismooth Muscle Antibody (Serum)	
PT (Plasma)	
Cholesterol (Serum)	
Hepatitis A Virus (Serum)	
HB$_s$Ag (Serum)	
HB$_s$Ab/anti-HB$_s$ (Serum)	
HB$_c$Ab/anti-HB$_c$ (Serum)	

(Continued)

LABORATORY TESTS	DIAGNOSTIC TESTS

DIAGNOSTIC TESTS

Gallbladder
X-ray of Abdomen
Cholecystography (Oral)
Cholangiography
  Intravenous
  Percutaneous
  T-Tube
ERCP
Ultrasonography of Gallbladder and Biliary System
Gallbladder Nuclear Study
HIDA Scan
CT: Gallbladder and Biliary System

Pancreas
Amylase (Serum) and P-type Isoenzyme
Amylase (Urine)
Lipase (Serum)
Secretin Test

ERCP
Ultrasonography of Pancreas
Hypotonic Duodenography
CT, Pancreas
Pancreatic Ultrasonography

Introduction

Because the liver, gallbladder, and pancreas are in close proximity, several diagnostic tests (i.e., computed tomography; ultrasound of the liver, gallbladder, and pancreas; and endoscopic retrograde cholangiopancreatography [ERCP]) are performed on two or three of these organs at the same time. However, assessment of these organs will be represented separately.

Liver Assessment
Laboratory Tests

Bilirubin (Serum): *Norms:*

PERSON	INDIRECT UNCONJUGATED	DIRECT CONJUGATED	TOTAL
Adult	0.1–1 mg/dL	0.1–0.3 mg/dL	0.1–1.2 mg/dL
	1.7–17.1 µmol/L (SI units)	1.7–5.1 µmol/L (SI units)	1.7–20.5 µmol/L (SI units)
Child older than 6 months	Same as adult	Same as adult	0.2–0.8 mg/dL
Newborn			1–12 mg/dL

Bilirubin is derived from hemoglobin and results from the breakdown of red blood cells (RBCs). There are two forms of bilirubin in the body: indirect or unconjugated and direct or conjugated.

Indirect or Unconjugated: Elevated indirect bilirubin is related to increased destruction of RBCs.

Erythroblastosis fetalis in newborns results from massive hemolysis of RBCs, resulting in a possible serum indirect bilirubin level of 20 mg/dL or greater. Other causes include sickle-cell anemia, drug toxicity, transfusion reaction caused by blood incompatibility, and autoimmune diseases.

Direct or Conjugated: Bilirubin is conjugated (transformed) by the liver and made water soluble. There are smaller amounts of conjugated bilirubin than unconjugated bilirubin in the blood. Only water-soluble bilirubin (conjugated) can be excreted in the urine. Causes of an increase in direct bilirubin are cirrhosis, biliary obstruction, infectious hepatitis, carcinoma of the pancreas, and drugs (e.g., oral contraceptives, sulfonamides, rifampin, aspirin, morphine, thiazides, and procainamide).

Transcutaneous Bilirubin: *(See Bilirubin.)*

The purpose is to check for the presence of hyperbilirubinemia in newborns.

Bilirubin (Urine): *Norm:* Negative to 0.02 mg/dL.

Unconjugated bilirubin (fat soluble) cannot be excreted in the urine because it is not water soluble. If urine bilirubin test is positive, then conditions causing conjugated hyperbilirubinemia are likely to be the cause.

Urobilinogen (Urine): *Norms:* Adult: Random: 0.3–3.5 mg/dL. 24-hour specimen: 0.05–2.5 mg/24 h. 0.09–4.23 µmol/24 h (SI units).

Conjugated bilirubin from bile is changed in the duodenum to urobilinogen. Decreased urobilinogen level might indicate severe liver damage, biliary obstruction, and/or severe inflammatory disease. Elevated levels may be indicative of hemolytic disease, early cirrhosis of the liver, toxic or infectious hepatitis.

Liver Enzyme Tests: As the result of liver damage by insult or disease, most of the liver enzymes are released into the bloodstream, resulting in increased enzyme levels. Some of these enzymes are also found in other organs and are considered nonspecific. Examples of the nonspecific enzymes are alkaline phosphatase and lactic dehydrogenase. Usually several liver enzyme tests are performed at the same time to confirm liver disorder. In Table 3.6 six liver enzyme tests compare the enzyme studies that are usually ordered to evaluate suspected liver diseases: alkaline phosphatase (ALP), alanine aminotransferase (ALT or SGPT), 5'-nucleotidase (5'NT), leucine aminopeptidase (LAP), LDH_5, and gamma-glutamyl transferase (GGT).

TABLE 3.6 Liver Enzyme Tests

ENZYME (SERUM)	REFERENCE VALUES	COMMENTS
Alkaline phosphatase (ALP) and isoenzyme	*Norms:* Adult: 42–136 U/L ALP_1 20–130 U/L Child: 40–115 U/L Older Child: 50–230 U/L	ALP is found mainly in bone and liver and also in intestine, kidney, and placenta. Because ALP is produced by several systems and cells in the body, its activity is classified as nonspecific; therefore, other liver function tests should be performed to confirm the diagnosis. In severe liver damage (i.e., cancer of liver, hepatocellular problems), serum ALP is greatly increased. ALP isoenzymes assist in identifying the origin of the problem. ALP_1 is of liver origin, and ALP_2 is of bone origin.
5'-Nucleotidase (5'-NT or 5'-N)	*Norm:* less than 17 U/L	5'-NT is specific to liver cells. ALP and 5'-NT are measured at the same time, because both enzymes are found in liver cells and are elevated in hepatocellular disease. However, serum ALP will be elevated in bone disease, but 5'-NT will *not* be increased.

(Continued)

TABLE 3.6 Continued

ENZYME (SERUM)	REFERENCE VALUES	COMMENTS
Leucine aminopeptidase (LAP)	*Norms:* 8–22 mU/mL, 12–33 IU/L, 75–200 U/mL, 20–50 U/L at 37°C (SI units)	LAP enzyme is found mainly in liver tissue. Serum LAP is elevated in liver disease (i.e., cancer of the liver, viral hepatitis, acute necrosis of the liver, and extrahepatic biliary obstruction). LAP, 5'-NT, and ALP tests are frequently ordered together to confirm liver disease. If only ALP is elevated and the other two enzymes are not, bone disease would be probable.
Alanine aminotransferase (ALT or SGPT)	*Norms:* 10–35 U/L 4–36 U/L at 37°C (SI units)	ALT/SGPT is found primarily in liver cells and is effective in diagnosing hepatocellular obstruction. AST/SGOT is found in liver cells; however, it is more specific to cardiac muscle and skeletal muscle. Serum ALT is slightly to moderately increased in cancer of the liver and cirrhosis. It is highly increased during viral hepatitis and drug hepatotoxicity.
Lactic dehydrogenase (LD/IDH) isoenzymes	*Norms:* Adult: 100–190 IU/L Isoenzyme LDH$_5$ 6–16% Child: 50–150 IU/L, 110–295 U/L	LDH is elevated in heart, lung, liver, and renal disease. To determine if the increased LDH is due to liver disease, LDH isoenzymes are measured. LDH$_5$ rises before jaundice occurs and falls before bilirubin level does.
Gamma-glutamyl transferase/transpeptidase (GGT/GGTP)	*Norms:* Adult: Male: 4–23 IU/L Female: 3–13 IU/L Average: 0–45 U/L	GGT/GGTP is found mostly in the liver and kidney and small amounts in heart muscle, spleen, and prostate gland. It is a more sensitive indicator for liver disease than other liver enzymes (i.e., ALP and AST/SGOT). Elevated GGT/GGTP occurs in cirrhosis of the liver, alcoholism, cancer of the liver, viral hepatitis, and acute pancreatitis.

Protein (Serum), Protein Electrophoresis: *Norms:* Adult: Total protein: 6–8 g/dL. Albumin: 3.5–5 g/dL. Globulin: 1.5–3.5 g/dL.

Serum protein is an indirect measure of albumin and globulin. Albumin and globulin are indicators of liver function and diseases. Protein electrophoresis gives the breakdown of albumin and globulin. The albumin level is decreased, and the gamma globulin level is elevated in cirrhosis of the liver. The α_2-globulin fraction is elevated in inflammatory disease of the liver and cancer of the liver. An elevated β-globulin might occur in biliary obstruction. In chronic liver disease the A/G ratio is reversed.

Ammonia (Plasma, Blood): *Norms:* Adult (depends on method used): 15–45 mcg/dL, 3.2–4.5 g/dL, or 32–45 g/L; 11–35 μmol/L (SI units). Child: 21–50 mcg/dL. Newborn: 64–107 mcg/dL.

Ammonia, a by-product of protein metabolism, is converted to urea by the liver. Ammonia levels are elevated in severe liver diseases (i.e., cirrhosis, acute hepatic necrosis, or when blood flow to the liver is altered).

Antimitochondrial Antibody (AMA) Serum: Negative at 1:5 dilution.

This test may be ordered to differentiate between persons having primary biliary cirrhosis and other liver disease.

Antismooth Muscle Antibody (ASTHMA) (Serum): Negative or less than 1:20; Positive: Greater than 1.20.

ASTHMA is associated primarily with autoimmune chronic active hepatitis (CAH). The titer is usually greater than 1:160 with CAH. Clients with primary biliary cirrhosis may have a slight titer elevation.

Prothrombin Time (Plasma): *Norms:* Adult: 11–15 seconds or 70–100%. PT levels might differ among institutions.

Prothrombin, factor II of the coagulation factors, is produced by the liver and requires vitamin K for its synthesis. Increase in PT time frequently occurs in liver disease.

Cholesterol (Serum) *Norms:* Adult: 150–240 mg/dL, less than 200 mg/dL (desired level); 3.9–6.5 mmol/L (SI units). Child: 130–185 mg/dL. Infant: 90–130 mg/dL.

Cholesterol is a blood lipid that is synthesized in the liver. In chronic liver disease, serum cholesterol could be decreased. In biliary obstruction and pancreatitis, serum levels could be increased.

Hepatitis A Virus (HAV) Serum: None detected.

Previously HAV was called "infectious hepatitis." It is usually transmitted by oral–fecal contact.

Hepatitis B Surface Antigen (HBsAg) (Serum): *Norm:* Negative.

A positive HBsAg is an indicator of acute hepatitis B, chronic active hepatitis, or a carrier of hepatitis B.

Hepatitis B Surface Antibody (HBsAb/anti-HBs): *Norm:* Negative.

A positive HBsAb test indicates a *previous* infection of hepatitis B virus. Years after an acute hepatitis B infection, the HBsAb test might still be positive.

Hepatitis B Core Antibody (HBcAb/anti-HBc) (Serum): *Norm:* Negative.

This test is performed following negative serum HBsAg and HBsAb results when hepatitis is suspected. A positive HBcAb might indicate a recent hepatitis B infection.

Diagnostic Tests

X-ray of Abdomen: A flat plate x-ray of the abdomen is used to detect abdominal masses in the liver, pancreas, stomach, and intestine. It could indicate small-bowel obstruction and ascites.

Ultrasonography, Ultrasound (Liver): This is a noninvasive procedure useful in locating cysts, abscesses, and tumors. Liver ultrasound can differentiate between obstructive and nonobstructive jaundice. It is useful with liver scanning to define the cold spots. This test is usually ordered for clients with jaundice of unknown cause and unexplained hepatomegaly.

Liver and Spleen Scan: In nuclear liver imaging, a radionuclide (e.g., technetium [Tc] compound [Tc-99m pertechnetate, Tc-99m sulfide]) is administered intravenously to determine the size and structure of the liver and to detect abnormalities. If the liver has less radionuclide uptake than the spleen, cirrhosis or chronic hepatitis could be suspected. If cold spots (areas that do not take up radionuclide) appear, cysts, abscesses, and tumors might be suspected. Follow-up diagnostic tests (i.e., ultrasound, CT scan, and/or biopsy) are needed to confirm diagnosis.

Computed Tomography (Liver): CT visualizes the liver and biliary tract with or without contrast medium. It can detect hepatic cysts, abscesses, tumors, and can differentiate between obstructive and nonobstructive jaundice. CT should be performed before or 4 days after barium studies. Ultrasound is cheaper than CT and can detect liver and biliary disorders equally well.

Percutaneous Liver Biopsy: Liver cells can be obtained for microscopic examination by needle biopsy. The needle is inserted through the skin to the liver. It is used to confirm diagnosis of hepatocellular diseases (i.e., cirrhosis, hepatitis, tumors). Liver biopsy should not be performed on clients with bleeding disorders or having obstructive jaundice caused by possible bile leakage.

Hepatic Angiography, Celiac and Mesenteric Arteriography: Hepatic angiography is used to evaluate cirrhosis and portal hypertension and to evaluate vascular damage after abdominal trauma.

Peritoneal Fluid Analysis: *Norm:* Clear, pale yellow, no to few RBC, no bacteria.

Peritoneal fluid is taken from the peritoneum area to determine the cause of excess peritoneal fluid. Excess ascites fluid in the peritoneal area can be caused by cirrhosis of the liver.

Gallbladder Assessment
Diagnostic Tests

X-ray of Abdomen: Flat plate x-ray of the abdomen can visualize gallbladder stones. The stones that are not calcified and are composed of cholesterol will not be seen. Therefore, contrast medium tests should be ordered.

Cholecystography (Oral), Gallbladder Series: Oral cholecystography is an x-ray test to visualize stones and to diagnose inflammatory disease and tumors of the gallbladder. The client ingests radiopaque iodinated dye tablets the night before. The dye is concentrated in the gallbladder 12–14 hours after ingestion. This test should be performed before or 2–4 days after upper gastrointestinal tract and small-bowel series, because the barium would hamper visualization.

Cholangiography (Intravenous, Percutaneous, and T-Tube or Postoperative): Cholangiography is an x-ray examination of the bile ducts using contrast medium either intravenously or percutaneously or through the T-tube. Table 3.7 describes the cholangiography tests used for visualizing the biliary ducts.

Endoscopic Retrograde Cholangiopancreatography: Through a fiberoptic endoscope, contrast medium (dye) is injected into the duodenal papilla to visualize the biliary tract for cause of obstructive jaundice. The use of ERCP has increased, since the development of the fiberoptic

TABLE 3.7   Cholangiography Tests

TESTS	COMMENTS
IV cholangiography	With IV cholangiography, contrast medium [e.g., meglumine iodipamide] is injected intravenously. The dye is filtered by the liver and passes into the gallbladder and biliary ducts for visualization. There are more reported side effects with the use of IV contrast media than with oral tablets. This test is not indicated if hepatocellular disease is highly suspected or serum bilirubin is greater than 3 mg/dL.
Percutaneous transhepatic cholangiography (PTHC)	A needle is passed through the skin to the liver and into a dilated bile duct. Contrast medium is injected. The purpose is to visualize the biliary tract and to determine the cause of obstructive jaundice.
T-tube or postoperative cholangiography	Dye is injected into the T-tube, which was inserted during surgery. Purpose is to check for retained gallstones in the common bile duct.

side-view endoscope. This test is used when other diagnostic tests fail to determine cause of jaundice (i.e., stones, tumors).

Ultrasonography, Ultrasound of the Gallbladder and Biliary System: Ultrasound of the gallbladder and biliary tract is useful for diagnosing cholelithiasis and cholecystitis and to differentiate between obstructive and nonobstructive jaundice. It can detect polyps and tumors. Advantages for the use of ultrasound include the fact that it is cheaper than CT scan with equal results, there is no risk of radiation, and no contrast media is used.

Gallbladder Nuclear Study: The use of cholecytokinin (CCK) may be used to promote emptying of the gallbladder. Low emptying values can suggest chronic cholecystitis.

HIDA Scan: Technetium 99m dimethylacetanilide iminodiacetic acid (Tc-99m HIDA) is injected intravenously to visualize the hepatobiliary system. It is useful in detecting biliary obstruction and also hepatocellular disease.

Computed Tomography of the Gallbladder and Biliary System: CT of the right upper quadrant includes the visualization of the liver, gallbladder, and biliary tract. It can detect stones in the gallbladder and biliary ducts. Although ultrasound is cheaper, CT is preferred for obese clients and for those who have livers high in the rib cage.

Pancreas Assessment

Laboratory and diagnostic tests for diabetes mellitus will be covered in the section on assessment of endocrine function.

Laboratory Tests

Amylase (Serum): *Norms:* Adult: 60–160 Somogyi unit/dL, 30–170 unit/L (SI units). Child: usually not done.

Amylase is a pancreatic enzyme that changes starch to sugar. In acute pancreatitis, serum amylase level is elevated 2–12 hours after onset and remains elevated for 2–3 days. Levels are also increased in biliary duct obstruction (e.g., gallstones). P-type isoenzyme is elevated with acute pancreatitis.

Amylase (Urine): *Norm:* Adult: 4–37 unit/L/24 h.

When serum amylase is slightly to moderately elevated and pancreatitis is suspected, a 24-hour urine amylase level may be ordered. Urine amylase level is useful to confirm the diagnosis of acute pancreatitis.

Lipase (Serum): *Norms:* Adult: 20–180 international unit/L, 114–286 unit/L, 14–280 unit/L (SI units). Child: 20–136 international unit/L at 37°C.

Lipase is a pancreatic enzyme that aids in the digestion of fats in the duodenum. Serum lipase level is elevated early in acute pancreatitis and remains elevated longer than serum amylase level.

Secretin Test: This test assesses pancreatic exocrine function and is helpful in diagnosing pancreatic tumor, obstruction of the pancreatic duct, and chronic pancreatitis. It is a 3-hour test and requires a double-lumen tube; one lumen is inserted into the duodenum for aspiration of duodenal secretions and the other lumen into the stomach for aspiration of gastric secretions. Three samples are collected for baseline determination. Then secretin is administered intravenously, and four more samples are collected.

Diagnostic Tests

Endoscopic Retrograde Cholangiopancreatography: At the duodenal papilla, ERCP visualizes the biliary tract and the pancreatic duct. This test can detect pancreatic tumor and stricture of the pancreatic duct caused by chronic pancreatitis. A complication that might result from this procedure is pancreatitis.

Ultrasonography, Ultrasound of the Pancreas: Ultrasound is helpful in the detection of pancreatic abscess, cysts, and tumors. It could support the diagnosis of pancreatitis after serum amylase and lipase levels have returned to normal.

Hypotonic Duodenography: The purpose of this test is to detect pancreatic and duodenal diseases (i.e., tumor at the head of pancreas, stricture caused by chronic pancreatitis, and small duodenal lesion). A catheter is passed through the nose to the duodenum, and barium sulfate and air are injected. Spot x-ray films are taken.

Computed Tomography of the Pancreas: CT of the pancreas is useful to distinguish between pancreatic tumors and cysts and to detect suspected pancreatitis. The use of oral or IV contrast media during the test provides a more detailed visualization of the pancreas. Recent barium studies could hamper visualization of the pancreas.

Pancreatic Ultrasonography: Ultrasound of the pancreas does not measure pancreatic function, but it can detect pancreatic abnormalities, such as pancreatic tumors, pseudocysts, and pancreatitis.

NURSING IMPLICATIONS WITH RATIONALE

- Explain that the purpose of the laboratory and diagnostic tests is to aid in diagnosing liver, gallbladder, and pancreatic disorders. Be specific with the explanation as indicated.
- Give an explanation, in detail if indicated, about the laboratory and diagnostic procedures. Provide a written instruction sheet to reinforce verbal instructions. Emphasize the importance of the client's compliance to the test procedures. Stress that tests might need to be repeated if the procedure is improperly performed.
- Inform the client of any food, beverage, or drug restrictions. Each test should be checked for specific restrictions (*see Parts I and II*).
- Inform the health care provider if the client has had recent barium studies or if ultrasonography, CT, or ERCP is ordered. Barium sulfate can hinder visualization, and a 2- to 4-day waiting period after barium studies is usually required.
- Listen to the client's expressed anxiety concerning the tests and potential client problems. Clarification of test procedure might alleviate fear and anxiety and promote test compliance.
- Be prepared to repeat information to the client and family if the anxiety and/or fear level is determined to be high.
- Elicit from the client a history of any allergies to contrast medium (dye), iodine, or seafood.
- Monitor the client's vital signs before and following laboratory and diagnostic tests.
- Assess lower extremities and abdomen for signs of or changes in peripheral edema and/ or ascites.
- Notify the health care provider if the client's serum bilirubin is greater than 3 mg/dL prior to cholecystography or intravenous cholangiography. An elevated serum bilirubin can prevent contrast medium uptake and excretion.

- Check the laboratory results, and notify health care provider of abnormal test reports.
- Assess for bleeding from the nose, rectum, and skin. Liver disorders can cause prolonged prothrombin time resulting in bleeding tendencies.
- Check gag reflex for endoscopic procedures (e.g., ERCP), before giving fluids and food.

Gastrointestinal function

LABORATORY TESTS	DIAGNOSTIC TESTS
Upper GI	
Electrolytes (Serum)	Esophageal Studies
Gastrin (Serum)	Acid Perfusion (Bernstein Test)
Pepsinogen-I (Serum)	Esophageal Acidity
Prealbumin Antibody (Serum)	Esophageal Manometry
	Gastric Analysis Studies
	Basal Gastric Secretion
	Gastric Acid Stimulation
	Gastric Cytologic Examination
	Esophagogastroduodenoscopy
	Gastroscopy
	Esophagoscopy
	Barium Swallow
	Fluoroscopy
	Cineradiography
	Upper GI Series and Small Bowel
	Angiography Celiac and Mesenteric Arteriography
Lower GI	
CEA (Plasma)	X-ray of Abdomen
Carotene (Serum)	Barium Enema
Electrolytes (Serum)	Sigmoidoscopy
Antiparietal Cell Antibody	Colonoscopy
D-Xylose Absorption	Peritoneal Analysis/Paracentesis
Lactose Intolerance	Gastric Emptying Nuclear Study
Galactose-1-Phosphate Uridyl	Gastrointestinal Bleeding Nuclear Test
Transferase (GPUT)	Video Capsule Endoscopy (VCE)
Fecal Analysis	
Occult Blood	
Fat Content	
Ova and Parasites	
Fecal Fat	
Trypsin (Fecal)	
Rotavirus Antigen (Feces)	

Introduction

There are numerous gastrointestinal (GI) tests performed for assessing GI disorders. When the problem is of the esophagus, stomach, or duodenum, a series of upper GI tests (i.e., gastric analysis, upper GI series, and/or esophagogastroduodenoscopy) might be performed. When the problem is of the colon, a series of lower GI tests (i.e., fecal analysis, barium enema, proctosigmoidoscopy, and/or colonoscopy) might be performed.

Endoscopy is a method using an endoscope, a metal or fiberoptic tube, for visualizing abnormalities of the GI tract. Many upper and lower GI tests are classified as endoscopic tests or procedures. Tests for GI disorders are classified as upper GI and lower GI.

Upper GI Assessment

Laboratory Tests

Electrolytes: Potassium, Sodium, Magnesium (Serum): *Norms:* Adult: Potassium: 3.5–5.3 mEq/L. Sodium: 135–145 mEq/L. Magnesium: 1.5–2.5 mEq/L. Child: (*See individual tests.*)

Electrolytes are plentiful in the GI tract. Continuous vomiting or gastric intubation can cause a loss of the cations (i.e., potassium [K], sodium [Na], and magnesium [Mg]). Electrolyte replacement through IV fluids is essential to restore electrolyte balance and to prevent life-threatening problems (e.g., cardiac dysrhythmias). Serum electrolyte levels should be monitored, and any changes, decreases, or elevations should be reported immediately.

Gastrin (Serum): *Norms:* Adult: Fasting: less than 100 pg/mL. Nonfasting: 50–200 pg/mL.

Gastrin is a hormone secreted from the distal part of the stomach. This hormone stimulates the secretion of gastric juices, mainly hydrochloric acid (HCl). Serum gastrin levels are slightly to moderately elevated in clients having gastric ulcer or pernicious anemia and are highly elevated in clients with Zollinger-Ellison syndrome (pancreatic islet-cell tumor that secretes excess gastrin).

Pepsinogen-I (PG-I) Serum: *Norm:* 124–142 ng/mL.

Elevated pepsinogen-I is frequently present with duodenal ulcer. High PG-I level can be inherited as an autosomal dominant trait.

Prealbumin (PA) Antibody (Serum): 17–40 mg/dL.

This test is used primarily for nutritional assessment.

Diagnostic Tests

Esophageal Studies: One or more esophageal studies are usually performed for determining the cause of heartburn (pyrosis) and swallowing difficulty (dysphagia). Most of these tests check for the pH in the esophagus and esophageal sphincter pressure. Table 3.8 explains the purposes of three esophageal tests with abnormal results.

Gastric Analysis Studies: *Norms:* Basal (fasting): 1–5 mEq/h. Stimulation: 10–25 mEq/h.

Gastric analysis studies determine the quantity of gastric acid secreted between meals or feedings and during gastric acid stimulation. Stimulants used include histamine phosphate, betazole HCl (Histalog), pentagastrin, and caffeine. Table 3.9 describes the two tests performed for gastric analysis.

Gastric Cytologic Examination: Gastric aspiration for cytologic examination is obtained either during gastroscopy or after nasogastric catheter/tube insertion. If secretions aspirated through the tube are insufficient, then 100 mL of saline is instilled to facilitate specimen collection.

Esophagogastroduodenoscopy, Gastroscopy, Esophagoscopy: These endoscopic tests examine the esophagus, stomach, and duodenum to determine the cause of epigastric or substernal pain and hematemesis. They are among the most effective methods in diagnosing GI disorders (i.e., peptic ulcer [gastric or duodenal], esophageal varices, tumors, inflammatory conditions, and hiatal hernia, Mallory-Weiss syndrome) and for obtaining biopsy, foreign body, cells for cytology, or gastric acid secretions. Esophagogastroduodenoscopy should be done before or 2 days

TABLE 3.8 Esophageal Studies

TEST	REFERENCE VALUES	RESULTS
Acid perfusion (Bernstein test)		Epigastric or retrosternal pain that radiates to the back or arms is usually associated with myocardial infarction; however, these symptoms could be due to juices from the stomach backflowing into the esophagus. This test is useful to determine if chest pain or epigastric discomfort is caused by a cardiac condition or by esophagitis.
		Normal saline and hydrochloric acid (HCl) are dripped at different times into the esophagus. If the client has pain during the HCl drip, the test is a positive for esophagitis.
Esophageal acidity	*Norm:* pH greater than 5	This test measures the pH level of fluid in the lower esophagus. When clients complain of frequent heartburn, a pH electrode attached to a catheter is inserted through the mouth into the esophagus. If the intraesophageal pH is 1–3, gastroesophageal reflux (backflow of gastric acid into esophagus) caused by an incompetent sphincter is highly probable.
Esophageal manometry	*Norm:* 15–25 mm Hg (lower esophageal sphincter [LES])	Esophageal manometry measures esophageal sphincter and intraluminal pressures and records the sequence and duration of esophageal peristaltic contractions. When LES pressure is 0–5 mm Hg, incompetent or hypotensive sphincter is likely to be the cause; gastroesophageal reflux results. High LES pressure (greater than 50 mm Hg) could indicate hypertensive sphincter caused by achalasia, esophageal diverticula, or tumor.

TABLE 3.9 Gastric Analysis Tests

TEST	REFERENCE VALUES	RESULT
Basal gastric secretion	Basal (fasting): 1–5 mEq/h	No fluid or food for 8–12 hours before the test. High gastric acid levels suggest peptic ulcer (gastric or duodenal), and very high levels could be indicative of Zollinger-Ellison syndrome. Low levels might suggest gastric carcinoma.
Gastric acid stimulation	Stimulation: 10–25 mEq/h	Usually this test follows the basal gastric test. A stimulant such as betazole HCl (Histalog) or pentagastrin is administered. After 15 minutes, four to eight 15-minute specimens are taken. High levels suggest duodenal ulcer and very high levels indicate Zollinger-Ellison syndrome. Low levels might suggest gastric carcinoma.

after an upper GI series, because the barium sulfate retention would inhibit visualization. This test is useful to confirm a diagnosis, especially when contrast radiography procedures (e.g., upper GI series) fail to detect the GI problem.

Gastroscopy: This test, part of the esophagogastroduodenoscopy, can detect gastric disorders. A metal gastroscope could be used instead of the fiberoptic endoscope.

Esophagoscopy: It is used to visualize only the esophagus.

Barium Swallow: This diagnostic procedure is ordered to assess the pharynx and the esophagus for abnormalities. Usually it is part of the upper GI series, although it could be a separate test. The client swallows a thick mixture of barium sulfate, and the cineradiographic examination of the pharynx and fluoroscopic examination of the esophagus is performed. Barium swallow is useful for detecting esophageal strictures, tumors, polyps, ulcers, hiatal hernia, diverticula, and motility disorders.

Fluoroscopy: This can be part of the upper GI series. It is x-ray viewing from the time barium sulfate or meglumine diatrizoate (Gastrografin) is ingested and passes from the esophagus to the stomach. Fluoroscopic viewing can also take place during the barium enema test as the contrast agent goes through the large bowel.

Cineradiography: This is a filming method used for detecting esophageal motility problems.

Upper GI Series: The upper GI series uses barium sulfate or meglumine diatrizoate (Gastrografin) as the contrast medium to visualize abnormalities in the esophagus and stomach. Usually barium sulfate is more effective for visualizing the mucosa, and meglumine diatrizoate is preferred when perforation is suspected because it is a water-soluble agent. This test is useful for detecting causes of dysphagia (difficulty in swallowing), epigastric pain and discomfort, hematemesis, and melena. It is primarily used to diagnose gastric or duodenal ulcers, strictures, and tumors. Double-contrast studies (barium and air) give a better view of the mucosa for detecting polyps, early carcinoma, and gastritis.

Angiography, Celiac and Mesenteric Arteriography: This is an invasive procedure in which a catheter is threaded from the femoral artery to the celiac or mesenteric artery to detect the site of GI bleeding or to detect ischemic areas. Contrast medium is injected for visualization. When the GI bleeding site is identified, vasopressin is infused slowly to the site of bleeding. If vasopressin is not effective in stopping bleeding, then arterial embolization might be necessary. This test is performed when endoscopy and barium studies fail to determine the cause of a GI bleeding problem.

Lower GI Assessment
Laboratory Tests

Carcinoembryonic Antigen (CEA) (Plasma): *Norms:* Nonsmokers: less than 2.5 ng/mL. Smokers: less than 3.5 ng/mL.

High plasma CEA levels are found in clients with colorectal cancer. The test should not be the sole criterion for diagnosing colon cancer, because this antigen is relatively nonspecific. The usefulness of this test is to monitor plasma CEA levels following surgical intervention or therapeutic treatment for colon cancer. A decreased CEA level indicates effective response to surgery or treatment. A rise in plasma CEA later might indicate a recurrence of the cancer.

Carotene (Serum): *Norms:* Adult: 60–200 mcg/dL, 0.74–3.72 µmol/L (SI units). Child: 40–130 mcg/dL.

A decreased serum carotene could be a result of intestinal fat malabsorption. This could affect the absorption of fat-soluble vitamins.

Electrolytes: Potassium, Sodium, Magnesium (Serum): *Norms:* Adult: Potassium: 3.5–5.3 mEq/L. Sodium: 135–145 mEq/L. Magnesium: 1.5–2.5 mEq/L. Child: (*See individual tests.*)

Potassium, sodium, and magnesium are plentiful in the intestine as well as the stomach. Loss of intestinal secretions because of diarrhea or intestinal intubation could cause serum electrolyte deficits (i.e., hypokalemia, hyponatremia, hypomagnesemia).

Antiparietal Cell Antibody (APCA): Negative or less than 1:120 titer; Positive: 1:180 titer.

Parietal cells in the stomach secrete hydrochloric acid (HCl), which is needed for protein catabolism. This test is effective for detecting pernicious anemia and chronic gastritis.

D-Xylose Absorption (Serum and Urine): *Norms:* Adult: Serum: 25–40 mg/dL/2 h. Urine: greater than 3.5 g/5 h and greater than 5 g/24 h. Older Adult: Serum: 25–40 mg/dL/2 h. Urine: greater than 4g/5 h. Child: Serum: 30 mg/dL/1 h.

Good urine function is needed for this test. It evaluates absorption of D-xylose, a pentose sugar, in the small intestine. Eighty to 95% of the D-xylose dose is excreted in 5 hours. Decreased serum and urine levels could indicate malabsorptive disorder of the small intestine, jejunal enteritis, or jejunal diverticula.

Lactose Tolerance: *Norms:* Adult: blood glucose increase of 20 mg/dL/2 h.

This test is to identify clients who have a deficiency of the intestinal enzyme lactase. With a decreased intestinal lactase activity, lactose ingested (e.g., milk products) is inadequately absorbed. As a result of lactose deficiency, diarrhea, abdominal cramps, and flatus occur, especially after ingestion of milk and/or milk products.

Galactose-1-Phosphate Uridyl Transferase (GPUT): Negative: Quantitative: 18.5–28.5 unit/g in Hb. Deficiency of the enzyme: less than 5 unit/g in Hb; Carrier of the deficiency: 5–18 unit/g in Hb.

The galactose enzyme is needed to convert galactose to glucose during lactose metabolism. A deficiency of this enzyme can lead to galactosemia.

Fecal Analysis: Various studies can be performed on stool specimens (e.g., occult blood, fat content, and ova and parasites). Table 3.10 shows substances that are analyzed in feces.

TABLE 3.10 Fecal Analysis Studies

FECAL SUBSTANCES	VALUES	COMMENTS
Occult blood	Negative	When bleeding from the GI tract is not evident but is suspected, a stool sample is examined for occult (hidden) blood. Either microscopic examination or chemical tests (i.e., guaiac or orthotolidine) are used for identifying fecal occult blood.
Fat content	*Norm:* Less than 6 g/24 h	This can be a screening test when malabsorption syndrome is suspected. If fecal fat content is greater than 6 g/24 h, then malabsorption syndrome is the probable cause. A very small stool could cause false test results.
Ova and parasites	Negative	Ova and parasites (O&P) may be present in the intestine. Usually three stool specimens are evaluated to identify and to confirm the organism present, so that appropriate treatment can be ordered.

Fecal Fat (Stool): *Norm:* 2–7 g/24 h.

Fecal fat test is conducted to confirm the diagnosis of steatorrhea (malabsorption of fat). Clients with a high fat content in the stools are positive for steatorrhea.

Trypsin (Feces): Positive in small amounts.

With pancreatic insufficiency, the stool trypsin test is usually negative.

Rotavirus Antigen (Feces): The rotavirus can cause infectious diarrhea in infants and children less than 2 years old. Adults can also be infected with this virus.

Diagnostic Tests

X-ray of Abdomen: Flat x-ray films of the abdomen are ordered to identify abdominal masses of the stomach, liver, and intestine. Suspected abnormal findings are confirmed with other GI tests.

Barium Enema: This is a test that has been used for years in diagnosing lower bowel disorders. Barium sulfate is the contrast agent used, and when a more detailed visualization is needed, barium sulfate and air (double contrast) is given. Barium enema is ordered when clients complain of abnormal bowel habits, lower abdominal pain or cramps, blood in the stool, or changes in stool formation. This test is useful for diagnosing polyps and intestinal masses (e.g., tumors, diverticula, strictures, and ulcerations). Barium should not be used when perforation of the bowel is strongly suspected.

Sigmoidoscopy: For years, the sigmoidoscope (a rigid 10- to 12-inch instrument) was used to examine the rectum and sigmoid colon. The proctosigmoidoscope (fiberoptic endoscope) is the instrument of choice today for this test procedure.

Biopsy and Cytologic Examination: During a sigmoidoscopy, specimens can be obtained by the use of biopsy forceps, cytology brush, or culture swab.

Colonoscopy: This is another endoscopic procedure, and its use has markedly increased in recent years. It is an inspection of the large intestine (colon) using a long, flexible fiberscope (colonoscope). Colonoscopy can detect lesions in the proximal colon that would be missed by sigmoidoscopy. Biopsy forceps and cytologic brush can be used during this test. It should not be done before or 2 days after a barium enema because the barium sulfate would inhibit visualization.

Colonoscopy is effective in detecting early cancerous lesions, which have a good prognosis. It can detect advanced cancerous tumors and determine the extent of inflammatory tissue. Polyps can be removed with the use of an electrocautery snare during the colonoscopy.

Peritoneal Analysis/Paracentesis: Draining copious amounts of fluid from the peritoneal cavity is not done unless the large abdominal fluid volume is causing respiratory distress. Loss of large quantities of peritoneal fluid could cause severe fluid and electrolyte imbalance. Fluid samples may be requested for analyzing the fluid content (i.e., electrolytes, blood cells, sugar, protein, organisms, and cancer cells).

Gastric Emptying Nuclear Study: The radionuclide Tc-99m Ac–labeled eggs and juice is ingested by the client. This study is useful for diagnosing gastric obstruction and the cause of dysmotility.

Video Capsule Endoscopy (VCE): *Norm:* Normal mucosa of the small bowel.

VCE test can identify origin of GI bleeding and can detect Crohn disease.

Gastrointestinal Bleeding Nuclear Test: This nuclear test is used to detect the localization of gastrointestinal and nongastrointestinal bleeding sites.

NURSING IMPLICATIONS WITH RATIONALE

- Explain that the purpose for the laboratory and diagnostic tests is to aid in the diagnosis of esophagus, stomach, or colon disorders. Be more specific in the explanation if indicated.
- Give an explanation (in detail if indicated) about the laboratory and diagnostic procedures. Emphasize the importance of the client's compliance to the test procedures. Stress that tests might need to be repeated if the procedure was improperly performed.
- Inform the client of any food, beverage, or drug restrictions. Each test should be checked for specific restrictions (*see Parts I and II*).
- Inform the health care provider if the client has had recent barium studies (i.e., upper GI series, barium enema), especially if esophagogastroduodenoscopy, sigmoidoscopy, and colonoscopy are ordered. Barium sulfate can hinder visualization and a 2- to 4-day waiting period after barium studies is usually required.
- Listen to the client's expressed anxiety and fear concerning the tests and potential client problems. Clarification of the test procedure might alleviate fear and anxiety and promote test compliance.
- Monitor the client's vital signs before and after laboratory and diagnostic tests. Report significant changes.
- Obtain a stool specimen for occult blood analysis. Determine frequency of bowel movements.
- Assess for throat discomfort (i.e., soreness, swallowing difficulty after oral endoscopic procedure).
- Check gag reflex before giving fluids and food after endoscopic procedures.
- Check laboratory results, and report abnormal test findings.

Neurologic and musculoskeletal function

Introduction

With suspected neurologic disorders, a group of diagnostic tests is performed to confirm a diagnosis. When there are frequent headaches, the tests usually ordered to determine their origin include cerebrospinal fluid (CSF) examination, skull x-rays, and electroencephalography (EEG). If headaches intensify and persist, echoencephalogram, computed tomographic scan of the head, brain scan, or cerebral angiogram or MRI or PET might be requested. For seizure disorders, EEG, echoencephalography, and CT scan of the head are usually ordered. After acute head injury, skull x-rays are immediately taken. CT scan and MRI of the head might be requested. Musculoskeletal disorders are evaluated by using various diagnostic procedures (e.g., synovial fluid analysis, electromyography [EMG] arthrography, bone scan, and arthroscopy). Neurologic assessment will be presented first, and then musculoskeletal.

LABORATORY TESTS	DIAGNOSTIC TESTS
Neurologic	
CSF	X-rays
Pressure	Skull
Color	Lumbosacral Spine
WBC	EEG
Protein	Echoencephalography
Glucose	Electronystagmography (ENG)
Culture	Electroneurography (ENoG)
Cytology	Apnea Test
Amyloid Beta Protein Precursor	Brain Nuclear Scan
TDM—Anticonvulsants	Brain Perfusion Nuclear Scan
	CT, of the Head
	Cerebral Angiography, Arteriography
	MRI
	PET
	Electroneurography
	Myelography
	Thermography (Lumbar, Thoracic, and Cervical)
	Oculoplethysmography
	Oculovestibular Reflex Study (OVR Study)
Musculoskeletal	
Acetylcholine Receptor Antibody (AChR) (Serum)	X-ray, Bone and Joints
Muscle and Bone Enzyme Tests	Synovial Fluid Aspiration
ALD (Serum)	Arthrography
AST/SGOT (Serum)	Bone Scan
CPK/CK (Serum)	Bone Densitometry
Isoenzyme (CPK-MM)	Arthroscopy
Bone Enzymes—ALP	
N-Telopeptide Cross-Links (NTx)	EMG
Osteocalcin (Serum)	Muscle Biopsy
Pyridinium (PYD) (Serum)	MRI
Electrolytes (Ca) (Serum)	

Neurologic Assessment

Laboratory Tests

Cerebrospinal Fluid: *Norms:* (*See reference values in Part I.*)

Analysis of CSF usually includes color, pressure, white blood cell count, protein, chloride, glucose, culture, and cytologic cells. Table 3.11 lists the components found in CSF and the result of the analysis.

Amyloid Beta Protein Precursor (CSF): *Norms:* 450 units/L.

This CSF test aids in diagnosing Alzheimer disease. The amyloid beta protein is present in the senile plaques within the brain. It is believed that this type of protein may have neurotoxic effects to the brain cells.

Therapeutic Drug Monitoring (TDM): Anticonvulsants are ordered for seizure disorders (i.e., grand mal, psychomotor, and/or petit mal), and therapeutic drug levels should be closely monitored. The drug outline given below gives the name of anticonvulsant, type of seizure, therapeutic range, and toxic level for adults (child as indicated).

TABLE 3.11 Analysis of CSF

COMPONENT OF CSF	ABNORMAL RESULTS
Pressure	A pressure greater than 200 mm H_2O is considered abnormal and could be due to increased intracranial pressure caused by meningitis, subarachnoid hemorrhage, and tumors.
Color	Pink or red color could be due to subarachnoid or cerebral hemorrhage or a traumatic spinal tap. Yellow color might indicate old blood (4–5 days after cerebral hemorrhage).
WBC	WBC differential count may be ordered. An increased number of neutrophils could be indicative of bacterial meningitis or cerebral abscess. An increased number of lymphocytes could be indicative of viral meningitis or encephalitis.
Protein	In acute bacterial meningitis, protein levels could be greater than 250 mg/dL. Increased protein levels indicate infections or inflammatory processes (i.e., meningitis, encephalitis, and tumors).
Glucose	Glucose levels in CSF are 40–80 mg/dL, two-thirds of blood/plasma levels. When there is a decrease in CSF glucose, there is usually an increase of other cells (i.e., bacterial, tumor cells in the spinal fluid). A decrease in glucose, less than 40 mg/dL, might be indicative of bacterial meningitis, leukemia, or tumors.
Culture	A culture specimen of spinal fluid is withdrawn to determine the type of organism present.
Cytology	Slough cells from tumor sites in the brain or spinal column could flow into the spinal fluid. Examination of CSF for cancerous cells might be requested.

Diagnostic Tests

X-rays: *Skull:* Skull x-rays are usually ordered after head trauma to detect fracture of the skull. Skull x-rays are also useful to visualize primary and metastatic tumors of the skull, to confirm the existence of increased intracranial pressure, and to diagnose pituitary tumors. *Lumbosacral Spine:* Spinal x-rays are frequently ordered to determine the cause of pain radiating from back to leg(s). Spinal x-rays could show narrowed intervertebral disk spaces and/or calcified spurs in intervertebral foramina, which could be indicative of degenerated disks.

Electroencephalography, Electroencephalogram (EEG): EEG measures the electrical activity of the brain cells to determine abnormalities (e.g., cerebral lesions [tumor, hemorrhage, abscess]). It is useful in locating the cause of seizure disorders. Another use is to confirm cerebral death. It is not the test of choice for evaluating head injuries.

Echoencephalography, Ultrasonography of the Brain, Brain Echogram: Ultrasound of the brain, a noninvasive procedure, is helpful in detecting cerebral midline shifts characteristic of an intracranial hemorrhage. It is used in neonatal intensive care units, checking infants suspected of having intracranial hemorrhage. Follow-up studies using CT and radionuclides might be indicated.

DRUG NAME	SEIZURE DISORDER	THERAPEUTIC RANGE	TOXIC LEVEL
Carbamazepine	Grand mal	4–12 mcg/mL	Greater than 12–15 mcg/mL
Ethosuximide	Petit mal	40–100 mcg/mL	Greater than 100 mcg/mL
Phenytoin	Grand mal	Adult: 10–20 mcg/mL Child: 4–8 mg/kg/day	Adult: greater than 20 mcg/mL Child: 15–20 mcg/mL
Primidone	Grand mal and psychomotor	Adult: 5–12 mcg/mL Child: 7–10 mcg/mL	Adult: greater than 12–15 mcg/mL Child: greater than 12 mcg/mL
Valproic Acid	Grand mal and petit mal	Adult: 50–100 mcg/mL Child: same as adult	Adult: greater than 100 mcg/mL Child: same as adult

Electroneurography (ENoG) Electroneurography evaluates and identifies peripheral nerve injury or disease. A common cause is diabetic neuropathy. A stimulus is applied to the affected areas to determine the presence of peripheral nerve injury.

Electronystagmography (ENG): This test helps to determine if the problem/abnormality is in the brain stem, the temporal lobe of the cerebral cortex, auditory nerve, or vestibular-cochlear areas. If nystagmus does not occur with stimulation, the ENG test aids in determining the neurologic problem.

Apnea Test: This test is to evaluate the presence of spontaneous breathing when the client is taken off a ventilator. It is usually conducted when the client has severe brain injury.

Brain Nuclear Scan: Brain scans may be ordered for clients complaining of severe headaches or having frequent seizures. This test can detect intracranial lesions (i.e., abscess, tumors [benign or malignant], metastasis to the brain, subdural hematoma, aneurysms, and cerebrovascular accident [CVA]). A technetium compound, Tc-99m-O4 or Tc-99m-DTPA, is given intravenously prior to cranial scanning. The blood-brain barrier is disrupted at the pathologic lesion site, thus increasing the amount of radionuclide agent uptake.

Brain Perfusion Nuclear Test: This test may be used for diagnosing Alzheimer disease, brain death, and AIDS dementia. It helps to locate the seizure foci and locate the size of the cerebral ischemia.

Computed Tomography of the Head: CT of the head is useful for diagnosing cerebral lesions (i.e., tumors, hematomas caused by intracranial bleeding, abscess, cerebral infarction [obstruction], hydrocephalus, and cerebral edema). For detailed visualization of the lesion, IV contrast medium (iodinated dye) is used. CT scan of the head is replacing more invasive procedures (i.e., pneumoencephalography, cerebral angiography).

Cerebral Angiography, Arteriography: Iodinated contrast medium is injected into the carotid or vertebral artery, usually through the femoral or brachial artery, to visualize the cerebral blood vessels for abnormalities (i.e., occlusions, aneurysms, abnormal vascularization resulting from neoplasms [tumors]). This is an invasive procedure, and there are clients who are allergic to the contrast medium.

Magnetic Resonance Imaging: This is a sensitive test for detecting edema, hemorrhage, blood flow, tumors, and infection sites in the brain tissue. MRI is useful in detecting demyelinating diseases, such as multiple sclerosis.

Positron Emission Tomography: PET is an effective test in determining blood flow to the brain. Radiation from PET is about one-fourth of that received by CT. It is useful in studying the epilepsy focal areas, viable brain tissue after a CVA (stroke), brain tumor, migraine headaches, and parkinsonism and in differentiating between Alzheimer disease and other types of dementia.

Electroneurography, Nerve Conduction Studies: *Norms:* Normal conduction velocity: 50–60 meters/sec.

This test is useful in determining peripheral nerve injury. It measures the time required for a nerve impulse to travel from the proximal site to the distal site. The distance per time the nerve impulse takes to travel from the proximal site of stimulation (shock) to the muscle for its contraction is known as the *conduction velocity*. The conduction velocity frequently varies with different nerves.

Myelography, Myelogram: Myelography is a fluoroscopic and radiologic examination of the spinal subarachnoid space (spinal column). The purpose of this test is to identify herniated intervertebral disks, cysts, metastatic tumors, neurofibromas, and meningiomas and to detect spinal nerve root injury.

Thermography (Lumbar, Thoracic, and Cervical): Irritated nerve root and musculoligamentous spasm may be detected by the use of thermography. An abnormal thermogram could include asymmetrical heat patterns that would be indicative of nerve root injury. This test might be ordered for clients with severe or chronic back pain. Usually other diagnostic tests are ordered to aid in the diagnosis (i.e., electromyography [EMG], myelography).

Oculoplethysmography: This is a noninvasive test to evaluate carotid blood flow to the ophthalmic artery. It may be used in clients with CVA to determine the size of carotid occlusion. Oculoplethysmographic techniques could also be used in clients with asymptomatic bruits, symptoms of transient ischemic attacks (TIA), and syncope; for detecting occlusions; and for preventing CVA.

Oculovestibular Reflex Study (OVR study): *Norm:* Nystagmus with irrigation.

This test evaluates the vestibular area of the 8th cranial nerve. If there is no nystagmus, there is likely disease of the 8th cranial nerve or the labyrinth, such as Ménière syndrome.

Musculoskeletal Assessment
Laboratory Tests

Acetylcholine Receptor Antibody (AChR) (Serum): Negative or less than 0.02 to less than 0.03 nmol/L. This test is used in the diagnosis of myasthenia gravis (MG).

Muscle and Bone Enzyme Tests: Certain enzymes are present in muscles, such as aldolase, creatine phosphokinase (CPK/CK), and aspartate aminotransferase (AST or SGOT), and in bones, such as alkaline phosphatase (ALP) and isoenzyme ALP_2. Table 3.12 explains the uses of these enzyme tests.

N-Telopeptide Cross-Links (NTx) (Serum and Urine): *Serum:* Female: 6.2–19 nM BCE/L; male: 5.4–24.2 nM BCE/L. *Urine:* Female: 5–65 mM BCE/mmol creatinine; male: 3–51 mM BCE/mmol creatinine. This test is used to identify bone disease and osteoporosis.

Osteocalcin (Serum): Female: Premenopausal: 0.5–7.8 ng/mL; Male: 1.5–11.5 ng/mL. A test used to identify bone disease and osteoporosis.

TABLE 3.12 Enzyme Tests of Muscles and Bones

ENZYME (SERUM)	REFERENCE VALUES	RESULTS
Muscle:		
Aldolase (ALD)	*Norms:* Adults: less than 6 U/L 3–8 U/dL (Sibley-Lehninger) 22–59 mU/L at 37°C (SI units) Child: 6–16 U/dL	Aldolase is abundant in skeletal and cardiac muscles. Serum aldolase is elevated in muscular dystrophy but not in muscle diseases of neural origin (i.e., multiple sclerosis, myasthenia gravis).
Aspartate aminotransferase (AST or SGOT)	*Norms:* Adult: 8–38 U/L	AST/SGOT is less sensitive than CPK/CK for determining muscle disorder. This enzyme is assessed in suspected myopathic diseases.
Creatine phosphokinase (CPK/CK)	*Norms:* Adult: Male: 5–35 mcg/mL 30–180 IU/L; Female: 5–25 mcg/mL 25–150 IU/L Child: Male: 0–70 IU/L at 30°C Female: 0–50 IU/L at 30°C	CKP/CK is more sensitive than AST/SGOT for determining muscle disorder. Actually CPK/CK is a better indicator of cardiac diseases than muscle diseases; however, this enzyme is assessed in suspected myopathic diseases.
Isoenzyme:		
(CPK-MM)	94–100%	
Bone:		
Alkaline phosphatase (ALP)	Adult: 42–136 U/L	ALP is an enzyme produced primarily in the bone and liver. In bone disorders, ALP level is increased because of abnormal osteoblastic activity (bone cell production).
	Child: 50–230 U/L Infant: 40–300 U/L	High ALP levels can be found in children during prepuberty and puberty ages because of bone growth. Elevated ALP levels are found in cancer of the bone, Paget disease (osteitis deformans), healing fractures, multiple myeloma, osteomalacia.
Isoenzyme ALP$_2$	20–120 U/L	Isoenzyme ALP$_2$ is of bone origin.

Pyridinium (PYD) (Urine): Female: 15.3–33.6 nM/mm; Male: 10.3–33.6 nM/mm. Another test used to identify bone disease. It can also be ordered to determine the effects of the treatment for bone disease.

Electrolyte (Calcium) (Serum): *Norms:* Adult: 4.5–5.5 mEq/L, 9–11 mg/dL, 2.3–2.8 mmol/L (SI units). Child: 4.5–5.8 mEq/L, 9–11.5 mg/dL. Infant: 5–6 mEq/L.

Calcium is found abundantly in bones. Frequently in bone disorders, calcium leaves bones and becomes plentiful in circulating body fluid; thus, serum calcium level is elevated (hypercalcemia). Elevated calcium levels occur as the result of bone tumors, multiple myeloma, multiple fractures, and prolonged immobilization.

Diagnostic Tests

X-Rays of Bone and Joint: X-rays are frequently taken of bones and joints to determine the presence of disease (i.e., arthritis, spondylitis, bone lesions, and fractures).

Synovial Fluid Aspiration, Arthrocentesis: Samples of synovial fluid are aspirated from a joint cavity for analysis of cells (WBCs, rheumatoid arthritic cells, lupus cells), protein, glucose, and uric acid and for culture.

Arthrography, Arthrogram: Arthrography uses contrast medium and/or air (both: double contrast) to visualize joint structure. This test is able to detect tears, derangements of joints, and synovial cysts. X-rays are taken during the procedure.

Bone Scan: Radionuclide, technetium-labeled phosphate compounds (e.g., Tc-99m diphosphonate, given intravenously) are absorbed into bone tissue and concentrated in abnormal bone cells. The scanner can pick up hot spots months before x-rays can note abnormal bone areas. This procedure is primarily used to diagnose metastatic bone disease. Bone scans are also useful to monitor bone response to radiation therapy and/or chemotherapy. This test may be used for early detection of osteomyelitis and for detection of degenerative bone disorders.

Bone Densitometry: The bone density test is used to detect early osteoporosis by determining the density of the bone mineral content.

Arthroscopy: This is an endoscopic procedure usually performed in an operating room. An incision is made into the knee joint cavity, and a fiberoptic endoscope is inserted for visualization and/or removal of loose particles. It is an invasive procedure, but the findings are more inclusive than with other diagnostic tests. Biopsy of the synovium could be taken during this procedure.

Electromyography (EMG): EMG measures the electrical activity of muscles at rest and during voluntary muscle contraction. When the muscle is at rest, normally there is no electrical activity. Abnormal EMG results occur in neuropathic and myopathic disorders (i.e., peripheral neuropathy [diabetes mellitus, alcoholism], myasthenia gravis, muscular dystrophy, amyotropic lateral sclerosis [ALS]).

Muscle Biopsy: The purpose for the muscle biopsy is to provide histopathologic information that could be used in the diagnosis of myopathic disorders. EMG is usually performed at the affected muscle site prior to the biopsy.

Magnetic Resonance Imaging: MRI can be used to identify muscle disease and skeletal abnormalities.

NURSING IMPLICATIONS WITH RATIONALE

- Explain that the purpose of the laboratory and diagnostic tests is to aid in the diagnosis of brain, muscle, and/or bone disorders. Be specific with the explanation as indicated.
- Give an explanation of the test procedures, and emphasize the need for the client's compliance. The explanation might be brief or in depth, depending upon the client's ability to comprehend.
- Inform the client of any food, fluid, or drug restrictions (*see Parts I and II*).
- Elicit from the client or family member information about any allergies to dye (contrast medium), iodine, or seafood.

- Listen to the client's expressed anxiety about the tests and potential client problems. Clarification of the test procedure might alleviate fear and anxiety and promote test compliance.
- Assess muscle strength in all extremities. Weak or lacking muscle strength might indicate a neurologic (e.g., CVA) or muscular problem.
- Assess the client's ability to talk. Inability to communicate could hinder the client's compliance to the test regimen.
- Assist the client with ambulation as needed.
- Observe for seizures prior to or after test procedure.
- Monitor the client's vital signs before and following diagnostic procedures (i.e., cerebral angiography, myelography, lumbar puncture, pneumoencephalography, arthroscopy).

Endocrine function

LABORATORY TESTS	**DIAGNOSTIC TESTS**
Thyroid	
T_4 (Serum)	RAIU Test
T_3 (Serum)	Thyroid Scan
T_3 Resin Uptake	Thyroid Biopsy
Free T_4 Index	Ultrasonography of Thyroid
Thyroid Peroxidase (TPO) Antibody	
Calcitonin, Thyrocalcitonin (Plasma)	
TA (Serum)	
TSH (Serum)	
Provocative Tests	
TSH Stimulation Test	
Thyroid Suppression Test	
TRH Stimulation Test	
Parathyroid	
Electrolytes (Ca, P) (Serum)	Ultrasonography of Parathyroid
PTH (Serum)	
cAMP (Urine)	
Prednisone Suppression Test	
Adrenal	
Electrolytes (K, Na, Ca) (Serum)	X-ray of Sella Turcica
Adrenocorticotropic Hormone (Plasma)	Adrenal Angiography, Arteriography
Cortisol (Plasma)	Adrenal Venography
Cortisol (Urine)	Ultrasonography of Adrenal
Aldosterone (Serum)	CT Scan
Aldosterone (Urine)	
Catecholamines (Plasma)	
17-OCHS (Urine)	
17-KS (Urine)	
17-KGS (Urine)	
Pregnanetriol (Urine)	
VMA (Urine)	
Adrenal Provocative Tests	

LABORATORY TESTS	DIAGNOSTIC TESTS

ACTH Stimulation Test
ACTH Suppression Test
Dexamethasone Suppression Test
Metyrapone Suppression Test
Aldosterone Stimulation Test
Aldosterone Suppression Test

Pancreas (Beta Cell)
Electrolytes (K, Na) (Serum)
BUN (Serum)
Creatinine (Serum)
Acetone/Ketone Bodies (Serum, Plasma, Urine)
Chemstrip bG and Dextrostix
Glucose: FBS and PPBS (Blood)
Glucose Self-Monitoring (Blood)
Glucose Tolerance Test (Serum, Blood)
Insulin (Serum)
Insulin Antibody
Diabetes Mellitus Autoantibodies
C-Peptide (Serum)
Tolbutamide Tolerance Test

Introduction

Usually there is a battery of laboratory and diagnostic tests ordered for suspected endocrine disorders of the thyroid, parathyroid, adrenal, and pancreas (beta cell) glands. Laboratory tests include serum, plasma, blood, urine, and provocative tests. Provocative tests assess glandular function by stimulating or suppressing secretions. Diagnostic tests are ordered to confirm suspected glandular disorders.

Thyroid Assessment
Laboratory Tests

Thyroxine (T_4) (Serum): *Norms:* Adult: T_4 (RIA); 5–12 mcg/dL; T_4 by column: 4.5–11.5 mcg/dL; free T_4: 1–2.3 ng/dL. Child: 1–6 years: T_4: 5.5–13.5 mcg/dL; 6–10 years: T_4: 5–12.5 mcg/dL.

T_4, a major hormone secreted by the thyroid gland, is an effective indicator of thyroid function. Elevated serum T_4 levels are found in clients with hyperthyroidism, acute thyroiditis, and thyrotoxicosis. Decreased levels are found in clients with hypothyroidism. Most thyroxine is bound to thyroxin-binding globulin (TBG).

Triiodothyronine (T_3) (Serum): *Norms:* Adult: 80–200 ng/dL. Child: 6–12 years: 115–190 ng/dL.

T_3, a hormone of the thyroid, is more potent, shorter acting, and of less quantity than T_4. It is helpful in diagnosing thyrotoxicosis, especially when serum T_4 is in normal range. In hypothyroidism, serum T_3 levels may be within normal range; therefore, T_4 would be more reliable.

T_3 Resin Uptake: *Norms:* 25–35%.

This test indirectly measures free T_4 levels by determining protein-binding sites present for T_4. T_3 resin uptake and serum T_4 (RIA) give free T_4 index. In hyperthyroidism, there is a high T_3 resin uptake and the percentage is increased; in hypothyroidism, there is a low T_3 resin uptake and the percentage is decreased.

Free T_4 Index: *Norms:* Adult: 0.9–2.2 ng/dL.

Free T_4 index is unaffected by TBG and correlates more with the true hormonal status. It is difficult to measure T_4 directly, so T_3 resin uptake and serum T_4 give the free thyroxine index.

Calcitonin, Thyrocalcitonin (Plasma): *Norms:* Basal: Adult: male: less than 40 pg/mL; female: less than 25 pg/mL. Child: less than 70 pg/mL.

Calcitonin is a hormone secreted by the C cells of the thyroid gland. Calcitonin lowers calcium levels. Elevated plasma calcitonin levels could indicate medullary carcinoma of the thyroid.

Thyroid Antibodies, Thyroglobulin Antibodies (TA) (Serum): *Norms:* Adult: negative to 1:20, 0–50 ng/mL (RIA). Child: same as adult.

A high titer of thyroglobulin antibodies is indicative of thyroid autoimmune disease. In Hashimoto thyroiditis, the titer is high, 1:5,000. Titer can also be elevated in carcinoma of the thyroid and thyrotoxicosis.

Thyroid Peroxidase (TPO) Antibody: *Norm:* Negative.

Thyroid antibodies inhibit the synthesis of the thyroid hormone. TPO antibody test is the newest test for thyroid dysfunction. Thyroid peroxidase is essential for the synthesis of thyroid hormones thyroxine (T_4) and triiodothyronine (T_3).

Thyroid-Stimulating Hormone (TSH) (Serum): *Norms:* Adult: 0.35–5.5 micro-international unit/mL, less than 10 micro-unit/mL (RIA), less than 3 ng/mL.

TSH is secreted from the anterior pituitary gland in response to thyroid-releasing hormone (TRH) from the hypothalamus. Secretion of TSH is dependent on a negative feedback system that promotes the release of TRH when the level of T_4 is decreased; this in turn stimulates TSH secretion. An elevated TSH level and a decreased T_4 indicate hypothyroidism.

Thyroid Provocative Tests: These tests are useful for evaluating thyroid function.

TSH Stimulation Test, Thyroid Stimulation Test: This test is useful in distinguishing between primary, or thyroidal, hypothyroidism and secondary, or hypothalamopituitary, hypothyroidism. After an injection of TSH, radioactive iodine uptake (RAIU), serum TSH, and/or serum T_4 are measured. In primary hypothyroidism, the RAIU will remain about the same, TRH and TSH will be increased, and T_4 will show no response. In secondary hypothyroidism, the RAIU will increase about 10%, TRH and TSH will not be increased, and T_4 will rise greater than 1.5 mcg/dL.

Thyroid Suppression Test: Norms: Adult: 25% decrease in RAIU; T_4 less than 50% of baseline.

This test is useful to confirm borderline hyperthyroidism. Baseline RAIU and T_3 or T_4 levels are first obtained. The client is given T_4 or T_3 for 7 days. Normally TSH production should be depressed, thus decreasing RAIU and T_4. In hyperthyroidism, the RAIU and T_4 will *not* be decreased.

Thyrotropin-Releasing Hormone (TRH) Stimulation Test: The purpose of the TRH stimulation test is to differentiate between hypothalamic and pituitary insufficiency in clients with hypothyroidism with low serum TSH levels. This test can be used to confirm equivocal thyrotoxicosis, because free thyroid hormone suppresses pituitary production of TSH. A baseline value for serum TSH is obtained. TRH is injected intravenously, followed by serum TSH measurements. A serum TSH increase is indicative of hypothalamic disorder; however, no response in serum TSH is indicative of a pituitary disorder. Decreased TRH and TSH levels occur when aspirin and steroids are being taken.

Diagnostic Tests

Radioactive Iodine Uptake Test (RAIU): *Norms:* Adult: 2 hours: 1–13%; 6 hours: 2–25%; 24 hours: 15–45%.

The RAIU test is primarily used in detecting hyperthyroidism. I-131 or I-123 is given orally or I-125 is given intravenously. The client's thyroid gland is scanned at three different times to determine the concentration of radioactive iodine uptake in the thyroid gland. An elevated RAIU indicates hyperthyroidism or Graves disease. A low RAIU could mean hypothyroidism; however, if T_3 and T_4 are elevated, then it could be caused by thyrotoxicosis or chronic thyroiditis.

Thyroid Biopsy: The biopsy of the thyroid gland is usually performed to diagnose or to confirm the diagnosis of thyroid cancer. Also, this biopsy may be ordered to identify the cause of hyperthyroidism or an inflammatory thyroid disease.

Thyroid Scan: The purpose for thyroid scanning is to determine the size, structure, and position of the thyroid gland, to detect thyroid masses (e.g., tumors), and to evaluate thyroid function. Thyroid nodules are easily detected; cold spots could indicate hypofunction and thyroid tumor, and hot spots could indicate hyperfunction (i.e., Graves disease, thyrotoxicosis).

Ultrasonography of Thyroid, Thyroid Echogram, Thyroid Sonography: Ultrasound of the thyroid gland is helpful in distinguishing between solid and cystic nodules. It is a noninvasive procedure and is considered safe for pregnant women.

Parathyroid Assessment
Laboratory Tests

Electrolytes: Calcium and Phosphorus (Serum): *Norms:*

PERSON	CALCIUM	PHOSPHORUS
Adult	4.5–5.5 mEq/L	1.7–2.6 mEq/L
	9–11 mg/dL	2.5–4.5 mg/dL
Child	9–12 mg/dL	2.5–6 mg/dL
		7 mg/dL during bone growth

Parathyroid hormone (PTH) promotes calcium absorption from the gastrointestinal tract and promotes a release of calcium from bone when there is a deficit. If the client is in renal failure, the serum calcium level is usually low, and the serum phosphorus (phosphate) is elevated. Secondary hyperparathyroidism can occur because of low calcium levels stimulating the secretion of PTH. Decreased serum phosphorus level (hypophosphatemia) is associated with hyperparathyroidism and hypercalcemia. An elevated phosphorus level (hyperphosphatemia) is associated with hypoparathyroidism, hypocalcemia, and renal failure.

Parathyroid Hormone (Serum): *Norms:* Adult: Intact PTH: 11–54 pg/mL, 50–330 pg/mL (C-Terminal); 8–24 pg/mL (N-Terminal).

PTH is released according to serum calcium levels. Decreased circulating calcium stimulates PTH release, and elevated or normal circulating calcium inhibits PTH release. PTH levels might be elevated as the result of parathyroid hyperplasia or tumor. Decreased PTH level could be due to parathyroid trauma or postparathyroidectomy.

Cyclic Adenosine Monophosphate (Cyclic AMP, cAMP) (Urine): PTH promotes production of cAMP in the kidneys. After an IV infusion of PTH, urine cAMP is measured. In primary hyperparathyroidism, cAMP excretion is increased. Poor renal function can decrease cAMP excretion; thus, this test may not be the most accurate one for evaluating parathyroid function.

Prednisone/Cortisone Suppression Test: The purpose of this test is to determine the cause of hypercalcemia. Oral prednisone or cortisone is administered daily for 10–14 days. If the serum calcium level is lowered in clients with hypercalcemia, then the cause of elevated calcium level is not hyperparathyroidism but might be bone metastasis, sarcoidosis, or excess vitamin D. In hyperparathyroidism, prednisone or cortisone will not lower calcium levels.

Diagnostic Tests

Ultrasonography of the Parathyroid Gland: In ultrasound of the parathyroid gland, the echo pattern is of less amplitude than that of thyroid tissue. Enlargement of the gland(s) might be caused by hyperplasia or tumor growth.

Adrenal Assessment:
Laboratory Tests

Electrolytes (Potassium, Sodium, Calcium) (Serum): *Norms:* Adult: Potassium: 3.5–5.3 mEq/L. Sodium: 135–145 mEq/L. Calcium: 4.5–5.5 mEq/L, 9–11 mg/dL.

Steroids (e.g., cortisone, secreted from the adrenal gland) promote sodium retention and potassium excretion. Adrenal hyperfunction causes an elevated serum sodium level (hypernatremia), a decreased serum potassium level (hypokalemia), and a decreased serum calcium level (hypocalcemia). Adrenal insufficiency causes hyponatremia and hyperkalemia.

Adrenocorticotropic Hormone (ACTH) (Plasma): 7 AM–10 AM: 8–80 pg/mL; 4 PM: 5–30 pg/mL; 10 PM–midnight: less than 10 pg/mL.

Plasma ACTH is performed to determine whether a decreased plasma cortisol is due to adrenal cortex hypofunction or pituitary hypofunction. When the plasma cortisol is increased, ACTH release is inhibited, and when plasma cortisol is decreased, ACTH is released. ACTH stimulation and suppression tests are usually needed to confirm the diagnosis of adrenal disorders. Elevated ACTH could be due to pituitary tumors or nonpituitary ACTH-producing tumor (e.g., of the pancreas, lung, ovary), or it could be due to primary adrenal insufficiency in those with Addison disease. A decreased ACTH level in Addison disease could indicate hypofunction of the pituitary gland.

Cortisol (Plasma): *Norms:* Adult: 8 AM–10 AM: 5–23 mcg/dL, 138–635 nmol/L (SI units); 4 PM–6 PM: 3–13 mcg/dL, /dL, 83–359 nmol/L (SI units).

Cortisol is a potent glucocorticoid released from the adrenal gland. Cortisol levels are higher in the morning than in the afternoon. The diurnal variation ceases in early adrenal hyperfunction. In Addison disease, the plasma cortisol levels are decreased.

Cortisol (Urine): *Norm:* Adult: 24–108 mcg/24 h.

Urine cortisol levels usually reflect the secretion of cortisol. With an elevated plasma cortisol level, excess free cortisol enters the urine, increasing urine cortisol level. Elevated plasma and urine cortisol are signifiers of adrenal hyperfunction.

Aldosterone (Serum): *Norms:* Less than 16 ng/dL (fasting); 4–30 ng/dL (sitting). Child: 3–11 years: 5–70 ng/dL.

Aldosterone, a potent mineralocorticoid, promotes sodium reabsorption from the kidneys and potassium excretion. Thus, this hormone affects electrolyte balance, especially sodium and potassium. A 24-hour urine aldosterone level is more reliable than the serum aldosterone test. A decreased serum aldosterone level is indicative of adrenal hypofunction and an elevated level is indicative of adrenal hyperfunction. Serum aldosterone may be checked with serum renin; an elevated aldosterone and a decreased serum renin is usually due to primary hyperaldosteronism. If both serum aldosterone and serum renin are elevated, secondary hyperaldosteronism is suspected.

Aldosterone (Urine): *Norm:* Adult: 6–25 mcg/24 h.

The 24-hour urine aldosterone test eliminates diurnal variation that occurs with serum aldosterone. Decreased urine aldosterone levels can indicate adrenal hypofunction, and elevated levels can indicate primary or secondary hyperaldosteronism, stress, or adrenal hyperfunction.

Catecholamines (Plasma) (*See Plasma Catecholamines in Part I.*) *Epinephrine:* Supine: less than 50 pg/mL. *Norepinephrine:* Supine: 110–410 pg/mL.

Epinephrine, norepinephrine, and dopamine are the major catecholamine hormones secreted by the adrenal medulla. Elevated catecholamines, greater than 1,000 pg/mL, indicate pheochromocytoma.

17-Hydroxycorticosteroids (17-OHCS) (Urine): *Norms:* Adult: Male: 5–15 mg/24 h. Female: 3–13 mg/24 h. Child: lower than adults.

The 17-OHCS are a group of steroids, cortisone and hydrocortisone, excreted in the urine. Urine 17-OHCS and serum cortisol are frequently the tests of choice for assessing adrenal function. Elevated urine 17-OHCS level is indicative of adrenal hyperfunction (i.e., Cushing syndrome), and a decreased urine 17-OHCS is indicative of adrenal hypofunction (i.e., Addison disease).

17-Ketosteroids (17-KS) (Urine): *Norms:* Adult: Male: 5–25 mg/24 h. Female: 5–15 mg/24 h. Adolescent: 3–14 mg/24 h. (*For other reference values, see Part I.*)

The 17-KS are metabolites of male hormones secreted from the adrenal cortex and testes. Urine 17-KS levels are higher in males than females. An elevated urine 17-KS could indicate adrenal cortical hyperfunction (e.g., hyperplasia, Cushing syndrome, adrenal tumors), and a decreased urine 17-KS could indicate adrenal cortical hypofunction (e.g., Addison disease).

17-Ketogenic Steroids (17-KGS) (Urine): *Norms:* Adult: Male: 4–22 mg/24 h. Female: 2–15 mg/24 h. Adolescent: 2–9 mg/24 h.

The 17-KGS are a group of steroids that are used to assess adrenal cortical function. An elevated urine 17-KGS level occurs in adrenal hyperfunction, and a decreased level occurs in adrenal hypofunction.

Pregnanetriol (Urine) *Norms:* Adult: Male: 0.4–2.4 mg/24 h. Female: 0.5–2 mg/24 h. Child: 0–1 mg/24 h.

Pregnanetriol comes from adrenal corticoid synthesis. Elevated level is indicative of adrenal cortical hyperfunction (i.e., congenital hyperplasia, adrenal gland tumor).

Vanillylmandelic Acid (VMA) (Urine): *Norms:* Adult: 1.5–7.5 mg/24 h, 7.6–37.9 µmol/24 (SI units).

VMA is a by-product of catecholamines (epinephrine and norepinephrine). Elevated urine VMA levels might indicate adrenal medulla tumor. Certain foods and drugs can give false-positive test results.

Adrenal Provocative Tests: These tests help evaluate adrenal function.

ACTH Stimulation Test: With the administration of ACTH, the plasma cortisol level should double in 1 hour. If the plasma cortisol level remains the same or is lower, adrenal gland insufficiency or Addison disease is the cause.

ACTH Suppression Test: When a synthetic, potent cortisol, dexamethasone (Decadron), is given, the ACTH production should be suppressed. If an extremely high dose is needed for ACTH suppression, the cause is of pituitary origin, such as pituitary tumor.

Dexamethasone Suppression Test: Norms: Adult: Plasma Cortisol: 8 AM, less than 10 mcg/dL; 4 PM, less than 5 mcg/dL.

This is an overnight screening test to evaluate the pituitary feedback system and to determine the presence of adrenal hyperfunction (e.g., Cushing syndrome). Dexamethasone (Decadron), a potent adrenal steroid, is given at midnight, and plasma cortisol levels are measured at 8 AM and 4 PM (17-OHCS may be measured also).

With Cushing syndrome, the adrenals will continue to secrete cortisone despite the ACTH suppression by the pituitary gland.

Metyrapone Suppression Test: Norm: Adult: 17-OHCS should be twofold.

This test evaluates the pituitary feedback system and determines the presence of adrenal hyperfunction. Metyrapone is a potent blocker of cortisol production. After administration of metyrapone, cortisol production should decline, and a decreased plasma cortisol should increase the ACTH secretion. If urine 17-OHCS levels are markedly increased, adrenal hyperplasia is suspected. If there is not an increase in urine 17-OHCS, adrenal tumor might be suspected. Adrenocortical insufficiency (e.g., Addison disease) is a complication of this test.

Aldosterone Stimulation Test: Norms: Plasma aldosterone increases twofold to fourfold. Urine aldosterone increases twofold to threefold.

This provocative test using furosemide (Lasix) differentiates between adrenal disorder and essential hypertension. As body fluids deplete, aldosterone secretion increases and so does renin secretion. Increased plasma and urine aldosterone levels suggest primary aldosteronism, and decreased levels suggest hypoaldosteronism.

Aldosterone Suppression Test: Norms: Adult: approximately 50% decrease in secretion or excretion of aldosterone.

IV saline infusion expands extracellular fluid volume, thus decreasing aldosterone secretion. If aldosterone levels are not suppressed, primary hyperaldosteronism is suspected. After normal saline for 3–5 days, the plasma aldosterone level should decrease by approximately 70%.

Diagnostic Tests

X-Ray of Sella Turcica: X-raying this site can detect destruction of the sella turcica, which would be suggestive of an ACTH-producing tumor of the pituitary gland. An overproduction of ACTH caused by the pituitary tumor results in secondary adrenal hyperfunction (e.g., Cushing syndrome).

Adrenal Angiography, Arteriography: Radiopaque dye is injected into the adrenal arteries to visualize the adrenal gland and adrenal arterial system. This is an invasive test and should not be performed if the client is allergic to iodine or dye. This test will detect adrenal tumors and hyperplasia. If pheochromocytoma is suspected, beta- and alpha-adrenergic blockers should be given several days before the test to decrease the chance of hypertensive crisis.

Adrenal Venography: This test detects adrenal vein and adrenal disorders. Plasma cortisol levels from both adrenal glands are obtained to determine the involved gland causing Cushing syndrome (e.g., unilateral tumor). If cortisol levels are bilaterally elevated, then adrenal hyperfunction is caused by bilateral adrenal hyperplasia. If pheochromocytoma is suspected, then adrenal venous blood is tested for catecholamines.

Adrenal Ultrasonography, Sonography: Ultrasound is useful in detecting adrenal gland abnormalities (e.g., tumors).

Computed Tomography of the Adrenal Gland: CT scan determines the size and shape of the adrenal gland. It is useful in detecting adrenal abnormalities (e.g., tumors).

Pancreas (Beta Cell) Assessment
Laboratory Tests

Electrolytes (Potassium and Sodium) (Serum): *Norms:* Adult: Potassium: 3.5–5.3 mEq/L. Sodium: 135–145 mEq/L.

In diabetic ketoacidosis, serum potassium could be normal or elevated, depending on the client's state of body fluid balance. If severe dehydration is present because of polyuria and glycosuria, there would be elevated potassium value resulting from hemoconcentration secondary to dehydration.

The serum sodium level could be normal or low, depending on body fluid balance. Frequently sodium is lost with fluid as a result of osmotic diuresis because of increased blood sugar.

Blood Urea Nitrogen (Serum): *Norm:* Adult: 5–25 mg/dL.

In diabetic ketoacidosis with dehydration, the BUN is slightly to moderately elevated because of hemoconcentration. After hydration, the BUN should return to normal; if it does not, then renal disorder should be suspected.

Creatinine (Serum): *Norms:* Adult: 0.5–1.5 mg/dL, 53–106 µmol/dL (SI units). Child: 0.4–1.2 mg/dL.

A serum creatinine level greater than 2.5 mg/dL could be indicative of renal impairment. In diabetic ketoacidosis, BUN and creatinine levels are usually compared. If BUN is elevated and serum creatinine is in the normal range or less than 2.5 mg/dL, dehydration is likely to be the problem.

Acetone, Ketone Bodies (Serum, Plasma, Urine): *Norms:* Adult: Serum acetone: 0.3–2 mg/dL. Serum ketones: 2–4 mg/dL.

Ketone bodies, by-products of fat metabolism and fatty acids, are greatly increased during uncontrolled diabetes mellitus and starvation. Urine should also be checked with reagent strips or tablets for ketone bodies. Positive acetone and ketone tests are indicative of ketoacidosis.

Chemstrip bG, Dextrostix (Blood): Dextrostix has been a useful screening test for blood sugar for 20 years. In this method, a drop of blood is placed on the Dextrostix, and after 1 minute the strip is compared to a color chart with many ranges (40–240 mg). It is not as accurate as the Chemstrip bG. The use of Chemstrip bG for hospital and home blood sugar monitoring is popular and is considered accurate. Follow directions on set.

Glucose: Fasting Blood Sugar (FBS) and 2-Hour Postprandial Blood Sugar (PPBS), or Feasting: *FBS:* Serum/plasma: 70–110 mg/dL. Blood: 60–100 mg/dL. *PPBS:* Serum/plasma: less than 140 mg/dL/2 h. Blood: less than 120 mg/dL/2 h.

Insulin is needed for transportation of glucose into the cells. A decrease in insulin production increases blood glucose level. A decreased glucose level (hypoglycemia) frequently results from too much circulating insulin. An elevated glucose level greater than 200 mg/dL indicates not enough insulin, the condition known as diabetes mellitus.

Glucose Self-Monitoring (Blood): Glucose monitoring devices are available for accurately checking blood glucose levels.

Glucose Tolerance Test (GTT) (Serum, Blood): GTT is a test to diagnose diabetes mellitus. This test should not be performed if the fasting blood sugar is greater than 200 mg/dL.

Insulin (Serum): *Norms:* Adult: 10–250 micro-unit/mL; 5–25 micro-unit/mL.

Serum insulin and blood glucose levels are compared to determine the glucose disorder. If the serum insulin level is elevated or the insulin:glucose ratio is greater than 0.3, tumor or hyperplasia of the islet cells of the pancreas should be suspected.

Insulin Antibody: *Norm:* No insulin antibodies detected.

Insulin antibody test is ordered when a client with diabetes requires larger and larger insulin dosage. These antibodies are mainly of immunoglobulin G type (most common type) that can neutralize the insulin and prevent glucose metabolism.

Diabetes Mellitus Autoantibodies: *Norm:* No antibodies detected.

Autoimmune diabetes could be the result of a genetic or environmental occurrence. These antibodies occur in type 1 diabetes mellitus (DM) but not in type 2 DM.

C-Peptide (Serum): *Norm:* Fasting 0.8–1.8 ng/mL.

C-peptide is an inactive amino acid formed during the conversion of pro-insulin to insulin in the beta cells of the pancreas. It can indicate the presence of insulin antibodies in clients with diabetes who receive insulin.

Tolbutamide (Orinase) Tolerance Test: This test determines the insulin and glucose response to the hypoglycemic agent tolbutamide. After IV injection of tolbutamide, the blood glucose level should decrease and remain low for 30 minutes. Blood samples are drawn for baseline value and then 5, 10, 20, 30, 60, and 120 minutes after IV injection. Serum insulin may also be drawn. With a high serum insulin level and severe hypoglycemia resulting, insulinoma should be suspected. A diminished response could mean possible diabetes mellitus; thus, further studies would be necessary.

NURSING IMPLICATIONS WITH RATIONALE

- Explain that the purpose of the laboratory and diagnostic tests is to aid in diagnosing a thyroid, parathyroid, adrenal, or pancreatic disorder. Be more specific with explanation as indicated.
- Give an explanation, in detail if indicated, about the laboratory and diagnostic procedures. Emphasize the importance of the client's compliance with the test procedures. Stress that tests might need to be reordered if the procedure is improperly performed.
- Inform the client of any food, fluid, or drug restrictions. Each test should be checked for specific restrictions (*see Parts I and II*).
- Listen to the client's expressed anxiety about the tests and potential patient problems. Clarification of the test procedure might alleviate fear and anxiety and promote test compliance.
- Check laboratory results, and notify the health care provider of abnormal test reports.
- Observe for signs and symptoms of fluid volume deficit or excess, hypokalemia or hyperkalemia, and hypocalcemia or hypercalcemia. Fluid-volume deficit could result from hyperglycemia because of osmotic diuresis. Symptoms would be those of dehydration or shock. Fluid-volume excess could occur from excess secretion of antidiuretic hormone, which reabsorbs water from the distal renal tubules. Hypokalemia could result from excess aldosterone production. Hypocalcemia or hypercalcemia usually occurs from parathyroid and thyroid disorders.
- Monitor the client's vital signs before and after laboratory and diagnostic tests.
- Provide support to the client and family members during and after test procedure.

Reproductive function

LABORATORY TESTS

Female Reproductive

Estrogen (Serum and Urine)
Estrone (E_1) (Serum and Urine)
Estradiol (E_2) (Serum)
FSH (Serum and Urine)
LH (Serum)
Progesterone (Serum)
Pregnanediol (Urine)
Prolactin (Serum)
Sexual Assault

Male Reproductive

Antisperm Antibody Test
Testosterone (Serum)
Semen Examination
17-KS (Urine)
Cytogenetic Studies
Prostate-Specific Antigen (PSA)

Pregnancy

HCG (Serum and Urine)
Home Pregnancy Test Kits
HPL (Serum
Estriol (E_3) (Serum and Urine)
Estetrol (E_4) (Plasma)
Progesterone (Serum)
Pregnanediol (Urine)
Infertility Screen
Placental Growth Factor (PGF)
Pregnancy-Associated Plasma Protein-A
Amino Acid Screen (Urine)
AFP (Serum and Amniotic Fluid)
Genetic Defect Tests: Down Syndrome, Tay-Sachs Disease,
   Sickle-Cell Anemia, Galactosemia, Thalassemia, PKU
Chromosome Analysis
Rubella Antibody Detection
Mumps Antibody Test (Serum)
Rubeola Antibodies
Maternal Enzymes (Serum)
Blood Type, Rh Screen
L/S Ratio (Amniotic Fluid)
Nitrazine Paper Test
CPK/CK (Serum)
Renin (Plasma)

DIAGNOSTIC TESTS

Colposcopy
Laparoscopy
Dilation and Curettage (D & C)
Hysterosalpingography
Cytogenetic Studies
   Sex Chromatin Mass
   Chromosome Analysis
Pap Smear
Cervical Biopsy
Mammography
Uterotubal Insufflation Tests
Postcoital Tests
Thermography
Cervicography
Hysteroscopy
Saliva Ferning Test

Postcoital Test
Prostate Gland Biopsy
Prostate Ultrasonography
Scrotum/Testes Ultrasonography

Amniocentesis
Pelvic Ultrasonography
Fetal Nonstress Test (NST)
Fetoscopy
External Fetal Monitoring
Internal Fetal Monitoring
Breast Massage Stress Test
Fetal Biophysical Profile
Fetal Fibronectin (fFN)
Saliva Ferning Test

(Continued)

LABORATORY TESTS	DIAGNOSTIC TESTS
Albumin (Serum)	

Albumin (Serum)
Hormone Changes
Hematologic Changes
RPR (Serum)
Herpes Simplex Virus-2 (Serum)
Cytogenetic Studies
Chlamydia Test (Serum, Tissue Smear, Culture)
Cytomegalovirus Antibody (Serum)

Neonate
Glucose (Blood)
Cord Blood: Type and Rh
Bilirubin (Blood)
PKU (Serum and Urine)
TORCH Test
Severe Combined Immunodeficiency (SCID)
Trypsin (Feces)
Herpes Simplex Virus-2 (Serum)
Toxoplasmosis Antibody (Serum)

Introduction

The focus on reproductive function in this section is on reproductive processes and products involving both males and females. Certain tests in the discussion of the female reproductive function, such as cytogenetic studies, also apply to the male reproductive function and pregnancy. Laboratory tests for reproductive function include serum, plasma, urine, and amniotic fluid. The number of tests in pregnancy has greatly increased in the last 10–20 years.

Female Reproductive Assessment
Laboratory Tests

Estrogen (Serum): *Norms:* Early menstrual cycle: 60–200 pg/mL. Midmenstrual cycle: 100–600 pg/mL. Late menstrual cycle: 150–350 pg/mL. Postmenopausal: less than 30 pg/mL. Male: 40–115 pg/mL.

This test is useful for evaluating gonadal hypofunction in females, timing ovulation, and determining hormonally active tumors. Serum estrogen measures estrone (E_1) and estradiol (E_2), but also measures small amounts of estriol (E_3); therefore, it is *not* a test used in pregnancy to determine fetal well-being.

Estrogen (Urine): *Norms:* Female: Preovulation: 5–25 mcg/24 h. Follicular: 24–100 mcg/24 h. Luteal phase: 22–80 mcg/24 h. Postmenopausal: 0–10 mcg/24 h. Male: 4–25 mcg/24 h.

Urine estrogen test includes estrone (E_1), estradiol (E_2), and estriol (E_3). This 24-hour urine test is useful for diagnosing ovarian disorders, tumors, hypogonadism, hypopituitarism, and adrenal hyperplasia. It is not a test for assessing fetal well-being.

Estrone (E_1) (Serum and Urine): (*See values for estrone in Part I.*)

Estrone is a potent estrogen. A decreased estrone level can indicate ovarian failure or dysfunction.

Estradiol (E_2) (Serum): *Female:* Follicular phase: 20–150 pg/mL. Midcycle: 100–500 pg/mL. Luteal phase: 60–260 pg/mL. *Male:* 15–20 pg/mL. *Child:* 3–10 pg/mL.

E_2 evaluates gonadal dysfunction, such as amenorrhea syndromes and testicular tumors. It is decreased in primary amenorrhea and ovarian failure and is elevated in testicular tumors, ovarian tumors, and adrenal tumors.

Follicle-Stimulating Hormone (FSH) (Serum): *Norms:* Female: Preovulation, Postovulation: 4–30 milli-unit/mL. Midcycle: 10–90 milli-unit/mL. Luteal phase: 4–30 milli-unit/mL. Postmenopausal: 40–170 milli-unit/mL. Male: 4–25 milli-unit/mL. Child: 5–12 milli-unit/mL.

Serum FSH is useful for diagnosing infertility and menstrual disorders. FSH is responsible for developing ovarian follicles for ovulation. A decreased serum FSH can indicate anovulation, causing infertility or secondary hypogonadotropic state caused by panhypopituitarism or anorexia nervosa. Elevated serum FSH might indicate primary hypogonadism (Turner syndrome) or precocious puberty. It may be elevated in postmenopausal women.

Follicle-Stimulating Hormone (Urine): *Norms:* Female: Preovulation, Postovulation: 2–15 international unit/24 h. Midcycle: 8–60 international unit/24 h. Postmenopausal: 50–150 international unit/24 h. Male: 4–18 international unit/24 h. Child: less than 10 international unit/24 h.

A decreased urine FSH level might indicate neoplasms of the ovary, adrenal gland, or testes or anorexia nervosa. An elevated level could indicate gonadal failure caused by postmenopause, FSH-producing pituitary tumor, or Klinefelter syndrome.

Luteinizing Hormone (LH) (Serum): *Norms:* Female: Follicular: 3–30 milli-international unit/mL. Midcycle: 30–100 milli-international unit/mL. Postmenopausal: 40–100 milli-international unit/mL. Male: 5–25 milli-international unit/mL. Child: less than 10 milli-international unit/mL.

LH may determine the cause of menstrual disturbances, gonadal failure, and infertility. The FSH test is ordered with LH to check on causes of anovulation and infertility. An elevated LH level might indicate ovarian failure associated with Stein-Leventhal syndrome (which is polycystic ovary syndrome), Turner syndrome (ovarian dysgenesis), or postmenopause.

Progesterone (Serum): *Norms:* Preovulation: 20–150 ng/dL, 0.1–1.5 ng/mL. Midcycle: 250–2,800 ng/dL, 2–28 ng/mL.

Purposes of this test are to determine ovulation, to evaluate infertility problems, and to assess placental function. Serum progesterone levels are elevated at time of ovulation, including 5 days postovulation, in early pregnancy, and in adrenal tumors.

Pregnanediol (Urine): *Norms:* Female: Preovulation: 0.5–1.5 mg/24 h. Midcycle: 2–7 mg/24 h. Postmenopausal: 0.1–1 mg/24 h. Male: 0.1–1.5 mg/24 h. Child: 0.4–1 mg/24 h.

Pregnanediol is the major metabolite of progesterone. It is produced by the corpus luteum during the latter half of the menstrual cycle and by the placenta. A decreased level could be due to menstrual disorders, ovarian hypofunction, threatened abortion, tumors of the ovary or breast, lutein cell tumors of the ovary, or preeclampsia. Elevated level could be due to pregnancy, ovarian cyst, choriocarcinoma of the ovary, or adrenal hyperplasia.

Prolactin (Serum): *Norms:* Nonlactating female: 0–23 ng/dL. Pregnancy: rise of 10- to 20-fold.

This test is useful for detecting a suspected pituitary tumor. High prolactin levels, greater than 100 ng/dL, in a nonpregnant female could indicate pituitary adenoma. Hyperprolactinemia may be due to hypothyroidism, acromegaly, or hypothalamic disorders or may occur in clients with galactorrhea and amenorrhea.

Sexual Assault (Rape): When a woman (could be a man) has been physically and sexually assaulted, she should be professionally tested soon after the assault. Most health institutions have a kit, Sexual Assault Evidence Collection Kit (SAECK), with directions for testing persons who are sexually assaulted. A pelvic examination is usually performed to obtain sperm and other cells from the perpetrator.

Diagnostic Tests

Colposcopy: A colposcope is used to examine the vagina and cervix for precancerous lesions. Colposcopy is performed after an abnormal Pap test, to monitor treatment for dysplasia and cervical lesions, and to monitor females with vaginal and/or cervical tissue changes caused by their mothers taking diethylstilbestrol (DES) during pregnancy.

Laparoscopy: A laparoscope, a small fiberoptic telescope, is inserted through the abdominal wall for the purpose of detecting cysts, fibroids, adhesions, and pelvic masses and for diagnosing the cause of pelvic pain (i.e., endometriosis, pelvic inflammatory disease [PID]). This procedure may be used for tubal sterilization, ovarian biopsy, and removal of foreign bodies. Laparoscopy has decreased the number of surgical laparotomies performed.

Dilation and Curettage (D & C): D & C is performed to obtain cells from the endometrium of the uterus and for abnormal bleeding.

Hysterosalpingography: Ultrasonography has nearly replaced hysterosalpingography. However, this test is still useful for evaluating patency of the fallopian tubes. It is one of the infertility studies. The procedure uses contrast medium and fluoroscopic x-ray filming.

Cytogenetic Studies: Cytogenetic studies for analysis are performed on tissue, blood, bone marrow, and amniotic fluid. Sex chromatin and chromosome analysis are the two tests usually ordered when chromosomal abnormalities are suspected.

Sex Chromatin Mass: Sex chromatin mass or Barr chromatin body (clump of chromatin adhered to nuclear membrane in cells) is represented as an inactive X chromosome in females and not in males. With disturbances of gonadal development or function and/or with disturbance in reproductive function, sex chromosome defect (absence or an increased number of inactivated X chromosomes or Barr chromatin bodies) may be suspected. The purpose of the test is to screen for sex chromosome anomalies such as the following:

- Turner syndrome: poorly developed sex characteristics (amenorrhea, undeveloped breasts, sterility) in a female due to XO (no Barr body) or XX/XO mosaics (some with Barr body and some without).
- Klinefelter syndrome: poorly developed sex characteristics (small penis, testes, sterility) in a male due to presence of chromatin body of the Y chromosome with PXY (mostly), XXXY, or XXYY variants.

Buccal mucosa is obtained for sex chromosome study. If results are abnormal, chromosome analysis (karyotype) is indicated.

Chromosome Analysis: Blood, tissue, bone marrow, and amniotic fluid are used to identify chromosomal abnormalities (e.g., Down syndrome, congenital anomalies, genetic disorders, and proliferative diseases such as leukemias). Chromosomal karyotyping is used to identify abnormal sex chromosomes that can cause Turner syndrome (female) or Klinefelter syndrome (male).

Papanicolaou (Pap) Smear: This is a cytologic test to detect precancerous or cancerous cells of the cervix; it is also used to detect some infectious diseases, such as monilia. A positive Pap smear needs further diagnostic test (i.e., colposcopy or cervical biopsy) to confirm the Pap result.

Pap smears are generally performed during a pelvic examination and during the first prenatal visit if not done previously.

Cervical Biopsy: A cervical biopsy may be indicated for suspicious cervical lesions.

Mammography, Mammogram: This procedure is an x-ray examination of the breasts to detect cysts or tumors. Usually it can detect breast lesion(s) 2 years before the lesion is palpable.

Thermography: An infrared photographic test records heat energy from the skin surface of the breast. Increased breast surface temperature may be caused by increased vascularity resulting from a cancerous lesion.

Cervicography (Cervigram): Cervicography is a photographic method to record an image of the cervix. It can identify some cancerous lesions that were missed by Pap smears.

Hysteroscopy: Hysteroscopy visualizes the entire endometrial cavity of the uterus. It is more effective for viewing and obtaining endometrial pathology than the dilatation and curettage (D & C), in which blind scraping is performed.

Postcoital Test: This test (Sims-Huhner test) assists in the determination of infertility. It is performed during ovulation. It measures the motility of sperm cells in the endocervical mucus of a woman after intercourse. The possible cause of the infertility could be from an inadequate cervical mucus, lack of sperms, or antisperm antibodies.

Uterotubal Insufflation Test: This test (Rubin's test) is performed to determine the patency or occlusion of the fallopian tubes. The fallopian tubes are inflated with carbon dioxide. Today, the *hysterosalpingography test* is prescribed to determine fallopian tube patency.

Saliva Ferning Test: This test is a home ovulation test that gives approximate time of ovulation. It checks for drug saliva under the minimicroscope that is purchased with the kit. The dry saliva gives a frosted appearance, which is ferning. Estrogen occurs 3–4 days before ovulation and lasts 2–3 days after ovulation.

Male Reproductive Assessment
Laboratory Tests

Antisperm Antibody Test (Semen, Blood, Serum): *Norm:* Negative: 0.15%; moderately positive: 50%; strongly positive: 100%.

A positive antisperm antibody test can be a sign of infertility.

Testosterone (Serum): *Norms:* Adult: Male: 0.3–1 mcg/dL, 300–1,000 ng/dL. Child: Male (12–14 years): greater than 0.1 mcg/dL, greater than 1,000 ng/dL. Female: 0.03–0.1 mcg/dL, 30–100 ng/dL.

Testosterone, a male sex hormone, is mostly responsible for male sex characteristics and masculinity. The highest serum testosterone level occurs in the morning.

Decreased level could indicate a testicular disorder, Klinefelter syndrome, alcoholism, estrogen therapy, or hypopituitarism. An elevated level could indicate adrenal hyperplasia or tumor, benign prostatic hypertrophy (BPH), or adrenogenital syndrome in women.

Semen Examination: Semen content is useful for determining sperm count, volume of fluid, percentage of mature spermatozoa (sperms), and percentage of actively mobile sperm cells. This test is ordered to help identify the cause of infertility or to determine the effectiveness of sterilization after a vasectomy.

17-Ketosteroids (17-KS) (Urine): *Norms:* Adult: Male: 8–25 mg/24 h; over 65 years old: 4–8 mg/24 h. Female: 5–15 mg/24 h. Adolescent: Male: 3–15 mg/24 h.

17-KS are metabolites of male hormones from the adrenal cortex and testes. This test is useful in diagnosing adrenal cortex dysfunction and determining pituitary and gonadal hormone function. A decreased level could be indicative of hypogonadism and hypopituitarism. An elevated level could be indicative of adrenocortical hyperplasia or tumor, testicular tumor, hirsutism, or hyperpituitarism.

Postcoital Test: The test (Sims-Hubner test) assists in the cause of infertility. It examines the number and the motility of the sperm cells in the endocervical mucus of a woman after intercourse. It could detect the presence of antisperm antibodies in the cervical mucus.

Cytogenetic Studies: (*See Female Reproductive Assessment.*)

Prostate-Specific Antigen (PSA) (Serum): *Norms:* PSA less than 4 ng/mL; BPH: 4–10 ng/mL; Prostate cancer: 10–120 ng/mL; Total PSA: 2.5–4 ng/mL; Free PSA: greater than 1 ng/mL; % Free PSA: greater than 25%.

Diagnostic Tests

Prostate Gland Biopsy: When the PSA is 10 mg/mL or higher, a biopsy of the prostate gland may be performed to diagnose the presence of prostate cancer.

Prostate (Transrectal) Ultrasound: Ultrasound of the prostate gland is used to evaluate palpable prostate nodules and urinary problems related to benign prostatic hypertrophy, to detect early small prostate tumors, and for use of biopsy and/or radiation.

Scrotum/Testes Ultrasound: Ultrasound of the scrotum sac contents is helpful in diagnosing abscess, cyst, hydrocele, spermatocele, varicocele, testicular tumors, and chronic scrotal swelling.

Pregnancy Assessment
Laboratory Tests

Human Chorionic Gonadotropin (HCG) (Serum and Urine): HCG, glycoprotein hormone, is produced by the trophoblast cell of placental tissue. Serum and urine HCG are early tests for confirming pregnancy. HCG tests are positive in pregnant women only and *not* in nonpregnant women. HCG is present 10 days after egg implantation or 14–26 days after conception. It peaks within 8–12 weeks.

Home Pregnancy Test Kits: Pregnancy kits were first introduced in 1976, and today there are several commercially prepared kits available for home use (e.g., Gravindex [Ortho Diagnostics], Prognosis [Roche], Early Pregnancy Test [EPT; Warner/Chicott], Daisy 2 [Bio Dynamics Home Healthcare], and First Response [Tambrands]). Some tests can be used to detect pregnancy as soon as the day of the first missed menstrual period. False readings can occur. If tests results are negative and menses has not begun a week later, it is suggested that the home pregnancy test be repeated.

Human Placental Lactogen (HPL) (Serum): *Norms:*

WEEKS OF GESTATION	MCG/ML
8–27	less than 4.6
28–31	2.4–6
32–35	3.7–7.7
36–40	5–10

HPL is produced by the placenta throughout pregnancy. The test is valuable to determine fetal well-being but should not be used as the only test. If HPL value falls below 4 mcg/mL after

30 weeks, fetal distress might be present because of impaired placental function. If HPL value falls 50% during late pregnancy, fetal distress is apparent.

Estriol (E$_3$) (Serum and Urine): *Norms:*

SERUM		URINE	
Weeks of Gestation	ng/dL	Weeks of Gestation	mcg/24 h
25–28	25–165	16–24	2–6
29–32	30–230	25–28	6–28
33–36	45–370	29–32	6–32
37–38	75–420	33–36	10–45
39–40	95–450	37–40	15–60

E$_3$ is a major estrogenic compound produced largely by the placenta. It increases in maternal serum and urine after 2 months of pregnancy and continues at high levels until term. If toxemia, hypertension, or diabetes is present after 30 weeks of gestation, E$_3$ levels are monitored. A decline in serum or urine E$_3$ levels suggests fetal distress caused by placental malfunction. The test may be repeated to confirm a suspected situation. A cesarean section may be indicated.

Estetrol (E$_4$) (Plasma): *Weeks of Gestation:* 20–26 weeks: 140–210 pg/mL; 30 weeks: 350 pg/mL; 36 weeks: 900 pg/mL; 40 weeks: greater than 1,050 pg/mL.

A decreased estetrol level may indicate fetal distress and fetal malformation. Other tests to determine fetal distress should be done.

Progesterone (Serum): *Norm:* Pregnancy: greater than 2,400 ng/dL.

Progesterone is responsible for maintaining pregnancy after fertilization and for placental development. It has little value in evaluating fetal well-being but is useful in assessing placental function during pregnancy.

Pregnanediol (Urine): *Norms:* Pregnancy: 10–19 gestation weeks: 5–25 mg/24 h; 20–28 gestation weeks: 15–42 mg/24 h; 29–32 gestation weeks: 25–49 mg/24 h.

Pregnanediol measures the urinary metabolite of progesterone. At times urine pregnanediol may be of normal range even when fetal distress or fetal death has occurred

Infertility Screen: *Norms:* See values: Female: Luteinizing hormone values and follicle stimulating hormone values. Males: Antisperm antibody.

Infertility screen tests are a group of tests ordered for the female and male to determine cause(s) of infertility.

Placental Growth Factor (PGF): *Norms:* Nonpregnancy: less than 50 pg/mL; Pregnancy: 20 weeks: greater than 200 pg/mL.

Placental growth factor rises throughout pregnancy. During pregnancy, if the female has low or very low PGF, she is at risk for developing preeclampsia during pregnancy.

Pregnancy-Associated Plasma Protein-A (PAPP-A): *Norm:* Differs with various laboratories.

PAPP-A test is useful in predicating preeclampsia and various fetus development disorders, such as Down syndrome, Trisomy 18 and 21, and Turner syndrome.

Amino Acid Screen (Urine): *Norm:* Adult: 200 mg in 24 hours.

This test screens for elevated levels of amino acid in the urine (aminoaciduria), which can indicate inborn errors of metabolism.

α-1-Fetoprotein (AFP): *Norms:*

SERUM		AMNIOTIC FLUID	
Weeks of Gestation	ng/mL	Weeks of Gestation	mcg/mL
8–12	0–39		
13	6–31		
14	7–50	14	11–32
15	7–60	15	5.5–31
16	10–72	16	5.7–31.5
17	11–90	17	3.8–32.5
18	14–94	18	3.6–28
19	24–112	19	3.7–24.5
20	31–122	20	2.2–15
21	19–124	21	3.6–18

Usually serum AFP is done between 16 and 20 weeks of gestation to detect probability of twins, risk of premature delivery or an infant of low birth weight, or serious birth defects, such as open neural tube defect. It is a screening test, and if abnormal results occur, it should be repeated. If a high serum AFP level occurs, amniotic AFP may be done to diagnose neural tube defect in the fetus. Amniocentesis and ultrasound are required to confirm or to rule out the possible condition.

Genetic Defect Tests: Specific laboratory tests are designed to determine genetic disorders. Table 3.13 shows the defect, specimen, person from whom specimen was obtained, and findings.

Chromosome Analysis (Blood): *Norms:* Male: 44 autosomes + XY sex chromosome = 46; Female: 44 autosome + XX sex chromosome = 46.

Chromosome analysis is to determine abnormal chromosomes that are associated with genetic disease or the risk of developing a genetic disease.

Rubella Antibody Detection (Serum): *Norms:* Titer greater than 1:64 protection against rubella or German measles.

TABLE 3.13 Tests for Genetic Defects

DEFECT	SPECIMEN	PERSON	FINDINGS
Down syndrome	Amniotic fluid	Pregnant female	Trisomy 21 chromosome
Neural tube defects	Serum	Pregnant female	Increased serum AFP
	Amniotic fluid		Increased amniotic AFP
Tay-Sachs disease	Blood	Mother and father (as carriers)	Low level of enzyme hexosaminidase A
	Amniotic fluid	Pregnant female	
Sickle-cell anemia	Blood	Mother and father (as carriers)	Hemoglobin S cells
	Cord blood	Newborn	
Galactosemia	Amniotic fluid	Pregnant female	Presence of galactose
Thalassemia (Cooley or Mediterranean anemia)	Blood	Mother and father (as carriers)	Hemoglobin F cells
	Cord blood	Newborn	
Phenylketonuria (PKU)	Blood	Mother and father (as carriers)	Increased serum phenylalanine

The rubella antibody detection test is done prior to pregnancy or to check pregnant women during their first trimester of pregnancy at time of rubella exposure and again in 3–4 weeks.

Mumps Antibody Test (Serum): Negative or less than 1:8.

Mumps virus could cause orchitis, oophoritis, or meningoencephalitis. Adolescent males who contract mumps are at risk of becoming sterile.

Rubeola Antibodies (Serum): *Norms:* 0- to 4-fold titer. Positive: greater than 4-fold titer.

Rubeola (old-fashioned measles) is a contagious and communicable virus caused by the RNA paramyxovirus. This test is to determine the presence of the rubeola virus or measles.

Maternal Enzymes (Serum): During pregnancy there is an increase in maternal serum enzymes (i.e., heat-stable alkaline phosphatase [HSAP], diamine oxidase [DAO], and oxytocinase). Table 3.14 describes the maternal enzymes and their uses.

Blood Type and Rh Screening: *Norms:* Adult: Rh+ (positive); RH– (negative).

The Rh-negative pregnant female who carried a fetus that was Rh positive should receive Rho (D) immune globulin or RhoGAM by 72 hours after delivery or abortion to prevent Rh sensitization or Rh antibodies. This is important for prevention of erythroblastosis in future fetus. If the mother is Rh negative and unsensitized, some suggest that Rh immune globulin should be given at 28 weeks gestation.

Maternal blood type should be checked. If mother's type is O positive and the baby's type is A or B, there may be potential for ABO incompatibility after delivery.

Lecithin/Sphingomyelin (L/S) Ratio (Amniotic Fluid): *Norms:* Before 35 weeks of gestation: 1:1; after 35 weeks of gestation: 4:1. (L: 15–21 mg/dL; S: 4–6 mg/dL.)

L/S ratio is a predictor of fetal pulmonary maturity before delivery. Lecithin is primarily responsible for the formation of alveolar surfactant that lubricates the alveolar lining and inhibits alveoli collapse. A marked rise in amniotic lecithin after 35 weeks is normal, thus decreasing chances for having hyaline membrane in respiratory distress syndrome. Pulmonary maturity occurs earlier in African Americans than in Caucasians.

Nitrazine Paper Test: *Norms:* Intact membranes: pH 5–6 (yellow to olive green). Ruptured membranes: pH 6.5–7.5 (blue green to deep blue).

This is a paper test to determine if the amniotic membrane is intact or has ruptured. The pH of amniotic fluid is 7–7.5, whereas the pH of vaginal secretions is 4.5–5.5.

TABLE 3.14 Maternal Enzymes

MATERNAL ENZYME	COMMENTS
Heat-stable alkaline phosphatase (HSAP)	HSAP rises in concentration throughout pregnancy. A sudden rise in later pregnancy could indicate placental dysfunction and fetal distress or death. Usually a rise in HSAP occurs before a decrease in E_3.
Diamine oxidase (DAO)	This enzyme protects the pregnant female against histamine produced by the fetus. It rises during early pregnancy but tends to plateau during the third trimester.
Oxytocinase (cystylaminopeptidase)	Oxytocinase is produced by the placenta during pregnancy and inactivates oxytocin. It indicates placental function, not fetal well-being.

TABLE 3.15 Hormonal Changes During Pregnancy

HORMONE	CHANGES	COMMENTS
TBG	Increased markedly	Rise begins after fertilization and continues until 12 weeks of gestation. Failure of TBG rise might indicate hypothyroidism or estrogen deficiency.
T_4	Increased	T_4 rise is not as great as that of TBG.
Resin T_3 uptake	Decreased	T_3 uptake decreases slightly during pregnancy.
TSH	Normal	TSH remains normal in the euthyroid pregnant female.
ACTH	Decreased	Markedly decreased during first trimester of pregnancy.
Cortisol	Increased	Cortisol production slightly declines during pregnancy; however, the plasma half-life is increased. If cortisol value is in the normal range, adrenal hypofunction might be suspected.
Aldosterone	Increased	Aldosterone is increased throughout pregnancy, which increases plasma volume and sodium retention.
PTH	Increased	Reason unknown.

Creatine Phosphokinase (CPK/CK) (Serum): *Norms:* Female: 5–25 mcg/mL, 10–80 international unit/L.

Decreased CPK/CK level might occur during the second trimester of pregnancy.

Renin (Plasma): *Norm:* Upright: 1.6–4.3 ng/mL/h.

An elevated plasma renin level might occur during the first trimester of pregnancy, pre-eclampsia, and eclampsia. This could be due to a kidney problem.

Albumin (Serum): *Norm:* 3.5–5 g/dL.

Albumin levels may decrease by 0.5–1 g/dL. This could be due to increased plasma volume or acceleration of albumin degradation.

Hormone Changes: Thyroid, parathyroid, and adrenal hormone alterations usually accompany pregnancy. Table 3.15 shows the increases and decreases of these hormones during pregnancy.

Hematologic Changes: Hematologic values should be monitored during pregnancy. Changes in laboratory values are expected. Table 3.16 shows the expected changes of hematologic tests.

Rapid Plasma Reagin (RPR) (Serum): *Norms:* Nonreactive.

The RPR test is a rapid screening test for syphilis. A positive RPR should be verified by VDRL and/or FTA-ABS tests.

Herpes Simplex Virus (Type 2) (HSV-2) (Serum): HSV-2 is sexually transmitted and infects the urogenital tract. It can also be transmitted to the newborn during vaginal delivery. Neonatal herpes can result in minor to severe complications (e.g., from skin rash or eye infection to central nervous disorder). If the mother has active HSV-2 at the time of birth, a cesarean delivery may be indicated.

Cytogenetic Studies: (*See Female Reproductive Assessment.*)

Chlamydia Test (Serum, Tissue Smear, Culture): *Serum:* Less than 1:16.

Chlamydia is a bacteria-like organism that resembles a virus. Chlamydia can be passed to the newborn during birthing and may result in blindness to the newborn if untreated. Untreated genital chlamydia infection could lead to sterility.

TABLE 3.16 Hematologic Changes During Pregnancy

BLOOD TESTS	CHANGES	COMMENTS
Red blood cells (RBCs)	Increased	RBC mass increases slightly during pregnancy even with increased plasma volume.
Hemoglobin and hematocrit	Decreased	Plasma volume increase causes hemodilution.
Platelets	Slightly decreased or normal value	Decreased platelet count could result from increased plasma volume.
Reticulocytes	Increased	There is a slight rise in reticulocytes during the second trimester of pregnancy.
White blood cells (WBCs)	Increased	Slightly elevated WBCs. During the last half of pregnancy, granulocytes increase and lymphocytes remain unchanged.
Fibrinogen	Increased	Fibrinogen level increases throughout pregnancy.
Plasminogen	Increased	Reason unknown.
Prothrombin time (PT) and partial thromboplastin time (PTT)	Slightly decreased or normal	Reason unknown.
Erythrocyte sedimentation rate (ESR)	Increased	ESR increases markedly because of increase in fibrinogen level.
Folate (folic acid)	Decreased	Mother's tissues absorb more folic acid.
Vitamin B_{12}	Decreased	Mother's tissues absorb more vitamin B_{12}.
Iron	Decreased	Fetal use and increased plasma volume (hemodilution).

Cytomegalovirus Antibody (CMV) Serum: Negative to less than 0.30.

This virus belongs to the herpes virus family. If the pregnant woman is infected with CMV, the fetus may become infected. In infants, this virus could cause cerebral tissue malformation and/or damage.

Diagnostic Tests

Amniocentesis, Amniotic Fluid Analysis: The purposes for analysis of amniotic fluid are to detect chromosomal abnormalities such as Down syndrome (Trisomy 21), neural tube defects, sex-linked disorders, and fetal and pulmonary maturity. (*See Female Reproductive Assessment and Amniotic Fluid Analysis in Part II.*)

Pelvic Ultrasonography: The numerous uses for pelvic ultrasound are to detect multiple fetuses or fetal anomalies; to determine the location of the placenta (rule out placenta previa) or fetal and placenta locations during an amniocentesis; and to evaluate fetal viability, gestational age, and fetal growth. This test procedure is considered noninvasive because contrast media is *not* used.

Fetal Nonstress Test (NST): The NST as well as the contraction stress test (CST) are performed to evaluate the viability of the fetus and the function of the placenta to provide adequate blood flow. NST is a noninvasive test that monitors fetal heart rate with fetal movement. The CST can be an invasive test with the use of oxytocin, a uterine stimulant. The CST with oxytocin is usually not performed before 32 weeks.

Fetoscopy: This endoscopic procedure uses a fetoscope that is inserted through the abdominal wall into the uterine cavity for direct visualization and to obtain blood samples from the blood vessel in the umbilical cord. It is usually performed during the 18th week of gestation. This procedure is useful for detecting neural tube defect, sickle-cell anemia, and hemophilia.

External Fetal Monitoring: External fetal monitoring records the fetal heart rate and uterine contractions. It is considered a noninvasive test. It can be used as a nonstress test to determine fetal well-being during stressful and nonstressful conditions. Also, it can be used as a stress test using oxytocin to determine fetal well-being.

Internal Fetal Monitoring: This is an invasive procedure in which an electrode is attached to the scalp of the fetus to measure fetal heart rate and a catheter is placed in the uterine cavity to measure uterine contractions. Internal fetal monitoring is performed during labor after the membranes have ruptured. It is indicated when external fetal monitoring provides inadequate information.

Fetal Biophysical Profile: This test evaluates the fetal activity to determine the status of the fetus. It includes the fetal heart rate, breathing and body movements, muscle tone, and the volume of the amniotic fluid. It can denote fetal distress because of fetal hypoxemia.

Fetal Fibronectin (fFN): This test is to detect the cervicovaginal secretions during the first 22 weeks of pregnancy. fFN is secreted in early pregnancy to help in the attachment of the fertilized egg to the endometrium. There is a high risk of preterm (premature birth) if the fFN is present in the vaginal secretion after 34 weeks.

Breast Massage Stress Test: Breast massage is a relatively new contraction stress test (CST) for assessing fetal well-being in high-risk pregnancies. If a nonstress test is *not* effective in determining fetal well-being, then a CST is indicated. CST can be done using the standard stress test with IV infusion of oxytocin or breast massage.

Neonate Assessment
Laboratory Tests

Glucose (Blood): *Norm:* 40 mg/dL.
Neonatal hypoglycemia may occur 4–6 hours after birth. Chemstrip bG and Dextrostix are useful for monitoring blood glucose in the newborn. Blood sugar falls rapidly during the first few hours of life but stabilizes in 6 hours in the healthy newborn. Newborns who are at high risk (e.g., born of mothers with diabetes, erythroblastotic newborns, and pregnant women taking terbutaline) should have blood glucose monitored closely. In some institutions, Chemstrip bG is used as a routine screening test for all newborns.

Cord Blood At the time of birth, a blood sample from the umbilical cord is tested for blood type and Rh (factor) antibody titer.

Bilirubin: Neonatal (Blood): *Norms:* Less than 12 mg/dL. *Critical Range:* 15 mcg/dL.
Blood is drawn from the newborn's heel by means of a capillary pipette.
Neonatal jaundice could be due to erythroblastosis fetalis, hemorrhage, or physiologic jaundice (caused by increased RBC breakdown and immature liver cells). Repeated heel stick may be needed to monitor bilirubin levels in the newborn.

Phenylketonuria (PKU) (Urine) or Phenylalanine (Blood): *Norms:* 1–3 mg/dL (blood). *Critical Range:* Greater than 4 mg/dL.
Blood phenylalanine is checked 48–120 hours after birth following milk or protein feedings. A positive test indicates that the newborn lacks the enzyme needed to metabolize phenylalanine, an amino acid found in protein foods.

PKU testing of the urine is done between 2 and 4 weeks of life. Phenistix (Ames) is a dipstick for testing the infant's urine for PKU. Green color is an indicator of a positive PKU test.

Severe Combined Immunodeficiency (SCID): SCID is a screening blood test performed on infants 3 months or younger to determine the absence or deficiency of T-cells in the body. The T-cells are needed for immunity. With a deficiency or lack of T-cells, the infant cannot fight off viruses, bacteria, or fungus infection.

TORCH Test (TORCH Screen, TORCH Battery, TORCH Titer): TORCH stands for toxoplasma, rubella, cytomegalovirus, and herpes virus. It is used to determine the presence or exposure of a TORCH agent that could cause congenital or neonatal infections, which could result in central nervous system (CNS) impairment. The test identifies past infection, immunity, or recent infection. It can be done on pregnant women as well as newborns and infants. The number of TORCH testings has grown, with more than 20 TORCH kits produced for laboratory and health care providers' use. Accuracy of test results has been questioned, as there is often a variation in TORCH titers.

Trypsin (Feces): Positive in small amounts in the stool.

For a child with cystic fibrosis, the test result is negative at dilution greater than 1:10.

Herpes Simplex Virus-2 (HSV-2) (Serum): Negative or less than 1:10.

Herpes simplex virus-2 (HSV-2) is referred to as genital herpes, which primarily infects the genitourinary tract. HSV-2 is transmitted primarily through sexual contact, and the virus can infect the newborn during vaginal delivery. This can cause neonatal herpes.

Toxoplasmosis Antibody (Serum): No previous infection: less than 1:4.

Congenital form of toxoplasmosis occurs to the fetus when the mother is acutely infected with the *Toxoplasma gondii* (*T. gondii*) during pregnancy and passes the organism via placenta to the unborn child. *T. gondii* is transmitted via raw or poorly cooked meat or by feces from infected cats (litter box).

NURSING IMPLICATIONS WITH RATIONALE

- Explain that the purpose for the laboratory and diagnostic tests is to aid in establishing baseline data regarding previous male or female disease, existing disease, predisposition to disease, or complications in pregnancy.
- Give an explanation (in detail if indicated) about the laboratory and diagnostic procedures. Emphasize the importance of the client's compliance with the test procedure (*see procedures for individual tests in Parts I and II*).
- Assess the client's communication for verbal and/or nonverbal expressions of anxiety or fear concerning tests and/or potential sexual problems.
- Determine if the anxiety level needs to be reduced before the client will be able to absorb information concerning test procedure.
- Encourage expression of feelings through provision of private, calm environment; use quiet, steady speech patterns when interacting; and employ touch if appropriate.
- Be prepared to repeat information to the client and family briefly and clearly if the anxiety or fear level is determined to be high. Attempt not to appear irritated with the client's behavior; plan time to be with the client.
- Answer questions, or refer the questions to appropriate health professionals.
- Check laboratory results, and report the abnormal test findings.

Arthritic, collagen, and infectious and allergic conditions

LABORATORY TESTS

RHEUMATOID ARTHRITIS	LUPUS ERYTHEMATOSUS	INFECTIOUS, ALLERGIC
RA Factor	Lupus Erythematosus (LE) Cells	Bioterrorism Infectious Products
ESR/Sed Rate	ANA (Serum)	Cannabinoid (Urine)
CRP	Anti-DNA	Latex Allergy Testing
Complements C_3, C_4	Complements C_3, C_4	Legionnaire Antibody (Serum)
ASO (Serum)	Cryoglobulins	Lyme Disease Antibody (Serum)
Cryoglobulins (Serum)	RA Factor	Zika Virus
		West Nile Virus Antibodies (Serum & CSF)
Parvovirus B_{19} Antibody	Synovial Fluid Analysis	*Clostridium Difficile* Toxin Assay
Synovial Fluid Analysis	Hydroxyproline (Urine)	
		Fungal Antibody Test
		Allergen-Specific IgE
		Influenza A and B Titer
		HIV OraQuick Tests

Introduction

The majority of laboratory tests for arthritic and collagen disorders are to confirm the diagnosis or progression of rheumatoid arthritis and lupus erythematosus. Several of the same laboratory tests are ordered for both suspected conditions; these tests are complements C_3, C_4, and rheumatoid arthritis (RA) factor; cryoglobulins; and synovial fluid analysis.

New section added is infectious and allergic conditions, which includes tests for Lyme, Legionnaire, and West Nile diseases, and latex allergy testing.

Rheumatoid Arthritis
Laboratory Tests

Rheumatoid Factor (RF), Rheumatoid Arthritis (RA) Factor: *Norms:* Adult: less than 1:20 titer, greater than 1:80 positive for rheumatoid arthritis.

RA factor is a screening test used to detect antiglobulin antibodies in clients with suspected rheumatoid arthritis. It is not uncommon to have positive RA factor test results in clients with collagen diseases (e.g., lupus erythematosus). Approximately 75% of those with rheumatoid arthritis have a positive RA factor. Other tests are needed to confirm diagnosis.

Erythrocyte Sedimentation Rate (ESR, Sed Rate) (Serum): *Norms: (See reference values in Part I.)*

Sed rate, or ESR, is a nonspecific test that usually increases during an acute inflammatory process. Frequently the ESR is elevated in clients with rheumatoid arthritis; however, it is not the most reliable test. C-reactive protein (CRP) test is considered more useful than ESR.

C-Reactive Protein (CRP) (Serum): *Norms:* Not usually present; greater than 1:2 titer considered positive.

CRP is a nonspecific test similar to ESR; however, during an inflammatory process, CRP elevates sooner than ESR and returns to normal faster than ESR. This test is useful in monitoring the progression of rheumatoid arthritis.

Complements C_3 and C_4 (Serum): *Norms:* C_3: Adult: 83–177 mg/dL. C_4: Adult: 15–45 mg/dL.
Both C_3 and C_4 could be slightly elevated in clients with rheumatoid arthritis.

Antistreptolysin O (ASO) (Serum): *Norms:* Adult: less than 100 international unit/mL.
Serum ASO levels can be mildly elevated in clients with rheumatoid arthritis.

Cryoglobulins (Serum): *Norm:* Negative.
Cryoglobulins are proteins that are present in the immunoglobulins IgG and IgM. They may be present in rheumatoid arthritis and also in systemic lupus erythematosus.

Parvovirus B 19 Antibody (Serum): *Norm:* Negative.
A positive parvovirus B 19 has been associated with joint inflammation and joint arthritis.

Synovial Fluid Analysis: Examination of the synovial fluid for rheumatoid factor, complements, leukocytes (white blood cells), and glucose gives additional information about the possibility of the presence of rheumatoid arthritis. In rheumatoid arthritis, synovial fluid analysis could include a positive RA factor, decreased complements because of complement binding, slightly elevated leukocyte count, and decreased glucose level.

Lupus Erythematosus
Laboratory Tests

Lupus Erythematosus (LE) Cell Test: The LE cell test is an in vitro procedure used either to aid in the diagnosis of systemic lupus erythematosus (SLE) or to monitor the treatment for this condition. It is not the most reliable test; however, LE cells can be found in 60–80% of clients with SLE. If it is used for the purpose of diagnosing SLE, then other laboratory tests, such as antinuclear antibodies (ANA) and anti-DNA, should be ordered to confirm SLE.

Antinuclear Antibodies (ANA) (Serum): *Norm:* Negative.
The ANA test for assessing tissue-antigen antibodies is frequently used for diagnosing SLE. A positive titer can indicate SLE; however, other clinical conditions, such as rheumatoid arthritis, scleroderma, myasthenia gravis, and infectious mononucleosis, may have positive titers.

Anti-Deoxyribonucleic Acid (Anti-DNA): Anti-DNA, an antinuclear antibody, is almost always present in SLE and is in lupus nephritis 95% of the time. Anti-DNA values may fluctuate according to the remission and exacerbation of the disease.

Complements C_3 and C_4 (Serum): *Norms:* (*See complements under Rheumatoid Arthritis.*)
C_3 and C_4 of the complement system (group of 11 serum proteins) are measured during acute and/or chronic inflammatory process. In SLE, both serum C_3 and C_4 will be decreased.

Cryoglobulins (Serum): *Norm:* Negative.
Positive cryoglobulin findings may be reported in clients with SLE. Cryoglobulins are also present in other conditions, such as rheumatoid arthritis, multiple myeloma, and leukemia.

Rheumatoid Factor (RF, RA Factor) (Serum): *Norm:* 1:20–1:80 positive for collagen diseases.
Even though RA factor is a serum test used to detect antibodies in clients with rheumatoid arthritis, positive findings are common in clients with collagen disease (e.g., SLE, scleroderma).

Synovial Fluid Analysis: Examination of synovial fluid might reveal positive LE cells and decreased complement levels in patients with SLE.

Hydroxyproline (Urine): Adult: 15–42 mg/24 h, 0.4–4.5mg/2 h. Child: higher than adult.

Urine hydroxyproline levels increase with collagen breakdown such as with bone destruction. Levels are higher at night, in teenagers, and during the third trimester of pregnancy.

Infectious and Allergic Conditions
Laboratory Tests

Bioterrorism Infectious Products Tests: *Norm:* Negative for anthrax, botulism, and smallpox.

These three infectious products may be used in a bioterrorism act. If untreated, the infectious agent could cause death.

Cannabinoid (Marijuana) (Urine): *Norm:* Negative.

Test may require a signed consent form. It is used to check if the client has used marijuana or has marijuana toxicity.

Latex Allergy Testing (Serum): *Norm:* Negative or less than 0.35 international unit/mL based on EIA.

The test is used to determine if the client is allergic to latex products, which could include gloves, urinary catheters, and others.

Allergen-Specific IgE: *Norms:* Adult: <100 international units/mL; Children: neonates to 2 years old: <12 international units/mL; 2–5 years old: <40 international units/mL; 6–12 years old: <90 international units/mL.

An allergen is a substance that the person is allergic to, which causes an increase in IgE. This test is used to identify allergies to substances such as animal dander, foods, pollens, molds, dust, grasses, weeds, trees, insects, drugs, and miscellaneous substances. The person does not have an allergic reaction because the allergen is introduced into the blood sample and not the body.

Influenza A and B titer: *Norm:* Negative titer; <1.8 titer influenza immunization.

There are two main influenza viruses, A and B, that cause most major epidemics every 2–4 years. Virus A has two types and three subtypes of influenza virus. It spreads rapidly to many populations. Virus B is associated with sporadic epidemics mostly among children and young adults. The incubation period of influenza is brief and enters through the respiratory tract. Symptoms are fever, chills, sore throat, cough, muscular pain, GI upset, and headache.

HIV OraQuick Test: This home test is used to detect the presence of HIV in saliva. It has been FDA approved. It is 92% correct in detecting HIV carriers. It can rule out 99% of those who are not carrying the virus.

Legionnaire Antibody (Serum): *Norm:* Negative.

This test is used to diagnose the presence of Legionnaire disease. It is caused by a gram-negative bacillus causing an acute respiratory infection, such as severe, consolidated pneumonia.

Lyme Antibody (Serum): *Norm:* Titer: negative; less than 1:256.

It is used to detect the occurrence of Lyme disease. It is caused by a spirochete, *Borrelia burgdorferi*, that is carried primarily by the deer tick.

West Nile Virus Antibodies (Serum, CSF): *Norm:* Negative for IgM antibodies to flavivirus (10 days after flulike symptoms).

Clostridium Difficile **Toxin Assay (Stool):** *Norm:* Negative.

C. difficile is a gram-positive bacteria that releases necrotizing toxins. This bacteria can occur in the intestine, usually to those who are immunocompromised or those taking broad-spectrum antibiotics.

Fungal Antibody Tests (Serum, Cerebrospinal Fluid): *Norm:* Negative.

Fungal antibody testing detects antibodies present in fungal disease, such as blastomycosis, coccidioidomycosis, and histoplasmosis. This test is not for superficial fungal infections (mycosis) that appear on the skin, hair, or nails.

Zika Virus: *Norm:* Negative.

Zika virus is a mosquito-borne virus (*Aedes aegypti* mosquito) that was first reported in Brazil in 2015 and then in the United States in 2016. This virus can also be transmitted sexually between same and opposite sexes following the *Aedes aegypti* mosquito bite.

NURSING IMPLICATIONS WITH RATIONALE

- Explain the purpose of the laboratory tests.
- Give an explanation concerning the test procedures and the need for the client's compliance. The explanation might be brief or in depth, depending on the client's familiarity with the test.
- Inform the client of any food, fluid, or drug restrictions (*see Part I*).
- Assess urinary output in clients with SLE.
- Assess the client's ability to ambulate. Elicit from the client the times of day when mobility is not as much of a problem.
- Listen to the client's expressed anxiety concerning tests and potential clinical problems. Clarification of test procedures might alleviate fear and anxiety and promote test compliance.
- Be supportive of the client and family members and answer questions or refer the questions to appropriate professionals.

Shock

LABORATORY TESTS

Electrolytes (Serum)
Lactic Acid (Blood)
Anion Gap
Glucose (Blood, Plasma)
Osmolality (Serum)
CBC (Hgb, Hct, WBC, Platelets)
Type and Crossmatch (T&C) CT
ABGs
Enzymes (Cardiac)
BUN
Creatinine (Serum)
Protein (Total) (Serum)
Fibrin Degradation Products (Serum)
Euglobulin Lysis Time (Plasma)
PT and PTT
Urinalysis (Specific Gravity)
Urine Electrolytes

DIAGNOSTIC TESTS

ECG/EKG
Central Venous Pressure (CVP)
Pulmonary Arterial Pressure (PAP) and Pulmonary Capillary
  Wedge Pressure (PCWP)
X-rays, Chest or Abdominal
Computed Tomography (CT)

Introduction

Laboratory and diagnostic assessment of shock is extremely important for evaluation and management of shock syndrome. Laboratory studies, ordered immediately, usually include electrolytes, lactic acid/lactate, glucose, osmolality, complete blood count (CBC), type and crossmatch, and arterial blood gases. Other laboratory tests used to determine the state and progression of shock include serum enzymes, especially if cardiogenic shock is likely, blood urea nitrogen, creatinine, total protein, prothrombin time, and urine electrolytes. Diagnostic tests performed to determine cardiac and circulatory status are electrocardiogram (ECG), central venous pressure (CVP) or pulmonary arterial pressure (PAP), and x-ray. Later, computed tomography might be ordered.

Laboratory Tests

Electrolytes (Serum): Serum electrolytes—potassium, sodium, and calcium—are closely monitored during shock. Changes in electrolytes can occur quickly, such as in the levels of potassium and sodium. Table 3.17 shows the electrolytes associated with shock, with reasons for their decreases and increases.

Lactic Acid, Lactate (Blood): *Norm:* Adult: 0.5–2 mmol/L, 5–20 mg/dL.

Elevated blood lactic acid is related to cellular hypoxia. In shock, lactic acid/lactate levels increase greatly and quickly, greater than 5 mmol/L or greater than 25 mg/dL, before blood pressure (BP) falls and urine output decreases. Lactic acidosis occurs when blood lactic acid level is greater than 2.5 mmol/L or greater than 25 mg/dL. As lactic acid level increases, cells need more oxygen.

TABLE 3.17 Electrolyte Changes

ELECTROLYTE (SERUM)	REFERENCE VALUES	COMMENTS
Potassium (K)	3.5–5.3 mEq/L	During shock, potassium leaves the cells because of tissue injury and hypoxia. If urinary output is adequate, potassium is excreted by the kidneys, thus causing a serum potassium loss, or hypokalemia. If kidney shutdown occurs during shock, potassium builds up in the vascular fluid, causing serum potassium excess, or hyperkalemia.
Sodium (Na)	135–145 mEq/L	Serum sodium level can be normal, decreased, or elevated. During cellular damage, potassium shifts out of the cells and sodium shifts in, contributing to the serum sodium loss, or hyponatremia. Also, in massive tissue injury, sodium goes to the injured site. If the client is receiving liters of saline solutions and kidney shutdown occurs, serum sodium level is increased and hypernatremia occurs.
Calcium (Ca)	4.5–5.5 mEq/L	With massive tissue damage, calcium leaves the extracellular fluid and accumulates at the injured site, causing serum calcium deficit, or hypocalcemia. A calcium loss will increase cellular permeability, thus permitting electrolyte and fluid loss from cells.
Ionizing Calcium (iCa)	4.4–5 mg/dL, 2.2–2.5 mEq/L	Only ionized calcium can be used by the body. A decrease in iCa leads to tetany symptoms or neuromuscular irritability.
Chloride (Cl)	95–105 mEq/L	Chloride combines with sodium and potassium, and as these cations are lost, so is chloride. Result is hypochloremia.

Anion Gap: *Norm:* 10–17 mEq/L.

Anion gap is an interrelationship between serum electrolytes in determining metabolic acid–base imbalances. An elevated anion gap greater than 17 mEq/L is indicative of metabolic acidosis, a complication of shock. The formula for calculating anion gap is as follows:

$$(sodium + potassium) - (chloride + CO_2) = mEq/L$$

Glucose (Blood, Plasma): *Norms:* Adult: Blood: 60–100 mg/dL. Plasma: 70–110 mg/dL. Child: 60–100 mg/dL. Newborn: 30–80 mg/dL.

During acute trauma and shock, blood/plasma glucose levels could rise to 200 mg/dL. After correction of shock, hypoglycemia could result. An elevated glucose level occurs as the result of an increase in epinephrine and steroid response because of tissue damage.

Osmolality (Serum): *Norms:* Adult: 280–300 mOsm/kg. Child: 270–290 mOsm/kg.

Serum osmolality is an indicator of body fluid concentration, mainly the vascular fluid. If shock is due to massive fluid loss, serum osmolality is increased, and fluid replacement is necessary. Care should be taken not to administer massive fluids for mild shock, because overhydration could result. In overhydration, a low serum osmolality occurs.

Complete Blood Count (Blood): Abnormal hematology values in hemoglobin (Hgb/Hb), hematocrit (Hct), white blood cell count, and platelet count can occur in shock. Therefore, a CBC is taken in early shock and is monitored for changes during treatment and recovery. Table 3.18 shows the changes that can occur with these four blood values in shock.

Type and Crossmatch (T&C): Although the method for type and crossmatch is more expedient today, blood sample for T&C should be obtained immediately when blood loss and shock are determined.

TABLE 3.18 Complete Blood Count

HEMATOLOGY	REFERENCE VALUES	COMMENTS
Hgb	Male: 13.5–18 g/dL Female: 12–16 g/dL Child: 11–16 g/dL	Hemoglobin levels decrease after hemorrhage, but change may not occur until hours later.
Hct	Male: 40–54% Female: 36–46%	Hematocrit is an effective indicator of body fluid volume. If shock is due to a large fluid loss, increased hematocrit level occurs because of hemoconcentration. It usually takes 4–8 hours for the hematocrit to increase after fluid loss.
WBC	Adult: 5,000–10,000 µL Child, 2 years old: 6,000–17,000 µL	If WBC levels are slightly increased, the change could be due to tissue damage. If levels are markedly increased, the change could be due to infection.
Platelet count	Adult: 150,000–400,000 µL	Platelet count is monitored during and after blood loss and acute trauma. A low platelet count, thrombocytopenia, will cause bleeding. If platelet count is markedly decreased, hemorrhage might occur. Shock is intensified.

Arterial Blood Gases: *Norms:* Adult: pH: 7.35–7.45; $PaCO_2$: 35–45 mm Hg; PaO_2: 75–100 mm Hg; HCO_3: 24–28 mEq/L; BE: +2 or –2.

In shock, ABGs are helpful in evaluating respiratory and metabolic status. Normally metabolic acidosis occurs in shock as the result of tissue breakdown (release of acid metabolites from cells). Indicators of acidosis are pH less than 7.35, HCO_3 less than 24 mEq/L, PCO_2 of greater than 45 mm Hg. If the pH is less than 7.35 and the HCO_3 is less than 24 mEq/L, *metabolic* acidosis is present. If the pH is less than 7.35 and the $PaCO_2$ is greater than 45 mm Hg, *respiratory* acidosis is present.

Enzymes:CPK/CK, LDH/ID, AST/SGOT (Serum): *Norms:* (*See individual reference values in Part I.*)

Cardiac enzyme levels are obtained when cardiac damage is suspected and in cardiogenic shock. After a myocardial infarction, serum CPK/CK rises first, then serum AST/SGOT, and last LDH/ID.

Blood Urea Nitrogen: *Norm:* Adult: 5–25 mg/dL.

BUN should be assessed during shock. A BUN of 30–40 mg/dL could be indicative of fluid loss and dehydration. If the BUN is greater than 50 mg/dL and does not decrease substantially with the administration of IV fluids, kidney damage is highly suspected. Renal insufficiency or failure can result from prolonged shock.

Creatinine (Serum): *Norms:* Adult: 0.5–1.5 mg/dL. Older child: 0.4–1.2 mg/dL. Infant to 6 years: 0.3–0.6 mg/dL.

The laboratory test most effective in evaluating kidney function is serum creatinine. As kidney function diminishes, serum creatinine level rises. Creatinine level greater than 3 mg/dL is indicative of kidney disorder.

Protein (Total) (Serum): Total protein count is composed mostly of albumin and globulins. With severe body fluid loss, elevated serum protein (total) level could be present because of hemoconcentration.

Fibrin Degradation Products (FDP) (Serum): *Norm:* Adult: 2–10 mcg/mL.

FDP test indicates the activity of the fibrinolytic system. This test is performed when the client is hemorrhaging following a severe injury. An elevated FDP, greater than 10 mcg/mL, is usually indicative of disseminated intravascular coagulation (DIC).

Euglobulin Lysis Time (Plasma): *Norm:* No lysis.

This test measures the fibrinogen activity by measuring the interval between clot formation and euglobulin precipitation. If clot lysis is less than 1 hour, pathologic fibrinolysis is occurring.

Prothrombin Time and Partial Thromboplastin Time (Plasma): *Norms:* Adult: PT: 11–15 seconds; PTT: 60–70 seconds.

PT and PTT are ordered to evaluate clotting time. With prolonged PT and PTT times, bleeding can occur. These levels are usually monitored during shock.

Urinalysis/Specific Gravity (SG): In shock, clients frequently have a Foley catheter inserted, and so urine specific gravity can easily be checked. A specific gravity greater than 1.026 is indicative of fluid volume deficit (dehydration). In certain renal diseases (e.g., glomerulonephritis, polynephritis), the specific gravity is less than 1.005.

Urine Electrolytes (Potassium and Sodium): *Norms: Norm:* Adult: Potassium: 40–80 mEq/L/24 h (average). Sodium: 40–220 mEq/L/24 h.

In renal failure, the urine potassium and sodium levels could be increased (chronic failure) or decreased (acute failure). Urine electrolytes are frequently monitored.

Diagnostic Tests

Electrocardiography (ECG/EKG): ECG can detect cardiac changes occurring prior to or following shock. It is performed immediately in suspected cardiogenic shock.

Central Venous Pressure: *Norms:* Adult: 4–10 cm of H_2O.

CVP is monitored during shock to determine fluid imbalance. A decreased CVP is indicative of hypovolemia (fluid volume deficit), and an increased CVP is indicative of hypervolemia (fluid volume excess). As an indicator of left ventricular pressure, CVP is not as accurate as pulmonary arterial pressure (PAP) but is considered safer and accompanied by fewer complications.

Pulmonary Arterial Pressure (PAP) and Pulmonary Capillary Wedge Pressure (PCWP): *Norms:* Adult: PAP: 10–20 mm Hg mean, 20–30 mm Hg systolic, 10–15 mm Hg diastolic; PCWP: 4–12 mm Hg mean.

PAP indicates the pulmonary blood volume and the pulmonary vascular resistance. A low PAP is indicative of fluid volume deficit (hypovolemia) or vasodilation, and an elevated PAP is indicative of fluid volume overload or increased pulmonary vascular resistance, possibly due to pulmonary embolism. A decreased PCWP is indicative of fluid volume deficit (hypovolemia). An elevated PCWP can occur in fluid volume overload (hypervolemia) because of excess IV fluids or because of increased preload from fluid retention in cardiac failure. Increased afterload, vascular resistance to left ventricular ejection, will also increase PCWP.

X-rays: Chest or abdominal x-rays at a suspected trauma site might be helpful in detecting cause of shock.

Computed Tomography: Emergency CT might be ordered to determine cause of shock.

NURSING IMPLICATIONS WITH RATIONALE

- Explain the purpose of the laboratory and diagnostic tests briefly to the client and family members. A detailed explanation during a crisis might not be appropriate.
- Obtain a blood sample collection and send it to the laboratory immediately. Check that results are returned and report abnormal results.
- Monitor the client's intake and output and vital signs before and after laboratory and diagnostic tests and at specified times. Report changes immediately.
- Listen to the client's and family members' expressed anxiety and/or fear concerning the tests and the client's outcome from trauma.
- Assess for excess bleeding and apply pressure if appropriate. Report changes.
- Be supportive of the client and family members during and after the crisis.

Neoplastic conditions

LABORATORY TESTS

ADH (Serum)
ACTH (Plasma)
Bence-Jones Protein (Urine)
Bilirubin (Serum)
Breast Cancer Genetic Testing (Blood)
Breast Cancer Tumor Prognostic Markers
Bladder Cancer/Tumor Markers
Calcitonin (Serum)
Calcium (Serum)
Cancer Tumor Markers
Carcinoembryonic Antigen (Blood, Plasma)
Catecholamines (Plasma)
Ceruloplasmin (Serum)
Cold Agglutinins (Serum)
Complements C_3, C_4 (Serum)
Copper (Serum)
Cortisol (Plasma)
C-Reactive Protein (Serum)
Cryoglobulins (Serum)
Cytology: sputum, gastric washing, colon, pleural
    fluid, bronchial secretions, urine, Pap smear, CSF
Enzymes: ACP, ALP, ALT/SGPT, AST/SGOT, GGT, LD/
    LDH, LAP
ESR, Sed Rate (Blood)
Estradiol (E_2) (Serum)
Estrogen/Total (Serum and Urine)
FSH (Serum and Urine)
Gastrin (Serum)
Haptoglobin (Serum)
Hormones
HCG (Serum, Urine)
5-HIAA (Urine)
Human Papilloma Virus
Immunoglobins (Serum)
17-KS (Urine)
LH (Serum)
Melanin (Urine)
Occult Blood (Feces)
PTH
PTT (Plasma)
Platelet Count (Blood)
Pregnanediol (Urine)
Pregnanetriol (Urine)
Prolactin (Serum)
PSA (Serum)
Protein Electrophoresis (Serum)
Renin (Plasma)

DIAGNOSTIC TESTS

X-rays: chest, bone, GI series, barium enema, IVP,
    bronchography
Mammography
Thermography (Breast)
Lymphangiography
Endoscopy: bronchoscopy, esophagogastroscopy,
    sigmoidoscopy, colonoscopy, colposcopy,
    cystoscopy, ERCP
Electronystagmography
Thoracoscopy
Ultrasonography/Ultrasound
Nuclear Scans
Monoclonal Antibodies for Colon and Ovarian
    Cancers
Computed Tomography (CT)
Angiography/Arteriography
Biopsy
Bone Marrow Aspiration
MRI
Endoscopic Ultrasound (EUS)
Mammary Ductoscopy

LABORATORY TESTS	DIAGNOSTIC TESTS

Serotonin (Plasma)
Testosterone (Serum)
Thyroid Antibodies (Serum)
Uric Acid (Serum)
WBC/Leukocytes (Blood)

Introduction

Numerous laboratory and diagnostic tests are performed to identify and to confirm the presence of cancer (i.e., carcinomas, sarcomas, leukemias, lymphomas). One test only is not sufficient to diagnose cancer. Although most laboratory tests are ordered to determine the function of body organs and glands, there are many elevated and decreased test values associated with cancer. Usually diagnostic tests are necessary to confirm cancer site and diagnosis. In this section, abnormal laboratory values, elevated or decreased, as they relate to cancer are given instead of the norms for the test. Laboratory tests are arranged in alphabetic order. Refer to Part I for the reference values of these laboratory tests.

A summarized chart of laboratory and diagnostic tests used for diagnosing specific cancers follows the brief description of the tests.

Laboratory Tests

Antidiuretic Hormone (Serum): ADH may be elevated, greater than 5 pg/mL in syndrome of secretion of inappropriate antidiuretic hormone (SIADH) as a result of ectopic secretion by bronchogenic carcinoma.

Adrenocorticotropic Hormone (Plasma): Decreased plasma ACTH could occur in clients with cancer of the adrenal gland, and elevated plasma ACTH could occur in clients with pituitary tumor. ACTH could be elevated with any tumor that secretes ACTH ectopically (e.g., bronchogenic carcinoma).

Bence-Jones Protein (Urine): Increased Bence-Jones protein greater than 1 mg/dL is commonly found in the urine of clients with multiple myeloma, and increased levels are also associated with metastatic carcinoma, bone cancer, and leukemia.

Bilirubin: Total (Serum): Elevated serum total bilirubin greater than 1.2 mg/dL could occur in clients with tumors of the liver or liver metastasis. Elevated bilirubin level could occur in pancreatic carcinoma secondary to common duct obstruction.

Bladder Cancer/Tumor Markers: Urine: BTA: Negative to less than 13 units/mL; NMP 22: negative to less than 9 units/mL.

Bladder tumor antigen (BTA) and nuclear matrix protein 22 (NMP 22) are antigens/proteins produced by the bladder tumor cells that can be obtained from the urine.

Breast Cancer Genetic Testing (BRCA-1, BRCA-2) (Blood): *Norm:* Negative.

Positive BRCA-1 or BRCA-2 is predisposition to breast and ovarian cancers. Approximately 20–22% of families have members that have inherited the BRCA-1 or BRCA-2 gene.

Breast Cancer Tumor Prognostic Markers: *Norm:* See values in the text.

ER assay, DNA ploidy, S-phase fraction, cathepsin D, Her-2/neu oncoprotein, and p53 protein are cancer markers that can predict if more extensive therapy is needed to treat the presence of breast cancer.

Calcitonin (Hct) (Serum): A high serum calcitonin level, greater than 2,000 pg/mL, indicates thyroid medullary carcinoma.

Calcium (Serum): Hypercalcemia, elevated serum calcium level greater than 5.5 mEq/L or greater than 11 mg/dL, occurs in 10–20% of all cancer clients. Metastatic tumors can cause bone destruction, which elevates the serum calcium level. Common causes of hypercalcemia are metastatic breast cancer, multiple myeloma, ectopic secretion of parathyroid hormone, and bony metastasis.

Cancer Tumor Markers (CA 15-3, CA 19-9, CA 27.29, CA 50, CA 125. CA 549): *Norm:* See values in text.

These markers are used primarily to screen and diagnose the presence of possible cancer, to monitor the response of cancer treatment, and to determine the recurrence of cancer. CA 549 is a new marker to detect breast cancer recurrence and to monitor the response to treatment of breast cancer.

Carcinoembryonic Antigen (Blood, Plasma): CEA has been extracted from tumors in the gastrointestinal tract. CEA has been frequently found in clients with cancer of the large intestine and pancreas. Plasma CEA might be elevated in other cancers (e.g., esophagus, stomach, lung, breast, bladder, kidney, cervix, testes, and leukemia). CEA is used to evaluate the effectiveness of cancer therapies and to monitor clients in remission for early signs of recurrence. CEA will be increased before clinical symptoms are evident.

Catecholamines (Plasma): *(See Plasma Catecholamine in Part I.) Epinephrine:* Supine: less than 50 pg/mL. *Norepinephrine:* Supine: 110–410 pg/mL.

Fractional analysis of catecholamine levels is helpful for identifying certain adrenal medullary tumors.

Ceruloplasmin (Cp) (Serum): Cp is produced in the liver and binds with copper. An elevated serum ceruloplasmin level, greater than 50 mg/dL, could occur in clients with cancer of the bone, stomach, or lung and in clients with Hodgkin disease.

Cold Agglutinins (CA) (Serum): Elevated serum CA, greater than 1:16–1:32, might be present in lymphatic leukemia and multiple myeloma.

Complements C_3, C_4 (Serum): Elevated serum C_3 and C_4 could be found with malignant neoplasms of the esophagus, stomach, colon, rectum, pancreas, lungs, breast, cervix, ovary, prostate, and bladder.

Copper (Cu) (Serum): Elevated serum copper levels, greater than 140 mcg/dL in males and greater than 155 mcg/dL in females, might be present in cancer of the bone, stomach, large intestine, liver, and lung, and in Hodgkin disease and leukemias.

Cortisol (Plasma): Plasma cortisol level could be elevated with cancer of the adrenal gland.

C-Reactive Protein (CRP) (Serum): Positive CRP titer might occur with cancer of the breast with metastasis. Clients with Hodgkin disease might also have positive CRP titer.

Cryoglobulins (Serum): Positive cryoglobulin findings might be present in clients having Hodgkin disease, lymphocytic leukemia, or multiple myeloma.

Cytology: Cells that have been sloughed from neoplasms/tumors can be found in body secretions. These secretions are obtained from sputum, gastric washing, colon, pleural fluid, bronchial tract, urine, Pap smear, and cerebrospinal fluid (CSF) for cytologic examination.

Enzymes: When cancer affects organs that produce enzymes, enzyme values are checked. The enzyme *acid phosphatase (ACP)* is plentiful in the prostate gland, and an elevated serum ACP level usually indicates carcinoma of the prostate gland. If ACP is markedly elevated, metastasis to the bone is suspected. Also, elevated serum ACP can be associated with multiple myeloma and Paget disease. The enzyme *alkaline phosphatase (ALP)*, produced by the bone and liver, is usually elevated in clients with cancer of the bone and liver. An elevated ALP might occur in clients with multiple myeloma. *Alanine aminotransferase (ALT/SGPT)* and *aspartate aminotransferase*

(AST/SGOT) might be noted in clients with cancer of the liver. *Gamma-glutamyl (transpepti-dase) transferase (GGT)* could be elevated in cancer of the liver, kidney, pancreas, prostate, breast, lung, and brain. Elevated *lactic dehydrogenase (LD/LDH)* might occur in clients with cancer of the lung, bone, intestines, liver, breast, cervix, testes, kidney, stomach, and melanoma of the skin. Serum LDH could be elevated in acute leukemia. *Leucine aminopeptidase (LAP)* is an enzyme produced by the liver. Elevated serum LAP could indicate cancer of the liver.

Erythrocyte Sedimentation Rate (ESR, Sed Rate) (Blood): Clients with Hodgkin disease, multiple myeloma, and lymphosarcoma might have increased ESR.

Estradiol (E_2) (Serum): E_2 is useful in evaluating gonadal dysfunction. Elevated E_2 level in female, greater than 500 pg/mL, may be present in ovarian tumor, and elevated E_2 level in male, greater than 50 pg/mL, can indicate a testicular tumor.

Estrogen/Total (Serum and Urine-24-Hour): An elevated serum or urine estrogen test might indicate adrenocortical tumor, ovarian tumor, or some testicular tumor.

Follicle-Stimulating Hormone (FSH) (Serum and Urine): Decreased serum and urine FSH, less than 4 milli-unit/mL (serum), or 4 international unit/24 h (urine), could indicate tumor of the adrenal gland, testes, or ovary. Increased level could indicate FSH-producing pituitary tumor.

Gastrin (Serum): Elevated serum gastrin level, greater than 200 pg/mL, might be present in clients with malignant neoplasm of the stomach.

Haptoglobin (Serum): Elevated haptoglobin level, greater than 270 mg/dL, might be found in clients with cancer of the lung, large intestine, stomach, breast, or liver, and in clients with Hodgkin disease.

Hormones: Any hormone may be elevated with cancer, because many cancers secrete inappropriate hormones (ectopic hormone secretion) in response to bizarre differentiation of cancer cells.

Human Chorionic Gonadotropin (Serum, Urine): Usually positive HCG levels indicate pregnancy, but they might indicate hydatidiform mole or choriocarcinoma.

Human Papilloma Virus (HPV) (Cervical Specimen): *Norm:* Negative.

HPV has been the primary cause of cervical cancer. Some types of HPV do not progress to cancer. HPV testing may be obtained during the Pap procedure. High-risk strains HPV 16 and HPV 18 are the most carcinogenic and most prevalent to cervical cancer. Gardasil is a vaccine for all females and males ages 11 to 26 for preventing HPV.

5-Hydroxyindolacetic Acid (5-HIAA) (Urine): Elevated urine 5-HIAA, 10–100 mg/24 h, could indicate carcinoid tumors of the appendix and intestine. Usually these carcinoid tumor cells, which secrete excess serotonin, are of low-grade malignancy. When metastasis occurs, 5-HIAA could be greater than 100 mg/24 h. Food and certain drugs could give false-positive results. Several random or spot urine specimens should be tested.

Immunoglobulins (Ig) (Serum): Clients with lymphocytic leukemia could have decreased serum IgG, IgA, IgM levels. Clients with lymphosarcoma might have an increased IgM level.

17-Ketosteroids (17-KS) (Urine): Elevated urine 17-KS, greater than 25 mg/24 h (male), greater than 15 mg/24 h (female), could be associated with neoplasms of the adrenal gland, testes, and ovary.

Luteinizing Hormone (LH) (Serum): In pituitary and testicular tumors, LH is elevated.

Melanin (Urine): This test is to verify the presence or progression of a melanoma. With metastatic melanoma, melanin metabolites are usually found in high concentration in the urine.

Occult Blood (Feces): Hidden blood in the stools could indicate cancer in the upper or lower GI tract. Orthotoluidine (Occultest) is considered more sensitive than the guaiac test.

Parathyroid Hormone: PTH is secreted ectopically by many carcinomas (e.g., squamous cell lung cancer [most common cause], renal carcinoma, pancreatic carcinoma, and ovarian carcinoma). Also, PTH might be elevated in parathyroid carcinoma.

Partial Thromboplastin Time (Plasma): Increased PTT could be present in clients with myelocytic and monocytic leukemias.

Platelet Count (Blood): Decreased platelet count, less than 100,000 mm^3, may occur in clients with cancer of the bone, gastrointestinal tract, and brain, and in multiple myeloma, lymphatic, myelocytic, and monocytic leukemias. An elevated platelet count, greater than 400,000 mm^3, might occur in metastatic carcinoma. Many types of chemotherapy cause temporary thrombocytopenia.

Pregnanediol (Urine): Elevated urine pregnanediol, greater than 7 mg/24 h, may be present in choriocarcinoma of the ovary.

Pregnanetriol (Urine): Malignant neoplasm of the adrenal gland may have an elevated urine pregnanetriol, greater than 2.4 mg/24 h.

Prolactin (PRL) (Serum): In nonpregnant women and in men, an elevated prolactin level could indicate pituitary adenoma.

Prostate-Specific Antigen (PSA) Serum: *Norm:* 0–4 ng/mL.

PSA is slightly elevated in benign prostatic hypertrophy, 4–10 ng/mL; and in prostatic cancer the PSA level is greatly increased, 10–120 ng/mL.

Protein Electrophoresis (Serum): The following cancerous conditions could be reflected in protein fractions.

PROTEIN	DECREASED LEVEL	ELEVATED LEVEL
Albumin	Leukemia	
	Liver cancer (primary or metastatic)	
Globulin		
β	Lymphocytic leukemia	Malignant hypertensive
γ	Lymphosarcoma	Hodgkin disease
		Chronic lymphocytic leukemia
		Multiple myeloma

Renin (Plasma): Clients with cancer of the kidney may have an elevated plasma renin level.

Serotonin (Plasma): *Norm:* 50–175 ng/mL.

The primary purpose of this test is to confirm the diagnosis of carcinoid tumors of the argentaffin cells in the gastrointestinal tract. Ectopic production of serotonin can result from oat cell carcinoma of the lung, pancreatic tumors, and thyroid cancer.

Testosterone (Serum): Increased testosterone in women after menopause can be caused by malignant neoplasm of the breast.

Thyroid Antibodies (TA) (Serum): Elevated serum TA titer could indicate carcinoma of the thyroid gland.

Uric Acid (Serum): Elevated serum-uric acid, greater than 7.8 mg/dL, could occur in clients having lymphocytic, myelocytic, and monocytic leukemias, multiple myeloma, and in metastatic cancer (due to tumor lysis syndrome).

White Blood Cells/Leukocytes (Blood): An elevated total WBC count is frequently present in lymphocytic, myelocytic, and monocytic leukemias. A differential WBC count is ordered to determine the cause of disease. With an elevated lymphocyte count, the disease entities could be chronic lymphocytic leukemia, Hodgkin disease, or multiple myeloma. In monocytic leukemia, the monocyte count could be elevated. It is not uncommon to see the neutrophil count increased in myelocytic leukemia and Hodgkin disease. Leukocytes may be decreased in many forms of cancer (immunosuppression occurs by unknown mechanism). Chemotherapy and radiation frequently cause severe, temporary, decreased WBCs.

Diagnostic Tests

X-rays: X-rays are taken of various organs when malignant neoplasms and metastasis are suspected. Chest and bone x-rays are used to detect neoplasm in the lung and bone metastasis. Procedural x-rays taken of body organs include GI series, barium enema, intravenous pyelography, and bronchography.

Mammography: This is an x-ray examination of the breasts to detect cysts and tumors. Malignant tumors are irregular and poorly defined. They tend to be unilateral.

Thermography (Breast): Breast tumors cause increased metabolism, resulting in vascularity and increased breast-surface temperature. This test is used as a screening test; other diagnostic procedures are necessary to confirm breast cancer.

Mammary Ductoscopy: A mammary ductoscopy is performed for women who have complaints of nipple discharge. Most breast cancers begin in the cells of the breast milk ducts. A ductoscope is passed into the breast nipple. With water injected and a camera light, it can identify abnormal cells and those that are at the beginning stages of cancer.

Lymphangiography, Lymphangiogram: This test is an x-ray examination of the lymphatic system (i.e., lymphatic vessels and lymph nodes). It is used to identify lymphoma (e.g., Hodgkin disease) and metastasis to the lymph nodes. Lymphangiogram should not be performed on clients who are highly allergic to iodinated dye.

Electronystagmography (ENG): This test helps to determine if the problem or abnormality that occurs is in the brain stem or temporal lobe of the cerebral cortex, for example a brain stem lesion.

Endoscopy: Endoscopes, rigid (metal) or flexible fiberoptic, are used for direct visualization of body organs and body cavities to detect any abnormalities. The endoscopes are named for the organ that they are designed to view (e.g., colonoscope [colon], gastroscope [stomach], bronchoscope [lungs], cystoscope [bladder], colposcope [vagina and cervix]). The following endoscopic examinations are performed to detect neoplasms of the lung: bronchoscopy and mediastinoscopy; the esophagus and stomach: esophagogastroscopy; the colon: colonoscopy; the duodenum and pancreas: endoscopic retrograde cholangiopancreatography; the rectum and sigmoid: sigmoidoscopy; the vagina and cervix: colposcopy; and the bladder: cystoscopy. Peritoneoscopy is helpful in observing the peritoneum for effectiveness of treatment and recurrence of metastasis.

Thoracoscopy: This test can detect pleural or lung tumors and metastatic cancer in the lung or pleura area.

Ultrasonography, Ultrasound, Echography: This noninvasive test records echoes of sound from tissues of different densities. It is useful in detecting neoplasms of the brain, kidney, liver, pancreas, spleen, and thyroid. However, positive findings need to be confirmed by other diagnostic tests.

Nuclear Scans, Radioisotope Scan, Radionuclide Imaging: Nuclear scanning using radioactive isotopes or radionuclides is used to detect primary or metastatic cancer. If the radionuclide concentrates in the tumor, the involved area will show up as a dark spot or hot spot on the scintigram.

But if the tumor does not concentrate the radionuclide, then a light-colored area or cold spot is recorded. Radioisotope scans are useful for detecting metastatic tumor of the bone, tumors of the brain, lung, liver, spleen, and thyroid gland.

Monoclonal Antibodies for Colon and Ovarian Cancers: The radionuclide indium 111 is used to identify colon or ovarian cancer cells in areas of the body. The monoclonal 111 antibodies attach to the cancer cells, which can be detected with the use of a gamma camera.

Computed Tomography: CT is effective for detecting tumors of the brain, lung, liver, kidney, pancreas, and adrenals.

Angiography, Arteriography: Angiography is an examination of arteries leading to organs. This test is useful for detecting abnormal vascularization resulting from tumors. Cerebral angiography identifies brain tumors by the increased vascularization; pulmonary angiography can detect tumors of the lung; and renal angiography can identify kidney tumors.

Biopsy: Biopsy, excision of tissue, is a direct method for diagnosing cancer. Tissue specimens for microscopic examination can be obtained from the lung, liver, kidney, bone, thyroid, lymph nodes, skin, and bone marrow.

Bone Marrow Aspiration: Examination of the bone marrow detects abnormal cells. It is a useful test for diagnosing leukemias, lymphomas, and multiple myelomas.

Magnetic Resonance Imaging: MRI can detect small, primary, or metastatic tumors. It can distinguish solid masses from vascular structures better than CT. It is helpful in evaluating recurrent or residual masses. MRI is useful in supplementing CT.

Endoscopic Ultrasound (EUS): *Norm:* No irregular borders.

EUS is an imaging technique that allows fine visualization of structures outside the GI tract. This technique is mostly utilized for early detection of cancer, staging of cancer, and visualization of the biliary tree.

A summary of laboratory and diagnostic tests used in diagnosing cancer is outlined in Table 3.19.

TABLE 3.19 Tests Used to Diagnose Specific Cancers

CANCER	LABORATORY TESTS	DIAGNOSTIC TESTS
Leukemias	Bence-Jones protein CEA Cold agglutinins Cryoglobulins PTT Platelet count Protein fraction Uric acid WBC	Bone marrow aspiration/biopsy
Hodgkin disease	Ceruloplasmin Copper CRP Cryoglobulins ESR Haptoglobin Protein fraction WBC	Lymphangiography Lymph node biopsy Mediastinoscopy

CANCER	LABORATORY TESTS	DIAGNOSTIC TESTS
Multiple myelomas	Bence-Jones protein Calcium Cold agglutinins Enzymes: ACP, ALP Cryoglobulins ESR Melanin Platelet count Protein fraction Uric acid WBC	Bone marrow aspiration/biopsy
Stomach	CEA Ceruloplasmin C_3, C_4 Enzyme: LDH Copper Gastrin Haptoglobin	GI series Esophagogastroscopy
Colon	CEA C_3, C_4 Copper Enzyme: LDH Haptoglobin 5-HIAA Occult stool	Barium enema Colonoscopy Sigmoidoscopy ERCP Biopsy
Kidney, Bladder	C_3, C_4 Enzymes: GGTP, LDH Renin Bladder Cancer/Tumore Markers	IVP Cystoscopy Ultrasound Nuclear scan CT Angiography Biopsy
Lung	ADH ACTH Calcium CEA Ceruloplasmin Copper Cytology Enzymes: GGTP, LDH Haptoglobin	Bronchography Bronchoscopy Nuclear scan CT Angiography Mediastinoscopy Chest x-ray MRI Thoracoscopy
Liver	Bilirubin Ceruloplasmin Copper Enzymes: ALP, LAP, ALT/SGPT, AST/SGOT, GGTP Haptoglobin	Ultrasound Nuclear scan CT Biopsy EUS

(Continued)

TABLE 3.19 (Continued)

CANCER	LABORATORY TESTS	DIAGNOSTIC TESTS
Reproductive	Calcium CEA C_3, C_4 CRP Enzymes: ACP, GGTP Estradiol Estrogen FSH HCG 17-KS LH Pap smear Pregnanediol Testosterone	Mammography Thermography Colposcopy Biopsy Peritoneoscopy Mammary ductoscopy
Bone	Bence-Jones protein Calcium Ceruloplasmin Copper Enzymes: ALP, LDH	X-ray Biopsy
Brain	Enzyme: GGTP	Ultrasound Nuclear scan CT MRI Angiography Electronystagmography
Endocrine	ACTH Calcitonin Cortisol FSH 17-KS LH Pregnanetriol Prolactin Thyroid antibodies	Ultrasound Nuclear scan CT Biopsy

NURSING IMPLICATIONS WITH RATIONALE

- Explain the purpose for the laboratory and diagnostic tests.
- Provide a detailed explanation concerning the test procedures and the need for client's compliance. The explanation might be brief or in depth, depending on the client's familiarity with the test.
- Inform the client of any food, fluid, or drug restrictions. Each test should be checked for specific restrictions (*see Parts I and II*).
- Obtain specimen collection at specific times according to the procedures.
- Elicit from the client, or family members, client history and information about any allergies, especially to contrast medium (dye), iodine, or seafood.
- Monitor intake and output and vital signs before and after laboratory and diagnostic tests.

- Listen to the client's expressed anxiety or fear concerning the tests and potential clinical problems. Clarification of the test procedure might alleviate fear and anxiety and promote compliance. Assess communications for verbal or nonverbal expression of anxiety and fear.
- Assess the client's discomfort by eliciting from him or her the intensity, duration, and location of pain. Provide pain relief using positional changes and medication.
- Observe for bleeding caused by decreased platelet count and treatment regimen.
- Check laboratory results, and report the abnormal test results.
- Provide support to the client and family members during test procedure, treatment regimen, and in response to expressed fear and anxiety about physical condition and outcome.
- Repeat information to the client and family briefly and clearly if anxiety and/or fear level is determined to be high.

Hematologic conditions

LABORATORY TESTS

Complete Blood Count (CBC)
  RBC Count
  Hb (Hgb)
  Hct
  RBC Indices: MCV, MCH, MCHC, RDW
  WBC Count
  Differential WBC Count
Platelet Count
Platelet Aggregation
Platelet Antibody Test
Reticulocyte Count
Hb Electrophoresis
Erythrocyte Osmotic Fragility
Bleeding Time (Blood)
Coagulation Time (Blood)
Clot Retraction (Blood)
Fetal Hemoglobin
Fibrinogen (Plasma)
Fibrin Degradation Products (Serum)
Euglobulin Lysis Time
DIC Screening Tests
D-Dimer Test
Antineutrophil Cytoplasmic Antibody (ANCA)
Antithrombin III (Plasma)
Plasminogen (Plasma)

PT (Plasma)
PTT and APTT (Plasma)
Factors Assay (Coagulation Factors)
Blood Typing
Bone Marrow Aspiration
Lymph Node Biopsy
G-6-PD (Blood)
Haptoglobin (Serum)
Methemoglobin
Coomb's—Indirect (Serum)
Ferritin (Serum)
Iron (Serum)
IBC/TIBC (Serum)
Transferrin (Serum)
Bilirubin—Indirect (Serum)
Sickle-Cell Screening Test
Heinz Bodies
Folic Acid (Serum)
Vitamin B_{12} (Serum)
ESR (Sed Rate) (Blood)
Urobilinogen (Urine)
Zinc Protoporphyrin (ZPP) (Blood)

Introduction

Laboratory tests for hematologic conditions described in this section are done to diagnose anemias, such as microcytic (iron deficiency) and macrocytic (aplastic, hemolytic, pernicious) bleeding disorders and blood cell changes.

(For leukemias and multiple myeloma, see Neoplastic conditions.)

Laboratory Tests

Complete Blood Count: The six components of CBC are (1) the RBC count; (2) hemoglobin (Hb/Hgb); (3) hematocrit (Hct); (4) RBC (erythrocyte) indices: mean corpuscular volume (MCV), mean corpuscular hemoglobin (MCH), mean corpuscular hemoglobin concentration (MCHC), RBC distribution width (RDW); (5) WBC; and (6) differential WBC count. Usually a CBC is ordered to aid in the detection of anemias; to determine blood loss, hydration status, and as part of the routine hospital admission test; to evaluate blood cell status prior to surgery; and as part of a physical examination. The RBC count, Hb, Hct, and RBC index values are useful in determining the type of anemia (*see Part I on RBC indices*).

The differential WBC is necessary for determining the type of infection. During an acute bacterial infection, the body's first line of defense is neutrophils. An increased number of lymphocytes occurs in chronic bacterial and acute viral infections. Monocytes increase in number late in acute bacterial infections but continue to function during the chronic phase. Table 3.20 shows the norms for CBC tests and clinical problems associated with decreased and elevated levels.

TABLE 3.20 Hematologic Causes for Abnormal CBC Results

TYPE	REFERENCE VALUE	DECREASED LEVEL	ELEVATED LEVEL
RBC count	Adult: Male: 4.5–6 μL Female: 4–5 μL Elderly Male: 3.7–6 μL Female: 4–5 μL Child: 3.8–5.5 μL	Hemorrhage Anemias Hemodilution (overhydration)	Hemoconcentration (dehydration) Polycythemia vera
Hb	Adult: Male: 13.5–18 g/dL Female: 12–16 g/dL Elderly: Male: 11–17 g/dL Female: 11.5–16 g/dL Infant: 10–15 g/dL Child: 11–16 g/dL	Anemias: Iron deficiency Aplastic Hemocytic Acute blood loss Hemodilution	Hemoconcentration (dehydration) Polycythemia vera
Hct	Adult: Male: 40–54% Female: 36–46% Elderly: Male: 38–42% Female: 38–41% Child, 1–3 years: 29–40% Child, 4–10 years: 36–38%	Anemias: Aplastic Hemolytic Folic acid deficiency Pernicious Sickle cell	Hemoconcentration (dehydration) Polycythemia vera
RBC indices MCV	Adult: 80–98 μm^3 Elderly: Male: 74–110 μm^3 Female: 78–100 μm^3	Microcytic anemia: Iron deficiency	Macrocytic anemias: Aplastic Hemolytic Pernicious

TYPE	REFERENCE VALUE	DECREASED LEVEL	ELEVATED LEVEL

MCH	Adult: 27–31 pg
	Elderly:
	  Male: 24–33 pg
	  Female: 23–34 pg
		Microcytic,
		  hypochromic anemia
			Macrocytic anemias

MCHC	Adult: 32–36%
	  0.32–0.36 g/dL
	Elderly:
	  Male: 28–36%
	  Female: 30–36%
		Microcytic,
		  hypochromic
		  anemia
		Thalassemia	

RDW	11.5–14.5
	  Coulter S
			Anemias:
			  Iron deficiency
			  Folic acid deficiency
			  Pernicious
			  Sickle cell

WBC count	Adult: 5,000–10,000 µL
	Child, 2 years:
	  6,000–17,000 µL
	Elderly:
	  Male: 4,200–16,000 µL
	  Female: 3,100–10,000 µL
		Anemias:
		  Aplastic
		  Pernicious
			Anemias:
			  Hemolytic
			  Sickle cell

Differential
  WBC count
Neutrophils
	Adult: 50–70%
	Elderly: 45–75%
	Child: 35%
		Anemias:
		  Aplastic
		  Folic acid deficiency
		  Iron deficiency
			Anemia:
			  Acquired hemolytic

Basophils	Adult: 0.5–1% Elderly, Average: 1%		Anemia: Acquired hemolytic
Lymphocytes	Adult: 25–35% Elderly, Average: 30% Child: 38–50%	Anemia: Aplastic	

Monocytes	Adult: 4–6%
	Elderly, Average: 10%
		Anemia:
		  Aplastic
			Anemias:
			  Sickle cell
			  Hemolytic

Platelet Count: *Norm:* Adult: 150,000–400,000 µL (mm^3 or K/UL).

Thrombocytopenia (decreased platelet count) is associated with aplastic, iron deficiency, pernicious, folic acid deficiency, and sickle-cell anemias. Thrombocytosis (elevated platelet count) occurs in polycythemia vera.

Platelet Aggregation and Platelet Adhesion (Blood): *Norm:* 3–5 minutes.

Platelet aggregation measures the ability of platelets to adhere to one another. A decrease in platelet aggregation time will cause increased bleeding tendencies. Both platelet aggregation and platelet adhesion aid in diagnosing hereditary and acquired platelet diseases, such as von Willebrand disease.

Platelet Antibody Test (Blood): *Norm:* Negative.

Platelet antibodies frequently develop as the result of platelet antigens from transfused blood. This can cause thrombocytopenia because of the destruction of the platelets.

Blood Smear: Blood smear is used to determine abnormalities associated with blood cells. It is useful for examining the cause of a hematologic disease, for example, anemia (especially iron deficiency anemia) and leukemia.

Reticulocyte Count: *Norms:* Adult: 25,000–75,000 μL, 0.5–1.5% of all RBCs. Elderly: 0.4–3.6%. Child: 0.5–2% of all RBCs.

Reticulocytes are immature, nonnucleated RBCs that are formed in the bone marrow. A decreased reticulocyte count might be present in pernicious, folic acid, and aplastic anemias. A persistently low count could be suggestive of bone marrow hypofunction or aplastic anemia. An elevated reticulocyte count could be present in hemolytic and sickle-cell anemias and could be due to hemorrhage, hemolysis, or treatment of iron deficiency.

Hb/Hgb Electrophoresis: *Norms:* (*See values in Part I.*)

This test detects abnormal types of Hb (i.e., Hb S [sickle-cell anemia], Hb C [hemolytic anemia], and Hb F [thalassemia]).

Erythrocyte Osmotic Fragility: *Norm:* Adult: 0.30–0.46%.

This test determines the ability of RBCs to resist hemolysis (RBC destruction) in hypo-osmolar solutions. Osmotic fragility might be decreased in the anemias—iron deficiency, folic acid deficiency, sickle cell, thalassemia major and minor (Mediterranean anemia or Cooley anemia)—and also in polycythemia vera. Elevated osmotic fragility might be present in acquired hemolytic anemia.

Bleeding Time: *Norms:* Adult: 1–6 minutes (Ivy's method), 1–3 minutes (Duke's method).

The bleeding time test is useful in determining abnormal function of platelets. A prolonged bleeding time could be due to decreased platelet count, increased platelet destruction, platelet abnormality, vascular abnormalities, disseminated intravascular coagulation (DIC) disease, aplastic anemia, and factors V, VII, and XI deficiencies.

Coagulation Time, Lee-White Clotting Time (Blood): *Norm:* Adult: 5–15 minutes.

CT, frequently known as Lee-White clotting time, is one of the oldest tests of coagulation. A prolonged CT might be indicative of afibrinogenemia, hyperheparinemia, or severe coagulation factor deficiencies.

Clot Retraction (Blood): *Norms:* Adult: 1 hour: half its size; 4 hours: near completion; 24 hours: completely shrunken. Child: same as adult.

Clot retraction (shrunken clot) test is useful for detecting platelet disorder (platelet deficit or platelet abnormality). A decreased clot retraction (greater than 4–24 hours) could be indicative of thrombocytopenia (decreased platelets); thrombasthenia (platelet abnormality); or pernicious, folic acid deficiency, or aplastic anemia.

Fetal Hemoglobin (Hb F) (Blood): *Norms:* Adult: 0.2%. Child: Newborn: 60–90%; 1–5 mo: less than 70%; 6–12 mo: less than 5%; less than 1 year: less than 2%.

Elevated fetal hemoglobin is normal for an infant under 6 months old. After 6 months, hemoglobinopathy should be considered, which could be minor or major thalassemias.

Fibrin Degradation Products (Serum): *Norm:* Adult: 2–10 mcg/mL.

The FDP test, also known as fibrin split products (FSP), indicates the activity of the fibrinolytic system. This test is frequently done in an emergency when the client is hemorrhaging. An increased FDP, greater than 10 mcg/mL, is usually indicative of DIC caused by severe injury or trauma.

Fibrinogen (Plasma): *Norm:* 200–400 mg/dL.

TABLE 3.21 Disseminated Intravascular Coagulation (DIC) Screening Tests

TEST	POSITIVE RESULTS
Platelet count	greater than 400,000 µL
Bleeding time	greater than 6 minutes
PT	greater than 15 seconds
PTT	greater than 60 seconds
APTT	greater than 40 seconds
Factor I: fibrinogen	less than 100 mg/dL
Fibrin degradation products	greater than 10 mcg/dL
Euglobulin lysis time	1½–6 hours, or greater than 6 hours
Plasminogen	less than 2.5 U/mL, less than 20 mg/dL

Fibrinogen produces fibrin strands necessary for clot formation. A deficiency of fibrinogen results in bleeding. A low fibrinogen level may be due to DIC.

Euglobulin Lysis Time (Fibrinolysis Time) Test: *Norm:* Adult: 1½–6 hours.

This test evaluates the activity of the fibrinolytic system by determining the time from clot formation to clot lysis. It is useful in differentiating between primary fibrinolysis (e.g., cancer of prostate) and DIC. The lysis time is short in primary fibrinolysis and normal or prolonged in DIC.

Disseminated Intravascular Coagulation Screening Tests: This is a group of tests ordered for detecting the presence of DIC. Table 3.21 shows the screening tests used for suspected DIC.

D-Dimer Test (Blood): *Norm:* Negative for D-Dimer fragments; greater than 250 ng/mL; 250 mcg/L.

A fibrin degradation fragment, D-Dimer, occurs through fibrinolysis. This test confirms the presence of fibrin split products and is more specific for diagnosing disseminated intravascular coagulation than FSPs.

Antithrombin III (Plasma): *Norm/Average:* 75–135%.

The test is to detect genetic deficiency of AT-III, DIC, thrombophlebitis, AMI, and pulmonary embolism. Reference values can be increased following acute hepatitis, hyperglobulinemia, and vitamin K deficiency.

Plasminogen (Plasma): *Norm:* 2.5–5.2 unit/mL; 7–16 mg/dL.

Plasminogen test is useful in evaluating the fibrinolytic process, a breakdown of fibrin clots in prevention of coagulation. The level is decreased in DIC, advanced liver disease, and thrombolytic therapy.

Prothrombin Time: *Norms:* Adult: 11–15 seconds; 70–100%. Child: same as adult; INR: 2–3.

Prothrombin, factor II, is converted to thrombin by the action of thromboplastin, which is needed to form a clot. A prolonged PT time could be associated with afibrinogenemia, deficiencies of factors II, VII, and X. This test is useful for monitoring anticoagulant therapy.

Partial Thromboplastin Time, Activated Partial Thromboplastin Time (Plasma): *Norms:* Adult: PTT: 60–70 seconds; APTT: 20–35 seconds.

The PTT is useful for detecting clotting factors and platelet disorders. APTT is more sensitive than PTT. PTT and APTT are commonly used to monitor heparin therapy.

Factor Assay (Coagulation Factors): Factor assay determines the concentration of specific coagulating factors in the blood. Prolonged clotting time occurs when values of factors I, II, V, VII, VIII, IX, X, and XI are decreased.

Blood Typing (Type and Crossmatch): Blood typing and crossmatching is necessary to provide compatible blood to recipients. Major and minor antigens can be detected through blood typing.

Bone Marrow Aspiration (Biopsy): Bone marrow specimen is useful for evaluating hematopoiesis. The size, shape, and number of RBCs, WBCs, and megakaryocytes (platelet precursors) are examined to diagnose hematologic disorders (i.e., aplastic anemia, leukemia, Hodgkin disease, polycythemia vera, and multiple myeloma).

Lymph Node Biopsy: *Norm:* No pathology.

Lymph node(s) biopsy may be performed during a mastectomy to determine if the cancer cells have metastasized to the lymph nodes. Lymph node pathology may be checked for other cancers.

Glucose-6-Phosphate Dehydrogenase/G-6-PD (Blood): *Norms:* Adult (varies with method used): 8–18 international unit/g Hb, 125–281 unit/dL packed RBCs.

G-6-PD, an enzyme in RBCs, assists in glucose use in RBCs. A decreased amount of this enzyme causes hemolysis and hemolytic anemia.

Haptoglobin (Hp) (Serum): *Norms:* Adult: 60–270 mg/dL. Infant: 0–30 mg/dL, and then gradually increases.

Hp, a group of α_2-globulins, combines with free Hb during intravascular hemolysis. A decreased Hp level occurs in hemolytic anemia because of too much free Hb to bind. Also, a decreased level could occur in pernicious, folic acid deficiency, and sickle-cell anemias.

Antineutrophil Cytoplasmic Antibody (ANCA): *Norm:* Negative to less than 1:20 titer.

The ANCAs are autoimmune antibodies that respond to cytoplasmic components of neutrophil granules.

Methemoglobin (Hb M) (Blood): *Norms:* Less than 1.5% of total Hb; 0.06–0.24 g/dL; 9.2–37 µmol/L. Positive: greater than 20–70%; greater than 70% death.

Hb M occurs when the deoxygenated heme or iron portion of hemoglobin is oxidized to a ferric state; methemoglobinemia results. This problem can be due to chemicals, radiation, and certain drugs, such as nitrites and nitrates.

Coombs Indirect (Serum): *Norm:* Negative.

This test detects free antibodies in the client's serum and identifies certain red cell antigens. It is done in crossmatching blood for transfusion. Positive results mean incompatible crossmatched blood, anti-Rh antibodies, or acquired hemolytic anemia.

Ferritin (Serum): *Norms:* Male: 15–445 ng/mL. Female: 10–235 ng/mL.

Serum ferritin level is useful in evaluating the total storage of iron in the body. It can detect early iron deficiency anemia and anemias due to chronic disease.

Iron (Serum): *Norms:* Adult: 50–150 mcg/dL. Infant: 40–100 mcg/dL.

A decreased serum iron level frequently occurs in iron deficiency anemia. An elevated level might be present in hemolytic, pernicious, and folic acid deficiency anemias.

Iron-Binding Capacity (IBC) or Total Iron-Binding Capacity (TIBC) (Serum): *Norms:* Adult: 250–450 mcg/dL. Infant: 100–350 mcg/dL.

IBC is 2–3 times greater than the serum iron level. When serum iron is decreased, IBC is increased, and when serum iron is increased, IBC is decreased. A decreased IBC level is present in hemolytic, pernicious, and sickle-cell anemias. An elevated IBC level is present in iron deficiency anemia.

Transferrin (Serum): *Norms:* 200–430 mg/dL; 2–4.3 g/L (SI units).

Transferrin is responsible for transporting iron to the bone marrow for the purpose of hemoglobin synthesis. A decrease in transferrin occurs in anemias of chronic diseases, and an elevated level occurs in iron deficiency anemia.

Bilirubin Indirect (Serum): *Norm:* Adult: 0.1–1 mg/dL.

An elevated indirect bilirubin is associated with transfusion reaction and with sickle-cell, pernicious, and hemolytic anemias.

Sickle-Cell Screening Test: *Norm:* Negative.

Hb S, a crescent- or sickle-shaped cell, is present in sickle-cell disease when the RBC is deprived of oxygen. Hb electrophoresis is needed to confirm sickle-cell anemia.

Heinz Bodies (Blood): *Norm:* Negative: Absence of Heinz bodies; less than 30% Heinz bodies present.

Heinz bodies are small, irregular, decomposed particles on the hemoglobin that are normally removed by the spleen. Heinz bodies can cause hemolytic anemia (hemolysis of red blood cells [RBCs]) or hemoglobinopathy.

Folic Acid Folate (Serum): *Norms:* Adult: 5–20 ng/mL, greater than 2.5 ng/mL (RIA).

A decreased folic acid level is indicative of folic acid deficiency anemia. In pernicious anemia, the serum folic acid level might be elevated.

Vitamin B$_{12}$ (Serum): *Norms:* Adult: 200–900 pg/mL, 132–703 pmol/L (SI units).

Vitamin B$_{12}$ is essential for RBC maturation. A decreased vitamin B$_{12}$ level is indicative of pernicious anemia.

Erythrocyte Sedimentation Rate (ESR/Sed Rate) (Blood): *Norms:* (*See values in Part I.*)

ESR, a nonspecific test, measures the rate at which RBCs settle in unclotted blood. A decreased ESR could be present in sickle-cell anemia and polycythemia vera.

Urobilinogen (Urine): *Norms:* Adult: Random: 0.3–3.5 mg/dL; 24 hours: 0.05–2.5 mg/24 h.

Increased urine urobilinogen level could be present in hemolytic, pernicious, and sickle-cell anemias.

Zinc Protoporphyrin (ZPP) Blood: *Norms:* Adult and Child: 15–77 mcg/dL.

ZPP is a screening test to check for lead poisoning and iron deficiency. The test is positive for lead poisoning if the ZPP level is elevated.

NURSING IMPLICATIONS WITH RATIONALE

- Explain that the purpose for the laboratory tests is to identify the cause for the hematologic disorder.
- Give a detailed explanation concerning the test procedures and the need for the client's compliance. The explanation might be brief or in depth, depending upon the client's familiarity with the test.

- Inform the client of any food, fluid, or drug restrictions. Each test should be checked for specific restrictions (*see Part I*).
- Monitor the client's vital signs before, during, and after the laboratory test procedures. Check respiratory status and skin color, because oxygen deficit frequently results from a decreased hemoglobin.
- Listen to the client's expressed anxiety or fear concerning the tests and potential clinical problems. Clarification of the test procedure might alleviate fear and anxiety and promote compliance.
- Check laboratory results and report abnormal test reports.
- Be supportive of the client and family members during tests and treatment of hematologic disorders.

PART FOUR

Therapeutic Drug Monitoring (TDM)*

4

Selective drugs are monitored by serum and urine for the purposes of achieving and maintaining therapeutic drug effect and for preventing drug toxicity. Drugs with a wide therapeutic range (window), the difference between effective dose and toxic dose, are not usually monitored. Drug monitoring is important in maintaining a drug concentration–response relationship, especially when the serum drug range (window) is narrow, such as with digoxin and lithium. Therapeutic drug monitoring (TDM) is the process of following drug levels and adjusting them to maintain a therapeutic level. Not all drugs can be dosed and/or monitored by their blood levels alone.

Drug levels are obtained at peak time and trough time after a steady state of the drug has occurred in the client. Steady state is reached after 4–5 half-lives of a drug and can be reached sooner if the drug has a short half-life. Once steady state is achieved, serum drug level is checked at the peak level (maximum drug concentration) and/or at trough/residual level (minimum drug concentration). If the trough or residual level is at the high therapeutic point, toxicity might occur. Careful assessment is needed by both physical and laboratory means.

TDM is required for the following:

- Drugs with a narrow therapeutic index or range (window).
- When other methods for monitoring drugs are not effective, such as blood pressure (BP) monitoring.
- To determine when adequate blood concentrations are reached.
- To evaluate a client's compliance to drug therapy.
- To determine whether or not other drugs have altered serum drug levels (increased or decreased) that could result in drug toxicity or lack of therapeutic effects.
- To establish a new serum drug level when the dosage is changed.

Drug groups for TDM include analgesics, antibiotics, anticonvulsants, antineoplastics, bronchodilators, cardiac drugs, hypoglycemics, sedatives, and tranquilizers. To effectively

---

*Revised and updated by Ronald J. Lefever, RPh, Lead Pharmacist, Medical College of Virginia, Richmond, Virginia.

conduct TDM, the laboratory must be provided with the following information: the drug name and daily dosage, time and amount of last dose, time blood was drawn, route of administration, and client's age. Without complete information, serum drug reporting might be incorrect.

HIV drugs are primarily dosed based on the client's viral load or CD4 counts. Many of these drugs have dosage adjustments for renal and hepatic impairment.

DRUG	THERAPEUTIC RANGE	PEAK TIME	TOXIC LEVEL
acetaminophen (Tylenol)	10–20 mcg/mL	1–2½ h	greater than 50 mcg/mL Hepatotoxicity: greater than 200 mcg/mL
acetohexamide (Dymelor)	20–70 mcg/mL (should be dosed according to blood glucose levels)	2–4 h	greater than 75 mcg/mL
alcohol	Negative		Mild toxic: 150 mg/dL Marked toxic: greater than 250 mg/dL
alprazolam (Xanax)	10–50 ng/mL	1–2 h	greater than 75 ng/mL
amikacin (Amikin)	Peak: 20–30 mcg/mL	Intravenously: ½ h	Peak: greater than 35 mcg/mL
	Trough: equal or less than 10 mcg/mL	½–1½ h	greater than 10 mcg/mL
aminocaproic acid (Amicar)	100–400 mcg/mL	1 h	greater than 400 mcg/mL
aminophylline (see Theophylline)			
amiodarone (Cordarone)	0.5–2.5 mcg/mL	2–10 h	greater than 2.5 mcg/mL
amitriptyline (Elavil) + nortriptyline (parent and active metabolite)	110–225 ng/mL	2–4 h (and up to 12 h)	greater than 500 ng/mL
amobarbital (Amytal)	1–5 mcg/mL	2 h	greater than 15 mcg/mL Severe toxicity: greater than 30 mcg/mL
amoxapine (Asendin)	200–400 ng/mL	15 h	greater than 500 ng/mL
amphetamine:			
Serum	20–30 ng/mL		0.2 mcg/mL
Urine		Detectable in urine after 3 h; positive for 24–48 h	greater than 30 mcg/mL urine
aspirin (see Salicylates)			
atenolol (Tenormin)	200–500 ng/mL	2–4 h	greater than 500 ng/mL
beta carotene	48–200 mcg/mL	Several weeks	greater than 300 mcg/mL
bromide	20–80 mg/dL		greater than 100 mg/dL
butabarbital (Butisol)	1–2 mcg/mL	3–4 h	greater than 10 mcg/mL
butalbital	10–20 mcg/mL	½–1 h	greater than 40 mcg/mL
caffeine	Adult: 3–15 mcg/mL Infant: 8–20 mcg/mL		greater than 50 mcg/mL
carbamazepine (Tegretol)	4–12 mcg/mL	6 h (range 2–24 h)	greater than 9–15 mcg/mL
chloral hydrate (Noctec)	2–12 mcg/mL	1–2 h	greater than 20 mcg/mL
chloramphenicol (Chloromycetin)	10–20 mg/L		greater than 25 mg/L
chlordiazepoxide (Librium)	1–5 mcg/mL	2–3 h	greater than 5 mcg/mL
chlorpromazine (Thorazine)	50–300 ng/mL	2–4 h	greater than 750 ng/mL

DRUG	THERAPEUTIC RANGE	PEAK TIME	TOXIC LEVEL
chlorpropamide (Diabinese)	75–250 mcg/mL	3–6 h	greater than 250–750 mcg/mL
cimetidine (Tagamet)	Trough: 0.5–1.2 mcg/mL	1–1½ h	Trough: greater than 1.5 mcg/mL
clonazepam (Klonopin)	10–60 ng/mL	2 h	greater than 80 ng/mL
clonidine (Catapres)	0.2–2 ng/mL (Hypotensive effect)	2–5 h	greater than 2 ng/mL
clorazepate (Tranxene)	0.12–1 mcg/mL	1–2 h	greater than 1 mcg/mL
codeine	10–100 ng/mL	1–2 h	greater than 200 ng/mL
cyclosporine	100–300 ng/mL	3–4 h	greater than 400 ng/mL
dantrolene (Dantrium)	1–3 mcg/mL	5 h	greater than 5 mcg/mL
desipramine (Norpramin)	125–300 ng/mL	4–6 h	greater than 500 ng/mL
diazepam (Valium)	0.5–2 mg/L, 400–600 ng/mL Therapeutic	1–2 h	greater than 3 mg/L greater than 3,000 ng/mL
digitoxin (rarely administered)	10–25 ng/mL	Noticeable: 2–4 h Peak: 12–24 h	greater than 30 ng/mL
digoxin	0.5–2 ng/mL	PO: 6–8 h IV: 1½–2 h	2–3 ng/mL
Dilantin (see Phenytoin)			
diltiazem (Cardizem)	50–200 ng/mL	2–3 h	greater than 200 ng/mL
disopyramide (Norpace)	2–4 mcg/mL	2 h	greater than 4 mcg/mL
doxepin (Sinequan)	150–300 ng/mL	2–4 h	greater than 500 ng/mL
ethchlorvynol (Placidyl)	2–8 mcg/mL	1–2 h	greater than 20 mcg/mL
ethosuximide (Zarontin)	40–100 mcg/mL	2–4 h	greater than 150 mcg/mL
flecainide (Tambocor)	0.2–1 mcg/mL	3 h	greater than 1 mcg/mL
5-flucytosine	Peak: 100 mcg/mL Trough: 50 mcg/mL		125 mcg/mL 125 mcg/mL
fluoride			greater than 15 μmol/mL
fluoxetine	90–300 ng/mL	2–4 h	greater than 500 ng/mL
flurazepam (Dalmane)	20–110 ng/mL	0.5–1 h	greater than 1,500 ng/mL
folate	greater than 3.5 mcg/mL	1 h	
gentamicin (Garamycin)	Peak: 6–12 mcg/mL Trough: less than 2 mcg/mL	IV: 15–30 minutes	Peak: greater than 12 mcg/mL greater than 2 mg/mL
glutethimide (Doriden)	2–6 mcg/mL	1–2 h	greater than 20 mcg/mL
gold	1–2 mcg/mL	2–6 h	greater than 5 mcg/mL
haloperidol (Haldol)	5–15 ng/mL	2–6 h	greater than 50 ng/mL
hydromorphone (Dilaudid)	1–30 ng/mL	½–1½h	greater than 100 ng/mL
ibuprofen (Motrin, etc.)	10–50 mcg/mL	1–2 h	greater than 100 mcg/mL
imipramine (Tofranil) + desipramine (parent and active metabolite)	200–350 ng/mL	PO: 1–2 h IM: 30 minutes	greater than 500 ng/mL
isoniazid (INH, Nydrazid)	1–7 mg/mL (dose usually adjusted based on liver function tests)	1–2 h	greater than 20 mg/mL
kanamycin (Kantrex)	Peak: 15–30 mcg/mL	PO: 1–2 h IM: 30 minutes–1 h	Peak: greater than 35 mcg/mL Trough: greater than 10 mcg/mL

(continued)

DRUG	THERAPEUTIC RANGE	PEAK TIME	TOXIC LEVEL
lead	less than 20 mcg/mL Urine: less than 80 mcg/24 h		greater than 80 mcg/mL Urine: greater 125 mcg/ 24 h
lidocaine (Xylocaine)	1.5–5 mcg/mL	IV: 10 minutes	greater than 6 mcg/mL
lithium	0.8–1.2 mEq/L	½–4 h	greater than 1.5 mEq/L
lorazepam (Ativan)	50–240 ng/mL	1–3 h	greater than 300 ng/mL
maprotiline (Ludiomil)	200–300 ng/mL	12 h	greater than 500 ng/mL
meperidine (Demerol)	0.4–0.7 mcg/mL	2–4 h	greater than 1 mcg/mL
mephenytoin (Mesantoin)	15–40 mcg/mL	2–4 h	greater than 50 mcg/mL
meprobamate (Equanil, Miltown)	15–25 mcg/mL	2 h	greater than 50 mcg/mL
methadone (Dolophine)	100–400 ng/mL	½–1 h	greater than 2,000 ng/ mL or greater than 0.2 mcg/mL
methaqualone	1–5 mcg/mL		greater than 10 mcg/mL
methotrexate	less than 0.1 μmol/L after 48 h	1–2 h	1×10^6 at 48 h
methsuximide	less than 1 mcg/mL	1–4 h	greater than 40 mcg/mL
methyldopa (Aldomet)	1–5 mcg/mL	3–6 h	greater than 7 mcg/mL
methyprylon (Noludar)	8–10 mcg/mL	1–2 h	greater than 50 mcg/mL
metoprolol (Lopressor)	75–200 ng/mL	2–4 h	greater than 225 ng/mL
mexiletine (Mexitil)	0.5–2 mcg/mL	2–3 h	greater than 2 mcg/mL
morphine	10–80 ng/mL	IV: immediately IM: ½–1 h SC: 1–1½ h	greater than 200 ng/mL
netilmicin (Netromycin)	Peak: 0.5–10 mcg/mL Trough: less than 4 mcg/mL	IV: 30 minutes	Peak: greater than 16 mcg/mL greater than 4 mcg/mL
nifedipine (Procardia)	50–100 ng/mL	½–2 h	greater than 100 ng/mL
nortriptyline (Aventyl)	50–150 ng/mL	8 h	greater than 200 ng/mL
oxazepam (Serax)	0.2–1.4 mcg/mL	1–2 h	
oxycodone (Percodan)	10–100 ng/mL	½–1 h	greater than 200 ng/mL
pentazocine (Talwin)	0.05–0.2 mcg/mL	1–2 h	greater than 1 mcg/mL Urine: greater than 3 mcg/mL
pentobarbital (Nembutal)	1–5 mcg/mL	½–1 h	greater than 10 mcg/mL Severe toxicity: greater than 30 mcg/mL
phenmetrazine (Preludin)	5–30 mcg/mL (Urine)	2 h	greater than 50 mcg/mL (urine)
phenobarbital (Luminal)	15–40 mcg/mL	6–18 h	greater than 40 mcg/mL Severe toxicity: greater than 80 mcg/mL
phenytoin (Dilantin)	10–20 mcg/mL	4–8 h	greater than 20–30 mcg/mL Severe toxicity: greater than 40 mcg/mL
pindolol (Visken)	0.5–6 ng/mL	2–4 h	greater than 10 ng/mL
primidone (Mysoline)	5–12 mcg/mL	2–4 h	greater than 12–15 mcg/mL

DRUG	THERAPEUTIC RANGE	PEAK TIME	TOXIC LEVEL
procainamide (Pronestyl)	4–10 mcg/mL	1 h	greater than 10 mcg/mL
procaine (Novocain)	less than 11 mcg/mL	10–30 minutes	greater than 20 mcg/mL
prochlorperazine (Compazine)	50–300 ng/mL	2–4 h	greater than 1,000 ng/mL
propoxyphene (Darvon)	0.1–0.4 mcg/mL	2–3 h	greater than 0.5 mcg/mL
propranolol (Inderal)	greater than 100 ng/mL	1–2 h	greater than 150 ng/mL
protriptyline (Vivactil)	50–150 ng/mL	8–12 h	greater than 200 ng/mL
quinidine	2–5 mcg/mL	1–3 h	greater than 6 mcg/mL
ranitidine (Zantac)	100 ng/mL	2–3 h	greater than 100 ng/mL
reserpine (Serpasil)	20 ng/mL	2–4 h	greater than 20 ng/mL
salicylates (aspirin)	10–30 mg/dL	1–2 h	Tinnitus: 20–40 mg/mL Hyperventilation: greater than 35 mg/dL Severe toxicity: greater than 50 mg/dL
secobarbital (Seconal)	2–5 mcg/mL	1 h	greater than 15 mcg/mL Severe toxicity: greater than 30 mcg/mL
streptomycin	Peak: 5–20 mcg/mL Trough: less than 5 mcg/mL		greater than 40 mcg/mL greater than 40 mcg/mL
sulfadiazine	100–120 mcg/mL		greater than 300 mcg/mL
sulfamethoxazole	90–100 mcg/mL		greater than 300 mcg/mL
sulfapyridine	75–90 mcg/mL		greater than 300 mcg/mL
sulfisoxazole	90–100 mcg/mL		greater than 300 mcg/mL
theophylline (Theo-Dur, Aminodur)	10–20 mcg/mL	PO: 2–3 h IV: 15 minutes (depends on smoking or non-smoking)	greater than 20 mcg/mL
thiocyanate	4–20 mcg/mL		greater than 60 mcg/mL
thioridazine (Mellaril)	100–600 ng/mL 1–1.5 mcg/mL	2–4 h	greater than 2,000 ng/mL greater than 10 mcg/mL
timolol (Blocadren)	3–55 ng/mL	1–2 h	greater than 60 ng/mL
tobramycin (Nebcin)	Peak: 5–10 mcg/mL Trough: 1–1.5 mcg/mL	IV: 15–30 minutes IM: ½–1½ h	Peak: greater than 12 mcg/mL Trough: greater than 2 mcg/mL
tocainide (Tonocard)	4–10 mcg/mL	½–3 h	greater than 12 mcg/mL
tolbutamide (Orinase)	80–240 mcg/mL	3–5 h	greater than 640 mcg/mL
trazodone (Desyrel)	500–2500 ng/mL	1–2 weeks	greater than 4,000 ng/mL
trifluoperazine (Stelazine)	50–300 ng/mL	2–4 h	greater than 1,000 ng/mL
trimethoprim/sulfamethox-azole (TMP/SMX)	Peak: trimethoprim: greater than 5 mcg/mL Peak: sulfamethoxazole greater than 100 mcg/mL		
valproic acid (Depakene)	50–100 mcg/mL	½–1½ h	greater than 100 mcg/mL Severe toxicity: greater than 150 mcg/mL

(*continued*)

DRUG	THERAPEUTIC RANGE	PEAK TIME	TOXIC LEVEL
vancomycin (Vanocin)	Peak: 20–40 mcg/mL	IV: Peak: 5 minutes	Peak: greater than 80 mcg/mL
	Trough: 5–10 mcg/mL	IV: Trough: 12 h	
verapamil (Calan)	100–300 ng/mL	PO: 1–2 h	greater than 500 ng/mL
		IV: 5 minutes	
warfarin (Coumadin)	1–10 mcg/mL (dose usually adjusted by 1–2.5 × control)	1½–3 days	greater than 10 mcg/mL

HIV drugs are primarily dosed based on the client's viral load or CD_4 counts. Many of these drugs have dosage adjustments for renal and/or hepatic impairment.

DRUG	PEAK TIME (TMAX)	ELIMINATION HALF-LIFE (t½)	SPECIAL CONSIDERATIONS
Nucleoside/Nucleotide Reverse Transcriptase Inhibitors (NRTIs)			
abacavir (Ziagen)	0.7–1.7 h	1.5 h	Dose adjustment for hepatic impairment
abacavir + lamivudine + zidovudine (Trizivir)	See individual agents		
didanosine (Videx)	0.25–1.5 h	1.5 h	
emtricitabine (Emtriva)	1–2 h	10 h	
emtricitabine + tenofovir (Truvada)	1–2 h	10–17 h	
lamivudine (Epirvir)	0.9–3.2 h	5–7 h	Dose adjustment for renal impairment
lamivudine + abacavir (Epzicom)	See individual agents	1.5–7 h	abacavir t½ is 1.5 h and lamivudine t½ is 5–7 h. Dose adjustment for renal impairment
lamivudine + zidovudine (Combivir)	See individual agents		
stavudine (Zerit)	1–1.5 h	1.5 h (8 h with renal impairment)	
tenofovir (Viread)	1 h	17 h	Dose adjustment for renal impairment
zidovudine (Retrovir)	0.5–1.5 h	1 h (1–3 h with renal impairment)	
Non-Nucleoside Reverse Transcriptase Inhibitors (NNRTIs)			
delavirdine (Rescriptor)	1 h	2–11 h	
etravirine (Intelence)	2.5–4 h	41 h	NRTI and first-line NNRTI (delavirdine, efavirenz, or nevirapine) contra-indicated with either a detectable viral or an intolerance to current regimen
efavirenz (Sustiva)	3–5 h	40–55 h	
nevirapine (Viramune)	4 h	25–30 h	

DRUG	PEAK TIME (TMAX)	ELIMINATION HALF-LIFE (t½)	SPECIAL CONSIDERATIONS
Multiclass Combination Agents			
efavirenz + emtricitabine + tenofovir (Atripla)	See individual agents		
Protease Inhibitors (PIs)			
atazanavir (Reyataz)	2.5 h	7 h	
darunavir (Prezista)	2.5–4 h	15 h	Elimination t½ when coadministered with ritonavir
fosamprenavir (Lexiva)	1.5–4 h	7.7 h	
indinavir (Crixivan)	0.8 h	2 h (3 h with hepatic impairment)	
lopinavir + ritonavir (Kaletra)	4 h	5–6 h	
maraviroc (Selzentry)	0.5–4 h	14–18 h	NRTI and NNRTI are contraindicated with one or more PIs, or raltegravir or intolerance to current regimen
ritonavir (Norvir)	2–4 h	3–5 h	
tipranavir (Aptivus)	3 h	5.5–6 h	
Integrase Inhibitor			
raltegravir (Isentress)	3 h	9 h	

PART FIVE

School Health Services: Education, Screening, and Testing*

Fundamental to the success of all children is good physical and mental health. The goal of school health services is to remove health barriers to learning. Health and learning go hand in hand; when one falters, so does the other. The school nurse holds a unique and important position to that end. He or she needs physical, mental, social, emotional, and ethical capabilities in addition to a professional and educational nursing background to ensure the health needs of all students are provided for.

The school nurse provides direct student health services; conducts health and wellness programs for school personnel; is involved in program planning, development, management, and evaluation; and provides health education and counseling for students and their families. This requires a community-wide approach to the planning and implementation of services. School nurses steer uninsured families to access services and help navigate health care systems. The following must be considered in the approach:

- *Mortality:* trauma and violent causes, motor vehicle accident, homicide, suicide, malignancy, infections—meningitis and pneumonia, drug related.
- *Prevention:* data-reportable infections—sexually transmitted disease (STD), human immunodeficiency virus (HIV), attention deficit hyperactivity disorder (ADHD), drug and alcohol abuse, teen pregnancy, violence including cyberbullying and other bullying.
- *Chronic disorders:* asthma, seizure disorders, diabetes, cystic fibrosis, cerebral palsy, vision issues, hearing handicaps, mental disorders, and learning differences.
- *Other:* nutrition, pediculosis; scabies; ringworm; conjunctivitis; dental problems; nutritional, local conditions; managing environmental problems.

School Nurse Functions

A child-oriented focus with services based on identified student needs is key to a good health education program. Start by collecting data on local health problems (see Figure 5-1). Once

---

*Written by Anne M. Biddle, RN, BSN, NCSN, School Nurse, Newark Charter School, Delaware.

Last Name	First and Middle Name	M	F	Date of Birth	*

SCHOOL HEALTH RECORD - STATE OF DELAWARE

Parent or Guardian	Address		Home Phone
Family Physician	Phone	Family Dentist	Phone

School Pupil is Attending		
1	2	3

ILLNESS AND HEALTH PROBLEMS

Chicken Pox	▫	Frequent Colds	▫	Diabetes	▫
Measles	▫	Frequent Tonsillitis	▫	Convulsive Disorders	▫
Mumps	▫	Hearing Difficulty	▫	Heart Trouble	▫
Rubella	▫	Speech Difficulty	▫	Nephritis	▫
Whooping Cough	▫	Vision Difficulty	▫	Orthopedic Difficulty	▫
Rheumatic Fever	▫	Allergies	▫	Menstrual Difficulty	▫
Tuberculosis	▫	Asthma	▫	Other	▫

INJURIES-SURGERY   IMMUNIZATION RECORD (Dates)

	PRIMARY SERIES	BOOSTERS
D.P.T.		
D.T.		
M.M.R.		x x x x x x x x x x
Hep B		x x x x x x x x x x
Polio (Oral)		
Other		

VISION TESTING — W/O - Without Glasses / W - With Glasses

Grade	Date	R	L	Comments

TUBERCULIN TEST   OTHER TESTS

Date	Type	Result	Date	Type	Result

HEARING TESTING — V - Normal Range / X - Unsatisfactory

Grade	Date	R	L	Comments

REFERRAL AND TESTS
(Psychological, Mental, Hygiene, Speech, Social Service, Etc., Give Dates)

DENTAL REFERRALS AND CARE

ORTHOPEDIC SCREENING AND FOLLOW UP

*Color Code

BLACK - Convulsive Disorder	YELLOW - Vision	ORANGE - Allergies, Other
RED - Cardiac	GREEN - Orthopedic	PINK - Kidney

Figure 5-1 Example of School Health Record.

listed, prioritize and set goals and objectives, including parents and students at all levels. Networking with other community health workers enables sharing of successes and challenges with others' efforts. Good communication skills, legal and ethical knowledge, and familiarity with the budget process behoove the school nurse. As in business, the key is "knowing the student, so as to tailor a plan specific to the school and community."

Typically, the school health services offer a wide array of services in the course of a typical day, including the following:

- Health assessment.
  - Staff education (i.e., CPR/AED training).
  - Employee health, including workers' compensation assessment.
  - Work with community agencies to benefit children and parents (e.g., Basket Brigade, Soap for Hope, Children and Adults with Attention Deficit/Hyperactivity Disorder [CHADD], American Lung Association [ALA], American Diabetes Association [ADA]).
- Medical referral and follow-up.
- Vision screening/referral.
- Hearing screening/referral.
- Scoliosis screening/referral and follow-up.
- First aid.
- Immunization review and referral.
- Height, weight, BMI $\dfrac{\text{weight (lb)} \times 703}{\text{height (in)}^*}$
- Administration of medication.
- Special procedures (catheterization, blood glucose monitoring, peak flow meter, etc.).
- Teacher/nurse conferences.
- Health and puberty education.
- Individual health counseling.
- Mental health and well-being.
- Resource person in school/community (e.g., dental care and public health clinics).
- Evaluate nursing aspects of the school health program.

Hearing Screening

Among the diagnostic testing that the school nurse performs is hearing screening. A pure tone audiometer, which is calibrated annually, is used in a quiet room. It is important to eliminate ambient noises in a room with heavy drapes, carpeting, and solid-core doors. It is wise to test the audiometer, preferably on oneself, prior to testing, and to arrange the chairs so the student cannot view the equipment. Screening should be performed at 1,000, 2,000, and 4,000 hertz (Hz) with intensity level 20 dB (amplitude, or loudness) at each frequency (sound cycles per second). This level can be increased to 25 dB if there appears to be a fair amount of extraneous noise. Ears are assessed for hair, excess cerumen, or obstruction. When the student fails to respond at any

---

*BMI for age

Overweight:	>95 percentile
At risk for overweight:	85–95 percentile
Normal weight:	5–85 percentile
Underweight:	<5 percentile

frequency in either ear, failure is noted, and the student should be rescreened immediately and in 2 weeks if necessary. If both subsequent attempts result in failure, the student should be referred for appropriate follow-up and rescreened the following year. Excessive cerumen (wax) build-up is often a contributory cause of poor hearing. This is easily remedied with over-the-counter preparations for this purpose. Special equipment is available for students with significant limitations who are unable to test in the conventional method. These results are recorded on the School Health Record, and a parent should be notified and advised to seek an ENT referral. It is protocol to follow up with the family to ensure adequate care of a suspected hearing loss occurs.[1]

Normal hearing range is 1–15 decibels, while slight hearing loss (16–25 dB) can cause missed consonants, and moderate loss (41–65 dB) results in missing most speech sounds. No speech sounds or normal conversation are heard with severe loss (65–95 dB) and profound loss, where no sounds are heard, is considered greater than 95 dB. Students should be educated about hearing loss prevention with emphasis on noise-induced hearing issues connected to MP3 players, iPhones, ear buds, and others.

Vision Screening

Another test done routinely in the school is vision screening for near and far acuity, binocularity, and color. Various equipment is used for screening, such as a lighted chart, Sloan chart, graduated cards, occluder, and a quiet room with appropriate space available between student and chart. One eye is covered, with both eyes open. If corrective lenses are usually worn, all testing should be done wearing them. Some children learn to memorize the chart, so it is wise to test backward, using every other letter, and so on. Anything under 20/50 should be referred, or 20/40 if the student complains of trouble seeing the board or other visual concerns. Family history of visual impairment is often a significant factor to consider. School nurses are in an excellent position to assist families in financial need in obtaining corrective lenses.

Scoliosis: Postural Screening

School-age children are all rapidly growing, particularly in middle school, putting them at an increased risk for developing scoliosis. School nurses are often the ones to detect this curvature of the spine. The screening procedure includes assessment of symmetry, gait, movement, and pain.

- The nurse can take this time to ask if the student carries a backpack—how it is carried, what is the weight, and so on. Students should be informed that no more than 15% of their body weight should be carried; packs should be worn above the waist with a belt if possible. There are now many ergonomically designed models available, and rolling backpacks are a boon to backs. Although poor posture or disproportioned backpacks do not cause scoliosis, those predisposed can be aggravated by these factors.

Suspected deviations must be referred for Phase II rescreening, and all results must be recorded on the students' health records. This test is done yearly on all students. Again, prevention and early detection is the key to "getting it straight."

Vaccine Review

Before school entry, all children must have five DtaP vaccines (diphtheria, tetanus, acellular pertussis), four OPV (polio), four HIB (influenza), two MMR, one varicella (or proof of the disease), and three HBV (Hepatitis B). Currently, the HBV is required prior to entry into the seventh grade but is being given at birth routinely now. A lead screening is also done along with a purified protein derivative (PPD) test for tuberculosis (TB). If a student is at low risk for TB, a "paper screen" can be done by the school nurse. If all four answers are "no" as answered by parent/guardian, the student is considered to be no risk and a PPD test is not necessary. This has become a great time and hassle saver for student, family, and nurse.

In addition, the flu shot, pneumococcal, and hepatitis A vaccines may also be given according to local and state mandates. The bacterial meningitis vaccine is highly recommended for middle school students and usually for college freshmen who rate high in risk of contracting this deadly disease. Pertussis boosters are being given at 11–12 years of age, as this disease has also made a return to many areas. Human papilloma virus (HPV) vaccine is being given at the same age as well.

Obesity and Diabetes Assessment

Obesity has recently become a true epidemic in the school-age child. Reasons include sedentary lifestyles, more use of "screens" (computer, television, etc.), fast food eating, and high-fat, "empty-calorie" eating. Hence, it is vital to know more about diabetes than ever. Type 2 diabetes has reached epidemic proportions in our youth, a very unsettling fact. Some school nurses screen for acanthosis nigricans. The ADA has sited parameters for diagnosing diabetes as follows:

- Two fasting plasma glucose levels greater than 126 mg/dL if asymptomatic.
- Two random levels greater than 200 mg/dL if symptomatic.
- One high glucose level any time in someone who has diabetic symptoms.
- An oral glucose tolerance test showing a 2-hour postprandial result of greater than 200 mg/dL.

School nurses are in an opportune position to assist students and families with healthy food selections, increased physical activity, and education about the hazards of poor choices.

In summary, school nursing begins with prevention and the organization of a plan. It is vital to the student and tailors the care to the needs of the population. The population is not only the students in the school but the parents and families as well; hence, good communication skills are a must. The health and education covers physical, chronic, and acute, as well as mental health, which requires continual updating based on the needs of the community. Every year new disorders and treatments are discovered—staying abreast is the school nurse's responsibility. From child abuse, to asthma, to suicide, to legal and environmental issues, to bandages, and beyond, the school nurse holds an awesome responsibility and plays a pivotal role in health maintenance and prevention.

Bibliography

1. National Association of School Nurses (1998). *The Ear and Hearing: A Guide for School Nurses*. Scarborough, ME: National Association of School Nurses, Inc.
2. Adams, RM (1995). *School Nurse's Survival Guide*. Paramus, NJ: Prentice Hall.
3. Selekman, Janice (2012). *School Nurse: A Comprehensive Text*. Philadelphia: FA Davis.
4. National Association of School Nurses (NASN) (2010). *Definition of School Nursing*. http://www.nasn.org/Default.aspx?tabid=57.
5. National Association of School Nurses (NASN) (2011). *The Role of the School Nurse*. Position Statement.
6. National Association of School Nurses/American Nurses Association (NASN/ANA) (2005). *Scope and Standards of School Nursing Practice*, pp. 1–8. Silver Spring, Nursebooks.org.

APPENDIX A

Abbreviations

ABG	Arterial blood gas
ACA	Anticardiolipin antibody
ACE	Angiotensin-converting enzyme
AchR	Acetylcholine receptor antibody
ACP	Acid phosphatase
ACTH	Adrenocorticotropic hormone
ADH	Antidiuretic hormone
AFB	Acid-fast bacillus
AFP	Alpha-fetoprotein
AGBM	Antiglomerular basement membrane antibody
A/G ratio	Albumin/globulin ratio
AHF	Antihemophilic factor
AIDS	Acquired immune deficiency syndrome
ALD	Aldolase
ALP	Alkaline phosphatase
ALT	Alanine aminotransferase (same as SGPT)
$\alpha_1 AT$	Alpha-1-antitrypsin
AMA	Antimitochondrial antibody
ANA	Antinuclear antibodies
ANCA	Antineutrophil cytoplasmic antibody
ANH	Atrial natriuretic hormone
Anti-DNA	Anti-deoxyribonucleic acid

A

Apo	Apolipoproteins
APA	Antiphospholipid antibody
APTT	Activated partial thromboplastin time
ARC	AIDS-related complex
AS	Arsenic
ASO	Antistreptolysin O
AST	Aspartate aminotransferase (same as SGOT)
BE	Base excess
B_2M; BMG	Beta$_2$ microglobulin
BNP	Brain natriuretic peptide
BP	Blood pressure
BPH	Benign prostatic hypertrophy
BRCA-1 and -2	Breast cancer genetic testing
BUN	Blood urea nitrogen
C	Complement (e.g., complement C_3)
Ca	Calcium
CA	Cold agglutinins
CA 15-3 to CA 125	Cancer tumor markers
cAMP	Cyclic adenosine monophosphate
CAT	Computed axial tomography
CBC	Complete blood count
CEA	Carcinoembryonic antigen
CHO	Carbohydrate
CHS	Cholinesterase
Cl	Chloride
CMV	Cytomegalovirus antibody
CO	Carbon monoxide
CO_2	Carbon dioxide
Cp	Ceruloplasmin
CPK or CK	Creatine phosphokinase
CPK-BB	Creatine phosphokinase, brain
CPK-MB	Creatine phosphokinase, heart
CPK-MM	Creatine phosphokinase, skeletal muscle
Cr	Creatinine
CRF	Corticotropin-releasing factor
CRP	C-reactive protein
CSF	Cerebrospinal fluid

CT	Coagulation time
CT	Computed tomography
CTnI	Troponin I
CTnT	Troponin T
CTT	Computed transaxial tomography
Cu	Copper
CVD genetic test	Cardiovascular disease genetic test
D & C	Dilation and curettage
DIC	Disseminated intravascular coagulation
E_1	Estrone
E_2	Estradiol
E_3	Estriol
E_4	Estetrol
EBV	Epstein-Barr virus
ECG (EKG)	Electrocardiogram
ECF	Extracellular fluid
EDTA	Ethylenediaminetetraacetate
EEG	Electroencephalogram
ELISA	Enzyme-linked immunosorbent assay
EMG	Electromyography
ENoG	Lectroneurography
ENG	Electronystagmography
ERCP	Endoscopic retrograde cholangiopancreatography
ESR	Erythrocyte sedimentation rate
EUS	Endoscopic ultrasound
FBS	Fasting blood sugar
FDP	Fibrin degradation products
fFN	Fetal fibronectin
FSH	Follicle-stimulating hormone
FSP	Fibrin or fibrinogen-split product
FTA-ABS	Fluorescent treponemal antibody absorption
G-6-PD	Glucose-6-phosphate dehydrogenase
GGTP or GTP	Gamma-glutamyl (transferase) transpeptidase
GH	Growth hormone
GI series	Gastrointestinal series (upper)
HAA	Hepatitis-associated antigen
HAI or HI	Hemagglutination inhibition

HAV	Hepatitis A virus
Hb or Hgb	Hemoglobin
HB_cAb	Hepatitis B core antibody
HB_sAb	Hepatitis B surface antibody
HB_sAg	Hepatitis B surface antigen
HBD	Hydroxybutyric dehydrogenase
HCG	Human chorionic gonadotropin
HCO_3	Bicarbonate
Hct	Hematocrit
hCT	Calcitonin
HDL	High-density lipoprotein
HF	Heart failure
5-HIAA	5-Hydroxyindoleacetic acid
HIV	Human immunodeficiency virus
HLA	Human leukocyte antigen
Hp	Haptoglobin
HPL	Human placental lactogen
HPV	Human papilloma virus
HSV	Herpes simplex virus
HTLV-III	Human T-lymphotropic virus-III
IBC	Iron-binding capacity (see TIBC)
Ig	Immunoglobulin
IM	Intramuscular
INR	International normalized ratio
IV	Intravenous
IVP	Intravenous pyelography
K	Potassium
17-KS	17-Ketosteroid
KUB	Kidney, ureter, bladder
LAP	Leucine aminopeptidase
LAV	Lymphadenopathy-associated virus
LDH (LD)	Lactic dehydrogenase
LDL	Low-density lipoprotein
LE	Lupus erythematosus preparation
LH	Luteinizing hormone
L/S	Lecithin/sphingomyelin
MA	Microalbumin

MCH	Mean corpuscular hemoglobin
MCHC	Mean corpuscular-hemoglobin concentration
MCV	Mean corpuscular volume
Mg	Magnesium
MI	Myocardial infarction
Na	Sodium
NPO	Nil per os (nothing by mouth)
5′NT	5′Nucleotidase
NTx	N-Telopeptide cross-links
17-OHCS	17-Hydroxycorticosteroid
OVR study	Oculovestibular reflex study
P	Phosphorus
PA	Prealbumin antibody
$PaCO_2$	Partial pressure of carbon dioxide
PaO_2	Partial pressure of oxygen
PAP	Pulmonary arterial pressure
PAPP-A	Pregnancy Associated Plasma Protein-A
Pap smear	Papanicolaou smear
PCWP	Pulmonary capillary wedge pressure
PGF	Placental growth factor
pH	Negative logarithm of hydrogen ion concentration
PKU	Phenylketonuria
PPBS	Postprandial blood sugar (feasting blood sugar)
PRL	Prolactin
PSA	Prostate-specific antigen
PT	Prothrombin time
PTH	Parathyroid hormone
PTT	Partial thromboplastin time
PYD	Pyridinium
RA	Rheumatoid arthritis
RAIU	Radioactive iodine uptake
RBC	Red blood cell (erythrocyte)
RDW	Red blood cell distribution width
RF	Rheumatoid factor
RIA	Radioimmunoassay
RPR	Rapid plasma reagin
SaO_2	Oxygen saturation

SCID	Severe combined immunodeficiency
SGOT	Serum glutamic oxaloacetic transaminase (same as AST)
SGPT	Serum glutamic pyruvic transaminase (same as ALT)
SIADH	Syndrome of inappropriate antidiuretic hormone
SLE	Systemic lupus erythematosus
T_3	Triiodothyronine
T_4	Thyroxine
TA	Thyroid antibodies
TB	Tuberculosis
TBG	Thyroxine-binding globulin
TCA	Tricyclic antidepressants
TDM	Therapeutic drug monitoring
TIBC	Total iron-binding capacity (see IBC)
TPO	Thyroid Peroxidase Antibody
TRH	Thyrotropin-releasing hormone
T_3 RU	T_3 resin uptake
TSH	Thyroid-stimulating hormone
UA	Urinalysis
URI	Upper respiratory infections
VCE	Video capsule endoscopy
VCT	Venous clotting time
VDRL	Venereal Disease Research Laboratory
VLDL	Very low-density lipoprotein
VMA	Vanillylmandelic acid
VS	Vital signs
WBC	White blood cell (leukocyte)
ZPP	Zinc protoporphyrin

Laboratory Test Groups: Panels and Profiles

Groups of laboratory tests, identified as panel, profiles, and sequential analyzers (SMAs), are useful for diagnosing and assessing clinical problems. Tests are usually grouped as general tests for determining health status and organ and disease panels/profiles. Laboratories, private or in health care institutions, develop test groups according to their equipment for analyzing laboratory values. The majority of these tests require either one 7- or 10-mL red-top tube of blood.

Today, the SMA group name is infrequently used. *Panel*, *profile*, and *chem* are the terms usually used to refer to groups of laboratory tests. Medicare may not pay for groups that have a large number of tests because of their cost. Laboratories and health care providers, including physicians, may select certain tests within the group to minimize cost and maximize Medicare payments. Numerous tests may be performed from one tube of blood.

General laboratory test groups

Basic Metabolic Panel (8)

BUN	Creatinine
Calcium	Glucose
Carbon dioxide (total)	Potassium
Chloride	Sodium

Comprehensive Metabolic Panel (14)

Albumin	BUN
Alkaline phosphatase	Calcium
AST/SGOT	Cholesterol

Bilirubin (total)
Glucose
LD/LDH
Potassium
Protein (total)

Creatinine
Sodium
Triglyceride
Urea nitrogen (BUN)

Profile 22

A/G ratio
Albumin
Alkaline phosphatase
ALT/SGPT
AST/SGOT
Bilirubin (total)
BUN
BUN/creatinine ratio
Calcium
Protein (total)
Sodium

Chloride
Cholesterol
CO_2 (content)
Creatinine
Globulin
Glucose
LD/LDH
Phosphorus
Potassium
Triglyceride
Uric acid

Chemistry Profile

Albumin
Alkaline phosphatase
AST/SGOT
Bilirubin (total)
BUN
Calcium

Creatinine
Glucose
LD/LDH
Phosphorus
Protein (total)
Uric acid

Profile 11

Albumin
Alkaline phosphatase
AST/SGOT
Bilirubin (total)
Calcium
Cholesterol

CPK/CK
LD/LDH
Phosphorus
Protein (total)
Uric acid

Electrolytes [LYTES]

(Might be ordered with SMA 12, chemistry profile, or profile 11.)

Chloride	Potassium
CO_2 content	Sodium

SMA 12-60

(Laboratory may select any 12 tests to program on their analyzer.)

Albumin	Cholesterol
Alkaline phosphatase	Glucose
AST/SGOT	LD/LDH
Bilirubin (total)	Phosphorus
BUN	Protein (total)
Calcium	Uric acid

Routine hematology and urine tests

Complete Blood Count [CBC]

WBC count and differential:	Hematocrit
Neutrophil	Hemoglobin
Band	Platelets
	RBC count
Segment	RBC indices
Basophils	MCV
Eosinophils	MCH
Lymphocytes	MCHC
Monocytes	RDW

Urinalysis

Appearance	pH
Bacteria	Protein
Casts	RBC
Color	Specific gravity (SG)
Glucose	WBC
Ketones	

Organ and disease panel and profile

Anemia Panel/Profile

CBC with RBC indices	Reticulocyte count
Folate/folic acid	TIBC
Hemoglobin electrophoresis	Vitamin B_{12}
Iron	

Arthritis Panel/Profile

ANA	ESR
ASO	Phosphorus
Calcium	Rheumatoid factor
CRP	Uric acid

Bone/Joint Panel/Profile

Albumin	Protein (total)
Alkaline phosphatase	Synovial fluid analysis
Calcium	Uric acid
Phosphorus	

Cardiac Panel/Profile

AST/SGOT	Potassium
CPK/CK and isoenzymes	Tropinins
LDH/LD and isoenzymes	

Coagulation Panel/Profile

APTT and PT	Factor assay
Bleeding time	FDP
Clot retraction	Platelet count
Coagulation time/clotting time	PT
INR	

Coma Panel/Profile

Alcohol	Electrolytes
Ammonia	Glucose
Blood gases (pH, $PaCO_2$, HCO_3)	Lactic acid
BUN	Osmolality (serum and urine)
Creatinine	Salicylate
Drug-abuse toxicology screen	

Coronary Risk Panel/Profile

Cholesterol (total)

   HDL

   LDL

   VLDL

Glucose

Tropinins

Lipoprotein phenotyping

Phospholipids

Total lipids

Triglycerides

Diabetes Mellitus Panel/Profile

BUN

Cholesterol Creatinine

Electrolytes (K, Na, Cl, CO_2)

Glucose (fasting/2-hour feasting)

Glucose tolerance (*not* for high blood sugar)

Ketones (serum and urine)

Triglycerides

Drug Toxicology/Drug Abuse Panel/Profile

Acetaminophen

Amphetamines

Barbiturates

Benzodiazepines

Cocaine

Codeine

Meperidine (Demerol)

Meprobamate (Equanil)

Methadone

Morphine

Phenothiazines

Phenytoin (Dilantin)

Propoxyphene (Darvon)

Salicylates

Tricyclic antidepressants

Hepatic/Liver Panel/Profile

A/G ratio

Albumin

Alkaline phosphatase

ALT/SGPT

AST/SGOT

Bilirubin (total and direct)

Cholesterol

GGT/GGTP

LDH/LD

LDH isoenzymes

Protein (total)

PT

Hepatitis Panel/Profile

HA Ab IgM

HB_cAb or Anti-HB_c (antibody to
   hepatitis B core antigen)

HB_cAB IgM

HB_sAb (hepatitis B surface antibody) or
   Anti-HB_s (antibody to HB_sAg)

HB_sAg (hepatitis B surface antigen)

HB$_e$Ab (hepatitis B e
  (antibody) or Anti-HB$_e$
  (antibody to HB$_e$Ag)   Anti-HAV (antibody to hepatitis A
                                           virus [IgM])

HB$_e$Ag (hepatitis B e antigen)

Hypertension Panel/Profile

BUN   LDH/LD
Cholesterol   T$_4$
Creatinine   Renin
Electrolytes (K, Na, Cl, CO_2)   Triglycerides
Glucose   VMA

Lipid Panel/Profile

Cholesterol (total)   Lipids (total)
  HDL   Phospholipids
  LDL   Triglycerides
  LDL/HDL Ratio

Neonatal Panel/Profile

Albumin   Calcium
Bilirubin (total)   Electrolytes (K, Na, Cl, CO_2)
Blood type (ABO)   Glucose
BUN   Rh typing

Obstetric Panel/Profile

ABO/Rh   RPR (DX) w/reflex confirm
Antibody Scr RBCw/reflex   Hb$_s$AG w/reflex confirm
CBC   Rubella IgG Ab

Pancreatic Panel/Profile

Amylase   Glucose
Calcium   Lipase

Parathyroid Panel/Profile

Alkaline phosphatase   Phosphorus
Calcium (serum and urine)   Protein (total)
Magnesium

Prenatal Panel/Profile

Atypical antibody screen

Blood type (ABO)

CBC with differential

Rh typing

Hepatitis B surface antigen (HB_sAg)

RPR or VDRL

Rubella screen

Urinalysis

Pulmonary/Lung Panel/Profile

Blood gases (pH, $PaCO_2$, PaO_2, HCO_3)

CO_2 content

SaO_2

Renal Panel/Profile

Albumin

BUN

BUN: creatinine ratio

Creatinine (serum and 24-hour urine)

Creatinine clearance

Electrolytes (K, Na, Cl, CO_2)

Glucose

Protein (total and 24-hour urine)

Uric acid

Thyroid Panel/Profile

Calcitonin

Free thyroxine index (FTI or Free T_4)

T_4RIA

T_3RIA

T_3 resin uptake

TSH

TA

APPENDIX C

Health Problems with Laboratory and Diagnostic Tests

Various laboratory and diagnostic tests are ordered for diagnosing common clinical health problems. Sixty common health problems with frequently ordered laboratory and diagnostic tests are listed below:

1. **Alzheimer disease**
   Laboratory tests: amyloid beta protein, apolipoprotein, cerebrospinal fluid (CSF), ceruloplasmin, protein electrophoresis
   Diagnostic tests: CT of brain, MRI (brain), EEG, PET (brain)

2. **Amyotrophic lateral sclerosis (ALS)**
   Laboratory tests: complete blood count (CBC), vital signs, dyspnea, muscular weakness
   Diagnostic tests: electromyelography studies, MRI (neurography), biopsy of the muscle as indicated

3. **Anemia**
   Laboratory tests: complete blood count (CBC), RBC indices, reticulocyte, iron, total iron-binding capacity (TIBC), ferritin, folic acid, vitamin B_{12}, haptoglobin (HP), erythrocyte sedimentation rate (ESR)
   Diagnostic tests: bone marrow biopsy, Schilling test

4. **Angina pectoris**
   Laboratory tests: troponins, creatine phosphokinase (CPK), anticardiolipin antibody, antimyocardial antibody, homocysteine, lactate dehydrogenase isoenzymes, aspartate aminotransferase (AST), lipoproteins, troponins
   Diagnostic tests: echocardiography, cardiac catheterization, stress exercise test, Holter monitor, ECG (EKG), ultrasonography (heart), PET, nuclear scan of the heart

5. **Anorexia nervosa**
   Laboratory tests: electrolytes (especially potassium, sodium, chloride), transthyretin (prealbumin), thyroxine (T_4), triiodothyronine (T_3), estradiol, luteinizing hormone, lipoprotein

6. **Appendicitis**
   Laboratory tests: complete blood count (CBC), differential leukocyte count, vital signs, urinalysis, blood culture
   Diagnostic tests: ultrasonography, CT (computed tomography)

7. **Arteriosclerosis (atherosclerosis)**
   Laboratory tests: lipid profile (cholesterol [LDL, HDL], triglycerides), platelet count, homocysteine, international normalized ratio (INR), C-reactive protein, anticardiolipin antibody
   Diagnostic tests: stress test, Doppler ultrasonography flow studies, CT (computed tomography)

8. **Arthritis**
   Laboratory tests: antinuclear antibody (ANA), C-reactive protein (CRP), culture (synovial fluid), antistreptolysin O, complement (total), lupus test, rheumatoid factor (RF), ESR, uric acid
   Diagnostic tests: x-ray of the bone

9. **Asthma**
   Laboratory tests: arterial blood gases (ABGs), culture (sputum), CBC allergen-specific IgE, eosinophil
   Diagnostic tests: pulmonary function tests, pulse oximetry, chest x-ray

10. **Brain tumor (malignant or benign)**
    Laboratory test: cerebrospinal fluid analysis
    Diagnostic tests: cerebral angiography, biopsy of the brain tissue, electroencephalography, MRI, positron emission tomography (PET)

11. **Breast cancer**
    Laboratory tests: breast cancer tumor tests (BRCA-1 and BRCA-2), cancer tumor markers (CA 15.3 and CA 27.29 most common, also CA 50, CA 125, CA 549), carcinoembryonic antigen (CEA), Her-2/neu oncogene, estrogen, estradiol, prolactin, progesterone, follicle-stimulating hormone (FSH)
    Diagnostic tests: mammography, mammary ductoscopy, biopsy (stereotactic-breast), ultrasonography, MRI, PET, ultrasonography of breast

12. **Bronchitis (acute and chronic)**
    Laboratory tests: arterial blood gases (ABGs), complete blood count (CBC), bronchial culture
    Diagnostic tests: x-ray of the lungs, bronchoscopy, pulmonary function tests, CT scan

13. **Celiac disease**
    Laboratory tests: complete blood count (CBC), chemistry (metabolic) panel, fecal fat stool, D-xylose absorption
    Diagnostic tests: GI studies, small bowel biopsy

14. **Cerebrovascular accident (CVA)**
    Laboratory tests: CBC, serum cholesterol, cerebrospinal fluid, PT, comprehensive metabolic panel
    Diagnostic tests: CT brain scan, nuclear brain scan, MRI, cerebral angiography, PET, oculoplethysmography, ECG, EEG, Doppler ultrasonographic (carotid)

15. **Cholecystitis (acute)**
Laboratory tests: CBC, direct bilirubin, serum alkaline phosphatase
Diagnostic tests: gallbladder and biliary ultrasound, CT of the gallbladder, cholangiogram, nuclear gallbladder scan

16. **Cirrhosis of the liver**
Laboratory tests: liver enzyme tests: alkaline phosphatase (ALP), gamma-glutamyltransferase (GGT), alanine aminotransferase (ALT/SGPT) 5′nucleotidase (5′N), total and direct bilirubin, serum protein, serum albumin, prealbumin assay, CBC, platelet aggregation, prothrombin time (PT), serum electrolytes, plasma ammonia, antimitochondrial antibody, zinc, zinc protoporphyrin, antismooth muscle antibody (ASMA)
Diagnostic tests: nuclear liver scan, CT of the liver, liver biopsy, hepatic angiography, biopsy, peritoneal fluid analysis

17. **Colorectal cancer**
Laboratory tests: serum electrolytes, CA 19.9, CA 50, carcinoembryonic antigen, fecal analysis for occult blood, colorectal cancer allelotyping for chromosomes, 17 p and 18 q
Diagnostic tests: colonoscopy, sigmoidoscopy, barium enema, biopsy, CT

18. **Cystic fibrosis**
Laboratory tests: chloride (sweat), sputum culture, electrolytes, D-xylose absorption test, trypsin
Diagnostic tests: chest x-rays, pulmonary function tests

19. **Cystitis**
Laboratory tests: urinalysis, culture (urine), BUN, serum creatinine, CBC
Diagnostic tests: cystoscopy, cystometry, ultrasound (kidney), CT (kidney), nuclear scan (kidney)

20. **Deep-vein thrombophlebitis (DVT)**
Laboratory tests: CBC PT, PTT/APTT, plasminogen assay, fibrinogen, antithrombin III
Diagnostic tests: Doppler ultrasonography, venography, MRI, CT

21. **Dementia**
Laboratory tests: CBC, lipid levels, cerebrospinal fluid, Venereal Disease Research Laboratory (VDRL)
Diagnostic tests: brain scan, CT (brain), MRI, transcranial Doppler ultrasonography

22. **Diabetes mellitus (DM)**
Laboratory tests: CBC, serum/blood FBS (fasting blood sugar or blood glucose), and postprandial blood sugar (PPBS or feasting blood sugar), glucose self-monitoring, hemoglobin A_1c, insulin and insulin antibody, glucagon, serum electrolytes, serum acetone, ABGs, oral glucose tolerance test, serum BUN, osmolality, lactic acid
Diagnostic test: ECG

23. **Eclampsia (toxemia) of pregnancy**
Laboratory tests: CBC, electrolytes, glucose, creatinine, BUN, uric acid, albumin (urine), protein (quantitative), PTT, INR (international ratio), lipoproteins, placental growth factor (PGF), pregnancy-associated plasma protein-A (PAPP-A)
Diagnostic test: blood pressure monitoring

24. **Emphysema**
    Laboratory tests: ABGs, serum alpha-1-antitrypsin, CBC, electrolytes
    Diagnostic tests: chest x-ray, pulmonary function tests, nuclear lung scan, thoracoscopy, sputum cytology

25. **Endocarditis**
    Laboratory tests: blood cultures, RBC indices, WBC count, ESR, ANA, C_2 and C_4 complements, CRP, RF, creatinine
    Diagnostic test: ECG (EKG), echocardiography, blood culture, transesophageal ultrasonography

26. **Fever, unknown origin**
    Laboratory tests: blood culture, urine culture, CBC differential WBC, mycobacteria specimen (culture), TB culture
    Diagnostic test: chest x-ray

27. **Glomerulonephritis**
    Laboratory tests: chemistry (metabolic) panel, protein (urine), culturette for streptococcus, urinalysis, albumin/globulin ratio, complement C_3 and C_4, anti-DNA, antistreptolysin 0 titer
    Diagnostic tests: kidney biopsy, IV pyelography

28. **Gout**
    Laboratory tests: chemistry (metabolic) panel, uric acid (blood and urine)
    Diagnostic tests: synovial fluid analysis

29. **Gynecologic problems**
    Laboratory tests: estrone (E_1), estrogen, estradiol (E_2), prolactin
    Diagnostic tests: biopsy, cervicography, colposcopy, hysteroscopy

30. **Heart failure (HF): (Old term: Congestive heart failure [CHF])**
    Laboratory tests: CBC, electrolytes, serum and urine osmolality, comprehensive metabolic panel, cardiac enzymes (CPK, LDH, AST, and isoenzymes), atrial natriuretic peptide (ANP), brain natriuretic peptide (BNP), troponin 1 and troponin T, ESR
    Diagnostic tests: ECG (EKG), x-ray of the heart and chest, cerebral vascular pressure (CVP), echocardiography, nuclear scan (MUGA), PET, pulmonary capillary wedge pressure (PCWP), ventriculography

31. **Heart palpitations**
    Laboratory tests: CBC, arterial blood gases (ABCs), troponins
    Diagnostic tests: ECG (EKG), echocardiography, Holter monitor, stress tests

32. **Helicobacter pylori**
    Laboratory tests: Helicobacter pylori test (office), *Helicobacter pylori* antigen test (stool), stool culture, pepsinogen test
    Diagnostic tests: gastroscopy, gastric analysis tests

33. **Hepatitis**
    Laboratory tests: hepatitis A (HAV) antibody, hepatitis profile, hepatitis B surface antigen (HbsAG), CBC, bilirubin (total, direct, indirect, urine) urobilinogen, alkaline phosphatase
    Diagnostic tests: CT (liver), ultrasound (liver), biopsy (liver), nuclear scan (liver)

34. **Hodgkin disease**
    Laboratory tests: CBC, differential WBC, chemistry (metabolic) panel, platelet count, protein electrophoresis, C-reactive protein, D-xylose absorption tests, cryoglobulin, T and B lymphocyte assay, liver enzyme tests
    Diagnostic tests: bone marrow aspiration, biopsy of the lymph node(s), CT (chest and abdomen), chest x-ray

35. **Hypertension**
    Laboratory tests: electrolytes, BUN, creatinine, BUN/creatinine ratio, aldosterone, renin, catecholamines, thyroid tests, urinalysis
    Diagnostic tests: blood pressure monitoring, ECG, echocardiography

36. **Infertility**
    Laboratory tests: female hormones (estrogen, progesterone), luteinizing hormone, follicle-stimulating hormone, prolactin, semen analysis, testosterone, chromosome analysis, infertility screen
    Diagnostic tests: hysterosalpingography, D & C (dilation and curettage), biopsy of the endometrium, cervical culture, gynecologic ultrasonography, postcoital tests (Sims-Huhner)

37. **Leukemia**
    Laboratory tests: complete blood count (CBC), differential WBC, platelet count, blood culture, cryoglobulin, T and B lymphocytes assay, BUN, creatinine (serum)
    Diagnostic tests: bone marrow aspiration, chest X-ray, abdominal ultrasonography

38. **Lung cancer**
    Laboratory tests: ABGs, sputum cytology, CA 15, CA 50, serotonin
    Diagnostic tests: chest x-ray, bronchoscopy, CT of the lungs, lung biopsy, MRI, mediastinoscopy, transesophageal ultrasonography, pulmonary function tests, nuclear scan of the bone and brain

39. **Melanoma**
    Laboratory tests: complete blood count (CBC), histopathology, hepatic analysis, melanin (urine)
    Diagnostic tests: biopsy of the skin site, computed tomography of area, lymph node biopsy, chest x-ray, cerebral CT, positron emission tomography (PET)

40. **Meningitis**
    Laboratory tests: blood cultures, cerebrospinal fluid (CSF), sputum, WBC, electrolytes, CBC, cryptococcal antigen, bacterial and viral culture
    Diagnostic tests: cerebrospinal fluid for culture and pressure (lumbar puncture), CT scan of the brain, MRI, x-ray of the skull

41. **Multiple sclerosis (MS)**
    Laboratory tests: cerebrospinal fluid analysis, protein electrophoresis
    Diagnostic tests: MRI, CT scan, electromyography (EMG), EEG

42. **Myocardial infarction, acute (AMI)**
    Laboratory tests: cardiac enzymes: CPK and CPK isoenzymes (CPK-MB), aspartate aminotransferase (AST/SGOT), lactic dehydrogenase (LDH), and LDH isoenzymes with LDH_1 greater than LDH_2, CBC, lipoproteins, cholesterol, triglycerides, LDL, HDL,

serum electrolytes, PT, PTT/APTT, INR, serum and urine myoglobin, anticardiolipin antibody, antimyocardial antibody, serum/blood glucose, ESR, ABGs, AMA, homocysteine, troponins (troponin 1 and troponin T)

Diagnostic tests: cardiac catheterization, x-ray of the heart and chest, stress exercise test, ECG (EKG), nuclear heart scan (MUGA), positron emission tomography (PET), pacemaker monitoring, echocardiography

43. **Obstructive bowel disorder**

Laboratory tests: CBC, differential WBC count, electrolyte analysis, chemistry (metabolic) panel, urinalysis, stool for occult blood

Diagnostic tests: x-ray of the abdomen, ultrasonography flow studies of the abdomen, barium enema

44. **Osteoporosis**

Laboratory tests: serum calcium, serum phosphorus, serum ALP, protein electrophoresis, estrogen, osteocalcin, thyroid function tests

Diagnostic tests: x-ray of the bone, bone density scan, nuclear bone scan

45. **Ovarian cancer**

Laboratory tests: CBC, CA 15, CA 72, CA 125, chemistry (metabolic) panel, endothelial growth factor, electrolytes

Diagnostic tests: GYN ultrasonography, x-ray of the abdomen

46. **Pancreatitis (acute)**

Laboratory tests: serum and urine amylase, serum lipase, serum alcohol, gamma-glutamyl transpeptidase, leucine aminopeptidase, serum electrolytes, trypsin

Diagnostic tests: CT and ultrasound of the pancreas, endoscopic retrograde cholangiopancreatography, MRI

47. **Peptic ulcer**

Laboratory tests: serum electrolytes, *Helicobacter pylori*, pepsinogen, CBC, occult blood, serum amylase

Diagnostic tests: upper GI series, gastric analysis studies, gastric acid stimulation test, esophagogastroduodenoscopy, biopsy of GI tissue

48. **Pharyngitis/sinusitis**

Laboratory tests: culture of the pharynx, culture from nasal secretions, CBC

Diagnostic tests: sinus CT, x-ray (facial area), sinus endoscopy

49. **Pneumonia**

Laboratory tests: ABGs, CBC, sputum culture, blood culture

Diagnostic tests: chest x-ray, pulmonary function tests, bronchoscopy, oximetry, thoracentesis, nuclear lung scan

50. **Pregnancy and fetal distress**

Laboratory tests: alpha fetoprotein, estrone (E_1), estriol (E_3), estetrol (E_4), fetal hemoglobin, CBC, ferritin, human chorionic gonadotropin, methemoglobin, pregnanediol, progesterone, PAPP-A, PGF, folic acid (folate), severe combined immunodeficiency (SCID)

Diagnostic tests: pregnancy test, fetal nonstress test, contraction stress test, fetoscopy, fetal fibronectin, fetal monitoring, fetal biophysical profile, obstetric ultrasonography

51. **Prostatic disorders (cancer, benign prostatic hypertrophy [BPH], prostatitis)**
    Laboratory tests: prostate-specific antigen (PSA), total and free % PSA, acid phosphatase (ACP)/prostatic acid phosphatase (PAP), CBC, ALP, CA 15.3, urinalysis
    Diagnostic tests: digital examination, ultrasonography, biopsy of the prostate gland, nuclear bone scan, CT

52. **Pulmonary embolism (PE)**
    Laboratory tests: CBC, PT, PTT/APTT, INR, ABGs, ESR, plasminogen
    Diagnostic tests: chest x-ray, nuclear lung (perfusion) scan, pulmonary angiography, CT, MRI, Doppler ultrasonographic studies, echocardiography, ECG (EKG), venography

53. **Renal failure (RF)**
    Laboratory tests: serum BUN, serum creatinine, urinalysis, serum and urine osmolality, BUN/creatinine ratio, ABGs, CBC, electrolytes, beta$_2$ microglobulin, antiglomerular basement membrane (anti-GBM), urine protein
    Diagnostic tests: kidney, ureter, and bladder (KUB) x-ray, nuclear renal scan, renal angiography, kidney biopsy, kidney ultrasonography, MRI, intravenous pyelography

54. **Rheumatoid arthritis (RA)**
    Laboratory tests: rheumatoid arthritis (RA) factor, CBC, antinuclear antibody (ANA), antimitochondrial antibody (AMA), anti-DNA, C-reactive protein (CRP), complements C_3 and C_4, sed rate or ESR, protein electrophoresis, antistreptolysin-O titer, electrolytes
    Diagnostic tests: synovial fluid analysis, x-ray of joints, nuclear bone scan

55. **Systemic lupus erythematosus (SLE or lupus)**
    Laboratory tests: lupus erythematosus cell test (LE cell test), anti-DNA, C-reactive protein (CRP), antinuclear antibody (ANA), antiphospholipid antibody, complements C_3 and C_4, CBC, sed rate or ESR, protein electrophoresis, urinalysis
    Diagnostic tests: ECG (EKG), kidney biopsy

56. **Thrombophlebitis**
    Laboratory tests: APTT, INR, CBC, differential WBC
    Diagnostic tests: MRI, Doppler thoracic ultrasonography, venography

57. **Thyroid disorders**
    Laboratory tests: triiodothyronine (T_3), thyroxine (T_4), thyroid antibodies (TA), thyroglobulin antibodies, thyroid-stimulating hormone (TSH), triiodothyronine resin uptake (T_3RU), serum electrolytes, TPO antibodies
    Diagnostic tests: nuclear scan of the thyroid, CT and ultrasound of the thyroid, radioactive iodine (RAI) uptake

58. **Tuberculosis**
    Laboratory tests: culture of sputum for acid-fast (AF) bacteria, tuberculin skin tests (Mantoux test), urinalysis for TB
    Diagnostic tests: x-ray of the chest, CT of chest, nuclear scan of the chest

59. **Ulcerative colitis**
    Laboratory tests: CBC, serum electrolytes, protein electrophoresis, occult blood (stool), prothrombin time (PT), erythrocyte sedimentation rate (ESR)

Diagnostic tests: colonoscopy, barium enema, biopsy of the colon, cytologic study of the GI tract, x-ray of the abdomen

60. Uterine cancer

Laboratory tests: CBC, CA 125

Diagnostic tests: Pap smear, biopsy of the endometrium, D & C, ultrasonography (GYN), CT (pelvis)

APPENDIX D

Laboratory Test Values for Adults and Children

The laboratory tests and their reference values for adults and children are listed according to the laboratory sections that analyze the specimens. The personnel from the laboratory and nuclear medicine departments frequently work together in obtaining blood specimens to be tested by the radioimmunoassay (RIA) method. So that the client does not receive several venous punctures, the laboratory personnel will collect enough blood for all laboratory tests, including RIA.

Arterial blood gases are analyzed in either the pulmonary function laboratory, critical care units, or chemistry section of the laboratory. The cerebrospinal fluid tubes are distributed to the appropriate laboratory sections (i.e., hematology, chemistry, or microbiology).

Reference values differ from laboratory to laboratory, so nurses should refer to the published laboratory values used in their hospitals or private laboratories to check for any differences.

D

REFERENCE VALUES

Hematology	Color-Top Tube	Adult	Child
Antithrombin III	Blue or red	75–137% (average)	
Bleeding time		Ivy's method: 3–7 minutes Duke's method: 1–3 minutes	Same as adult
Blood smear	Blood drop or lavender		
Carboxyhemoglobin (CO)— see Chemistry			
Clot retraction	Red	1–24 hours	Same as adult
Coagulation time (CT)		5–15 minutes; average: 8 minutes	Same as adult
Complete blood count (CBC)	Lavender	See CBC in text	
D-Dimer test	Blue	Negative; positive: greater than 250 ng/mL	
Erythrocyte sedimentation rate (ESR)	Lavender	Less than 50 years old (Westergren): Male: 0–15 mm/h Female: 0–20 mm/h Greater than 50 years old (Westergren): Male: 0–20 mm/h Female: 0–30 mm/h Wintrobe method: Male: 0–9 mm/h Female: 0–15 mm/h	Newborn: 0–2 mm/h 4–14 years old: 0–10 mm/h
Euglobulin lysis time	Blue	No lysis	
Factor assay	Blue		Same as adult
I Fibrinogen		200–400 mg/dL	
II Prothrombin		Minimum for clotting: 75–100 mg/dL	
III Thromboplastin		Minimum hemostatic level: 10–15% concentration	
IV Calcium		Variety of substances	
V Proaccelerin labile factor		4.5–5.5 mEq/L or 9–11 mg/dL	Same as adult
		Minimum hemostatic level: 50–150% activity; 5–10% concentration	
VI		Not used	
VII Proconvertin stable factor		Minimum hemostatic level: 65–135% activity; 5–15% concentration	
VIII Antihemophilic factor (AHF)		Minimum hemostatic level: 55–145% activity; 30–35% concentration	

Test	Tube color	Normal value	Children
IX Plasma thromboplastin component (PTC, Christmas factor)		Minimum hemostatic level: 60–140% activity; 30% concentration	
X Stuart factor, Prower factor		Minimum hemostatic level: 45–150% activity; 7–10% concentration	
XI Plasma thromboplastin antecedent (PTA)		Minimum hemostatic level: 65–135% activity; 20–30% concentration	
XII Hageman factor		0% concentration	
XIII Fibrinase, fibrin stabilizing factor (FSF)		Minimum hemostatic level: 1% concentration	
Fetal hemoglobin (Hb F)	Lavender	0.2%	Newborn: 60–90% 1–5 months: less than 70% 6–12 months: less than 5% greater than 1 year old: less than 2%
Fibrin degradation products (FDP)	Blue	2–10 mcg/mL	
Fibrinogen	Blue	200–400 mg/dL	Not usually done Newborn: 150–300 mg/dL Child: same as adult
Galactose-1-phosphate uridyl transferase (GPUT)	Lavender	Negative Quantitative: 18.5–28.5 units/g; less than 5 units/g in Hb Carrier of deficiency: 5–18 units/g of Hb	
Hematocrit (Hct)	Lavender	Male: 40–54%; 0.40–0.54 SI units Female: 36–46%; 0.36–0.46 SI units	Newborn: 44–65% 1–3 years old: 29–40% 4–10 years old: 31–43%
Hemoglobin (Hb or Hgb)	Lavender	Male: 13.5–17 g/dL Female: 12–15 g/dL	Newborn: 14–24 g/dL Infant: 10–17 g/dL Child: 11–16 g/dL
Hemoglobin Aic	Lavender	4.5–7.5% of Hb	
Hemoglobin electrophoresis	Green Lavender		
A_1		95–98% total Hb	
A_2		1.5–4%	
F		less than 2%	Newborn: 50–80% total Hb Infant: 2–8% total Hb Child: 1–2% total Hb
C		0%	
D		0%	
S		0%	

REFERENCE VALUES

Hematology	Color-Top Tube	Adult	Child
Heinz bodies	Lavender	Negative: less than 30% of Heinz bodies present	
Lymphocytes (T & B) assay	Lavender (2 tubes)	T cells: 60–80%, 600–2,400 cells/µL; B cells: 4–16%, 50–250 cells/µL	
Methemoglobin	Lavender Green	Normal: less than 1.5% total Hb; 0.06–0.24 g/dL; 9.2–37 µmol/L; positive: greater than 20–70%	
Osmotic fragility: erythrocyte		% Hemolysis	Same as adult

% SALINE (NaCl)	FRESH BLOOD (3 HOURS)	INCUBATED AT 37°C (24-HOUR BLOOD)
0.30	75–100	85–100
0.35	90–98	75–100
0.40	50–95	65–100
0.45	5–45	55–95
0.50	0–5	40–85
0.55	0	15–65
0.60	0	0–40

Hematology	Color-Top Tube	Adult	Child
Partial thromboplastin time (PTT)	Blue	PPT: 60–70 seconds; APTT: 25–40 seconds	
Plasminogen	Blue	7–16 mg/dL	
Platelet aggregation and adhesion	Blue	Aggregation in 3–5 minutes	
Platelet antibody test	Blue	Negative	
Platelet count (thrombocytes)	Lavender	150,000–400,000 µL (mean, 250,000 µL) (mm^3, K/µL also); SI units: 0.15–0.4 10^{12}/L	Premature: 100,000–300,000 µL; Newborn: 150,000–300,000 µL; Infant: 200,000–475,000 µL
Prothrombin time (PT)	Blue or black	11–15 seconds or 70–100%; Anticoagulant therapy: 2–2.5 times the control in seconds or 20–30%	Same as adult

Test	Tube color	Adult value	Pediatric value
RBC indices (mil/μL)	Lavender	Male: 4.6–6 Female: 4–5	Newborn: 4.8–7.2 Child: 3.8–5.5
MCV (cuμ)		80–98	Newborn: 96–108 Child: 82–92
MCH (pg)		27–31	Newborn: 32–34 Child: 27–31
MCHC (%)		32–36	Newborn: 32–33 Child: 32–36
RDW (Coulter S)		11.5–14.5	
Reticulocyte count	Lavender	0.5–1.5% of all RBCs 25,000–75,000 μL (absolute count)	Newborn: 2.5–6.5% of all RBCs Infant: 0.5–3.5% of all RBCs Child: 0.5–2% of all RBCs
Sickle-cell screening	Lavender	0	0
White blood cells (WBC)	Lavender	4,500–10,000 μL	Newborn: 9,000–30,000 μL 2 years old: 6,000–17,000 μL; 10 years: 4,500–13,500 μL
White blood cell differential	Lavender		
Neutrophils		50–70% of total WBCs	29–47%
Segments		50–65%	
Bands		0–5%	
Eosinophils		0–3%	0–3%
Basophils		1–3%	1–3%
Lymphocytes		25–35%	38–63%
Monocytes		2–6%	4–9%
Immunohematology (blood bank)			
Coombs direct	Lavender	Negative	Negative
Coombs indirect	Red	Negative	Negative
Crossmatching	Red	Absence of agglutination (clumping)	Same as adult
Rh typing	Red	Rh+ and Rh–	Same as adult

REFERENCE VALUES

Chemistry	Color-Top Tube	Adult	Child
Acetaminophen	Red	Therapeutic: 5–20 mcg/mL; 31–124 µmol/L (SI units) Toxic: greater than 50 mcg/mL; greater than 305 µmol/L (SI units) greater than 200 mcg/mL, possible hepatotoxicity	Therapeutic: same as adult
Acetone (ketone bodies) adult	Red	Acetone: 0.3–2 mg/dL; 51.6–344 µmol/L (SI units); Ketones: 2–4 mg/dL	Newborn: slightly higher than adult Infant and child: same as adult
Acetylcholine receptor antibody (AchR)	Red	Negative, less than 0.02 to less than 0.03 nmol/L	
Acid phosphatase (ACP)	Red	Less than 2.6 ng/mL; 0–5 U/L	
Adrenocorticotropic hormone (ACTH)	Lavender	7–10 AM: 8–80 pg/mL; 4 PM: 5–30 pg/mL; 10 PM to midnight: less than 10 pg/mL	
Alanine aminotransferase (ALT, SGPT)	Red	10–35 U/L	Same as adult
Albumin	Red	4–36 U/L at 37°C (SI units)	Infant: could be twice as high
Alcohol	Red	3.5–5 g/dL	
Aldolase (ALD)	Red	0%	
	Red	3–8 U/dL (Sibley-Lehninger) 22–59 m U/L at 37°C (SI units)	Infant: 12–24 U/dL Child: 6–16 U/L
Aldosterone	Red or green	Fast: less than 16 ng/dL; 4–30 ng/dL (sitting position)	3–11 years: 5–70 ng/dL
Alkaline phosphatase (ALP)	Red	42–136 U/L	Infant: 40–300 U/L Child: 40–115 U/L Older child: 50–230 U/L
Allergen-specific IgE	Red	78–200 mg/dL	Newborn: 145–270 mg/dL Neonates to 2 years: less than 12 international units/mL 3–5 years old: less than 40 international units/mL 6–12 years old: less than 90 international units/mL
	Red or gray	Less than 100 international units/mL	
ALP₁		20–130 U/L	
ALP₂		20–120 U/L	

Alpha-1-antitrypsin — Red — 0.78–2 g/L — Infant and child: same as adult

Alpha-fetoprotein (AFP)

WEEKS OF GESTATION	SERUM (ng/mL)	AMNIOTIC FLUID (mcg/mL)
14	7–50	11–32
15	7–60	5.5–31
16	10–72	5.7–31.5
17	11–90	3.8–32.5
18	14–94	3.6–28
19	24–112	3.7–24.5
20	31–122	2.2–15

Amikacin — Red — Therapeutic:
Peak: 15–30 mcg/mL
Trough: less than 10 mcg/mL
Toxic: greater than 35 mcg/mL

Amitriptyline (Elavil) — Red — Therapeutic range: 125–200 ng/mL
Toxic level: greater than 500 ng/mL

Ammonia — Green — 15–45 mcg/dL
11–35 µmol/L (SI units) — Newborn: 64–107 mcg/dL
Child: 21–50 mcg/dL

Amylase — 30–170 µ/L
Isoenzymes: S: 45–70%
P: 30–55%

Angiotensin-converting enzyme (ACE) — Red or green — 11–67 U/L

Anion gap — 10–17 mEq/L

Antidiuretic hormone (ADH) — Lavender — 1–5 pg/mL

Antineutrophil cytoplasmic antibody (ANCA) — Red — Negative, less than 1:20 — Not usually performed

Antisperm antibody — Semen / Blood / Serum (red) — Adult: negative for agglutinating antibody
Moderately positive: 50%
Strongly positive: 100%

REFERENCE VALUES

Chemistry	Color-Top Tube	Adult	Child
Antithrombin III	Blue or red	75–135% (average)	
Apolipoproteins (Apo)	Plasma (lavender)	Apo A-1: see test	
	Serum (red)	Apo B: see test	
	Gray or red	Ratio Apo A-1/Apo B: see test	
Arsenic (AS)	Hair, toenails, serum, blood, urine	0.6–2 mg/dL (plasma) (*See Arsenic in text*)	0.6–1.6 mg/dL (plasma)
Arterial blood gases—*See Others*			
Ascorbic acid (vitamin C)	Red	34–114 µmol/L (SI units, plasma)	Newborn: 4 times normal level
		0.2–2 mg/dL (blood)	
		12–114 µmol (SI units, serum)	
Aspartate aminotransferase (AST, SGOT)		0–35 U/L	Child: same as adult
		Average: 8–38 U/L	
Atrial natriuretic peptide (ANP)	Lavender	20–77 pg/mL	
		16–60 units/mL at 30°C	
		8–33 units/L at 37°C (SI units)	
Barbiturate, phenobarbital		0	0
		Therapeutic: 10–30 mcg/mL	15–30 mcg/mL
		Toxic: greater than 60 mcg/mL	
Beta₂ microglobulin	Blood (lavender)	Adult: less than 2 mcg/dL; 1–2.4 mg/L (SI units)	
	Serum (red)	Elderly: 0.25 mg/dL	
	Urine	Adult: less than 120 mcg/24 h	
Bilirubin (indirect)	Red	0.1–1 mg/dL	
		1.7–17.1 µmol/L (SI units)	
Bilirubin (total and direct)	Red	Total: 0.1–1.2 mg/dL; 1.7–20.5 µmol/L (SI units)	Newborn, total: 1–12 mg/dL; 17.1–205 mol/L (SI units)
		Direct (conjugated): 0.1–0.3 mg/dL; 1.7–5.1 µmol/L (SI units)	Child, total: 0.2–0.8 mg/dL

Test	Specimen/Tube	Adult	Children
Bioterrorism infectious products (anthrax, botulism, smallpox)	Culture: Blood, sputum, stool	Adult: negative	Children: negative
Blood urea nitrogen (BUN)	Red	5–25 mg/dL	Infant: 5–15 mg/dL
Brain natriuretic peptide (BNP)	Red	Desired: less than 100 pg/mL; positive: greater than 100 pg/mL	
Breast cancer genetic (BRCA-1 and BRCA-2)	Blood (lavender or blue)	Adult: negative	
Breast cancer tumor prognostic markers	Breast tissue	Adult: 6 markers; see test	
Bromide	Green	0 Therapeutic: less than 80 mg/dL Toxic: greater than 100 mg/dL	0
BUN/creatinine ratio	Red	10:1–20:1	
Calcitonin	Green or lavender	Male: less than 40 pg/mL Female: less than 25 pg/mL	Newborn: usually higher Child: less than 70 pg/mL
Calcium (Ca)	Red	4.5–5.5 mEq/L 9–11 mg/dL	Newborn: 3.7–7 mEq/L; 7.4–14 mg/dL Infant: 5–6 mEq/L; 10–12 mg/dL
Ionized calcium (iCa)		2.3–2.8 mmol/L (SI units) 4.4–5.9 mg/dL 2.2–2.5 mEq/L 1.1–1.24 mmol/L	Child: 4.5–5.8 mEq/L; 9–11.5 mg/dL
Cancer tumor markers (CA 15-3, CA 19-9, CA 27.29, CA 50, CA 125, CA 549)	Serum (red)	Normal: CA 15-3: less than 30 units/mL; less than 30 kU/L (SI units) CA 19-9: less than 37 units/mL; less than 37 kU/L (SI units) CA 27.29: less than 37 units/mL; less than 37 kU/L (SI units) CA 50: less than 17 units/mL; less than 17 kU/L (SI units) CA 125: less than 35 units/mL; less than 35 kU/L (SI units) CA 549: less than 10 units/mL; less than 10 kU/L (SI units)	
Cannabinoid (marijuana)	Urine	Negative: less than 50 ng/mL	

REFERENCE VALUES

Chemistry	Color-Top Tube	Adult	Child
Carbamazepine	Red	Therapeutic: 4–12 mcg/mL; 16.9–50.8 μmol/L (SI units); Toxic: greater than 12–15 mcg/mL; greater than 50.8–69 μmol/L (SI units)	
Carbon dioxide–combining power (CO_2)	Green	22–30 mEq/L; 22–30 mmol/L (SI units)	20–28 mEq/L
Carbon monoxide (CO); Carboxyhemoglobin (may be done in hematology)	Lavender	Less than 2.5% saturation of Hb; 2–9% saturation of Hb (smokers)	Same as adult
Cardiovascular disease genetic test	Plasma (lavender); Serum (red)	Negative: no angiotensinogen gene	
Carotene	Red	60–200 mg/dL; 0.74–3.72 μmol/L (SI units)	40–130 mcg/dL
Catecholamines	Green or lavender	Positive for pheochromocytoma: greater than 1,000 pg/mL	
Epinephrine		Supine: less than 50 pg/mL; Sitting: less than 60 pg/mL; Standing: less than 90 pg/mL	
Norepinephrine		Supine: 110–410 pg/mL; Sitting: 120–680 pg/mL; Standing: 125–700 pg/mL	
Dopamine		Supine and standing: less than 87 pg/mL	
Ceruloplasmin (Cp)	Red	18–45 mg/dL	Infant: less than 23 mg/dL or normal; Child: 30–65 mg/dL
Chlordiazepoxide (Librium)	Red	Therapeutic level: 1–5 mcg/mL; Toxic: greater than 6 mcg/mL	
Chloride (Cl)	Red	95–105 mEq/L; 95–105 mmol/L (SI units)	Newborn: 94–112 mEq/L; Infant: 95–110 mEq/L; Child: 98–105 mEq/L; Infant: 90–130 mg/dL

Test	Tube color	Values	
Cholesterol	Red	Desirable level: less than 200 mg/dL; Moderate risk: 200–240 mg/dL; High risk: greater than 240 mg/dL	2–19 years: Desirable level: 130–170 mg/dL; Moderate risk: 171–184 mg/dL; High risk: greater than 185 mg/dL; Same as adult
Cholinesterase	Green	0.5–1 units (RBC); 3–8 units/mL (plasma); 6–8 IU/L (RBC); 8–18 IU/L at 37°C (plasma)	
Copper (Cu)	Red or green	Male: 70–140 mcg/dL; 11–22 µmol/L (SI units); Female: 80–155 mcg/dL; 12.6–24.3 µmol/L (SI units); Pregnancy: 140–300 mcg/dL	Newborn: 20–70 mcg/dL; Child: 30–190 mcg/dL; Adolescent: 90–240 mcg/dL
Cortisol	Green	8 AM–10 AM: 5–23 mcg/dL; 138–635 nmol/L (SI units); 4 PM–6 PM: 3–13 mcg/dL; 83–359 nmol/L (SI units)	8 AM–10 AM: 15–25 mcg/dL; 4 PM–6 PM: 5–10 mcg/dL
C-peptide	Serum (red)	Fasting: 0.8–1.8 ng/mL; 0.27–0.63 mmol/L (SI units)	
Creatine phosphokinase (CPK)	Red	Male: 5–35 mcg/mL; 30–180 IU/L, 55–170 units/L at 37°C (SI units); Female: 5–25 mcg/mL; 25–150 IU/L; 30–135 units/L at 37°C (SI units)	Newborn: 65–580 IU/L at 30°C; Child: Male: 0–70 IU/L at 30°C; Female: 0–50 IU/L at 30°C
Creatinine	Red	0.5–1.5 mg/dL; 45–132.3 µmol/L (SI units)	Newborn: 0.8–1.4 mg/dL; Infant: 0.7–1.7 mg/dL; 2–6 years: 0.3–0.6 mg/dL, 24–54 µmol/L (SI units); 7–18 years: 0.4–1.2 mg/dL, 36–106 µmol/L (SI units)
Cryoglobulins	Red	Negative	
Cyanide	Lavender or green	Therapeutic: 50–200 ng/mL; Serum: lethal: greater than 0.1 mg/L or 3.7 µmol/L (SI units); smoker: 0.006 mg/L; Blood: lethal: greater than 1 mg/L or 36 µmol/L (SI units); smoker: 0.04 mg/L	
Dexamethasone suppression test	Green	Cortisol: 8 AM: less than 10 mcg/dL	

REFERENCE VALUES

Chemistry	Color-Top Tube	Adult	Child
Diabetes mellitus autoantibodies	Red	No antibody detection	
Diazepam (Valium)	Red	Therapeutic: 400–600 ng/mL; 0.5–2 mg/L; Toxic: greater than 1,000 ng/mL; greater than 3 mg/L	
Digoxin	Red	Therapeutic: 0.5–2 ng/mL; 0.5–2 nmol/L (SI units) Toxic: greater than 2 ng/mL; greater than 2.6 nmol/L (SI units)	Therapeutic: infant: 1–3 ng/mL; 1–3 nmol/L (SI units) Toxic: greater than 3.5 ng/mL
Diltiazem (Cardizem)		Toxic: greater than 200 ng/mL	
Disseminated intravascular coagulation (DIC) screening test		See Part III, Hematologic Conditions	
Doxepin (Sinequan)		Therapeutic range: 150–250 ng/mL Toxic level: greater than 500 ng/mL	
D-xylose absorption	Red	25–40 mg/dL/2h Elderly: same as adult	30 mg/dL/1 h
Estetrol (E$_4$)	Red	Pregnancy:	

SERUM

		pg/mL
Estetrol (E$_4$)	Weeks of Gestation	
	20–26	140–210
	30	350
	36	900
	40	greater than 1,050
Estradiol (E$_2$)	Female:	3–10 pg/mL
	Follicular: 20–150 pg/mL	
	Midcycle: 100–500 pg/mL	
	Luteal: 60–260 pg/mL	
	Postmenopausal: less than 30 pg/mL	
	Male: 15–50 pg/mL	
Estriol (E$_3$)	Pregnancy:	

SERUM

Test	Tube Color	Adult Values	Weeks of Gestation	ng/dL	Children
Estrogen	Red	Female: Early menstrual cycle: 60–200 pg/mL Midmenstrual cycle: 120–440 pg/mL Male: 40–155 pg/mL	25–28 29–32 33–36 37–38 39–40	25–165 30–230 45–370 75–420 95–450	1–6 years: 3–10 pg/mL 8–12 years: less than 30 pg/mL
Estrone (E₁)	Red	Follicular phase: 30–100 pg/mL; ovulatory phase: greater than 150 pg/mL; luteal phase: 90–160 pg/mL; postmenopausal: 20–40 pg/mL Male: 10–50 pg/mL			1–10 years: less than 10 pg/mL
Ethosuximide	Red	Therapeutic: 40–100 mcg/mL; 283–708 μmol/L Toxic: greater than 100 mcg/mL; greater than 708 μmol/L (SI units)			Therapeutic: 2–4 per/mg/kg/day Toxic: same as adult or higher
Fasting blood sugar (FBS) (See values in text)	Gray or red	70–110 mg/dL (serum)			Newborn: 30–80 mg/dL Child: 60–100 mg/dL
Feasting blood sugar (See Postprandial blood sugar)		60–100 mcg/dL (blood)			
Fecal fat	Stool	Quantitative: Adult: 2–7 g/24 h 7–25 mmol/day (SI units)			Child (less than 1 year old): 1 g/24 h Newborn: 20–200 ng/mL
Ferritin	Red	Female: 10–235 ng/mL 10–235 mcg/L (SI units) Male: 15–445 ng/mL 15–445 mcg/L (SI units)			Infant: 30–200 ng/mL 1–16 years: 8–140 ng/mL
Folate (folic acid) (may be done by nuclear medicine)	Red	3–16 ng/mL (bioassay) greater than 2.5 ng/mL (RIA; serum) 200–700 ng/mL (RBC)			Same as adult

REFERENCE VALUES

Chemistry	Color-Top Tube	Adult	Child
Follicle-stimulating hormone (FSH)	Red	Pre-ovulation: 4–30 mU/mL Midcycle: 10–90 mU/mL Postmenopausal: 40–170 mU/mL	5–12 mU/mL
Gamma-glutamyl transferase (GGT)	Red	Male: 4–25 mU/mL Male: 4–23 IU/L Female: 3–13 IU/L; 4–33 units/L at 37°C (SI units)	
Gastrin	Red or lavender	Fasting: less than 100 pg/mL	Not usually done

Gentamicin	Red	Therapeutic:
		  Peak: 5–10 mcg/mL
		  Trough: less than 2 mcg/mL
		  Toxic: greater than 12 mcg/mL	

Glucagon	Lavender	50–200 pg/mL	
Glucose-6-phosphate dehydrogenase (G-6-PD) (may be done in hematology)	Lavender or green	8–18 IU/gHb 125–281 units/dL (packed RBC) 251–511 units/dL (cells) 1,211–2,111 mIU/mL (packed RBC)	Same as adult
Glucose—fasting blood sugar (See fasting blood sugar)			
Glucose tolerance test (GTT) (See values in text)	Gray or red		
Growth hormone	Red	Male: less than 5 ng/mL Female: less than 10 ng/mL	less than 10 ng/mL
Haloperidol (Haldol)	Red	Therapeutic range: 3–20 ng/mL Toxic: greater than 50 ng/mL	
Heroin	Urine	Normal: negative; Positive: greater than 2 ng/mL	
Hexosaminidase	Red	Total: 5–20 units/L A: 55–80%	
HIV OraQUICK test	Saliva	Negative	
Homocysteine	Red	4–17 μmol/L (fasting)	
Human chorionic gonadotropin (HCG)	Red	Nonpregnant female: less than 0.01 IU/mL	

PREGNANT (WEEKS)	VALUES
1	0.01–0.04 IU/mL
2	0.03–0.10 IU/mL
4	0.10–1 IU/mL
5–12	10–100 IU/mL
13–25	10–30 IU/mL
26–40	5–15 IU/mL

WEEKS OF GESTATION	mcg/mL
8–27	4.6 mcg/mL
28–31	2.4–6 mcg/mL
32–35	3.7–7.7 mcg/mL
36–40	5–10 mcg/mL

Test	Tube	Values
Human immunosuppressive virus (HIV)	Red	
Human leukocyte antigen (HLA)	Green	Negative: See text
Human papilloma virus	Serum (red)	Histocompatibility match
Human placental lactogen (HPL)	Red or green	Absence of HPV
Imipramine (Tofranil)	Red	Toxic level: greater than 500 ng/mL; Therapeutic range: 150–300 ng/mL
Immunoglobulins—see *Serology*	Red	
Infertility screen	Red	See LH and FSH tests (female) and Antisperm Antibody test (male)
Influenza A and B titer	Red or red/gray	Negative titer: less than 1.8 titer influenza immunization
Insulin antibody	Red	No insulin antibodies
Insulin		5–25 µU/mL
International normalized ratio (INR)	Black	2–3
Iron	Red	50–150 mcg/dL; 10–27 µmol/L (SI units)
Iron-binding capacity (IBC, Red TIBC)	Red	250–450 mcg/dL; 6 months–2 years: 40–100 mcg/dL, Newborn: 100–270 mcg/dL; Infant (6 months–2 years): 100–350 mcg/dL, Child: same as adult
Kanamycin	Red	Therapeutic: Peak: 15–30 mcg/mL, Trough: 1–4 mcg/mL, Toxic: greater than 35 mcg/mL

REFERENCE VALUES

Chemistry	Color-Top Tube	Adult	Child
Lactic acid	Green	Arterial blood: 0.5–2 mmol/L; less than 11.3 mg/dL Venous blood: 0.5–1.5 mmol/L; 8.1–15.3 mg/dL Critical: greater than 5 mEq/L; greater than 45 mg/dL	
Lactic dehydrogenase (LDH/ID)	Red	100–190 IU/L; 70–250 units/L	Newborn: 300–1,500 IU/L Child: 50–150 IU/L
LDH isoenzymes	Red		
LDH_1		14–26%	
LDH_2		27–37%	
LDH_3		13–26%	
LDH_4		8–16%	
LDH_5		6–16%	
Lactose tolerance test	Gray	20–50 mg/dL rise from fasting blood glucose	
Latex allergy testing (serum)	Red	Negative, less than 0.35 IU/mL Toxic: greater than 0.35 IU/mL	
Lead	Lavender or green	10–20 mcg/dL 20–40 mcg/dL (acceptable) Toxic: greater than 40 mcg/dL	10–20 mcg/dL 20–30 mcg/dL (acceptable)
LE cells (Lupus)	Red or green	Negative	
Lecithin/sphingomyelin ratio (L/S; amniotic fluid)		1:1 before 35 weeks of gestation L: 6–9 mg/dL S: 4–6 mg/dL 4:1 after 35 weeks of gestation L: 15–21 mg/dL S: 4–6 mg/dL	
Leucine aminopeptidase (LAP)	Red	8–22 m units/mL, 12–33 IU/L; 20–50 U/L at 37°C (SI units)	

Test	Specimen (tube)	Reference values	Additional
Leukoagglutinin test	Blood (lavender) Serum (red)	Negative: no dye uptake	
Lidocaine	Red	Therapeutic: 1.5–5 mcg/mL; 6–22.5 μmol/L (SI units) Toxic: greater than 6 mcg/mL	
Lipase	Red	20–180 IU/L; 114–286 units/L 14–280 mU/mL 14–280 units/L (SI units)	Infant: 9–105 IU/L at 37°C Child: 20–136 IU/L at 37°C
Lipoproteins (see Cholesterol, Phospholipids, and Triglycerides)			
Lithium	Red	0 Therapeutic: 0.8–1.2 mEq/L Toxic: greater than 2 mEq/L	0
Luteinizing hormone (LH)	Red or lavender	Female: Pre-ovulation: 5–30 mIU/mL Midcycle: 50–150 mIU/mL Postmenopause: greater than 35 mIU/mL Male: 5–25 mIU/mL	6–12 years: less than 10 mIU/mL 13–18 years: less than 20 mIU/mL
Magnesium (Mg)	Red	1.5–2.5 mEq/L; 1.8–3 mg/dL	Newborn: 1.4–2.9 mEq/L Child: 1.6–2.6 mEq/L
Myoglobin	Red	12–90 mcg/L; 12–90 ng/mL	
Netilmicin		Therapeutic: Peak: 0.5–10 mcg/mL Trough: less than 4 mcg/mL Toxic: greater than 16 mcg/mL	
Nifedipine	Red	Therapeutic: 50–100 ng/mL Toxic: greater than 100 ng/mL	
Nortriptyline (Aventyl)	Red	Therapeutic range: 50–150 ng/mL Toxic level: greater than 200 ng/mL	
N-telopeptide cross-links (Ntx)	Serum (red)	Female: 6.2–19 nM BCE/L Male: 5.4–24.2 nM BCE/L	
	Urine	Female: 5–65 nM BCE/L creatinine Male: 3–51 nM BCE/L creatinine	
5'Nucleotidase (5'N)	Red	Less than 17 units/L	
Osmolality	Red	280–300 mOsm/kg	270–290 mOsm/kg

REFERENCE VALUES

Chemistry	Color-Top Tube	Adult	Child
Osteocalcin	Serum (red) Check with the institution	Female: premenopausal: 0.5–7.8 ng/mL; 0.5–7.8 mcg/L (SI units) Postmenopausal: 1.2–11 ng/mL; 1.2–11 mcg/L (SI units) Male: 1.5–11.5 ng/mL; 1.5–11.5 mcg/L (SI units)	
Parathyroid hormone (PTH)	Red	PTH: 11–54 pg/mL; C Terminal PTH: 50–330 pg/mL; N-Terminal PTH: 8–24 pg/mL	
Pepsinogen I	Red	124–142 ng/mL	Premature: 20–24 ng/mL Less than 1 year: 72–82 ng/mL 1–2 years: 90–106 ng/mL 3–6 years: 80–104 ng/mL 7–10 years: 77–103 ng/mL 11–14 years: 96–118 ng/mL Toxic: greater than 15–20 mcg/mL; 56–79 µmol/L (SI units)
Phenothiazines (*see Part I*)	Red	Therapeutic: 10–20 mcg/mL; 39.6–79.3 µmol/L (SI units) Toxic: greater than 20 mcg/mL greater than 79.3 µmol/L (SI units)	
Phenytoin (Dilantin)	Red	150–380 mg/dL	
Phospholipids	Red		
Phosphorus (P) (inorganic)	Red	1.7–2.6 mEq/L 2.5–4.5 mg/dL	Newborn: 3.5–8.6 mg/dL Infant: 4.5–6.7 mg/dL Child: 4.5–5.5 mg/dL
Placental growth factor (PGF)	Red	Nonpregnant: less than 50 pg/mL Pregnant: greater than 200 pg/mL in 20 weeks	
Postprandial blood sugar (feasting: PPBS)	Blood/plasma (gray)	Adult: Serum and plasma: less than 140 mg/dL/2hr; less than 7.8 mmol/L (SI units)	Child: Serum: less than 140 mg/dL; less than 6.7 mmol/L (SI units)
	Serum (red)	Whole blood: less than 120 mg/dL/2 h; less than 6.7 mmol/L (SI units) Elderly: Serum: less than 160 mg/dL; less than 8.9 mmol/L (SI units) Whole blood: less than 140 mg/dL; less than 7.8 mmol/L (SI units)	

Test	Tube	Values
Potassium (K)	Red	3.5–5.3 mEq/L 3.5–5.3 mmol/L (SI units) Infant: 3.6–5.8 mEq/L Child: 3.5–5.5 mEq/L
Pregnancy-associated plasma protein-A (PAPP-A)	Red	Values differ among laboratories
Primidone	Red	Therapeutic: 5–12 mcg/mL; 23–55 μmol/L (SI units) Therapeutic: child less than 5 years: 7–10 mcg/mL 30–45 μmol/L (SI units) Toxic: greater than 12–15 mcg/mL, greater than 55–69 μmol/L (SI units) Toxic: greater than 12 mcg/mL; greater than 55 μmol/L (SI units)
Procainamide	Red	Therapeutic: 4–8 mcg/mL; 17–34 μmol/L (SI units) Toxic: greater than 10 mcg/mL; greater than 102 μmol/L (SI units)
Progesterone	Red	Female: Follicular: 0.1–1.5 ng/mL Luteal: 2–28 ng/mL Pregnancy: First trimester: 9–50 ng/mL Second trimester: 18–150 ng/mL Third trimester: 60–260 ng/mL Male: less than 1 ng/mL
Prolactin (PRL)	Red or lavender	Female: Nonpregnant: Follicular: 0–23 ng/mL Luteal: 0–40 ng/mL Postmenopausal: less than 12 ng/mL Pregnancy: First trimester: less than 80 ng/mL Second trimester: less than 160 ng/mL Third trimester: less than 400 ng/mL Male: 0.1–20 ng/mL Pituitary adenoma: greater than 100–300 ng/mL
Propranolol (Inderal)	Red	Therapeutic: 50–100 ng/mL; 193–386 nmol/L (SI units) Toxic: greater than 150 ng/mL
Prostate-specific antigen (PSA)	Red	Normal: 0–4 ng/mL BPH: 4–10 ng/mL Prostate cancer: 10–120 ng/mL

REFERENCE VALUES

Chemistry	Color-Top Tube	Adult	Child
Prostate specific antigen		Total PSA: normal: 2.5–4 ng/mL Free PSA: normal: greater than 1 ng/mL % Free PSA: normal: greater than 26 %	
Protein	Red	6–8 g/dL	Premature: 4.2–7.6 g/dL Newborn: 4.6–7.4 g/dL Infant: 6–6.7 g/dL Child: 6.2–8 g/dL
Protein electrophoresis	Red	Albumin: 3.5–5 g/dL; 52–68% of total protein	Premature: 3–4.2 g/dL Newborn: 3.5–5.4 g/dL Infant: 4.4–5.4 g/dL Child: 4–5.8 g/dL
		Globulin: 1.5–3.5 g/dL; 32–48% of total protein	
Quinidine	Red	Therapeutic: 2–5 mcg/mL; 0.2–15.4 µmol/L (SI units) Toxic: greater than 6 mcg/mL; greater than 18.5 µmol/L (SI units)	
Renin	Lavender	Normal sodium diet: supine: 0.2–2.3 ng/mL upright: 1.6–4.3 ng/mL. Restricted salt diet: upright: 4.1–10.8 ng/mL	3–5 years: 1–6.5 ng/mL 5–10 years: 0.5–6 ng/mL
Rubeola antibodies	Serum (red)	Negative: less than 4-fold titer Positive: greater than 4-fold titer	

Salicylate	Red	0
		Toxic:
		  Mild: greater than 30 mg/dL
		  Severe: greater than 50 mg/dL
			0
			Toxic: greater than 25 mg/dL

		Therapeutic: 15–30 mg/dL	
SARS		Normal WBC; no coronavirus antibody	
Serotonin	Lavender	50–175 ng/mL; 10–30 mcg/dL; 0.29–1.15 µmol/L (SI units)	
Sodium (Na)	Red	135–145 mEq/L 135–142 nmol/L (SI units)	Infant: 134–150 mEq/L Child: 135–145 mEq/L
T_3	Red	80–200 ng/dL	Newborn: 90–170 ng/dL Child: 6–12 years: 115–190 ng/dL

Test	Tube	Adult values	Pediatric / other values
Testosterone	Red or green	Male: 0.3–1 mcg/dL; 300–1,000 ng/dL Female: 0.03–0.1 mcg/dL; 30–100 ng/dL	Male adolescent: greater than 0.1 mcg/dL Male: 12–14 years old: greater than 100 ng/dL
Theophylline	Red	Therapeutic: Adult: 5–20 mcg/mL; 28–112 µmol/L (SI units) Elderly: 5–18 mcg/mL Toxic: Adult: greater than 20 mcg/mL; greater than 112 µmol/L (SI units) Elderly: same as adult	Therapeutic: Premature: 7–14 mcg/mL Neonate: 3–12 mcg/mL Child: same as adult Toxic: Premature: greater than 14 mcg/mL Neonate: greater than 13 mcg/mL Child: same as adult
Thyroid-binding globulin (TBG)	Red or green	10–26 mcg/d	
Thyroid Globulin Antibodies	Red	No antibodies	
Thyroid Peroxidase (TPO) Antibodies	Red	Negative	
Thyroxine (T_4)	Red	4.5–11.5 mcg/dL (T_4 by column) 5–12 mcg/dL (T_4 RIA) 1–2.3 ng/dL (thyroxine iodine)	Newborn: 11–23 mcg/dL 1–4 months: 7.5–16.5 mcg/dL 4–12 months: 5.5–14.5 mcg/dL 1–6 years: 5.5–13.5 mcg/dL 6–10 years: 5–12.5 mcg/dL
Transferrin	Red	200–430 mg/dL; 2–4.3 g/L (SI units) pregnancy (full term): 300 mg/dL	Newborn: 125–275 mcg/dL
Transferrin percent saturation	Red	Male: 30–50% Female: 20–35%	
T_3 resin uptake (may be done by nuclear medicine)	Red	25–35% relative % uptake	Not usually done
Tricyclic antidepressants—*see Part I*			
Triglycerides	Red	10–150 mg/dL 0.11–2.09 mmol/L (SI units)	Infant: 5–40 mg/dL Child: 10–135 mg/dL
Troponins	Blood (green)		
Cardiac troponin 1	Serum (red)	Normal: 0.1–0.5 ng/mL; 0.1 mcg/L (SI units) Positive myocardial injury: greater than 2 ng/mL; greater than 2 mcg/L (SI units)	

REFERENCE VALUES

Chemistry	Color-Top Tube	Adult	Child
Cardiac troponin T		Normal: less than 0.2 ng/mL; less than 0.2 mcg/L (SI units)	
Uric acid	Red	Male: 3.5–8 mg/dL Female: 2.8–6.8 mg/dL	2.5–5.5 mg/dL
Valproic acid	Red	Therapeutic: 50–100 mcg/mL; 347–693 μmol/L Toxic: greater than 100 mcg/mL; greater than 693 μmol/L (SI units)	Therapeutic: same Toxic: same
Vancomycin	Red	Therapeutic range: Peak: 20–40 mcg/mL Trough: 5–10 mcg/mL Toxic level: greater than 40 mcg/mL	
Verapamil	Red	Therapeutic: 100–300 ng/mL; 0.08–0.3 mcg/mL Toxic: greater than 300 ng/mL; greater than 0.3 mcg/mL	
Vitamin A	Red	30–95 mcg/dL; 1.05–3 μmol/L (SI units); 125–150 IU/dL	1–6 years: 20–43 mcg/dL 0.7–1.5 μmol/L (SI units) 7–12 years: 26–50 mcg/dL 13–19 years: 26–72 mcg/dL
Vitamin B₁	Red	10–60 ng/mL; 5.3–8 mcg/dL	
Vitamin B₆	Lavender	5–30 ng/mL; 20–120 nmol/L (SI units)	
Vitamin B₁₂	Red	200–900 pg/mL	Newborn: 160–1,200 pg/mL
Vitamin C (see Ascorbic acid)			
Vitamin D₃	Red or green	1,23 dihydroxy: 20–76 pg/mL 25-hydroxy: 10–55 ng/mL	3–15 mcg/mL; 0.3–1 mg/dL
Vitamin E	Red	5–20 mcg/mL 0.5–1.8 mg/dL 12–42 μmol/L (SI units)	7–23 μmol/L (SI units)
West Nile virus antibodies	Serum (red) CSF	Negative	
Zika virus	Red	Negative	
Zinc	Navy blue	60–150 mcg/dL 11–23 μmol/L (SI units)	
Zinc	Urine	150–1,250 mcg/24 h	
Zinc protoporphyrin (ZPP)	Green or lavender	15–77 mcg/dL	
		Average: less than 35 mcg/dL, less than 0.56 μmol/L (SI units)	Same as adult

REFERENCE VALUES

Serology	Color-Top Tube	Adult	Child
Adenovirus antibody	Red	Negative	Negative
Anticardiolipin antibody	Red	Negative	
Anticentromere antibody	Red	Positive: greater than 1:40 for human epithelial type 2 cells (HEp-2) cells	
Anti-DNA	Red	Less than 1:85	Less than 1:60
Antiglomerular basement membrane antibody (AGBM)	Red	Negative	
Antimitochondrial antibody (AMA)	Red	Negative at 1:5	
		Positive: greater than 1:160	
Antimyocardial antibody	Red	None detected	
Antinuclear antibodies (ANA)	Red	Negative at 1:20 dilution	Negative
Antiparietal cell antibody (APCA)	Red or gray	Negative: less than 1:120 titer	
		Positive: 1:180 titer	
Antiscleroderma antibody	Red	Negative: borderline: 20–25 units; positive: greater than 25 units	
Antismooth muscle antibody (ASMA)	Red	Negative or less than 1:20	
		Positive: greater than 1:20 titer	
Antistreptolysin O (ASO)	Red	100 IU/mL; less than 160 Todd units/mL	Newborn: similar to mother's 2–5 years: less than 100 IU/mL 12–19 years: less than 200 IU/mL; less than 200 Todd U/mL
Candida antibody test	Red	Negative; positive: greater than 1:8 titer	
Carcinoembryonic antigen (CEA) (may be done by nuclear medicine)	Red or lavender	Less than 2.5 ng/mL (nonsmokers) Less than 3.5 ng/mL (smokers)	Not usually done
Chromosomal analysis	Green	Men: 44 autosomes + XY sex chromosomes Female: 44 autosomes + XX sex chromosomes Total: 46 chromosomes for men and female	
Chlamydia test	Red	Less than 1:16	
Cold agglutinins (CA)	Red	1:8 antibody titer	
Complement (total)	Red	75–160 units/mL; 75–160 kU/L (SI units)	Same as adult
Complement C_3	Red	Male: 80–180 mg/dL; 0.8–1.8 g/L (SI units) Female: 76–120 mg/dL; 0.76–1.2 g/L (SI units)	Not usually done

REFERENCE VALUES

Serology	Color-Top Tube	Adult	Child
Complement C$_4$	Red	15–45 mg/dL; 150–450 mg/L (SI units)	Not usually done
C-reactive protein (CRP)	Red	0	0
Cryoglobulins	Red	Up to 6 mg/dL	Negative
Cytomegalovirus (CMV) antibody	Red	Negative to less than 0.30	
Encephalitis virus antibody	Red	Titer: less than 1:10	
Enterovirus group	Red	Negative	
Febrile agglutinins	Red	Febrile group: titers *Brucella:* less than 1:20 *Tularemia:* less than 1:40 *Salmonella:* less than 1:40 *Proteus:* less than 1:40	Same as adult
FTA-ABS (fluorescent treponemal antibody absorption)	Red	Negative	Negative
Haptoglobin	Red	60–270 mg/dL 0.6–2.7 g/L (SI units)	Newborn: 0–10 mg/dL Infant: 1–6 months: 0–30 mg/dL, then gradual increase
HB$_c$ Ab	Red	Negative	Negative
HB$_s$ Ab	Red	Negative	Negative
Helicobacter pylori	Red	Negative	
Hepatitis A virus (HAV)	Red	None detected	
Hepatitis B surface antigen (HB$_s$ Ag)	Red	Negative	Negative
Herpes simplex virus (HSV)	Red	less than 1:10	
Heterophile antibody	Red	less than 1:28 titer	Same as adult

Immunoglobulins (Ig)	Adult	1–3 YEARS OLD	7–11 YEARS OLD
Total Ig	900–2,200 mg/dL	400–1,500 mg/dL	700–1,700 mg/dL
Total Ig	900–2,200 mg/dL		
IgG	800–1,800 mg/dL	300–1,400 mg/dL	600–1,450 mg/dL
IgG	800–1,800 mg/dL		
IgA	100–400 mg/dL	20–150 mg/dL	50–200 mg/dL
IgM	50–150 mg/dL	20–100 mg/dL	30–120 mg/dL
IgD	0.5–3 mg/dL		

Test		Adult	Child
Legionnaire antibody test	Red	Negative	Same as adult
Lyme antibody test	Red	Titer less than 1:256	
Mumps antibody	Red	Negative or less than 1:8 titer	
Parvovirus B19 antibody	Red	Negative	
Prealbumin antibody	Red	17–40 mg/dL	
Rabies antibody test	Red	IFA: less than 1:16	
Rapid plasma reagin (RPR)	Red	Negative	Negative
Rheumatoid factor (RF)	Red	less than 1:20 titer	Not usually done
Rubella antibody detection (HAI or HI)	Red	less than 1:8 titer susceptible 1:10–1:32 titer, past rubella exposure 1:32–1:64 titer, immunity greater than 1:64 titer, definite immunity	Same as adult
Severe combined immunodeficiency (SCID)	Red	Normal: presence of T-cells	Not usually done
Thyroid antibodies (TA)	Red	Negative or less than 1:20 titer	
TORCH test	Red	Negative	Negative
Toxoplasmosis antibody test	Red	No infection: less than 1:4 Infected: greater than 1:256	
Venereal Disease Research Laboratory (VDRL)	Red	Negative	Negative
West Nile virus antibodies	Red	Negative	Negative

REFERENCE VALUES

Microbiology	Adult	Child
Antibiotic susceptibility (sensitivity)	Sensitive to antibiotic Intermediate to antibiotic Resistant to antibiotic	Same as adult
Cultures (blood, sputum, stool, throat, wound, and urine)	No pathogen	Same as adult
Fungal organisms (mycotic infections)	No pathogen or under 8	Same as adult
Malarial smear	Negative	Negative
Occult blood (feces)	Negative	Negative
Parasites and ova (feces)	Negative	Negative
Trypsin (feces)	Negative at dilutions greater than 1:10	
Rotavirus antigen (feces)	Negative	

REFERENCE VALUES

Urine Chemistry	Adult	Child
Aldosterone	6–25 mcg/24 h	Not usually done
Amino acid screen	200 mg/24 h	
Amylase	4–37 units/L/2 h	Not usually done
Ascorbic acid tolerance (4-, 5-, or 6-hour sample)	Oral: 10% of administered amount IV: 30–40% of administered amount	Not usually done
Bence-Jones protein	Negative to trace	Same as adult
Bilirubin and bile	Negative to 0.02 mg/dL	Same as adult
Bladder cancer markers	Negative to less than 33 units/mL	
Calcium (Ca)	100–250 mg/24 h (average calcium diet) 2.50–6.25 mmoL/24 h	Same as adult
Cannabinoid (marijuana)	Negative	
Catecholamines	Less than 100 mcg/24 h Less than 0.59 µmoL/24 h (SI units) 0–14 mcg/dL (random)	Lower level than adult—weight difference
Creatinine	Male: 20–26 mg/kg/24 h; 0.18–0.23 mmol/kg/24 h (SI units) Female: 14–22 mg/kg/24 h; 0.12–0.19 mmol/kg/24 h (SI units)	
Creatinine clearance	85–135 mL/min	Similar to adult
Epinephrine	Less than 20 ng/24 h	
Norepinephrine	Less than 100 ng/24 h	
Cortisol	24–105 mcg/24 h	
Estriol (E_3)	Pregnant:	

WEEKS OF GESTATION	mg/24 h
25–28	6–28
29–32	6–32
33–36	10–45
37–40	15–60

Test	Values	Pediatric
Estrogens (total)	Female: Preovulation: 5–25 mcg/24 h Follicular phase: 24–100 mcg/24 h Luteal phase (menstruation): 22–80 mcg/24 h Postmenopause: 0–10 mcg/24 h Male: 4–25 mcg/24 h	less than 12 years: 1 mcg/24 h greater than 12 years: same as adult
Estrone (E$_1$)	Female: Follicular phase: 4–7 mcg/24 h Ovulatory phase: 11–30 mcg/24 h Luteal phase: 10–22 mcg/24 h Postmenopausal: 1–7 mcg/24 h	
Follicle-stimulating hormone (FSH)	Follicular: 2–15 IU/24 h Luteal phase: 4–20 IU/24 h Menopause: greater than 50 IU/24 h	less than 10 mIU/24 h (prepubertal)
Human chorionic gonadotropin (HCG)	Positive for pregnancy: no agglutination Negative for pregnancy: agglutination	Usually not done
17-Hydroxycorticosteroids (17-OHCS)	Male: 3–12 mg/24 h Female: 2–10 mg/24 h	Infant: less than 1 mg/24 h 2–4 years: 1–2 mg/24 h 5–12 years: 2–6 mg/24 h
5-Hydroxyindolacetic acid (5-HIAA)	Random: negative 24 hours: 2–10 mg/24 h	Usually not done
Hydroxyproline	14–42 mg/24 h 0.4–4.5 mg/2 h	Higher than adult
Ketone bodies (acetone)	Negative	Negative
17-Ketosteroids (17-KS)	Male: 5–25 mg/24 h Female: 5–15 mg/24 h Greater than 65 years: 4–8 mg/24 h	Infant: 1 mg/24 h 1–3 years: less than 2 mg/24 h 3–6 years: less than 3 mg/24 h 7–10 years: less than 4 mg/24 h 10–12 years: Male: less than 6 mg/24 h Female: less than 5 mg/24 h Adolescent: Male: less than 3–15 mg/24 h Female: less than 3–12 mg/24 h 3–6 years: less than 3 mg/24 h Greater than 65 years: 4–8 mg/24 h

Test		
Melanin	Negative	
Myoglobin	None detected	
Opiates	Negative	
Osmolality	50–1,200 mOsm/kg	Newborn: 100–600 mOsm/kg
	Average: 200–800 mOsm/kg	Child: same as adult
Phenylketonuria (PKU)	Not usually done	PKU: negative (positive when serum phenylalanine is 12–15 mg/dL)
		Guthrie: negative (positive when serum phenylalanine is 4 mg/dL)
		Same as adult
Porphobilinogen	Random: negative	
	24 hours: 0–2 mg/24 h	
Porphyrins coproporphyrins	Random: 3–20 mcg/dL	0–80 mcg/24 h
	24 hours: 50–160 mcg	
Uroporphyrins	Random: negative, 24 hours: less than 30 mcg	10–30 mcg/24 h
Potassium (K)	25–120 mEq/24 h	17–57 mEq/24 h
	25–120 mmol/24 h (SI units)	
Pregnanediol	Male: 0.1–1.5 mg/24 h	0.4–1 mg/24 h
	Female: 0.5–1.5 mg/24 h (proliferative phase); 2–7 mg/24 h (luteal phase); 0.1–1 mg/24 h (postmenopausal)	
	Pregnancy:	

7–10 years: less than 4 mg/24 h
10–12 years:
Male: less than 6 mg/24 h
Female: less than 5 mg/24 h
Adolescent: Male: less than 3–15 mg/24 h
Female: less than 3–12 mg/24 h

GESTATION WEEKS	mg/24 h
10–19	5–25
20–28	15–42
29–32	25–49

Test		
Pregnanetriol	Male: 0.4–2.4 mg/24 h	Infant: 0–0.2 mg/24 h
	Female: 0.5–2 mg/24 h	Child: 0–1 mg/24 h
Protein	0–5 mg/dL/24 h	

Protein	Negative	Negative
Glucose	Negative	Negative
Ketones	Negative	Negative
RBC	1–2/low-power field	Rare
WBC	3–4	0–4
Casts	Occasional hyaline	Rare
Pyridinium (PYD)	Female: 15.3–33.6 nM/mm Male: 10.3–33.6 nM/mm	
Sodium (Na)	40–220 mEq/24 h	Same as adult
Uric acid	250–500 mg/24 h (low-purine diet)	Same as adult
Urinalysis		
pH	4.5–8	Newborn: 5–7 Child: 4.5–8
Specific gravity (SG)	1.005–1.03	Newborn: 1.001–1.02 Child: same as adult
Vitamin B_1	100–200 mcg/24 h	

REFERENCE VALUES

Others	Adult	Child
Urobilinogen	Random: 0.3–3.5 mg/dL 0.05–2.5 mg/24 h 0.5–4 Ehrlich units/24 h 0.09–4.23 µmol/24 h (SI units)	Same as adult
Vanillylmandelic acid (VMA)	1.5–7.5 mg/24 h 7.6–37.9 µmol/24 h (SI units)	Same as adult
Bleeding time	Ivy's method: 3–7 minutes	Same as adult
Arterial blood gases (ABGs)		
pH	7.35–7.45	7.36–7.44
$PaCO_2$	35–45 mm Hg	Same as adult
PaO_2	75–100 mm Hg	Same as adult
HCO_3	24–28 mEq/L	Same as adult
BE	+2 to −2 (±2 mEq/L)	Same as adult

REFERENCE VALUES

Others	Adult	Child
Cerebrospinal fluid (CSF)		
Pressure	75–175 mm H_2O	50–100 mm H_2O
Cell count	0–8 mm^3	0–8 mm^3
Protein	15–45 mg/dL	15–45 mg/dL
Chloride	118–132 mEq/L	120–128 mEq/L
Glucose	40–80 mg/dL	35–75 mg/dL
Culture	No organism	No organism
Chloride (sweat)	Less than 60 mEq/L	Less than 50 mEq/L
Semen examination	60–150 mm/mL	Not usually done
	Volume: 1.5–5 mL	
	Morphology: greater than 75% mature spermatozoa	
	Motility: greater than 60% actively mobile spermatozoa	
Amyloid beta protein precursor (CSF)	Positive 450 units/L	
Viral culture (blood, biopsy, CSF, sputum, stool, urine)	Negative	

Bibliography

Abbas AK, Lichtman AH (2006). *Basic Immunology, Updated Edition 2006–2007*, 2nd ed. Philadelphia: WB Saunders/Elsevier.

American Diabetes Association: Standards of medical care in diabetes (2011). *Diabetes Care*, 34 (Suppl 1): S 11–61.

Availability of rapid HIV tests extended (2003, March 10). *Nursing Spectrum*, 12(5): 32.

Barzoloski-O'Connor B (2003, June 16). SARS—The latest menacing microbe. *Nursing Spectrum*, 12(12 PA): 16–18.

Bernstein AD, et al. (2000). The revised naspe/BPEG generic code for antibradycardia, adaptive-rate and multisite pacing. *PACE*, 25: 260–264.

Bisson J, Younker J (2006). Correcting arterial blood gases for temperature: Is it clinically significant? *Nursing in Critical Care*, 11(5): 232–238.

Brantley SL, Langdon JR (2011). The ABC's of ABCs. *Support Line*, 33(3): 13.

Braun L (2010). How inflammatory markers refine CV risk status. *American Nurse Today*, 5(5): 30, 31.

Brenner DJ, Hall EJ (2007). Computed tomography—An increasing source of radiation exposure. *New England Journal of Medicine*, 357 (22): 2277–2284.

Brenner H, et al. (2011). Protection from colorectal cancer after colonoscopy. *Annual Internal Medicine*, 154: 22–30.

Brown R (2006, July 13). 1-pill HIV cocktail approved by FDA. *The News Journal.* Wilmington, DE.

Carter T (2003, March 4). Studies say sex not main cause in Africa. *The Washington Times*, A-1, A-11.

Castle PE, et al. (2009). Five-year experience of human papilloma virus DNA and Papanicolaou test co-testing. *Obstetric Gynecology*, 113: 595–600.

CDC (2001). HIV/AIDS surveillance report, 13(2).

CDC (2002, March 11). Need for sustained HIV prevention among men who have sex with men. National Center for HIV, STD and TB Prevention Division of HIV/AIDS Prevention, pp. 1–3, www.cdc.gov/hiv/pubs/facts/msm.htm

CDC (2003, June 16). FAQs: Frequently asked questions about HIV and HIV testing. National HIV Testing Resources, CDC National Prevention Information Network (NPIN), pp. 1–4, www.hivtest.org/subindex.cfm?FuseAction=FAQ

CDC. Rapid HIV testing of women in labor and delivery (2003, April 25). CDC for HIV, STD, and TB Prevention. Divisions of HIV/AIDS Prevention, pp. 1–3, www.dcd.gov/hiv/pubs/rt-women.htm

Chernecky CC, Berger BJ (eds.) (2013). *Laboratory Tests and Diagnostic Procedure*, 6th ed. Philadelphia: WB Saunders/Elsevier.

Delbeke D, Martin WH (2001). Positron emission tomography imaging in oncology. *Radiologic Clinics of North America*, 39(5): 883–918.

Dershem B, Agruss J, Schwelnus E (2006, October 9). Tips to avoid blood redraws. *Nursing Spectrum*, 15(21).

Durkin S (2005, May 16). C-reactive protein: Inflammatory marker or predictor of outcomes. *Advance for Nurses*, 23(24).

Enfuvirtide (Fuzeon) for HIV infection (2003, June 23). *The Medical Letters*, 45(159): 49, 50.

Esch JF, Frank SV (2001, June). Drug resistance and nursing practice. *American Journal of Nursing*, 101(6): 30–36.

Fahey FH (2001). Positron emission tomography instrumentation. *Radiologic Clinics of North America*, 39(5): 919–930.

Fischbach FT, Dunning MB (2015). *A Manual of Laboratory and Diagnostic Tests*, 9th ed. Philadelphia: Wolters Kluwer.

Flake KJ (2000). HIV testing during pregnancy. Building the case for voluntary testing. *AWHONN Lifelines*, 4 C: 13–16.

Froom Pl, Barak M (2010). False elevated prothrombin international normalized ratio values. *American Journal of Pathology*, 134(1): 86–89.

Fulcher AS, Turner MA (2002). MRI cholangiopancreatography. *Radiologic Clinics of North America*, 40(6): 1363–1376.

Garg K (2002). CT of pulmonary thromboembolic disease. *The Radiologic Clinics of North America*, 40(1): 111–122.

Gebbie KM (2001, June). Privacy: The patient's right. *American Journal of Nursing*, 101(6): 69, 71, 72.

Gregory EK (1998). *The Ear and Hearing. A Guide for School Nurses*. Scarborough, ME: National Association of School Nurses.

Hanas RJG (2010). 2010 consensus statement on the worldwide standardization of the hemoglobin A1c measurement. *Diabetes Care*, 33(8): 1903, 1904.

Hatoum H, Cook NR, Nelson JJ (2008). Lipoprotein-associated phospholipase A2 activity improves risk discrimination of incident coronary heart disease among women. *American Heart Journal*, 361(3): 516–522.

Henry J. Kaiser Family Foundation (2002, July). The HIV/AIDS epidemic in the United States. HIV/AIDS Policy Fact Sheet (developed as part of AIDS at 20: A National HIV/AIDS Policy Initiative Joint initiative of the Henry J. Kaiser Family Foundation and the Ford Foundation), www.kff.org/AIDSat20

High triglyceride (2002). *Mayo Clinic Health Letter*, 20(9): 7.

Hoefner BM (2005, December). Serum tumor markers. Part I: Clinical utility. *MLO Medical Laboratory Observer*, 37(12): 20, 22–24, www.mlo-online.com

Homocysteine (2002). *Mayo Clinic Health Letter*, 20(9): 6.

IBC has meant fewer repeat smear test (2006). *Pulse*, 66(5): 23–25.

Improving bone density (2003). *Mayo Clinic Health Letter*, 21(2): 7.

Is it the "new cholesterol"? About homocysteine (2000). *The Cleveland Clinics*, 2(6): 4, 5.

Iskandrian AE, Chaudhry FA (2000). Stress echocardiography and stress nuclear testing. Part I. *A Journal of Cardiovascular Ultrasound and Allied Technology*, 17(5): 463–469.

Johnsen C (1999, June 1). Hepatitis C: The showdown epidemic. *Nursing Spectrum*, 8(11): 14–16.

Kalichman SC (2003). *The Inside Story on AIDS: Experts Answer Your Questions*. Washington, DC: American Psychological Association.

Kee JL (2014). *Laboratory and Diagnostic Tests with Nursing Implications*, 9th ed. Upper Saddle River, NJ: Pearson.

Kee JL, Hayes ER, McCuistion L (2014). *Pharmacology: A Patient-Centered Nursing Approach*, 8th ed. Philadelphia: Saunders/Elsevier.

Kee JL, Paulanka B, Polek C (2010). *Fluids and Electrolytes with Clinical Implications*, 8th ed. New York: Delmar Publishers.

Kirton CA, Talotta D, Zwolski V (eds.) (2001). *Handbook of HIV/AIDS*. St. Louis: CV Mosby, Elsevier.

LeBlond RF, DeGowin RL, Brown DD (2004) *DeGowin's Diagnostic Examination*, 8th ed. New York: McGraw-Hill.

Leonard T (2006, June 4). Misery likely to continue for many more decades. *Sunday News Journal*, Wilmington, DE.

Mallery S, VanDam J (2000). Advances in diagnostic and therapeutic endoscopy. *Medical Clinics of North America*, 84(5): 1059–1079.

McClatchey KD (ed.) (2002). *Clinical Laboratory Medicine*, 2nd ed. Philadelphia: Lippincott, Williams & Wilkins.

McGuinness G, Naidich DP (2002). CT of airways disease and bronchiectasis. *The Radiologic Clinics of North America*, 40(1): 3–10.

McPherson RA, Pincus MR (2011). *Henry's Clinical Diagnosis Management by Laboratory Methods*, 22nd ed. Philadelphia: Saunders/Elsevier.

Mettler FA, Guiberteau MJ (2012). *Essentials of Nuclear Medicine Imaging*, 6th ed. Philadelphia: Saunders/Elsevier.

Mottram C (2012). *Ruppel's Manual of Pulmonary Function Testing*, 10th ed. St. Louis: Mosby/Elsevier.

Nanda NC, Miller A, Puri VK, et al. (2000). Assessment of myocardial perfusion by power contrast agent. *A Journal of Cardiovascular Ultrasound and Allied Technology*, 17(5): 457–460.

National Association of School Nurses (2010). Definition of school nursing, http://www.nasn.org/Default.aspx?tabid-57

National Association of School Nurses (2011). The role of the school nurse (position statement).

National Center for HIV, STD, and TB Prevention, Divisions of HIV/AIDS Prevention (2003, April 13). *HIV and AIDS: Are you at risk?* pp. 1–5, www.cdc.gov/hiv/pubs/brochure/astrisk.htm

Nicolaides KH, Wright D, Poon LC, Snygelaki A, Gil MM (2013). First trimester contingent screening for trisomy 21 by biomarkers and maternal blood cell free DNA testing. *Ultrasound Obstetrics Gynecology*, 42: 41–50.

Norton M, Brar H, Weiss J, et al. (2012). Non-invasive chromosomal evaluation (NICE) study results of a multicenter, prospective, cohort study for detection of fetal trisomy 21 and trisomy 18. *American Journal of Obstetrics Gynecology*, 7(2): 137, 138.

Nuzhat AA, Shah JN, Kochman ML (2002). Endoscope ultrasonography and endoscopic retrograde cholangiopancreatography imaging for pancreaticobiliary pathology: The gastroenterologist's perspective. *Radiologic Clinics*, 40(6): 1377–1396.

Pagana KD, Pagana TJ, Pagana TN (2015). *Mosby's Diagnostic and Laboratory Test Reference*, 12th ed. St. Louis: Mosby/Elsevier.

Pap smear tests by nurses doubled (2008). *Australian Nursing Journal*, 15(10): 13–15.

Pavlovick-Davis SJ (2003, February 10). Human growth hormone—Pharmaceutical fountain of youth? *Nursing Spectrum*, 12(3 PA): 16–18.

Preston DC, Shapiro BE (2002, May). Needle electromyography: Fundamentals, normal and abnormal patterns. *The Neurologic Clinics of North America*, 20(2): 361–369.

Reiter PL, Linnan LA (2011). Cancer screening behaviors of African-American women enrolled in a community-based prevention trial. *Journal of Women's Health*, 20(3): 429–438.

Remer EM, Baker ME (2002). Imaging of chronic pancreatitis. *The Radiologic Clinics of North America*, 40(6): 1229–1242.

Roman M, Thimothee S, Vidal JE (2008). Arterial blood gases, *MEDSURG Nursing*, 17(4): 268, 269.

Ross E (2002, July 9). New medicine effective against drug-resistant HIV: T-20 studies show treatment could save lives. Conference: Barcelona, Spain. *The News Journal*, Wilmington, DE.

Ruholl L (2006). Arterial blood gases. Analysis and nursing responses. *MEDSURG Nursing*, 18(6): 343–351.

Rydstrom C, Tornberg S (2006). Cervical cancer incidence and mortality in best and worst of worlds. *Scandinavian Journal of Public Health*, 34(3): 295–303.

Sacks DB, Arnold M, Bakris GL, et al. (2011). Guidelines and recommendations for laboratory analysis in the diagnosis and management of diabetes mellitus. *Clinical Chemistry*, 57(6): e1–e47.

Selekman J (2012). *School Nurse: A Comprehensive Test.* Philadelphia: F. A. Davis.

Selig PM (1996). Pearls for practice: Management of anticoagulation therapy with the international normalized ratio. *Journal of American Academy of Nursing Practitioners*, 8(2): 77–80.

Silver LD, Farley TA (2011). Sodium and potassium intake. Mortality effects and policy implications. *Archives of Internal Medicine*, 171: 1191, 1192.

Smart SC, Sagar KB (2000). Diagnostic and prognostic use of stress echocardiography in stable patients. *A Journal of Cardiovascular Ultrasound and Allied Technology*, 17(5): 465–473.

Spinner A (2006, September 25). Less stress, more nursing care for infants. *Nursing Spectrum*, 15(21).

Thacker SB (2003, May 2). HIPAA privacy rule and public health: Guidance from CDC and Human Services. *MMWR*, 52(1): 1–12.

Thompson MA, Aberg JA, Cahn P, et al. (2010). Antiretroviral treatment of adult HIV infection. 2010 Recommendations of the International AIDS Society USA Panel. *Journal of the American Medical Association*, 304: 321–333.

Trzcianowska H, Martensen E (2001, June). HIV and AIDS: Separating fact from fiction. *American Journal of Nursing*, 10(6): 53–59.

Ungvarski PJ (2001). The past 20 years of AIDS. *American Journal of Nursing*, 101(6): 26–29.

U.S. Food and Drug Administration (2002, November 7). FDA approves new rapid HIV test kit. *FDA News (PO2-49)*, pp. 1–2, www.fda.gov/bbs/topics/NEWS/2002/NEW00852.html

VanLeeuwen AM, Poelhuis-Leth D, Bladh MR (2011). *Davis' Handbook of Laboratory and Diagnostic Tests with Nursing Implications*, 4th ed. Philadelphia: F. A. Davis.

Virtual colonoscopy: Not quite as good as the "real" thing (2002). *The Cleveland Clinics*, 4(12): 1–6.

Vitamin C (2000). *The Cleveland Clinics*, 2(6): 7.

Weiner S (2003, June 2). School nurse—Never a dull moment. *Nursing Spectrum*, 12(11 PA): 10.

Weintraub NL, Collins SP, Pang PS (2010). Acute heart failure syndromes: Emergency department presentation, treatment, and disposition: Current approaches and future aims: A scientific statement from the American Heart Association. *Circulation*, 122: 1975–1996.

Whole body CT: Looking for trouble (2003). *The Cleveland Clinics*, 5(7): 1, 7.

Wilbourn AJ (2002). Nerve conduction studies: Types, components, abnormalities, and value in localization. *The Neurologic Clinics of North American*, 20(2): 305–338.

Wilhelm SM, Kale-Pradhan PB (2011). Estimating creatinine clearance: A meta-analysis. *Pharmacotherapy*, 31(7): 658–664.

Wolfe LC (2012). The profession of school nursing. In: J. Selekman (ed.), *School Nursing: A Comprehensive Test.* Philadelphia: F. A. Davis.

Zurlinden J (2002, April 8). HIV update. *Nursing Spectrum*, 11 (7 PS).

Index